REDISCOVERING CANCER

REDISCOVERING CANCER

From Mechanism to Therapy

Edited by
Sayali Mukherjee, PhD
Somali Sanyal, PhD
Sonia Chadha, PhD

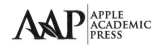

Apple Academic Press Inc.
3333 Mistwell Crescent
Oakville, ON L6L 0A2 Canada

Apple Academic Press Inc.
9 Spinnaker Way
Waretown, NJ 08758 USA

First issued in paperback 2021

Exclusive worldwide distribution by CRC Press, a member of Taylor & Francis Group
No claim to original U.S. Government works

ISBN-13: 978-1-77463-171-3 (pbk)
ISBN-13: 978-1-77188-690-1 (hbk)

Library and Archives Canada Cataloguing in Publication

Rediscovering cancer : from mechanism to therapy / edited by Sayali Mukherjee, PhD, Somali Sanyal, PhD, Sonia Chadha, PhD.
Includes bibliographical references and index.
Issued in print and electronic formats.
ISBN 978-1-77188-690-1 (hardcover).--ISBN 978-1-351-16656-0 (PDF)
1. Cancer. 2. Cancer--Etiology. 3. Cancer--Prevention.
4. Cancer--Treatment. I. Mukherjee, Sayali, editor II. Sanyal, Somali, editor III. Chadha, Sonia, editor

RC261.R43 2018   616.99'4   C2018-903221-9   C2018-903222-7

Library of Congress Cataloging-in-Publication Data

Names: Mukherjee, Sayali, editor. | Sanyal, Somali, editor. | Chadha, Sonia, editor.
Title: Rediscovering cancer : from mechanism to therapy / editors, Sayali Mukherjee, Somali Sanyal, Sonia Chadha.
Description: Oakville, ON ; Waretown, NJ : Apple Academic Press, 2018. |
Includes bibliographical references and index. |
Identifiers: LCCN 2018024997 (print) | LCCN 2018025644 (ebook) | ISBN 9781351166560 ()
| ISBN 9781771886901 (hardcover : alk. paper) | ISBN 9781351166560 (eBook)
Subjects: | MESH: Neoplasms
Classification: LCC RC263 (ebook) | LCC RC263 (print) | NLM QZ 200 | DDC 616.99/4--dc23
LC record available at https://lccn.loc.gov/2018024997

Apple Academic Press also publishes its books in a variety of electronic formats. Some content that appears in print may not be available in electronic format. For information about Apple Academic Press products, visit our website at **www.appleacademicpress.com** and the CRC Press website at **www.crcpress.com**

CONTENTS

ABOUT THE EDITORS

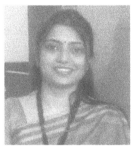

Sayali Mukherjee, PhD
*Amity Institute of Biotechnology, Amity University
Uttar Pradesh, Lucknow, India*

Sayali Mukherjee, PhD, is an Assistant Professor at the Amity Institute of Biotechnology, Amity University Uttar Pradesh, Lucknow, India. She completed her PhD from the Chittaranjan National Cancer Institute, Kolkata India, registered under Jadavpur University in Life Sciences. She received a NET-CSIR Research Fellowship. During her PhD she has worked on the toxicological and carcinogenic effects of air pollutants on human health. After completing her PhD, she has worked on stem cell culture as a Research Associate at the Jawaharlal Nehru Centre for Advanced Scientific Research (JNCASR), Bangalore, India. Presently she is working on immunological and biochemical aspects of oral cancer and oral diseases. She has several publications in peer-reviewed journals of national and international repute.

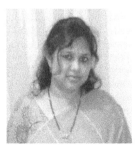

Somali Sanyal, PhD
*Amity Institute of Biotechnology, Amity University
Uttar Pradesh, Lucknow, India*

Somali Sanyal, PhD, is an Assistant Professor at Amity Institute of Biotechnology, Amity University Uttar Pradesh, Lucknow, India. She received her PhD from the Karolinska Medical University, Stockholm, Sweden. During her PhD she has worked on molecular epidemiology of urinary bladder cancer. After her PhD she worked as a postdoctoral fellow at the Karolinska Medical University, Stockholm, Sweden. Later on she moved to the Central Drug Research Institute, Lucknow, India, as a Research Associate. Her current research focuses on genetic aspects of head and neck, oral, and gall bladder cancer. She has published several research articles in journals of national and international repute.

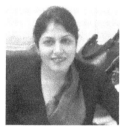

Sonia Chadha, PhD
Amity Institute of Biotechnology, Amity University Uttar Pradesh, Lucknow, India

Sonia Chadha, PhD, is presently working as a faculty member at the Amity Institute of Biotechnology, Amity University Uttar Pradesh, Lucknow, India. She completed her PhD from the Central Drug Research Institute, Lucknow, India, in biochemistry. During her PhD she has worked on the interaction of rat polymorphonuclear leukocyte derived free radical generation and nitric oxide in normal and in various pathological conditions. She has pursued her PDF from the National Environmental Engineering Research Institute (NEERI), Nagpur, India, where she worked on cytochrome P450. Her research interests include biochemical and molecular aspects of cancer and hypertensive disorders. She has several publications in national and international peer-reviewed journals.

LIST OF CONTRIBUTORS

Sen Abhik
Centre For Neurodegenerative Diseases, Blanchette Rockefeller Neurosciences Institute, West Virginia University, USA

Divakar Aman
Toxicological Division, CSIR–Central Drug Research Institute, Lucknow–226031, Uttar Pradesh, India

Mukherjee Apurba
Department of Environmental Carcinogenesis & Toxicology, Chittaranjan National Cancer Institute, 37, S.P. Mukherjee Road, Kolkata–700026, India

Sarkar Chandrani
Department of Pathology, The Ohio State University, 1645 Neil Avenue Columbus OH 43210, USA

Chakroborty Debanjan
Department of Pathology, The Ohio State University, 1645 Neil Avenue, Columbus OH 43210, USA

Datta Dipak
Biochemistry Division, CSIR–Central Drug Research Institute, Lucknow–226031, India

Tandon Divya
Toxicology Division, CSIR–Central Drug Research Institute, Lucknow–226031, India

Ravegnini Gloria
Department of Pharmacy and Biotechnology, Via Irnerio 48, Bologna, 40126, Italy

Dewangan Jayant
Toxicology Division, CSIR–Central Drug Research Institute, Lucknow–226031, India

Biswas Jaydip
Department of Environmental Carcinogenesis & Toxicology, Chittaranjan National Cancer Institute, 37, S.P. Mukherjee Road, Kolkata–700026, India

Gaur Vivek Kumar
CSIR–Indian Institute of Toxicology Research, M.G. Road, Lucknow, India

Pandey Prabhash Kumar
Toxicological Division, CSIR–Central Drug Research Institute, Lucknow–226031, Uttar Pradesh, India

Rath Srikanta Kumar
Toxicology Division, CSIR–Central Drug Research Institute, Lucknow–226031, India

Singh Anup Kumar
 B Biochemistry Division, CSIR–Central Drug Research Institute, Lucknow–226031, India

Srivastava Janmejai Kumar
Amity Institute of Biotechnology, Amity University Uttar Pradesh, Lucknow Campus, Lucknow–226028, Uttar Pradesh, India

K. Lohitesh
Department of Biological Sciences, Birla Institute of Science and Technology, Pilani, Rajasthan–333031, India

Banerjee Madhuchanda
Department of Zoology, Midnapore College (Autonomous), West Bengal, India

Roy Madhumita
Department of Environmental Carcinogenesis & Toxicology, Chittaranjan National Cancer Institute, 37, S.P. Mukherjee Road, Kolkata–700026, India

Meeran Syed Musthapa
Department of Biochemistry, CSIR–Central Food Technological Research Institute, Mysore, India

Hrelia Patrizia
Department of Pharmacy and Biotechnology, Via Irnerio 48, Bologna, 40126, Italy

Mandal Deba Prasad
Department of Zoology, West Bengal State University, Berunanpukuria, Malikapur, North-24 Parganas, Barasat, Kolkata–700126, West Bengal, India

Chaturvedi Priyank
Biochemistry Division, CSIR–Central Drug Research Institute, Lucknow–226031, India

Angelini Sabrina
Department of Pharmacy and Biotechnology, via Irnerio 48, Bologna, 40126, Italy

Khan Sajid
Laboratory of Cancer Epigenetics, Division of Endocrinology, CSIR–Central Drug Research Institute, Lucknow, India–226031

Mishra Sakshi
Toxicological Division, CSIR–Central Drug Research Institute, Lucknow–226031, Uttar Pradesh, India

Shukla Samriddhi
Laboratory of Cancer Epigenetics, Division of Endocrinology, CSIR–Central Drug Research Institute, Lucknow, India–226031

Gupta Sanjay
Department of Urology, Case Western Reserve University, 10900 Euclid Avenue, Cleveland, Ohio, USA

Mukherjee Sayali
Amity Institute of Biotechnology, Amity University Uttar Pradesh, Lucknow Campus, Lucknow–226028, Uttar Pradesh, India

Siddique Shabana
Cancer Care Ontario, 620 University Avenue, Toronto, Ontario, Canada

Bhattacharjee Shamee
Department of Zoology, West Bengal State University, Berunanpukuria, PO Malikapur, Kolkata–700126, Wset Bengal, India

Sanyal Somali
Amity Institute of Biotechnology, Amity University Uttar Pradesh, Lucknow Campus, Lucknow–226028, Uttar Pradesh, India

Srivastava Sonal
Toxicology Division, CSIR–Central Drug Research Institute, Lucknow–226031, India

Chadha Sonia
Amity Institute of Biotechnology, Amity University Uttar Pradesh, Lucknow Campus, Lucknow–226028, Uttar Pradesh, India

Biswas Souvick
Department of Environmental Carcinogenesis & Toxicology, Chittaranjan National Cancer Institute, 37, S.P. Mukherjee Road, Kolkata–700026, India

Chakraborty Sreeparna
West Virginia University, USA

Dash Subhra
Department of Biological Sciences, Birla Institute of Science and Technology, Pilani, Rajasthan–333031, India

Mukherjee Sudeshna
Department of Biological Sciences, Birla Institute of Science and Technology, Pilani, Rajasthan–333031, India

Yadav Suresh
Amity Institute of Biotechnology, Amity University Uttar Pradesh, Lucknow Campus, Lucknow–226028, Uttar Pradesh, India

Mukherjee Sutapa
Department of Environmental Carcinogenesis & Toxicology, Chittaranjan National Cancer Institute, 37, S.P. Mukherjee Road, Kolkata–700026, India

LIST OF ABBREVIATIONS

ABC	ATP-binding cassette
ACE	angiotensin-converting enzyme
ACT	adoptive cell therapy
ADCC	antibody-dependent cell-mediated cytotoxicity
ADCs	antibody-drug conjugates
AGO2	argonaute 2
AHH	aryl hydrocarbon hydroxylase
AICARFT	amino-4'-imidazolecarboxamide ribonucleotide transformylase
AIDS	acquired immune deficiency syndrome
AIF	apoptosis inducing factor
ALK	anaplastic lymphoma kinase
ALS	amyotrophic lateral sclerosis
ALT	alternative lengthening of telomeres
AML	acute myeloid leukaemia
AML	acute myelogenous leukaemia
AP	apurinic/apyrimidinic
AP	accelerated phase
APC	adenomatous polyposis coli protein
APC/C	anaphase-promoting complex/cyclosome
ARHGAP18	Rho GTPase activating protein 18
ATM	ataxia telangiectasia mutated
ATRIP	ATR-interacting protein
BAC	bacterial artificial chromosome
BCCs	basal cell carcinomas
BCG	Bacille Calmette-Guérin
BCRP	breast cancer resistance protein
BER	base excision repair
BP	blastic phase
BPH	benign prostatic hyperplasia
BRCA1	breast cancer 1
CAD	caspase activated DNase

CAFs	cancer-associated fibroblasts
CAK	CDK-activating kinase
CAM	cell adhesion molecules
CBP	CREB-binding protein
CDK	cyclin-dependent kinase
cdk2	cell division-stimulating protein
CDKs	cyclin-dependent kinases
CHIP	carboxy-terminus of Hsc70 interacting protein
Chk1	checkpoint kinase 1
cIAPs	cellular inhibitors of apoptosis proteins
CID	caspase-independent cell death
CIN	chromosomal instability
CIN	cervical intraepithelial neoplasia
CKIs	cyclin-dependent kinase inhibitors
CLKs	CDK-like kinases
CML	chronic myelogenous leukemia
CML	chronic myeloid leukemia
CMMRD	constitutional mismatch repairdeficiency syndrome
CP	chronic phase
CpGs	cytosine-guanosine dinucleotides
CRC	colorectal cancer
CSCs	cancer stem cells
CT	computed tomography
CTCs	circulating tumor cells
CTD	C-terminal domain
DADS	diallyl disulfide
DAS	diallyl sulfide
DATS	diallyl trisulfide
DBD	DNA-binding domain
DCs	dendritic cells
DDD	dichlorodiphenyldichloroethane
DDE	dichlorodiphenyldichloroethylene
DDR	DNA damage response
DDT	dichlorodiphenyltrichloroethane
DEHP	di-2-ethylhexyl-phthalate
DHFR	dihydrofolate reductase
DISC	death-inducing signaling complex
DKC1	dyskeratosis congenita 1

DNA	deoxyribonucleic acid
DNA-PK	DNA-dependent protein kinase
DNMTs	DNA methyltransferases
DSBs	double-stranded breaks
dsDNA	double-stranded DNA
EC	epicatechin
ECM	extracellular matrix
ECTR	extra-chromosomal telomeric repeat
EGC	epigal-locatechin
EGCG	epigallocatechin gallate
EGF	epidermal growth factor
EGFR	epidermal growth factor receptor
EMT	epithelial to mesenchymal transition
EPCs	endothelial progenitor cells
EPR	enhanced permeability and retention
ER	endoplasmic reticulum
ER	estrogen receptor
ERE	estrogen-responsible element
ESCC	esophageal squamous cell cancer
EZH2	enhancer of zeste homologue 2
FACS	fluorescence activated cell sorting
FADD	fas-associated death domain
FAK	focal adhesion kinase
FAP	familial adenomatous polyposis
FDA	Food and Drug Administration
FdUMP	fluorodeoxyuridine monophosphate
FGF	fibroblast growth factor
FGFR-1	fibroblast growth factor receptor 1
FKBPL	FK506-binding protein-like
Flt-1	fms like tyrosine kinase-1
GAPs	GTPase-activating proteins
GARFT	glycinamide ribonucleotide transformylase
GDF	growth and differentiation factor
GEF	guanine nucleotide exchange factor
GG-NER	global genome NER
GIST	gastrointestinal stromal tumor
GPR56	G-protein coupled receptor 56
GSH	glutathione

GSK3β	glycogen synthase kinase 3β
GSKs	glycogen synthase kinases
GSTs	glutathione S-transferase
HAT	histone acetyl transferase
HCAs	heterocyclic amines
HCC	hepatocellular carcinoma
HDAC	histone deacetylase
HDR	homology directed recombination
HER	hydroxyethylrutosides
hGH	human gonadotropic hormone
HGP	human genome project
HIF	hypoxia inducible factor
HIV	human immunodeficiency virus
HNC	head and neck cancer
HNPCC	hereditary non-polyposis colorectal cancer
HPV	human papilloma virus
HR	homologous recombination
HtrA2	high temperature requirement A2
IAP	indoor air pollution
IAPs	inhibitors of apoptosis proteins
IARC	International Agency for Research on Cancer
IBM	IAP-binding motif
ICAM-1	intercellular adhesiom molecule-1
IFNs	interferons
IFNγ	interferon-gamma
IGF-1	insulin-like growth factor 1
IL-10	interleukin-10
IL6	interleukin 6
ILs	interleukins
iPSC	induced pluripotent stem cells
ISM1	isthmin1
JNK	Jun N-terminal kinase
KHSV	Kaposi sarcoma herpes virus
KICS	KSHV inflammatory cytokine syndrome
KLF4	Krüppel-like factor 4
LCLs	lymphoblastoid cell lines
LDHB	lactate dehydrogenase B
LMP	permeabilization of lysosomal membrane

MALDI-TOF	matrix-assisted laser desorption/ionisation time-of-flight mass spectrometry
MAP	MUTYH-associated polyposis
MAPK	mitogen activated protein kinase
MBD	methyl-CpG binding domain
MCD	multicentric castleman disease
mCRC	metastatic colorectal cancer
MDR1	multidrug resistance protein 1
MDS	myelodysplastic syndromes
MDSC	myeloid-derived suppressor cells
MELT	Met-Glu-Leu-Thr
MET	mesenchymal-epithelial transition
mHCC	metastatic hepatocellular carcinoma
MLS	mitochondrial targeting signal
MM	multiple myeloma
MMPs	matrix metalloproteinases
MMR	mismatch repair
MMRN2	multimerin-2
MOMP	mitochondrial membrane potential
MPF	maturation-promoting factor
Mps1	monopolar spindle 1
mRNAs	messenger RNAs
MRP1	multidrug resistance-associated protein 1
MSCs	mesenchymal stem cells
MSI	microsattelite instability
MT	metallothionein
mTOR	mammalian target of rapamycin
NADM	non-AIDS-defining malignancies
NER	nucleotide excision repair
NF-κB	nuclear factor κB
NGS	next-generation sequencing
NHEJ	non-homologous end joining
NK	natural killer
NOD	non obese diabetic
NPC	nuclear pore complex
NPs	nanoparticles
NSCLC	non-small cell lung cancer
OCPs	organochlorine pesticides

Oct-1	octamer transcription factors
OD	oligomerization domain
OLA	oligonucleotide ligation assay
OSCC	oral squamous cell carcinoma
PAE	porcine aortic endothelial
PAGE	polyacrylamide gel electrophoresis
PAH	polycyclic aromatic hydrocarbons
PCBs	polychlorinated biphenyls
PCNA	proliferating cell nuclear antigen
PCR	polymerase chain reaction
PD-1	programmed death-1
PD-L1	programmed death ligand-1
PDAC	pancreatic ductal adenocarcinoma
PDGF	platelet-derived growth factor
PECAM	platelet/endothelial cell adhesion molecule
PEDF	pigment epithelium-derived factor
PEL	primary effusion lymphoma
PF4	platelet factor 4
PGE2	prostaglandin E2
Pgp	P glycoprotein
PH	pleckstrin-homology
PHDs	propyl hydroxylases
PI-3	phosphatidylinositol-3
PI3Ks	phosphatidylinositol 3-kinases
PIN	prostatic intraepithelial neoplasia
PIP3	phosphatidylinositol-3, 4 and 5-triphosphate
PKC	protein kinase C
PLGF	placental growth factor
PLK1	polo-like kinase 1
POLb	polymerase
POPs	persistent organic pollutants
PP2A	protein phosphatase 2A
PRC1	polycomb repressive complex 1
PRC2	polycomb repressive complex 2
PSGL-1	P-selectin glycoprotein ligand-1
PTEN	phosphatase and tensin homolog
PTH	parathyroid hormone
PTM	post-translational modifications

PVC	polyvinyl chloride
QD	quantum dots
RASGRF	RAS guanine-releasing factor
RB	retinoblastoma gene
RB1	retinoblastoma tumor susceptibility gene
RFPL3	ret finger protein like 3
RNA	ribonucleic acid
RNA pol II	RNA polymerase II
ROS	reactive oxygen species
RPA	replication protein A
SAC	spindle assembly checkpoint
SAC	S-allyl cysteine
SAM	S-adenosylmethionine
SBE	single base extension
SCC	squamous cell carcinoma
SCID	severe combined immunodeficient
SDF1	stromal cell derived factor 1
SIL	squamous intraepithelial lesions
SIRT1	sirtuin 1
SMC1	structural maintenance of chromosome 1
SNP	single nucleotide polymorphism
SNS	sympathetic nervous system
SOCS-3	suppressor of cytokine signaling-3
SOS	son of sevenless
SSCP	single strand conformation polymorphism
ssDNA	single-stranded DNA
TA	transactivation domains
TAA	tumor-associated antigen
TAD	transactivation domain
TAMs	tumor associated macrophages
TAp73	tumor protein 73-alpha
TC-NER	transcriptionally coupled NER
TCE	trichloroethylene
TERT	telomerase reverse transcriptase
TFIIH	transcription factor II human
TGF	transforming growth factor
TGF-β	tumor growth factor-β
TH1	T helper 1

TIA	transient ischemic attack
TIMPs	tissue inhibitors of matrix metalloproteinases
TME	tumor microenvironment
TMZ	temozolomide
TNBC	triple-negative breast cancer
TNF-α	tumour necrosis factor
TPO	thrombopoietin
TRADD	TNF receptor-associated death domain
TRPV	transient receptor potential vanilloid
TS	thymidylate synthase
TSA	trichostatin A
TSGs	tumor suppressor genes
TSP-1	thrombospondin 1
TSP-2	thrombospondin 2
Ub	ubiquitin
UTR	untranslated region
UV	ultraviolet ray
VCAM	vascular cell adhesion molecule
VEGF	vascular endothelial growth factor
VEGFR-1	VEGF receptor-1
VHL	von Hippel-Lindau
VPF	vascular permeability factor
WHO	World Health Organization
WRN	Werner syndrome protein
XPD	xenoderma pigmentosum group D
XRCC1	x-ray repair cross-complementing 1
ZNF24	zinc finger protein 24

PREFACE

Rediscovering Cancer: From Mechanism to Therapy is an attempt to comprehensively summarize cancer, a cumulative disorder responsible for a high rate of mortality. In this book our main approach has been to capture a snapshot of the ongoing research in the field of cancer. Deciphering the molecular mechanism of cancer is the present thrust area of research, which will help in finding better targets for drug therapy. This book is an amalgamation of basic and applied areas in cancer biology. Most of the available books deal with a specific type of cancer or a particular aspect of cancer, like only mechanism or therapy or drug targets. It is the first of its kind in bringing together molecular mechanism and cancer therapeutics under the same cover.

This book includes chapters on the molecular mechanism, etiology, prognosis, detection, and treatment of cancer, and has been contributed to by experts in their respective fields. Emphasis has been given on the intricate mechanism behind the deregulation of cell division, disruption of cell cycle check points, mutation in oncogenes and tumor suppressor genes, apoptosis and erratic cell signaling. The book discusses in detail topics such as angiogenesis and tumor microenvironment, which are increasingly receiving attention, especially in the field of neoplastic vascularization and metastasis. Cancer stem cells are a hot topic in the field of oncology. This book includes chapters detailing the current understanding and the future perspective of cancer stem cells. Overall, it covers the present knowledge and future direction on the field of cancer research. The book has been written in a lucid language supported by illustrations and tables and will be an asset to students, researchers and professionals worldwide.

Rediscovering Cancer: From Mechanism to Therapy also deals with therapeutic aspect of cancer. Chapters related to immunotherapy, chemotherapy and use of chitosan-based nanoparticles for cancer therapy have been included in the book. Recently, much emphasis is being placed on preventive measures for cancer. In this regard we have also included chapters on chemoprevention.

We are grateful to everyone who has assisted in one way or the other in the making of this book. We are thankful to our authors who have promptly responded to our many requests for alterations with forbearance. We are thankful to our families for their support and encouragement during the several phases of writing, re-writing, editing and reviewing. And finally we cannot help but thank our publishers who have encouraged us and accepted willingly our failure to meet our initial deadline and provided us with sufficient time to enable the completion of this book.

—Sayali Mukherjee,
Somali Sanyal,
Sonia Chadha

PART I

MOLECULAR MECHANISMS UNDERLYING INITIATION, PROMOTION, AND PROGRESSION OF CANCER

CHAPTER 1

GENETIC INSTABILITY IN CANCER

GLORIA RAVEGNINI, PATRIZIA HRELIA, and SABRINA ANGELINI

Department of Pharmacy and Biotechnology, Via Irnerio 48, Bologna, 40126, Italy, Tel.:+39 0512091787, E-mail: s.angelini@unibo.it

CONTENTS

ABSTRACT

Cancer is an uncontrolled and deregulated growth of cells. According to the specific tissue "hit" by cancer, there are peculiar and distinctive traits that may characterize the disease. However, different types of cancers share specific properties that are practically in common among all of them. These features, the so-called hallmarks of cancer, among others, mainly consist of uncontrolled proliferative signaling, antiapoptotic cascade, evasion from immunity, angiogenesis, and genomic instability. Genomic instability increases the rate of these alterations and, consequently, promotes the selection for growth and motility advantage that may lead to carcinogenesis. In general, genetic instability indicates a set of events that can lead to unscheduled alterations, temporary or permanent, within the genome. Genetic instability can be grouped into two main categories: at the nucleotide level and at the chromosomal level. Instability at the nucleotide level involves changes in the DNA sequence and leads to alterations of one or a few base pairs. Chromosomal instability (CIN) is a "state of numerical and/or structural chromosomal anomalies in cells," resulting in gains or losses of whole chromosomes, inversions, deletions, duplications, and translocations of large chromosomal segments.

In recent years, it has been recognized that the development of cancer involves a series of epigenetic changes across the genome as well as genetics. Epigenetics can be retained as a link between genotype and phenotype, as it may modify the final outcome of an allele, gene, and chromosome without altering the DNA sequence. Epignetic modifications, discussed here, may be classified into three main groups: i) DNA methylation, ii) histone alterations, and iii) microRNAs.

1.1   INTRODUCTION

Cancer is referred as an uncontrolled and deregulated growth of cells. According to the specific tissue "hit" by cancer, there are peculiar and distinctive traits that may characterize the disease. However, different types of cancers share specific properties that are practically in common among all of them. These features, the so-called hallmarks of cancer, among others, mainly consist of uncontrolled proliferative signaling, antiapoptic cascade, evasion from immunity, angiogenesis, and genomic instability [1]. For the first time, in 1976, genomic instability was proposed as a driving force in carcinogenesis [2]. Indeed, a normal cell requires a number of genetic changes to become tumorigenic. Genomic instability increases the rate of these alterations, and consequently, subsequent selection for growth and motility advantage may lead to carcinogenesis [3]. In general, genetic instability indicates a set of events that can lead to unscheduled alterations, temporary or permanent, within the genome. To better describe genetic instability, we can group it into two main categories: at the nucleotide level and at the chromosomal level.

1.2 GENETIC INSTABILITY AT THE NUCLEOTIDE LEVEL

Instability at the nucleotide level involves changes in the DNA sequence and leads to alterations of one or a few base pairs [4]; this kind of instability is rare in human cancers, but when it happens, it may cause dramatic consequences [4]. Also included in this category is microsatellite instability (MSI),which is caused by defects in the mismatch repair pathway. With regard to DNA repair machinery, the main response for defects at the nucleotide level is the DNA repair pathway. In normal cells, during "healthy" replication processes, mutations, representing an important source of variability between generation, occurs at a rate of 10^{-10} per base pair/cell division [5]. Two separate processes control the error rate: DNA polymerization (and associated proofreading by the polymerase) and repair. The repair machinery intervenes to correct sequence errors generated by polymerases or by exogen insults, including UV light, X-rays, and genotoxic chemicals [6, 7] To date, at least three types of repair have been well-described:

- nucleotide excision repair (NER),
- base excision repair (BER),
- DNA mismatch repair (MMR).

1.2.1 NUCLEOTIDE EXCISION REPAIR (NER)

The NER pathway is characterized by a broad specificity and operates to repair DNA damage caused by ultraviolet irradiation, alkylating and oxidizing agents, or chemotherapeutic drugs, forming bulky, helix distorting adducts.

NER is a well-defined multistep process that involves more than 30 proteins. It is very important to maintain the DNA integrity, and defects in this pathway are associated with severe disorders, including xeroderma pigmentosum, Cockayne syndrome, and trichothiodystrophy syndrome; these disorders share high sensitivity to UV irradiation, heavy cancer incidence, and multi-system immunological and neurological disorders [8, 9] To date, two sub-pathways are recognized, namely the global genome NER (GG-NER) and the transcriptionally coupled NER (TC-NER). The GG-NER examines the entire genome for helix distortion, associated with nucleotide changes, while the TC-NER is activated when RNA polymerase II is stalled due to a lesion in the template strand [8–10]

The first step of NER is the recognition of the DNA damage. The main player in this crucial phase is Xeroderma Pigmentosum complementation group C protein (XPC) associated with and stabilized by RAD23B [8]. Subsequently, the XPC/RAD23B complex binds to the damaged DNA, RAD23B dissociates from the complex, and the transcription initiation factor IIH (TFIIH) is recruited together with XPG endonuclease; at this point, TFIIH with its helicase activity widens the double helix close to the lesion, and other proteins are recruited including XPD, XPB, XPA, and the heterodimer XPF-ERCC. This heterodimer is arranged by Replication Protein A (RPA) to the broken strand to create a 5' incision; then, XPG excises a 22 to 30-nucleotide-long strand comprising the lesion. Finally, the DNA polymerase acts to fill the gap, and DNA ligase seals the nick [8].

1.2.2 BASE EXCISION REPAIR (BER)

The BER pathway is the primary mechanism for repairing small, non-bulky DNA lesions caused by oxidative base lesions, such as 8-oxoG and formamidopyrimidines. Additionally, BER corrects DNA damage from endogenous metabolic processes including alkylation, deamination, reactive oxygen species (ROS), and hydrolysis [11]. This system is primarily involved in the repair of modified nucleotides that have suffered relatively minor damage. Recently, it has been reported a germline mutations in MUTYH, a protein involved in BER, greatly increases the risk of MUTYH-associated polyposis (MAP), an autosomal recessive form of inherited colorectal cancer [12]. In general, we can categorize BER in short-patch, when only a new nucleotide is integrated in the place of the damaged base, or in long-patch, when two to six new nucleotides are incorporated [11] In the first phase, a glycosylase is involved; actually, a battery of glycosylases is involved in BER, which are involved depending on the specific type of lesion, as uracil DNA n-glycosylase, thymine DNA glycosylase, methyl purine DNA glycosylase, 8-oxoguanine glycolyse 1, or endonuclease three homolog 1. In general, there is mono- or bifunctional DNA glycosylase. The first one (mono) has glycosylase activity only and needs another enzyme (usually APE1) to create the incision, whereas the second one (bi) has both the activities and creates both base excision and incision [11] More in general, the glycosylase recognizes and cuts the damaged nucleotide to form an abasic site called apurinic/apyrimidinic (AP) site. AP sites, which generate single-strand breaks (SSBs), are highly mutagenic and the correct repair is critical. SSB harbors a 3'-αβ unsaturated aldehyde or 3'-phosphate based on the specific glycosylase that formed the AP site; the SSB requires removal of the altered 3'-terminal groups prior to polymerization and/or ligation. At this point, APE1 removes the 3'-terminal group, and nucleotide replacement is guaranteed by polymerase (POLb) [11].

1.2.3   MISMATCH REPAIR AND MICROSATELLITE INSTABILITY

The MMR is a multiprotein, highly conserved process with a pivotal and essential role in maintaining genomic stability by recognizing and repairing errors arising during DNA replication, and inhibiting recombination between homologous sequences [13]. MMR is a mechanism that intervenes at the postreplicative level and can take out mismatches among bases and insertion/deletion loops created within the DNA synthesis [13]

The main enzymes involved in this pathway are the heterodimers MSH2/MSH6 (MutSα) and MSH2/MSH3 (MutSβ), and the MLH1/PMS2 complex. In human cells, MSH2–MSH6 and MSH2–MSH3 heterodimers recognized base-base and insertion/deletion mispairs; in a further step, we observe MLH1/PMS2 complex recruitment, which degrades the mutated portion and begins the resynthesis [14]. The MMR system is very important, and its defects reflect in a severe phenotype, known as MSI [13, 14]. MSI is characterized by length modifications within repeated sequences, called microsatellites, resulting in mutations in cancer-related genes.

Germline mutations in MMR genes have been identified as responsible for inherited cancer syndrome; in particular, mutation in MLH1, MSH2, MSH6, and PMS2 may result in two hereditary tumor syndromes: the Lynch syndrome, formerly known as hereditary nonpolyposis colorectal cancer (HNPCC) and the constitutional mismatch repair deficiency syndrome (CMMRD), typical of childhood [15]. The Lynch syndrome is an autosomal dominant disorder, characterized by a high risk of different cancers, primarily colorectal cancer (CRC, accounting for about 2% of all CRCs) and extra-colorectal cancer, including cancer of the endometrium, stomach, ovaries, small intestine, renal pelvis, ureter and bladder, brain, and pancreas, breast cancer, prostate cancer, and sarcomas. The risk of a specific type of cancer mainly depends on sex differences and on the MMR-mutated gene [15]. Specifically, Richman has recently reported that 42% of patients have mutations in MLH1, 33% in MSH2, and 18% in MSH6; in addition, a very small subset of patients with Lynch syndrome is characterized by epimutations of MLH1[13]. CMMRD is a very rare disease caused by homozygous MMR gene mutations. To date, it counts more than 169 patients from 105 distinct families in the literature [13, 16]. In some aspects, it recalls neurofibromatosis type I, exhibiting cutaneous phenotype (café-au-lait macules). CMMRD is extremely severe with a high mortality rate mostly related to multiple childhood cancers, including hematological malignancies, brain tumors, Lynch syndrome-associated tumors, and embryonic tumors.

1.3   INSTABILITY AT THE CHROMOSOMAL LEVEL

As reported by Venkatesan et al. [17], CIN is a "state of numerical and/or structural chromosomal anomalies in cells," resulting in gains or losses of whole chromosomes, inversions, deletions, duplications, and translocations of large chromosomal segments. It is well known that CIN is linked with accelerated aging, cancer, or other genetic disorders [17]. Aneuploidy, a condition associated with the gains or losses of whole chromosomes or parts of them, leading to genomic imbalances, occurs in about 85% of human cancers, and several pathways may be responsible for the origin of CIN [18, 19].

To date, several pathways and processes have been implicated in CIN. Among the others, the most important are:

- mechanisms involved in centromere and telomere stability,
- cell cycle checkpoint pathways,
- sister chromatid cohesion,
- centrosome duplication.

In the next section, we will describe these pathways in detail.

1.3.1   CENTROMERE AND TELOMERE STABILITY

1.3.1.1   Centromere Stability

The centromere is a specific chromosome site essential in chromosome segregation. Indeed, to maintain genetic integrity, eukaryotic cells must segregate their chromosomes properly to opposite spindle poles before cell division, and the centromere is crucial to this process [20]. In particular, the principal function of centromere is to help the assembly of kinetochore, which attaches the chromosome to spindle microtubules [21]. Cell cycle represents an ordered progression of events, during which, prior to mitosis, the centrosome duplicates, generating two cells, each containing one centrosome [22]. Given the pivotal role of centromere, the inability to accurately segregate duplicated chromosomes between two daughter cells may translate into cells characterized by anomalous numbers of chromosomes [22].

What seems extremely important to avoid aneuploidy is the proper centrosome dynamics in ensuring faithful segregation [22]. Indeed, on the one hand, delayed centrosome separation enables chromosome missegregation, promoting merotelic attachments in the early prometaphase. Merotelic kinetochore attachment is a type of error that occurs when a single kinetochore is attached to microtubules arising from both spindle poles [23]. In this phase, immature kinetochores have not yet recruited all the proteins important for correct kinetochore–microtubule attachments, growing the possibility of merotelic attachments and/or diminishing the efficiency at which merotelic attachments are discovered and solved. On the other hand, late centrosome disengagement is associated with spindle asymmetry in the metaphase, which may also facilitate misattachments prior to the anaphase. Accelerated centrosome separation may result in merotelic attachments in the early prometaphase. Like delayed disengagement, accelerated centrosome separation has been associated with spindle asymmetry in the metaphase, which is expected to promote merotelic attachments shortly before anaphase onset. Unresolved merotelic attachments lead to underdeveloped chromosome [22].

It has been observed that both delayed and accelerating timing of segregation, without centromere amplification, are correlated with tumorigenesis. In this view, it seems that p53 is responsible for proper timing of centrosome disjunction by negatively regulating Aurora A mitotic kinase activity [24].

In mammalian cells, Aurora A regulates a number of cellular targets, including stress-responsive transcription factors and the p53 tumor suppressor. Aurora A may phosphorylate p53, causing its degradation and inhibiting its transcriptional activity. However, it remains to better clarify how p53 regulates Aurora A. In particular, p53 seems to negatively regulate Aurora A, suggesting the existence of a tight network of reciprocal regulation between Aurora A and p53 [25].

In this view, tumors with p53 mutations or loss of function may be characterized by whole chromosome gain or loss resulting from early centrosome disjunction and establishment of asymmetric mitotic spindles [22]. As a consequence, p53 appears to be the prototypical gene commonly altered in cancer that may also force CIN.

1.3.1.2 Telomere Stability

Mammalian telomeres consist of thousands of repetitions of tandem sequence "5-TTAGGG-3" presented at the end of chromosomes and are characterized by two main tasks. First, they can discriminate between chromosome ends and DNA double-strand breaks, thereby preventing unwanted DNA damage signaling and genome instability. The second one is the prevention of genetic information loss by providing a mechanism that is essential in maintenance of telomere length during replication [26].

During replication, the general chromosomal DNA replication machinery cannot fully copy the DNA out to the extreme ends of the linear chromosomes. For this reason, throughout the replication cycles, chromosome ends are subject to erosion [27]. However, the eukaryotic cells may compensate the loss of genetic material with the enzyme telomerase, human telomerase reverse transcriptase (hTERT), that can add telomeric repeat sequences to the ends of chromosomes [27]. Besides this activity, telomerase expression is quite low and repressed in the majority of somatic cells, leading to telomere reduction over the life course, which in turn lead to aging.

Interestingly, in about 85% of human cancers, TERT expression is reactivated [28], and the experiment of knocking down TERT resulted in a high decrease in cell proliferation and growth [28]. The main cause of TERT reactivation is due to point mutations in the promoter region that expose new potential binding sites for enhancers or transcriptional regulator factors, with a consequent increased TERT mRNA [28, 29]. However, several types of sarcoma have been described to have different lengthening of telomeres (ALT) without telomerase activity, demonstrating the existence of nontelomerase-based ALT mechanisms for telomere maintenance [30]; ALT is a recombination-based mechanism involving homologous recombination and is found in 10–15% of human cancers [31]. ALT activity is most common in mesenchymal cancers, including bone (62%), soft tissues (32%), and neuroendocrine systems (40%) [31].

Despite the fact that the majority of cancers are mainly characterized by high levels of TERT or ALT mechanism, in some cases, the loss of telomeric repeat sequences or deficiencies in telomeric proteins may culminate in chromosome fusion and force chromosome instability that eventually contributes to human cancer [31].

1.3.2   CELL CYCLE CHECKPOINT PATHWAYS

Among all the proteins that are associated with chromosome instability, there are numerous cell cycle regulators, including BRCA1 and 2, RB, MDM2, p53, and many others [32].

To date, the exact mechanism through which these proteins are involved or take part in CIN has not been clarified; however, it is believed that there are three possible modalities: i) cell cycle regulators may directly cooperate in maintaining chromosome separation reliability during mitosis; ii) deregulation of cell cycle events farther of the M phase (for example, centrosome duplication during the S phase) may indirectly stimulate the faulty segregation of chromosome during the following mitosis; and iii) disruption of cell cycle checkpoints may allow cells with missegregated chromosomes to proceed in cell cycle, thereby promoting tumor development [32].

One of the best examples of cell cycle regulators involved in CIN is pRB. The retinoblastoma tumor susceptibility gene (*RB1*) was one of the early discovered tumor suppressor genes [33], and more recently, different studies have demonstrated that loss of pRB activity promotes genomic instability. These studies have associated the pRB functional inactivation to various types of genomic alterations, including increase in ploidy on both chromosomal and subchromosomal – local amplifications, chromosome arm gains and losses – levels, and consistently high rates of chromosome separation errors resulting in CIN [33]. In particular, pRB inactivation determines defect during mitosis, and these seem less severe than those in the G1 phase; these alterations determine damages at chromosome segregation fidelity, resulting in excessive centrosomes, centromeric defects, and formation of micronuclei [33].

1.3.3   SISTER CHROMATID COHESION

During the S phase, the synthesis phase, new DNA molecules are created, which, in their chromatinized form, are called sister chromatids. The two sister chromatids are joined forming one chromosome during the G2 phase and mitosis phases – prophase, prometaphase, and metaphase. Once they reach the anaphase and are moved toward the opposite spindle poles of the mother cell, the sister chromatids are separated from each other [34]. The physical connection between the sister chromatids is called sister chromatid cohesion and is responsible for the correct events that occur through the S phase to the metaphase. With no cohesion, the sister chromatids could not be segregated in the correct manner, resulting in an asymmetry among the two daughter cells, and with a consequent aneuploidy that often is incompatible with life [33].

Sister chromatid cohesion is guaranteed by a set of evolutionarily conserved proteins that form a complex known as cohesion [35], consisting of two SMC subunits, SMC1 and SMC3, and two additional subunits Scc3 and Mcd1/Scc1. Keeping in mind these forewords, the disruption of this cohesion and the subsequent chromatid splitting depend on the orchestrated action of the cyclin-dependent kinase (CDK) activity and the mitotic spindle checkpoint [36].

The cohesin complex is regulated by specific proteins such as shugoshin 1 (hSgo1) and separase that proteolytically degraded the complex when the anaphase must begin [35]. Inhibition of these proteins determines increase in the number of tetraploid cells. On the other hand, the same effect (i.e., tetraploidy) also arises in cells that overexpress either Separase or Securin, the protein that blocks cohesin breakage. The increase in tetraploidy indicates that cohesion defects have a decisive influence in the development of CIN [35].

Barber and collaborators showed that genes involved in Sister Chromatid Exchange (SCE) are common mutated somatically and this leads to chromosome instability in colorectal cancers [37]. Similarly, Iwaizumi et al. analyzed 46 colon cancer tissues and observed that 47.8% hSgo1 was significantly downregulated in comparison with the normal tissue. These Sgo1-downregulated tumors had a higher variation in centromere numbers. In an in vitro study using HCT116 cell line, it has been shown that hSgo1-knockdown cells proliferated slowly due to a G2/M arrest and apoptosis block; in addition, markers of CIN in the form of aneuploidy and micronuclei were observed [37].

1.3.4   CENTROSOME DUPLICATION

The centrosome is a small non-membranous organelle usually located at the periphery of the nucleus. Its primary function is to anchor microtubules. The presence of two centrosomes per cell at mitosis is critical for the formation of bipolar mitotic spindles [39]. Centrosomes contain a pair of centrioles that duplicate during the S phase of the cell cycle to produce two centrosomes that function as mitotic spindle poles during cell division.

At the end of the telophase, the daughter cell must inherit one spindle pole. Thus, a tiny but firm regulation of the processes is necessary to govern the equal segregation of centrosomes during the cell cycle [40].

Because a frequent association between centrosome abnormalities and karyotype aberrations and disease progression is observed, centrosome amplification is considered as one of the major causes of CIN in cancer [18]. Furthermore, centrosome abnormalities have been implicated in CIN and aneuploidy in cancer [41, 42].

These defects, referred to as centrosome amplification, include size increase due to alterations in proteins such as centrin and pericentrin or protein number increase. Centrosome amplification is not merely an observer in CIN phenomenon; rather, centrosome amplification directly promotes incorrect chromosome segregation and that may then facilitate the development of more malignant phenotypes [41].

1.4   EPIGENETIC MODIFICATIONS IN CIN

In recent years, it has been recognized that the development of cancer involves a series of *epigenetic* changes across the genome as well as genetics.

The term "epigenetics" was first introduced in 1941 by Conrad Waddington to define a "branch of biology which studies the causal interactions between genes and their products, bringing the phenotype into being" [43]. In general, epigenetics can be retained as a link between genotype and phenotype, as it may modify the final outcome of an allele, gene, and chromosome without altering the DNA sequence [43]. Epigenetic modifications can be grouped in three main groups: (i) DNA methylation, (ii) histone alterations, and (iii) microRNAs.

1.4.1   DNA METHYLATION

DNA methylation is implicated in many cellular processes and regulates embryonic development, transcription, chromatin structure, X-chromosome inactivation, genomic imprinting, and chromosome stability [44].

DNA methylation occurs principally in the short sequence of CG dinu-cleotides known as CpG islands. Many human cancers have been related to aberrant DNA methylation or mutations in the DNA methylation pathway; usually, malignant cells show foremost disruptions in their DNA methyla-tion profiles, which manifest as hypermethylation of gene promoters, global hypomethylation, and increased proportion of mutation at methylated CpG dinucleotides. Indeed, in normal cells, the preponderance of the CpG islands is unmethylated, permitting the transcription of their linked genes. In cancer cells, hypermethylation of these regions implicates loss of gene expression. Extensive studies in the epigenetic field have allowed to identify, in differ-ent form of cancers, many genes with aberrant promoter hypermethylation. Among these, the most important are P16INK4a; P15INK4a; RB; P14ARF; DNA repair genes, including BRCA1, MGMT, and MLH1; genes govern-ing apoptosis, for instance, DAPK and TMS1; genes governing metasta-sis, for example, E-cadherin and CD-44; and genes governing angiogenesis such as TSP-1 and TIMP-3 [41]. However, we have to keep in mind that the methylation status is a cancer-specific trait and the same gene can be hypermethylated in one type of tumor and remain unmethylated in another one; this is the case of GSTP1 that appears hypermethylated in about 90% of prostate cancers, while is mainly unmethylated in acute leukemia [41]. Besides hypermethylation, in many cancers, genome hypomethylation is also common. Indeed, aberrant hypomethylation is believed to contribute to cancer progression by triggering oncogenes such as H-RAS, BORIS/CTCFL, FGFR1, and c-MYC [41].

1.4.2   HISTONE MODIFICATIONS

Chromatin consists of repeating units called nucleosomes and represents the packaged form of DNA present in the eukaryotic cell. Each nucleosome consists of DNA that is wrapped tightly around a group of conserved, highly basic proteins known as histones. Histones can be altered by different pro-cesses such as methylation, acetylation, phosphorylation, and ubiquitina-tion. These changes that involve the modification of the 15- to 30-amino acid N-terminal histone tails alter chromatin condensation [43].

These epigenetic modifications may impact the interaction between DNA and the proteins and then may be "read" as chromatine alteration state. The role of histone modification and chromatin remodeling in the carcinogenic process is a rapidly growing research area. To date, cancers have been associated with histone acetylation and methylation. For example, in prostate cancer, the histone deacetylase (HDAC) family of enzymes impacts the expression of genomic regions by enhancing the binding histone-DNA backbone. Modulating the role of HDAC enzymes may alter the regulation of oncogenes and tumor suppressor genes, and, as a consequence, neoplastic proliferation [45].

In general, the mechanisms at the basis of the regulation of pivotal cellular processes by histone post-translational modifications (PTM) are not clearly understood; however, they can be generally divided into two main groups: i) PTMs on histone proteins affect inter/intra-nucleosomal interactions and their binding to DNA by steric hindrance or charge interactions and ii) PTMs on histone proteins may inhibit or facilitate chromatin binding of various proteins [46].

Histone modifications, therefore, represent an additional level of high and sophisticated gene regulation. As a consequence, they can affect genome integrity and, in case of defects in this machinery, cancer development and progression occur.

1.4.3   MICRORNAS

MicroRNAs are a class of 18- to 24-nucleotide-long noncoding RNAs with epigenetic functions in posttranscriptional regulation of gene expression, via mRNA degradation or sequestering and translational repression. Thus, microRNAs play a pivotal role in several cell processes, and their altered expression is involved in human diseases, including cancer as well as developmental defects and inherited diseases. To date, over 1,400 microRNAs encoded by the human genome have been discovered. These microRNAs frequently target many genes related to cancer development or prevention, so that every microRNA can modulate many different targets, and at the same time, a single gene can be modulated by multiple microRNAs [47].

Loss of expression or mutations of features involved in microRNA biogenesis might lead to alterations in microRNA processing, stability, and targeting, and having deleterious consequences in the organism, including cancer development. The potential role of microRNAs in cancer development and progression is suggested by their contribution in the regulation of cell proliferation and apoptosis, and by modulating the expression of tumor suppressor genes and oncogenes. Moreover, to support their involvement in tumor development, approximately 50% of microRNAs are located at "fragile sites" in the genome, and these sites are often amplified or deleted in cancer [48].

In light of the association between microRNAs and cancer, they have been divided into two main groups: oncogenic and tumor-suppressive. In tumorigenesis, the loss of tumor-suppressive microRNAs promotes the expression of target oncogenes, while increased expression of oncogenic microRNAs can suppress target tumor suppressor genes [47]. Overall, downregulated microRNAs lead to an increased expression of oncogenes, while the upregulated ones cause suppression of tumor suppressor genes, indicative of the role of microRNAs as both tumor suppressors and oncogenes.

However, the role of microRNAs as tumor suppressor or oncogene is not univocal and strictly defined; indeed, microRNAs have differential expression in cancers according to the different tissues, as a result of hundreds of targets affecting horde of transcripts in cancer-related signaling pathways. The research field of microRNAs in cancer is relatively young and partially unexplored; for these reasons, a better understanding of the role of microRNAs in the molecular pathogenesis of cancer, treatment response, and modification in the current delivery systems is highly needed and would help in translation of these bench-based (laboratory – basic research) microRNA discoveries to the clinics.

1.5   SUMMARY

- 1 Hallmarks of cancer, among others, mainly consist of uncontrolled proliferative signaling, antiapoptic cascade, evasion from immunity, angiogenesis, and genomic instability.
- 2 Genetic instability indicates a set of events that can lead to unscheduled alterations, temporary or permanent, within the genome.
- 3 Genetic instability can be grouped into two categories: at the nucleotide level and at the chromosomal level.
- 4 Instability at the nucleotide level involves changes in the DNA sequence and leads to alterations of one or a few base pairs.
- 5 CIN is a "state of numerical and/or structural chromosomal anomalies in cells," resulting in gains or losses of whole chromosomes, inversions, deletions, duplications, and translocations of large chromosomal segments.

- 6 Epigenetic alterations are also involved in cancer development and progression.

KEYWORDS

- **cancer**
- **chromosomes**
- **DNA damage**
- **epigenetics**
- **genetic instability**

REFERENCES

1. Macheret, M., & Halazonetis, T. D., (2015). *Annu. Rev. Pathol.*, *10*, 425–448.
2. Nowell, P. C., (1976). *Science*, *194*(4260), 23–28.
3. Hanahan, D., & Weinberg, R. A., (2000). *Cell*, *100*(1), 57–70.
4. Lengauer, C., Kinzler, K. W., & Vogelstein, B., (1998). *Nature*, *396*(6712), 643–649.
5. Ferguson, L. R., Chen, H., Collins, A. R., Connell, M., Damia, G., Dasgupta, S., Malhotra, M., Meeker, A. K., Amedei, A., Amin, A., Ashraf, S. S., Aquilano, K., Azmi, A. S., Bhakta, D., Bilsland, A., Boosani, C. S., Chen, S., Ciriolo, M. R., Fujii, H., Guha, G., Halicka, D., Helferich, W. G., Keith, W. N., Mohammed, S. I., Niccolai, E., Yang, X., Honoki, K., Parslow, V. R., Prakash, S., Rezazadeh, S., Shackelford, R. E., Sidransky, D., Tran, P. T., Yang, E. S., & Maxwell, C. A., (2015). *Semin. Cancer Biol.*, *35 Suppl.*, S5–S24.
6. Kunkel, T. A., (1995). *Curr. Biol.*, *5*(10), 1091–1094.
7. Sia, E. A., Jinks-Robertson, S., & Petes, T. D., (1997). *Mutat. Res.*, *383*(1), 61–70.
8. Marteijn, J. A., Lans, H., Vermeulen, W., & Hoeijmakers, J. H. J., (2014). *Nat. Rev. Mol. Cell Biol.*, *15*(7), 465–481.
9. Petruseva, I. O., Evdokimov, A. N., & Lavrik, O. I., (2014). *Acta Naturae*, *6*(1), 23–34.
10. Roos, W. P., Thomas, A. D., & Kaina, B., (2016). *Nat. Rev. Cancer*, *16*(1), 20–33.
11. Maynard, S., Schurman, S. H., Harboe, C., De Souza-Pinto, N. C., & Bohr, V. A., (2009). *Carcinogenesis*, *30*(1), 2–10.
12. Cheadle, J. P., & Sampson, J. R., (2007). *DNA Repair (Amst).*, *6*(3), 274–279.
13. Richman, S., (2015). *Int. J. Oncol.*, *47*(4), 1189–1202.
14. Yamamoto, H., & Imai, K., (2015). *Arch. Toxicol.*, *89*(6), 899–921.
15. Sijmons, R. H., & Hofstra, R. M. W., (2016). *DNA Repair (Amst).*, *38*, 155–162.
16. Lavoine, N., Colas, C., Muleris, M., Bodo, S., Duval, A., Entz-Werle, N., Coulet, F., Cabaret, O., Andreiuolo, F., Charpy, C., Sebille, G., Wang, Q., Lejeune, S., Buisine, M. P., Leroux, D., Couillault, G., Leverger, G., Fricker, J. P., Guimbaud, R., Mathieu-Dramard, M., Jedraszak, G., Cohen-Hagenauer, O., Guerrini-Rousseau, L., Bourdeaut,

F., Grill, J., Caron, O., Baert-Dusermont, S., Tinat, J., Bougeard, G., Frébourg, T., & Brugières, L., (2015). *J. Med. Genet.*, *52*(11), 770–778.

17. Venkatesan, S., Natarajan, A. T., & Hande, M. P., (2015). *Mutat. Res. Genet. Toxicol. Environ. Mutagen.*, *793*, 176–184.

18. Cosenza, M. R., & Krämer, A., (2015). *Chromosome Res.*, *24*(1), 105–126.

19. Giam, M., & Rancati, G., (2015). *Cell Div.*, *10*, 3.

20. Tanaka, T. U., Clayton, L., & Natsume, T., (2013). *EMBO Rep.*, *14*(12), 1073–1083.

21. Cheeseman, I. M., & Desai, A., (2008). *Nat. Rev. Mol. Cell Biol.*, *9*(1), 33–46.

22. Nam, H. J., Naylor, R. M., & Van Deursen, J. M., (2015). *Trends Cell Biol.*, *25*(2), 65–73.

23. Gregan, J., Polakova, S., Zhang, L., Tolić-Norrelykke, I. M., & Cimini, D., (2011). *Trends Cell Biol.*, *21*(6), 374–381.

24. Nam, H. J., & Van Deursen, J. M., (2014). *Nat. Cell Biol.*, *16*(6), 538–549.

25. Wu, C. C., Yang, T. Y., Yu, C. T. R., Phan, L., Ivan, C., Sood, A. K., Hsu, S. L., & Lee, M. H., (2012). *Cell Cycle*, *11*(18), 3433–3442.

26. Xu, L., Li, S., & Stohr, B. A., (2013). *Annu. Rev. Pathol.*, *8*, 49–78.

27. Blackburn, E. H., Epel, E. S., & Lin, J., (2015). *Science*, *350*(6265), 1193–1198.

28. Akincilar, S. C., Unal, B., & Tergaonkar, V., (2016). *Cell. Mol. Life Sci.*

29. Killela, P. J., Reitman, Z. J., Jiao, Y., Bettegowda, C., Agrawal, N., Diaz, L. A., Friedman, A. H., Friedman, H., Gallia, G. L., Giovanella, B. C., Grollman, A. P., He, T. C., He, Y., Hruban, R. H., Jallo, G. I., Mandahl, N., Meeker, A. K., Mertens, F., Netto, G. J., Rasheed, B. A., Riggins, G. J., Rosenquist, T. A., Schiffman, M., Shih, I. M., Theodorescu, D., Torbenson, M. S., Velculescu, V. E., Wang, T. L., Wentzensen, N., Wood, L. D., Zhang, M., McLendon, R. E., Bigner, D. D., Kinzler, K. W., Vogelstein, B., Papadopoulos, N., & Yan, H., (2013). *Proc. Natl. Acad. Sci. USA.*, *110*(15), 6021–6026.

30. Matsuo, T., Shimose, S., Kubo, T., Fujimori, J., Yasunaga, Y., & Ochi, M., (2009). *Anticancer Res.*, *29*(10), 3833–3836.

31. Dilley, R. L., & Greenberg, R. A., (2015). *Trends in Cancer*, *1*(2), 145–156.

32. Thompson, S. L., Bakhoum, S. F., & Compton, D. A., (2010). *Curr. Biol.*, *20*(6), R285–R295.

33. Manning, A. L., & Dyson, N. J., (2011). *Trends Cell Biol.*, *21*(8), 433–441.

34. Peters, J. M., & Nishiyama, T., (2012). *Cold Spring Harb. Perspect. Biol.*, *4*(11).

35. *Chromosome Res.*, (2009). *17*(2), 229–238.

36. López-Saavedra, A., & Herrera, L. A., (2010). *Mutat. Res.*, *705*(3), 246–251.

37. Barber, T. D., Mc-Manus, K., Yuen, K. W. Y., Reis, M., Parmigiani, G., Shen, D., Barrett, I., Nouhi, Y., Spencer, F., Markowitz, S., Velculescu, V. E., Kinzler, K. W., Vogelstein, B., Lengauer, C., & Hieter, P., (2008). *Proc. Natl. Acad. Sci. USA.*, *105*(9), 3443–3448.

38. Iwaizumi, M., Shinmura, K., Mori, H., Yamada, H., Suzuki, M., Kitayama, Y., Igarashi, H., Nakamura, T., Suzuki, H., Watanabe, Y., Hishida, A., Ikuma, M., & Sugimura, H., (2009). *Gut*, *58*(2), 249–260.

39. Fukasawa, K., (2005). *Cancer Lett.*, *230*(1), 6–19.

40. Li, J. J., & Li, S. A., (2006). *Pharmacol. Ther.*, *111*(3), 974–984.

41. Shinmura, K., Kurabe, N., Goto, M., Yamada, H., Natsume, H., Konno, H., & Sugimura, H., (2014). *Mol. Biol. Rep.*, *41*(10), 6635–6644.

42. Ganem, N. J., Godinho, S. A., & Pellman, D., (2009). *Nature*, *460*(7252), 278–282.

43. Ravegnini, G., Sammarini, G., Hrelia, P., & Angelini, S., (2015). *Toxicol. Sci.*, *148*(1), 2–13.

44. Meng, H., Cao, Y., Qin, J., Song, X., Zhang, Q., Shi, Y., & Cao, L., (2015). *Int. J. Biol. Sci.*, *11*(5), 604–617.

45. Kaushik, D., Vashistha, V., Isharwal, S., Sediqe, S. A., & Lin, M. F., (2015). *Ther. Adv. Urol.*, *7*(6), 388–395.

46. Khan, S. A., Reddy, D., & Gupta, S., (2015). *World J. Biol. Chem.*, *6*(4), 333–345.

47. Choi, J. D., & Lee, J. S., (2013). *Genomics Inform.*, *11*(4), 164.

48. Mishra, S., Yadav, T., & Rani, V., (2016). *Crit. Rev. Oncol. Hematol.*, *98*, 12–23.

CHAPTER 2

ONCOGENESIS AND TELOMERASE ACTIVITY IN CANCER

SUTAPA MUKHERJEE, MADHUMITA ROY, and JAYDIP BISWAS

Department of Environmental Carcinogenesis & Toxicology, Chittaranjan National Cancer Institute, 37, S. P. Mukherjee Road, Kolkata 700 026, India, E-mail: sutapa_c_in@yahoo.com

CONTENTS

ABSTRACT

Cell division is an important mechanism of all living cells for maintaining normal growth. Most cells can divide for a limited period of time, which is regulated by telomere length. Telomeres are repetitions of DNA sequences (TTAGGG) situated at the ends of chromosomes and are protected by a six telomere-associated protein complex or shelterin. Shelterin aids in telomere capping because of which telomere can maintain stability and integrity of the chromosome. The ends of telomere create unique problems during DNA replication or due to oxidative damage and results in shortening of telomere repeat, the critical shortening of which induces replicative senescence. A complex and critical role of telomere biology is observed during the oncogenesis process. In more than 85% of cancer cells, telomerase, a ribonucleoprotein reverse transcriptase is overexpressed or its activity is dysregulated. Therefore, telomerase has emerged as a target for cancer therapeutics. Reactivation of telomerase is a common phenomenon of cancer stem cells and circulating tumor cells, which accelerates tumor metastasis. The enzyme consists of two components: the catalytic part is the human telomerase reverse transcriptase or hTERT and the RNA component is hTR. The underlying molecular mechanisms of telomerase regulation are very complicated; it can be controlled at multiple levels, including transcriptional, translational, and posttranslational levels. Some of the factors like transcription factors, hormones, cytokines, oncogenes, and epigenetic factors are intricately associated with hTERT regulation at the transcriptional level. Therefore, effective strategies need to be evolved to inhibit telomerase. Deactivation or inhibition of telomerase particularly by dietary natural phytochemicals with much lesser toxicity might ensure a rational approach in the therapy of cancer.

2.1 INTRODUCTION

Abnormal proliferation and cellular immortalization is a unique feature of cancer, which can be achieved by altered expression of several proteins, including the reverse transcriptase enzyme telomerase. Telomerase plays an essential role in maintaining chromosomal integrity stability by synthesizing telomeric DNA. Lack of telomerase imparts gradual shortening of telomeres as the enzyme DNA polymerase fails to replicate the chromosomal end, thereby resulting in cell cycle arrest or death. In humans, mortality due to shortening of telomere length may occur due to three probable factors. They are i) repression of telomerase before birth in normal somatic tissues, ii) existence of shortened telomere throughout life, or iii) progenitor cells expressing telomerase in a regulated manner [1]. Because of these three factors, telomeres behave like a mitotic clock and confer normal cells to divide for a finite period. Excessively shortened telomere compels chromosomal fusion and if not evaded by the enzyme telomerase could give rise to chromosomal instability and ultimately cell death. The facts of nonrequirement of telomerase in normal somatic tissues and essentiality of the enzyme for proliferation of tumor cells have established telomerase as a potential target for anticancer therapy.

2.2 TELOMERE AND ITS IMPORTANCE

Telomere, located at the linear chromosomal end, is a heterochromatin and exerts protective function on the chromosome [2]. Telomeres are like the plastic tips at the end of the shoelaces, protecting DNA ends from damages [3]. Long tracts of double-stranded G-rich repeats form telomere, extending up to 9–15 kb in case of humans. Projection of single-stranded repeats from the 3" end of about 30–300 nt long, known as G-tail, is a predominant feature of telomere end [4].

The question comes in mind why are telomeres important? Telomeres allow cells to distinguish chromosome ends from broken DNA and prevent chromosome fusions by nonhomologous end joining (NHEJ), thus providing a means for "counting" cell division. Vertebrate telomere comprises up to thousands of hexanucleotide repeats, bounded by a group of six proteins, which form a complex, termed as shelterin. Shelterin is composed of double-stranded TTAGGG repeats binding proteins 1 and 2 (TRF1 and TRF2). TRFs in turn recruit a protein POT1 or "protection of telomeres protein 1," TIN2 or "TRF1-interacting nuclear factor 2," TPP1 or "tripeptidyl peptidase I," and RAP1 or "Ras-related protein 1," each of which have clear defined functions [5]. Shelterin complex functions by preventing chromosomal end fusion, homologous recombination (HR), and degradation as it forms a protective T-loop lariat structure. The TRF2 protein helps in the formation of T-loop structure. Single-stranded 3' overhang loop invades double-stranded telomeric DNA involving TRF-2 and masks the linear ends of the chromosome from DNA damage response (DDR) machinery [4, 6]. The proteins TRF1 and TRF2 identify the TTAGGG duplex and bind to it. The single-strand binding protein POT1 binds the G-rich 5'-3' telomeric DNA strand. TIN2 and TPP1 aid in bridging TRF1/TRF2 with POT1 and stabilize telosome structure by connecting the telomere duplex with the single-stranded G-rich tail. Therefore, the TIN2 protein forms a bridge between TRFs and POT1-TPP1. TRF2 also forms attachment with hRap1, which suppresses

NHEJ by interacting with DNAPK-C [7]. Interaction between TRF1/TRF2 and TIN2 afford protection to TRFs from being degraded by tankyrase [5]. Interaction between POT1 and TRF2 prevents DDR induced by ataxia telangiectasia and Rad3-related protein (ATR) and ataxia telangiectasia mutated (ATM) and thus protect telomeres. The shelterin complex therefore functions as an inhibitor by preventing activation of telomeric DNA damage. Suppression of the activity of TRF2 protein results in DDR, leading to the activation of both p53 and ATM, which in turn induces inappropriate telomeric end-to-end fusions by the NHEJ machinery [5]. The shelterin proteins possess three distinct features that discriminate them from the nonshelterin telomere-associated proteins. These features are a) they are distinctively enriched at telomeres, b) they are present throughout the cell cycle at telomeres, and c) their functions are limited to telomere maintenance [8]. The shelterin complex allows or prevents telomerase to function on telomere by delivering signal related to telomere length. DNA polymerase, a key enzyme in replication process, fails to copy telomeric DNA as it is distal to the site of the last primase. This results in shortening of telomeric TTAGGG repeats and is termed as end replication problem. Telomeres therefore shorten with each S phase. Several other factors like oxidative damage and other processing events are also implicated in telomere shortening [9]. About 50–100 bp DNA remains unreplicated at the 3' end for each set of DNA replication, resulting in the loss of 50–100 bp and thereby progressive shortening of telomeres [10]. Shortening of telomere occurs from 10–15 kb (germ line) to 3–5 kb after 50–60 doublings. Repeated shortening ultimately limits the proliferative potential of somatic cells with aging. Telomeres reaching a critically short length are detected by the DNA repair systems, which ultimately induce death responses. Thus, telomere shortening represents a "molecular clock" as proposed by an American anatomist Leonard Hayflick [9] who explained the limited lifespan of cells in culture, otherwise termed as "Hayflick limit." Moreover, successive shortening of telomeres with each cell division activates p53-dependent checkpoint, leading to apoptosis or senescence [11]. Genomic instability at multiple levels occurs due to dysfunctional telomeres induced by progressive telomere shortening. Cells having critically short telomeres failed to enter permanent cell cycle arrest and activate the NHEJ pathway, thereby resulting in fusion of the chromosomal ends and subsequent breakage-fusion bridge cycles, eventually leading to a pro-cancer genotype [12]. Therefore, telomere dysfunction, telomere attrition may promote carcinogenesis by causing oncogenic chromosomal rearrangements, genomic instability, and cumulative risk of cancer progression. Role of different subunits of shelterin is represented in Table 2.1.

2.2.1 FACTORS MEDIATING THE FUNCTION OF SHELTERIN COMPLEX

Shelterin complex imparts its roles on telomere function by transient recruitment of some accessory factors that are often termed as nonshelterin proteins [8, 13], for example, MRN (Mre11-Rad50-NBS1), a protein complex that is implicated in recombination, telomeric overhang processing, and telomere length control by activating the checkpoint kinase (ATM) in response to DNA damage. TRF1 and TRF2 are known to recruit this complex to telomeres [13]. TRF2 also employs a shelterin accessory factor Apollo, which is a nuclease that protects human telomeres in the S phase, i.e., during or after their replication [14]. TRF1 recruits another poly-ADP-ribose polymerase or tankyrase 1 to telomere, which is responsible for telomere length regulation [15]. Tankyrase by effectively removing TRF1 from telomeres regulates telomeric length. This enzyme also plays a crucial role in Wnt signaling pathway and immortalization [16]. PIN2/TERF1-interacting telomerase inhibitor 1 protein, also known as PINX1, functions as a telomerase inhibitor. The domain in PINX1 responsible for the interaction with TRF1 is termed as TBM. PINX1 negatively regulates telomerase activity by binding directly to either hTERT or hTR [17]. Reports indicated that PINX1 by providing a link between TRF1 recruitment to telomere and telomerase inhibition inhibits elongation of telomere and thus sustains telomere homeostasis [18]. Shel-

TABLE 2.1   Function of Different Subunits of Shelterin Complex [25]

Subunits	Function
TRF1	Binds the TTAGGG duplex
TRF2	Forms T-loop structure by invading 3'overhang loop to double stranded telomereic DNA
TIN2	Binds TRFs 1 and 2; connects the telomere duplex with the single stranded G-overhang.
RAP1	Binds with TRF2; suppresses non-homologous end joining
TPP1	Recruits telomerase, recruits POT1
POT1	Binds single stranded overhang; Information from double-strand region is passed on to the single-strand region

terin also contributes to the repression of homology-directed recombination (HDR) at telomeres. Evidence showed that sister telomere exchanges (T-SCEs) are notable in the absence of either TRF2 or both POT1 proteins, but most importantly in cells lacking Ku70/80 [19]. Another shelterin-associated factor nucleostemin, a novel family of nucleolar GTP-binding proteins, promotes degradation of TRF1 by binding to it [20]. Nucleostemin decreases binding of TRF1 to telomeric DNA and reduces the association between telomere and TRF1 [20]. Another protein, namely GNL3L or guanine nucleotide-binding protein-like 3, is a GTP-binding nucleo-cytoplasmic shuttling protein that binds TRF1 in the nucleoplasm and accelerates the homodimerization and association of TRF1 to telomere. GNL3L reinforces TRF1 by diminishing ubiquitylation and FBX4 binding [21]. PIN1 protein or peptidyl-prolyl cis-trans isomerase NIMA-interacting 1 protein is an essential novel controller of TRF1 stability and telomere maintenance [22]. Inhibition of PIN1 accelerates binding of TRF1 on telomeres, leading to continuous shortening of telomere in human cells. A member of the F-box family of proteins or FBX4 protein targets PIN2/TRF1 and induces proteasomal degradation mediated by ubiquitination, thereby causing continuous elongation of telomeres in human cells [23]. A multisubunit DNA binding complex comprising six subunits, termed as origin recognition complex or ORC, assists in maintaining telomere integrity by enabling efficient replication of telomere DNA, thus preventing telomere circle formation [5, 24]. Another two important shelterin-associated proteins, PNUTS or phosphatase nuclear targeting subunit and MCPH1 or microcephalin 1, directly interact with TRF2 and controls length of telomere and telomeric DDR [25]. In a recent study, the expression profile of a set of nonshelterin genes replication protein A1(*RPA1*), DNA damage repair pathways protein (MRN genes), and Dyskeratosis Congenita 1, Dyskerin (DKC1) has been studied in patients with multiple myeloma. Disparity, in the expression profile of these genes, was correlated with telomere shortening and higher expression of telomerase [26]. Rad51, another protein by functioning as inducer of repair of DNA double-strand breaks, facilitates telomere replication, telomere maintenance, and capping. BRCA2, a key component of the HR pathway, acts as a suppressor of telomere shortening, in association with RAD51 [27, 28]. Shelterin, therefore, forms a complex platform for chromosome end protection and replication. Functions of some nonshelterin proteins are tabulated in Table 2.2.

TABLE 2.2 Function of Shelterin Complex-Associated Factors [13]

Proteins/Factors	Function
MRN	Aids in recombination, telomeric
(Mre11-Rad50-NBS1)	Overhang processing and telomere length control
Apollo (a nuclease)	Protects human telomeres in S phase
	i.e. during or after their replication
Tankyrase 1	Regulates telomere length and sister chromatid separation;
(a poly-ADP-ribose poly-merase)	Involves in Wnt signaling pathway and immortalization
PINX1 (PIN2/TERF1-interacting telomerase inhibitor 1)	Negatively regulates telomerase activity; prevent telomere elongation
Ku70/80	Represses of HDR
	(homology directed recombination)
Nucleostemin	Reduces the association between telomere and TRF1
GNL3L (guanine nucleo-tide-binding protein-like 3)	Binds TRF1; accelerates homodimerization and telomeric association of TRF1
PIN1 (Peptidyl-prolyl cis-trans isomerase NIMA-interacting 1)	Regulates TRF1 stability and telomere maintenance
FBX4 (F-box family of proteins)	Elongation of telomeres; ubiquitin-mediated degradation of PIN2/TRF1
ORC (Origin Recognition Complex)	Maintains telomere integrity;
	protects telomere
PNUTS (Phosphatase nuclear targeting subunit)	Controls telomere length
MCPH1 (Microcephalin 1)	Involves in telomere protection
RAD51	Repair of DNA double strand breaks telomere maintenance and capping

2.3 TELOMERASE, STRUCTURE, AND REGULATION

Telomerase, an RNA dependent DNA polymerase, helps to solve the end-replication problem by synthesizing new telomeres [11]. Reactivation of telomerase universally correlates with continuous cell growth, which is one of the hallmarks of advanced malignancies. Telomerase is detected in almost all malignant cases and may predict poor outcome [9]. Telomerase is therefore considered as an important biomarker and a potential target for cancer diagnostics and therapeutics. Telomerase is a reverse transcriptase by virtue of its action of copying RNA into DNA. This enzyme consists of a telomere RNA component, known as TERC or hTR, containing 451 nucleotides (including CAAUCCCAAUC telomere template) and a protein component telomerase reverse transcriptase (TERT) of 1132 amino acid sequence with reverse transcriptase motifs encoded by the hTERT gene located on chromosome 5p15.33. The hTERT expression is required to transform normal cells into cancer cells and is considered as a hallmark of tumorigenesis. The hTERT promoter is capable of promoting both constitutive hTERT genes, selectively in cancer cells and sparing normal cells. Most tumors or virtually all types of cancers express telomerase as it is required for long-term maintenance of telomeres, thereby long-term survival of cells [29]. TERT by utilizing the (3'-CAAUCCCAAUC-5') template region of TERC adds TTAGGG sequence of DNA repeats to 3' telomeric strands. A very strong correlation exists between telomerase expression and the presence of detectable hTERT mRNA [30]. Apart from two core components, several other proteins associate with the holoenzyme, including telomerase cajal body protein 1 [31, 32], the four H/ACA-motif RNA binding proteins dyskerin or NAP57, NHP2, NOP10, and Gar1 [33] and two ATPase proteins pontin and reptin [34]. Regulation of telomerase is very complex and involves multiple levels of control. Transcriptional regulation of the catalytic subunit TERT is the major determinant and crucial stage affecting telomerase activity. It has been suggested that hTERT can be regulated at both post-transcriptional and post-translational level. Moreover, reports are also available for transcriptional regulation of TR.

2.3.1   TRANSCRIPTIONAL REGULATION OF TERT

Multiple mechanisms regulate the gene encoding hTERT. Cooperation between multiple regulatory proteins is required for the activation of hTERT transcription. However, post-translational regulation of TERT also aids in regulation of telomerase activity. It is well documented that hTERT is expressed during early development; however, in normal somatic cells, the expression of TERT is very poor or absent barring proliferating cells and renewal tissues [9]. By transfecting hTERT promoter luciferase reporter, higher expression of hTERT was observed; this reflects telomerase activity asserting the involvement of TERT promoter in enzyme regulation [35]. The telomerase transcript containing 16 exons can be spliced into multiple isoforms, of which the major isoforms studied in cultured cancer cells involve exons 6–9 that encode part of the reverse transcriptase domain. Alternative splicing of mRNA is observed in TERT gene expression. Different variants of alternatively spliced TERT have been observed in the testis, colonic crypt, and other organs, suggesting a complex regulation of the TERT gene [36]. Ten splice variants of TERT have been identified so far, of which the α splice site and the β site are the most relevant ones [35, 37]. Subcellular localization of splicing factors, when varies, results in regulation of alternate splicing of the TERT gene [35]. Various factors have been reported to regulate TERT transcription. For example, TGF-β1 regulates TERT transcription through alternate splicing and induces rapid degradation of the TERT transcript. In contrast, c-Myc binds to E-boxes of the hTERT promoter and activates the TERT gene. This is a common feature observed in cancer [52]. Some of the factors regulating hTERT transcription are discussed in the following subsections.

2.3.1.1   Cellular Transcription Factors

Transcription factors like c-Myc and Sp1are known to regulate *hTERT* promoter. Involvement of HIF 1α in hTERT regulation has been reported. Activating enhancer-binding protein-2 or AP-2, family of transcription factors, the common regulator of gene expression, is reported as a transcriptional activator of the TERT promoter [38]. E26 transformation-specific or ETS family of transcription factors activate hTERT transcription [39]. Wilm's suppressor protein or WT1 protein binds to the hTERT promoter and negatively regulates hTERT expression. Repression of hTERT transcription is accomplished by some other protein factors like MZF-2, which is a zinc finger transcription factor, and also by suppressor proteins p53, pRb, E2F, and Mad1 [40].

2.3.1.2   Hormones

Androgen hormone has been shown to regulate the hTERT gene in human prostate cancer cells [41]. Estrogen via binding of ligand-activated estrogen receptor-α (ERα) to the estrogen-responsible element (ERE) of the hTERT promoter activates hTERT transcription. Apart from this, estrogen also activates hTERT expression via post-transcriptional mechanisms by stimulating nuclear accumulation of hTERT via its phosphorylation mediated by Akt signaling [38]. Progesterone, another female hormone exerts, effects on hTERT mRNA expression breast cancer cells with progesterone receptor-positive [38]. Short-term exposure activates hTERT transcription, but exposure for an extended period antagonizes estrogen, thereby inhibiting hTERT transcription. An autocrine human gonadotropic hormone (hGH) regulates telomerase activity by stabilizing hTERT mRNA in human mammary carcinoma cells, an effect mediated by binding of poly(C)-binding proteins $\alpha CP1$ and $\alpha CP2$ to specific *cis*-regulatory sequences in the 3'-UTR of hTERT mRNA [42]. Cholesterol-activated receptor C_k, a receptor protein, regulates transcription of the hTERT gene in peripheral blood mononuclear cells of human origin [43].

2.3.1.3 Cytokines

STAT3, a key transcription factor involved in the cytokine signaling pathway, regulates hTERT expression in both normal and cells [44]. IL-2, IL-7, and IL-8 are some critical cytokines that are involved in cell proliferation and self-renewal process and are known to increase telomere length by activating hTERT gene expression [39, 45]. TGF-β is a cytokine involved in the repression of hTERT transcription [46], probably by interaction of Smad3, c-Myc, and the hTERT gene [47] and through inhibition of E2F [48].

2.3.1.4 Oncogenes

BMI-1, a member of the Polycomb family, is an important oncogene product that can regulate hTERT expression. Uncontrolled expression BMI-1 ultimately activates hTERT transcription[49]. Some of the oncogenes like HER2/Neu, Ras, and Raf activate transcription of hTERT via the MAP kinase pathway [50]. CCAAT/enhancer-binding protein or CEBP-α and β are involved in genetic regulation of TERT during carcinogenesis [51]. Human papillomavirus type 16 oncoprotein E6 is a well-known activator of TERT gene transcription [52].

2.3.1.3   Epigenetic Regulation of hTERT Transcription

The hTERT promoter contains a cluster of CpG sites that are thought to be involved in DNA methylation. TERT promoter methylation at CpG sites has been studied, although the findings are contradictory. Some groups suggested an association between methylation and gene silencing [38], while others revealed invasion, lymph node metastasis, and poor prognosis [53]. Epigenetic status of the endogenous hTERT locus and chromatin environment plays pivotal roles in normal human somatic cells and genesis [54, 55]. Combination of DNA methylation and histone modifications, two important epigenetic mechanisms, regulates hTERT in hepatocellular carcinoma [56]. Increased DNA methylation in the hTERT promoter region in numerous cancers has been documented. Inhibition of HDAC differentially regulates TERT transcription and protein stability in cancer [57].

2.3.2   TRANSLATIONAL REGULATION OF TERT

The expression of hTERT is an essential determining factor of human telomerase activity. Regulation of telomerase activity at the post-translational level is observed via reversible phosphorylation of TERT at specific serine/threonine or tyrosine residues [36]. Some of the proteins, like protein kinase C (PKC) and Akt/protein kinase B (PKB), phosphorylate the hTERT protein, thereby upregulating telomerase activity. Ubiquitination is also known to influence telomerase activity. Overexpression of the ubiquitin ligase enzyme MKRN1 culminated in TERT degradation, because of which telomerase activity decreases and consequently leads to shortening of telomeres [35]. PKCα phosphorylates both TERT and human telomerase associated protein 1 or hTEP1. Protein phosphatase 2A (PP2A) dephosphorylates TERT at serine and/or threonine residue and thereby negatively regulates TERT expression [58]. Upregulation of telomerase activity without altering TERT protein expression by interleukin 6 (IL-6) and insulin-like growth factor 1 (IGF-1) is achieved through PI3K/Akt/NFκB signaling [36]. C-ABL protein (cellular form of the Abelson leukemia virus tyrosine kinase) and BCR (breakpoint cluster region protein) fusion product BCR-ABL phosphorylates telomerase and regulates the enzyme at the transcription as well as posttranslational level [59]. Another observation revealed that C terminus of Hsc70-interacting protein (CHIP) aids in the maintenance of hTERT in the cytoplasm, which thus negatively regulates telomerase activity by blocking entry of TERT to the nucleus [60].

2.3.3 REGULATION OF TR AT THE TRANSCRIPTIONAL AND POSTTRANSCRIPTIONAL LEVEL

Telomerase RNA, a small nucleolar RNA-like RNA (snoRNA-like RNA), controls the synthesis of telomeric DNA and thereby stabilizes chromosomes [61]. The telomerase RNA gene *hTERC*, located on chromosome 3q21-q28, encodes RNA component of telomerase. *hTERC* is transcribed by RNA polymerase II and, after processing at the 3' end, produces a mature transcript of 451 nucleotides (including the CAAUCCCAAUC telomere template). Unlike other RNAs, the mature form of hTR is formed by exonucleolytic cleavage by the H/ACA domain. Further cleavage is prevented by dyskerin associated with the RNA [62]. The human telomerase RNA (hTR) is composed of 5'-terminal pseudoknot domains that help in associating telomeric template sequence with hTERT. Apart from pseudoknot domain, hTR possesses another domain, namely H/ACA domain, which is crucial for the accumulation, enzymatic activity, and correct localization of telomerase RNP [63]. The H/ACA scaRNA domain of hTR binds with the four H/ACA core proteins. The ribonucleoprotein dyskerin or NAP57 (located at the X chromosome and encoded by the *DKC1* gene) is an inevitable protein essential for folding and stability of RNA part of telomerase and is an important protein component of the basic human telomerase enzyme complex [64]. Dyskerin, which forms a tetrameric complex with NOP10, NHP2, and the chaperone NAF1, binds to hTR co-transcriptionally [62]. Association of hTR with this complex is crucial for hTR accumulation. Transcription of hTR is regulated by some important transcription factors like Sp1, HIF-1α, etc., whereas factors like Sp3 repress hTR transcription. Epigenetic regulation plays an important role in repression of hTR expression [65]. Pseudouridylation, which is an important posttranscriptional modification, plays in important role in functional activity of hTR [66]. Tumor microenvironment also exerts its influence on telomerase gene regulation. Hypoxia induces transcriptional activity of endogenous hTR promoter [67].

2.3.4 HTERT AND HTR TRANSPORTATION TO THE NUCLEUS

Import of hTERT to the nucleus after synthesis is required for assembly of this protein with the RNA component (TERC) to become catalytically active telomerase. Multiple proteins are required for transportation and proper assembly of hTR and hTERT to telomeres. The molecular chaperone protein HSP90 and p23 help in maintaining hTERT conformation, thereby enabling nuclear translocation [68]. For nuclear import, the hTERT protein possesses a bipartite nuclear localization signal (NLS; residues 222–240) [69]. Importin 7, a soluble nuclear transport factor, is required for the efficient importation of hTERT from the cytoplasm to the nucleus. Another protein, Nup358, a nucleoporin and a member of nuclear pore complex (NPC), forms cytoplasmic filaments with NPC. Both these proteins (Importin 7 and Nup358) promote nuclear translocation of the hTERT protein to the nucleus [70]. Akt, a serine/threonine specific protein kinase phosphorylates hTERT at serine 227 residue and enhances the binding for importin α and accelerates hTERT translocation [69]. Multiple nuclear structures regulate displacement of TR and TERT. TR is present in cajal bodies (CBs) throughout the cell cycle that aids in translocation of the enzyme toward telomeres [71]. CBs may function in biogenesis and/or RNP assembly, RNA modification, and maturation (e.g., cap hypermethylation of hTR) at the posttranscriptional level. The notion has been reinforced by increased accumulation of hTR in CBs during the S phase of cell division, when telomeric DNA synthesis takes place [63]. Accumulation of hTR in CBs facilitates recruitment of telomerase to telomeres and ultimately telomere elongation [32]. TERT on the contrary is located in distinct nucleoplasmic foci. Translocation of TERT to nucleoli is an important event at the early S phase, whereas cajal bodies containing TR are known to accumulate within the nucleolus. TERT-dependent hTR telomere localization is an important event for the maintenance of telomere [72] In humans, telomerase has been reported to be associated with most telomeres at the S phase of the cell cycle [71, 73].

2.4 TELOMERASE FUNCTION

The enzyme telomerase is composed of a catalytic protein domain named TERT and an RNA part known as telomerase RNA component (TERC) or telomerase RNA (TR). Synthesis of telomere involves TERT protein that by using the small template region of TERC catalyzes reverse transcription. Telomerase activity is usually negative in normal somatic cells, differentiated cells, and post-mitotic cells. Normal cells, therefore, lose telomeres progressively until a few short telomeres become uncapped and the ends get associated with each other, leading to generation of a DNA damage signal and ultimately replicative senescence or replicative aging [9], which is commonly termed as an M1 stage or a cellular growth arrest. These cells remain in the quiescent stage in absence of any genetic alterations. Specific genetic and epigenetic alterations in normal human cells may advance to continuous proliferation, bypassing replicative senescence and eventually entering a second growth arrest state termed as a crisis stage. Alarmingly truncated telomeres lead to chromosome bridge breakage fusion, resulting into apoptosis or may affect health and lifespan at multiple levels [74]. Sometimes, shorter telomeres can mediate interchromosomal fusion followed by genomic instability, thereby contributing to the development of cancer [74]. Two mechanisms of cell growth restriction (senescence and crisis) existing in human cells are considered as initial anticancer protection mechanism [75]. Human cells can remain in this crisis period with cell growth being balanced by death, until a rare cell acquires a "turned on" control button, namely the enzyme telomerase, which can rejuvenate the telomere and allow the cells to divide endlessly [9] Continuous growth of telomeres due to increased telomerase activity is generally considered as a critical step in the progression of cancer [9]. Reactivation of telomerase expression in cancer is primarily due to transcriptional activation of TERT, which include reactivation of the TERT promoter [76]. TERT promoter reactivation involves multiple changes like mutation and chromosomal rearrangements [77, 78]. Another responsible factor for telomerase reactivation is mutations in the noncoding promoter region of TERT in two key positions C250T and C228T, as observed in 19% of cancer cells [78]. High telomerase activity is found in various proliferative cells, stem cells, intestinal stem cells, hematopoietic progenitor cells, activated lymphocytes, hair follicles, and cancer cells. Telomerase are found with detectable level in some adult cells like epithelial cells, fibroblasts, and endothelial cells. Association of HPV oncogenes (E6 and E7) with TERT promoter mutation has been frequently observed in Indian cervical and oral squamous cell carcinomas [79].

2.5 TELOMERASE ACTIVITY IN DIFFERENT CANCERS

Regulation at the level of transcription of hTERT is the major determinant of telomerase activity. Although TERT is expressed in stem cells, it is naturally silenced upon differentiation. Increased telomerase activity is frequent in different types of cancer, including colon, lung, liver, breast, leukemia, lymphoma, and prostate cancer [80]. Inhibition of telomerase activity may give rise to cellular senescence, growth retardation, and apoptosis, suggesting a fruitful drive to treat cancer [81]. Several researchers have shown telomerase activity in pancreatic and other types of cancers. Higher telomerase activity has been encountered in 95% of pancreatic adenocarcinoma cases [82]. In gastrointestinal cancers, very high telomerase activity has been observed, rendering telomeres and telomerase as potential targets for cancer therapy. Dysregulation of telomerase activity has been observed in some of the following cancers.

2.5.1 ESOPHAGEAL CANCER

Esophageal cancer carries a poor prognosis due to its relapse at advanced stages. Esophageal squamous cell cancer (ESCC) and esophageal adenocarcinoma (EAC) are two noticeable types of esophageal cancer. Telomere shortening has been observed in the early process of esophageal carcinogenesis [83], which might lead to chromosomal instability [84]. Activation of telomerase in esophageal cancer has been reported to occur early during cancer progression and is regulated on the transcriptional level. Epidermal growth factor receptor (EGFR) signaling furthermore activates telomerase through transcriptional as well as posttranscriptional regulation. Activation of the EGFR-signaling pathway in the cellular model of esophageal carcinoma enhances telomerase activation via phosphorylation and translocation of p21 supporting an additional role of telomerase in progression besides telomere elongation [85]. Activation of telomerase has been frequently detected in Barrett's esophagus, a type of gastro-esophageal reflux disease due to overexpression of hTERT and constitutes a useful biomarker for early detection of esophageal dysplasia and adenocarcinoma [86]. Another study revealed that HR activity is deregulated in Barrett's EAC. Elevated telomerase and HR activity are implicated in telomere maintenance. Therefore, targeting HR and telomerase has the potential to prevent growth in Barrett's adenocarcinoma [87].

2.5.2 GASTRIC CANCER

People with shorter telomeres in peripheral blood lymphocytes have chances of developing gastric cancer. Telomere length in DNA of peripheral leuko-cytes has been reported to reflect cumulative oxidative stress due to several factors like positivity for *Helicobacter pylori*, cigarette smoking, and intake of dietary fruits [88]. About 10–25% gastric cancers are identified due to defects in mismatch repair of DNA, resulting in microsatellite instability and thereby genomic instability. In such gastric cancer cases, alternative lengthening of telomeres (ALT) to maintain telomere length is a familiar event [89]. The underlying mechanisms of telomerase activation in gastric cancer remain elusive. Repeated mutations in the TERT promoter are asso-ciated with augmentation in TERT expression and activation of telomerase in patients with gastric cancer [90]. Another study showed that similar to esophageal cancer, the activation of Akt by EGFR signaling enhanced the expression of hTERT and telomerase activity in gastric cancer tissues. Sur-vival rates of patients with high p-Akt and high hTERT were poorer than those of other patients [91].

2.5.3 COLORECTAL CANCER

Shortening of telomere in colorectal cancer (CRC) is a common phenom-enon particularly during the preneoplastic stage and leads to chromosomal instability. hTERT levels increase with the adenoma–carcinoma stages with the highest level in carcinoma [92]. hTERT can promote cancer metastasis by stimulating epithelial to mesenchymal transition in CRC [93]. Another research team observed that colon and rectal cancer cells have different telomerase and MLH1 profiles that may be responsible for differences in biological and clinical behavior and progression of cancer [94]. TRF1, an inhibitor of telomerase and a negative regulator of telomere, is found to be overexpressed in CRC with appreciably shortened telomeres [95]. Colorec-tal polyps exhibiting shortened telomeres are likely to develop telomere dysfunction, driving genomic instability and progression toward malig-nancy [96]. In a cohort of 137 CRC patients, prognostic value in terms of hTERT expression has been evaluated. Bertorelle et al. in their study showed that CRC patients with high levels of hTERT messenger RNA (mRNA) in their cells had a significantly higher risk of death [95]. Hypermethylation of hTERT is correlated with high telomerase activity in CRC [97].

2.5.4   HEPATOCELLULAR CARCINOMA

Chronic liver inflammation is a frequent feature observed in hepatocellular carcinoma (HCC) leading to fibrosis and finally cirrhosis induced by several factors like hepatitis virus infection, alcohol consumption, nonalcoholic fatty liver disease, and other environmental factors. Progressive shortening of telomeres in HCC has been detected from cirrhotic to dysplastic nodules of low and high grade [89]. Telomere dysfunction and certain other cause-specific changes appear during cirrhosis and HCC [98]. Telomerase activation in hepatic precancerous lesions has been demonstrated by several groups. It is, however, a debatable issue whether telomerase activation supports liver regeneration or culminates in hepatocarcinogenesis [99]. Another observation by Oh et al. [100] has revealed increased hTERT mRNA expression with the progression of hepatocarcinogenesis, which is associated with significant induction in the transition between low- and high-grade dysplastic nodules. Frequent mutation in the hTERT promoter is the earliest genetic event indicated in cirrhotic preneoplastic lesions and is also the most frequent genetic alteration in hepatocellular carcinomas, occurring as a result of both the cirrhotic or noncirrhotic liver [101]. Somatic TERT mutation is therefore considered as a predictive biomarker of conversion of premalignant lesions into HCC [102, 103].

2.5.5   PANCREATIC CANCER

In more than 80% of the pancreatic ductal adenocarcinoma (PDAC), higher telomerase activity is evident. Mutation of the KRAS gene is the main driving force for the development of pancreatic cancer, and other subsequent effectors of RAS, such as MEK and ETS transcription, ultimately upregulate hTERT and are intricately associated with telomerase regulation in PDAC [104]. In PDAC cell line, enhanced hTERT expression induces cancer stem cell activity due to CD133 overexpression and EGFR activation, thereby promoting proliferation with high metastatic potential [105].

2.5.6   HEMATOLOGIC MALIGNANCIES

Shortening of telomeres, activation of telomerase, and marked change in the expression of telomere-associated proteins are some of the frequent characteristics observed in various hematologic malignancies, which are associated with ultimate disease progression due to resistance to chemotherapy [106]. Hematopoetic cells may develop genetic instability due to gradual telomere erosion leading to aplastic anemia, increased risk of myelodysplastic syndrome, acute myeloid leukemia, and some other hematological diseases. Characterization of telomeric length in hematopoetic cells therefore could be a potential clinical marker of hematologic neoplasia and may determine the prognosis of disease [107]. Telomere maintenance and telomerase activation pathway therefore are distinctive features of cancer including hematological cancer. Telomerase inhibition in preclinical and clinical studies has shown remarkable efficacy in different types of malignancies [108]. Role of telomerase in different types of hematological cancers is as follows.

2.5.6.1   Acute Leukemia

Acute leukemia (AL) is distinguished by abnormal multiplication of myeloid precursor cells (acute myeloid leukemia, AML) or lymphoblast cells (acute lymphoblastic leukemia, ALL). Patients with AL commonly show a feature like diminished telomere length, with corresponding chromosomal instability. Aberrant karyotype with significantly shorter telomere length has been observed among AL patients compared to normal karyotype in normal subjects. A report from Capraro et al. showed specific telomere dysregulation among each leukemia subtype that depends on phenotypic and karyotypic features, which determine the treatment response to particular therapeutics and survival [109]. However, shorter telomere length and higher telomerase activity have been observed in late stage AML patients or in patients in relapsed stage [106, 110].

2.5.6.2   Chronic Myeloid Leukemia

Role of telomere/telomerase in the biology of progression of disease in malignant stem disorder can be best understood in chronic myeloid leukemia (CML). BCR/ABL fusion genes with the corresponding expression of the BCR-ABL fusion protein with elevated tyrosine kinase activity is a major characteristic feature of CML. Several studies have revealed changes in telomere length and telomerase activity in both chronic phase (CP) and blastic phase (BP). Increased telomerase activity has been unveiled in the bone marrow cells of CML patients during development of the disease. Tyrosine kinase activity of BCR-ABL fusion protein increases telomere shortening due to generation of reactive oxygen species [106]. Accelerated telomere shortening was observed during progression of the disease from the CP to the BP. A correlation between accelerated telomere shortening with leukemia progression, risk score, and response to treatment has been established in CML [111]. The work done by Braig et al. further indicated that targeting telomerase might influence cellular senescence with a concomitant inhibition of promoting/progressing effect of BCR-ABL [111]. Pronounced shortening of telomeres in chromosome Y and chromosome 21 may lead to secondary chromosomal abnormality. Alterations of individual telomeric length and subsequent cellular proliferation has been reported during clonal selection of early CML stage [112, 113].

A study by Samassekou et al. [114] reported a high frequency of circular extra-chromosomal telomeric repeat (ECTR) during the CP stage of CML, which is a specific hallmark of activation of ALT pathway, suggesting its requirement at early stages of leukemogenesis. However, later stage CML displays activated telomerase proposing a state of progression from ALT to telomerase, manifesting a transformation of the CP to the blast crisis phase. Altered expressions of shelterin proteins were frequently observed in patients with CML progression. Increased expression of TRF1 and TRF2 was observed in the CP and accelerated phase (AP) in CML patients [106]. TRF1 overexpression may induce reduction in telomere length in CML patients [106]. Altered mRNA splicing of the hTERT gene might determine the functional level of hTERT and therefore conservation of telomeres and may direct disease progression [115].

2.5.6.3   Myelodysplastic Syndromes (MDS)

Myelodysplastic syndromes (MDS), characterized by features of dysplasia in hematopoietic cells, are disorders having the tendency to progress toward AL [106]. Mononuclear cell populations isolated from patients with MDS exhibited very high telomerase activity [106]. However, hematopoietic cells from MDS patients express low level of telomerase [116]. Loss of telomere ends up with mutations and disease progression by impelling genetic abnormalities [116]. Myeloid cells (CD15+) and lymphocytes (CD19+) of MDS patients have much shortened telomeres [117]. In a study, Lange et al. measured telomere lengths of individual chromosomes and confirmed gradual reduction in telomere length as a basic criterion for affecting hematopoietic cells in patients with MDS except in an monosomy 7 [118].

2.5.6.4 T-Cell Leukemia

Several lines of evidence established that human T-cell leukemia virus type I or HTLV-1, an agent of T cell leukemia, converts normal T cells to leukemic cells [116]. Despite the presence of high activity of telomerase, telomere length is short in cells infected with HTLV-1 [119], which is correlated with poorer prognosis. Therefore, telomerase activation may be considered as worthwhile markers for predicting disease progression. The effect of HTLV-1-coded Tax protein on hTERT remains debatable. Some study showed a negative effect of Tax on the hTERT promoter [116]. Another study on contrary showed that Tax through the nuclear factor κB (NF-κB) signaling pathway mediated by Sp1 and c-Myc, positively influence endogenous hTERT promoter [116]. It was reported that Tax activates hTERT promoter in T cells which are in quiscent stage vis a vis represses activity in T cells which are in proliferating stage; indicating its dual role in regulating hTERT. [120]. Several factors are also responsible for increased transcription of hTERT particularly during the late stage of leukemogenesis [116].

2.5.6.5 Multiple Myeloma (MM)

Multiple myeloma (MM), a disorder of plasma cells, is distinguished by the clonal expansion of cells, resulting in anemia, renal insufficiency, and bone disease. Telomere lengths are reported to be reduced in MM cells compared to normal age-matched control [121]. A gene expression profile study involving MM patient samples also revealed that myeloma and plasma cells maintain short telomeres that enable cells to divide continuously [122]. Telomerase activity was considered as a hallmark for proliferative capacity and mass plasma cells [121]. Preclinical data also showed that inhibition of telomerase is a novel therapeutic approach in MM [123].

2.5.6.6 B Cell Malignancies

Progressive accumulation of leukemia clone leads to B-cell chronic lympho-cytic leukemia (B-CLL) [116]. Telomere shortening is an important indica-tive feature of B-CLL. Evidence-based study revealed a strong impact of telomere length and telomerase activity in B-CLL patients; this is observed as slightly higher telomerase activity at the onset of disease than in normal subjects and increased activity among patients in advanced stage as well as poor prognosis. B-CLL patients can be identified with definite biologi-cal characteristics and treatment outcome based on comprehensive analy-ses of telomeres and telomerase [124]. A study using B cells isolated from untreated CLL patients showed shortening of relative telomere length com-pared to that in control; this suggests that the telomere/telomerase system is impaired in the early stages of CLL [125]. Another study proposed that telomere shortening and deprotection in the early stage of B-CLL is an out-come of shelterin alteration and dysregulation [126]. A very recent study demonstrated contribution of hTERT in preserving EBV latency (a prereq-uisite criterion for EBV-driven cell transformation) particularly through the NOTCH2 cellular pathway, thereby suggesting a significant role in immor-talization of lymphoblastoid cell immortalization [127]. The critical step of overcoming cellular senescence is accomplished by EBV through telomer-ase functioning of infected cells [128].

2.5.7 CERVICAL CANCER

Initiation and development of human cervical cancer are dependent on the activation of human telomerase reverse transcriptase (hTERT). The expres-sion level of Pin2/TRF1-interacting protein X1 (PINX1), a suppressor of hTERT, is diminished in cervical cancer cells with concomitant activation of telomerase. The underlying mechanism of PINX1 showed suppression of expression of PINX1 by HPV16 E6 via inhibiting p53 transcriptional activ-ity; this augmented telomerase activity in cervical cancer cells [129]. Hotspot mutation of TERT promoter either alone or in alliance with the HPV E6 and E7 proteins reactivates the enzyme and facilitates cervical carcinogenesis [79]. A study revealed re-expression of HPV16E2 in SiHa cells proceeded to increased expression of prosurvival genes like hTERT [130]. Another study that investigated the underlying mechanism of telomerase activation established a relation between activation of hTERT transcription and COX-2-PGE2-Sp1 expression in cervical cancer cells [131]. A study conducted by Petrenko et al. [132] showed that telomerase activity was found in 28% of adjacent normal tissue to CIN lesions and in 68% of CIN II-III. hTERT RNA was present in almost all CIN samples, thus indicating a correlation between the presence of HPV sequence and telomerase activation. The hTERT gene is enriched with CG regions. Core sequence of hTERT has the binding sites for transcriptional activators and repressors. The 5' region of the hTERT gene and its promoter are part of a large ~4 kb CpG island (-1800 to +2200, numbered relative to the ATG) and are the responsive region of CpG methylation. A study demonstrated a correlation between methylation of the CpG island in the hTERT promoter and deregulation of hTERT transcription in cervical cancer cells infected with HPV [133].

2.5.8 ORAL CANCER

The carcinogenesis process of oral squamous cell carcinoma (OSCC) is a highly complex process, which includes acquisition of genetic changes that lead to increased telomerase activity. The overexpression of hTERT is a common finding in OSCC [134]. Telomerase activation is considered as a biomarker in oral cancer cell proliferation [135]. In a previous study, telomerase activity was analyzed using salivary gland tissues (benign, malignant, and non-neoplastic) from patients, and the mRNA expression of hTERT and telomerase-associated proteins was examined. A strong correlation was observed between enzyme activity and mRNA expression, indicating telomerase as a potential marker in salivary gland carcinomas [136]. A recent study showed that hTERT has the potential to promote epithelial mesenchymal transition (EMT) by inducing the Wnt/β-catenin pathway that harmonize with the aggressiveness of OSCC in patients [137]. It was further observed that BMI-1 or (B lymphoma Mo-MLV insertion region 1 homolog), a protein that is overexpressed during cellular immortalization and EMT of oral epithelial cells, activates hTERT, which in turn plays a role in EMT [138]. A study conducted in an Indian laboratory revealed frequent hTERT promoter hotspot mutation among patients with OSCC [79]. Overexpression of EGFR activates telomerase by phosphorylating the hTERT protein via Akt in oral-esophageal carcinogenesis, thus suggesting a role of telomerase in the progression of tumor and in elongation of telomeres [85].

2.5.9 BREAST CANCER

It is well known that almost 100% breast adenocarcinoma cells express telomerase [139]. A mechanistic study of transcriptional regulation of telomerase has unveiled abundance of transcription factor sites in the TERT promoter [139]. The involvement of c-myc (a transcription factor involved in cellular immortalization) in telomerase regulation has been studied [139]. A study showed that Her2 and ER81 (a member of E26 transformation specific family) accelerate transcription of hTERT in breast cancer patients [140]. Another observation by Piscuoglio et al. revealed TERT alterations (promoter hotspot mutations and gene amplification) are the main driving force for the progression of Phyllodes tumors of breasts [141]. Several other studies reported upregulated telomerase activity in breast cancer tissues compared to that in adjacent normal tissues, and an association between high telomerase activity and poor response to chemotherapy has been documented among breast cancer cases [142]. Another important observation was that constitutively activated STAT3 binds to NF-κB, which in turn activates catalytic subunit of hTERT and thereby foster cancer stem cell phenotype in breast cancer [44]. Similarly, the Wnt pathway upregulates telomerase in human breast cancer cells [143]. Telomerase overexpression not only promotes survival of breast cancer cells but also impels resistance to anticancer agents [144].

2.5.10 LUNG CANCER

Telomere has been necessitated in the pathogenesis of a variety of lung diseases, like idiopathic pulmonary fibrosis, chronic obstructive pulmonary disease/emphysema, and lung carcinoma [145]. Studies that consider telomere as a prognostic marker for lung cancer risk are contradictory as reports indicate that both shorter and longer telomeres are associated with decreased overall survival [145]. Increased activity of telomerase is a recurrent event in lung cancer [146]. A positive correlation exists between telomerase activity and differentiation grade in non-small cell lung cancer (NSCLC) [147], resulting in poor prognosis of the disease. Oncogenic mutation of KRAS is reported to increase TERT mRNA expression and its activity in immortalized bronchial epithelial cells [148]. In nasopharyngeal carcinoma, lung cancer, and murine model of lung cancer, hTERT expression was found to be very high, and suppressor genes like Krüppel-like factor 4 (KLF4) and PINX1 downregulate telomerase activity in such cases [149, 150]. Another recent study has shown that transcriptional co-activators like CREB-binding protein (CBP) and ret finger protein like 3 (RFPL3) promote growth of lung cancer cells by activating hTERT [151,152]. A strong association between *TERT* polymorphism and EGFRmut[+] NSCLC has been established [153]. Accumulating evidence suggests that polymorphism of hTERT modulates IL-6 expression, an important cytokine responsible for the development of lung adenocarcinoma [154]. Another finding suggested that epidermal growth factor (EGF) upregulates telomerase activity by enhancing the binding of transcription factor ETS-2 with the hTERT promoter [155]. Promoter mutation of the hTERT gene leads to TERT mRNA upregulation, which is a more frequent event observed in malignant pleural mesothelioma [156].

2.5.11   PROSTATE CANCER

High telomerase activity is an important contributing factor in prostate carcinoma. Telomerase activity was detected in prostatic intraepithelial neoplasia (PIN), benign prostatic hyperplasia (BPH), in cases of atrophy, and in benign prostate glands. Prostate epithelial stem-like cells and progenitor fractions are reported to express high levels of telomerase activity, indicating that the enzyme is capable of maintaining benign prostatic hyperplasia (BPH) [157]. Mutation of the hTERT gene promoter is considered as a determining factor in the clinicopathological progression of urogenital cancer [158].

2.6   TELOMERASE ACTIVITY IN NORMAL AND CANCER STEM CELLS

Telomerase expression remains silent in most adult somatic tissues, which lead to gradual shortening of telomeres. However, telomeric DNA is actively regulated by numerous mechanisms in highly proliferative cells like germ cells, cancer cells, and pluripotent stem cells. Nuclear reprogramming ultimately restores telomere length and rejuvenates telomere status [159]. Telomerase and TERT are expressed during tumor evolution, starting from the cancer stem cells to circulating tumor cells and tumor metastases [160]. Several studies have confirmed extensive alternative splicing of TERT isoforms that leads to high expression of TERT in pluripotent stem cells [161].

This alternatively spliced subunit of TERT, having the ability to alter mitochondrial function and induce chromatin structure remodelling, participate in key signaling pathways like the Wnt/β-catenin pathway [161]. Normal stem cells are quiescent or slow growing with relatively long telomeres, whereas cancer stem cells universally express very high level of telomerase. Evidence showed the presence of telomere of shortened length in cancer stem cells, which probably indicated initiation of carcinogenesis [162]. Therefore, although proliferative descendants of stem cells of normal counterpart exhibit telomerase activity, the level is insufficient to maintain telomere length [162]. Cancer stem cells possess some characteristics like initiation of carcinogenesis, process of self-renewal, and the capacity to differentiate. Cancer cells would have to pass through critical shortening of telomeres that compels to upregulate telomerase so as to become immortal. For example, a subset of transiently amplified cells, which give rise to initiating cells, possess alarmingly shortened telomeres and culminates in genomic instability and eventual re-activation of telomerase [162]. A study revealed that NAD-dependent deacetylase SIRT1 levels are elevated in embryonic stem cells, suggesting a role for SIRT1 in pluripotency. In induced pluripotent stem (iPS) cells of murine model, SIRT1 is essential for post-reprogramming telomere elongation, which is mediated by c-myc-dependent regulation of murine TERT gene [163]. Telomerase upregulation/reactivation leads to the activation of multiple signaling pathways. A positive feedback loop probably exists between proteins targeting hTERT and TERT expression itself, which probably amplifies oncogenic pathways related to cancer stemness [164]. Several findings suggest the involvement of TERT functions independent from telomerase activity in the reprogramming process.

2.7 TELOMERASE THERAPEUTICS IN CANCER BY NATURAL MEANS

Reactivation of telomerase and telomere dysfunction as observed in almost all malignant cells and cancer stem cells has made the enzyme an attractive target for cancer therapy. Several strategies have been evolved to target telomerase, of which direct inhibition of the enzyme, telomerase interference, hTERT or hTERC promoter driven therapy, telomere-based approaches, and telomerase vaccines are noteworthy [81]. Several synthetic telomerase inhibitors are used for clinical trials. However, these inhibitors are not free from adverse toxic side effects. Therefore, deactivation or inhibition of enzyme by plant-derived compounds with little or no toxicity might assure a rational approach in cancer therapy. Several studies conducted worldwide have established the role of natural compounds in inhibiting or regulating telomerase activity in various cancers [165–167]. For example, natural iso-thiocynates are known to repress telomerase activity in many cancer cells like breast, cervical, and prostate cancer [168–170]. Curcumin, an Indian spice rich in polyphenol, extracted from plant turmeric *Curcuma longa* has been shown to inhibit telomerase activity in leukemia cells [171]. Both cur-cumin and isothiocyanates have reported to enhance therapeutic potential of anticancer chemotherapeutic drugs through downregulating telomerase; thus, it is tempting to speculate that these natural compounds by virtue of its inhibitory action on telomerase might prove useful in the prevention and therapy of cancer in conjunction with chemotherapeutics.

2.8 SUMMARY

- Chromosomal stability in mammalian cells largely depends on the proper maintenance of telomeres. Accumulation of chromosomal ab-normalities due to gradual shortening and improper functioning of telomere is implicated in human cancer.
- Telomere maintenance is achieved by an important reverse transcrip-tase enzyme telomerase that aids in extending telomeric repeats at the chromosomal end.
- Both telomeres and telomerase regulate a balance between genetic in-stability and senescence. Accelerated telomere shortening with pro-gressive cell division give rise to telomerase activation in cancer cells, predominantly in cancer stem cells.
- The potential of telomerase to maintain telomeric length is conditional as it depends on regulatory mechanisms of both hTERT and hTR at transcriptional, translational, and post-translational levels.
- Telomerase has emerged as a prospective prognostic indicator as well as a target for therapeutics in human malignancies.
- Several approaches have been developed to repress telomerase activity, both by synthetic and natural means. Currently, emphasis has been giv-en on the use of plant-derived dietary natural compounds in targeting telomerase because of their less toxic side effects and better efficacy.

- Exploitation of further knowledge of telomere biology is essential for early diagnosis and proper treatment of human malignancies. Furthermore, telomere-telomerase dynamics in cancer stem cells is an important area of research for the development of improved therapies to combat cancer.

KEYWORDS

- **cancer**
- **cancer stem cells**
- **phytochemicals**
- **shelterin**
- **telomerase**
- **telomere**

REFERENCES

1. Harley, C. B., (2008). Telomerase and cancer therapeutics. *Nat Rev Cancer, 8*(3), 167–179.
2. Bär, C., & Blasco, M. A., (2016). Telomeres and telomerase as therapeutic targets to prevent and treat age-related diseases. *F1000 Research, 5*(F1000 Faculty Rev), 89 doi: 10. 12688/f1000research. 7020. 1.
3. Blackburn, E. H., & Epel, E. S., (2012). Comment: Too toxic to ignore. *Nature, 490,* 169–171.
4. O'Sullivan, R. J., & Karlseder, J., (2010). Telomeres: protecting chromosomes against genome instability. *Nat Rev Mol Cell Biol., 3,* 171–181.
5. Diotti, R., & Loayza, D., (2011). Shelterin complex and associated factors at human telomeres. *Nucleus, 2*(2), 119–135.
6. Doksani, Y., Wu, J. Y., De Lange, T., & Zhuang, X., (2013). Super-resolution fluorescence imaging of telomeres reveals TRF2-dependent T-loop formation. *Cell, 155*(2), 345–356.
7. Arat, N. O., & Griffith, J. D., (2012). Human Rap1 interacts directly with telomeric DNA and regulates TRF2 localization at the telomere. *J. Biol. Chem., 287*(50), 41583–41594.
8. Sfeir, A., & De Lange, T., (2012). Removal of shelterin reveals the telomere end-protection problem. *Science, 42,* 301–334.
9. Shay, J. W., & Wright, W. E., (2011). Role of telomeres and telomerase in cancer. *Semin. Cancer Biol., 21*(6), 349–353.

10. Robin, J. D., Ludlow, A. T., Batten, K., Magdinier, F., et al., (2014). Telomere position effect: regulation of gene expression with progressive telomere shortening over long distances. *Genes Dev.*, *28*(22), 2464–2476.

11. Armanios, M., (2009). Syndromes of telomere shortening. *Annu. Rev. Genomics Hum. Genet.*, *10*, 45–61.

12. Jacobs, J. J. L., (2013). Loss of telomere protection: Consequences and opportunities. *Frontiers in Oncology*, *3*, 88.

13. Kalan, S., & Loayza, D., (2014). Shelterin complex in telomere protection: recent insights and pathological significance. *Cell Health and Cytoskeleton*, *6*, 11—26.

14. Wu, P., Van Overbeek, M., Rooney, S., & De Lange, T., (2010). Apollo contributes to G overhang maintenance and protects leading-end telomeres. *Mol Cell*, *39*, 606–617.

15. Li, B., Qiao, R., Wang, Z., Zhou, W., et al., (2016). Crystal structure of a tankyrase 1-telomere repeat factor 1 complex. *Acta Crystallogr. F. Struct. Biol. Commun.*, *72*(4), 320–327.

16. Riffell, J. L., Lord, C. J., & Ashworth, A., (2012). Tankyrase-targeted therapeutics: expanding opportunities in the PARP family. *Nature Reviews Drug Discovery*, *11*, 923–936.

17. Yonekawa, T., Yang, S., & Counter, C. M., (2012). PinX1 localizes to telomeres and stabilizes TRF1 at mitosis. *Mol Cell Biol.*, *32*(8), 1387–1395.

18. Soohoo, C. Y., Shi, R., Lee, T. H., Huang, P., Lu, K. P., & Zhou, X. Z., (2011). Telomerase inhibitor PinX1 provides a link between TRF1 and telomerase to prevent telomere elongation. *J. Biol. Chem.*, *286*(5), 3894–3906.

19. Kabir, S., Sfeir, A., & De Lange, T., (2010). Taking apart Rap1: an adaptor protein with telomeric and non-telomeric functions. *Cell Cycle*, *9*(20), 4061–4067.

20. Meng, L., Hsu, J. K., Zhu, Q., Lin, T., & Tsai, R. Y., (2011). Nucleostemin inhibits TRF1 dimerization and shortens its dynamic association with the telomere. *J. Cell Sci.*, *124*(21), 3706–3714.

21. Zhu, Q., Meng, L., Hsu, J. K., Lin, T., Teishima, J., & Tsai, R. Y., (2009). GNL3L stabilizes the TRF1 complex and promotes mitotic transition. *J. Cell Biol.*, *185*(5), 827–839.

22. Lee, T. H., Tun-Kyi, A., Shi, R., Lim, J., Soohoo, C., Finn, G., Balastik, M., Pastorino, L., Wulf, G., Zhou, X. Z., & Lu, K. P., (2009). Essential role of Pin1 in the regulation of TRF1 stability and telomere maintenance. *Nat. Cell Biol.*, *11*(1), 97–105.

23. Wang, C., Xiao, H., Ma, J., Zhu, Y., et al., (2013). The F-box protein β-TrCP promotes ubiquitination of TRF1 and regulates the ALT-associated PML bodies formation in U2OS cells. *Biochem. Biophys. Res. Commun.*, *434*(4), 728–734.

24. Deng, Z., Norseen, J., Wiedmer, A., Riethman, H., & Lieberman, P. M., (2009). TERRA RNA binding to TRF2 facilitates heterochromatin formation and ORC recruitment at telomeres. *Mol Cell.*, *35*(4), 403–413.

25. Kim, H., Lee, O. H., Xin, H., Chen, L. Y., Qin, J., Chae, H. K., Lin, S. Y., Safari, A., Liu, D., & Songyang, Z., (2009). TRF2 functions as a protein hub and regulates telomere maintenance by recognizing specific peptide motifs. *Nat. Struct. Mol Biol.*, *6*(4), 372–379.

26. Panero, J., Stella, F., Schutz, N., Fantl, D. B., & Slavutsky, I., (2015). Differential expression of non-shelterin genes associated with high telomerase levels and telomere shortening in plasma cell disorders. *PLoS One.*, *10*(9), e0137972.

27. Di Domenico, E. G., Mattarocci, S., Cimino-Reale, G., Parisi, P., Cifani, N., D'Ambrosio, E., Zakian, V. A., & Ascenzioni, F., (2013). Tel1 and Rad51 are involved

in the maintenance of telomeres with capping deficiency. *Nucleic Acids Res.*, *41*(13), 6490–6500.

28. Badie, S., Escandell, J. M., Bouwman, P., Carlos, A. R., Thanasoula, M., Gallardo, M. M., Suram, A., Jaco, I., Benitez, J., Herbig, U., Blasco, M. A., Jonkers, J., & Tarsounas, M., (2010). BRCA2 acts as a RAD51 loader to facilitate telomere replication and capping. *Nat. Struct. Mol Biol.*, *17*(12), 1461–1469.

29. Jafri, M. A., Ansari, S. A., Alqahtani, M. H., & Shay, J. W., (2016). Roles of telomeres and telomerase in cancer, & advances in telomerase-targeted therapies. *Genome Medicine*, *8*, 69.

30. Briatore, F., Barrera, G., Pizzimenti, S., & Toaldo, C., (2009). Increase of telomerase activity and hTERT expression in myelodysplastic syndromes. *Cancer Biol. Ther.*, *8*(10), 883–889.

31. Venteicher, A. S., Abreu, E. B., Meng, Z., Mc-Cann, K. E., Terns, R. M., Veenstra, T. D., Terns, M. P., & Artandi, S. E., (2009). A human telomerase holoenzyme protein required for Cajal body localization and telomere synthesis. *Science*, *323*(5914), 644–648.

32. Stern, J. L., Zyner, K. G., Pickett, H. A., Cohen, S. B., & Bryan, T. M., (2012). Telomerase recruitment requires both TCAB1 and Cajal bodies independently. *Mol Cell Biol.*, *32*(13), 2384–2395.

33. Egan, E. D., & Collins, K., (2010). Specificity and stoichiometry of subunit interactions in the human telomerase holoenzyme assembled *in vivo*. *Mol Cell Biol.*, *30*(11), 2775–2786.

34. Machado-Pinilla, R., Liger, D., Leulliot, N., & Meier, U. T., (2012). Mechanism of the AAA+ ATPases pontin and reptin in the biogenesis of H/ACA RNPs. *RNA*, *18*(10), 1833–1845.

35. Cifuentes-Rojas, C., & Shippen, D. E., (2012). Telomerase regulation. *Mutat. Res.*, *730*(1–2), 20–27.

36. Wojtyla, A., Gladych, M., & Rubis, B., (2011). Human telomerase activity regulation. *Mol Biol. Rep.*, *38*, 3339–3349.

37. Wong, M. S., Wright, W. E., & Shay, J. W., (2014). Alternative splicing regulation of telomerase: a new paradigm? *Trends Genet.*, *30*(10), 430–438.

38. Zhao, Y., Cheng, D., Wang, S., & Zhu, J., (2014). Dual roles of c-Myc in the regulation of hTERT gene. *Nucleic Acids Res.*, *42*(16), 10385–10398.

39. Ramlee, M. K., Wang, J., Toh, W. X., & Li, S., (2016). Transcription regulation of the human telomerase reverse transcriptase (hTERT) Gene Saretzki, G., ed. *Genes*, *7*(8), 50.

40. Hara, T., Mizuguchi, M., Fujii, M., & Nakamura, M., (2015). Krüppel-like factor 2 represses transcription of the telomerase catalytic subunit human telomerase reverse transcriptase (hTERT) in human T cells. *J. Biol. Chem.*, *290*(14), 8758–8763.

41. Jacob, S., Nayak, S., Kakar, R., Chaudhari, U. K., et al., (2016). A triad of telomerase, androgen receptor and early growth response 1 in prostate cancer cells. *Cancer Biol. Ther.*, *17*(4), 439–448.

42. Emerald, B. S., Chen, Y., Zhu, T., Zhu, Z., Lee, K. O., Gluckman, P. D., & Lobie, P. E., (2007). AlphaCP1 mediates stabilization of hTERT mRNA by autocrine human growth hormone. *J. Biol. Chem.*, *282*(1), 680–690.

43. Sikand, K., Kaul, D., & Varma, N., (2006). Receptor Ck-dependent signaling regulates hTERT gene transcription. *BMC Cell Biology*, *7*, 2. DOI: 10. 1186/1471–2121–7–2.

44. Chung, S. S., Aroh, C., & Vadgama, J. V., (2013). Constitutive activation of STAT3 signaling regulates hTERT and promotes stem cell-like traits in human breast cancer cells. *PLoS One.*, *8*(12), e83971.

45. Brazvan, B., Farahzadi, R., Mohammadi, S. M., et al., (2016). Key immune cell cytokines affects the telomere activity of cord blood cells in vitro. *Advanced Pharmaceutical Bulletin*, *6*(2), 153–161.

46. Tian, M., Neil, J. R., & Schiemann, W. P., (2011). Transforming growth factor-β and the hallmarks of cancer. *Cell Signal*, *23*(6), 951–962.

47. Li, H., & Liu, J. P., (2007). Mechanisms of action of TGF-beta in cancer: evidence for Smad3 as a repressor of the hTERT gene. *Ann. New York Acad. Sci.*, *1114*, 56–68.

48. Lacerte, A., Korah, J., Roy, M., Yang, X. J., Lemay, S., & Lebrun, J. J., (2008). Transforming growth factor-beta inhibits telomerase through SMAD3 and E2F transcription factors. *Cell Signal*, *20*(1), 50–59.

49. Qiao, B., Chen, Z., Hu, F., Tao, Q., & Lam, A. K., (2013). BMI-1 activation is crucial in hTERT-induced epithelial-mesenchymal transition of oral epithelial cells. *Exp. Mol Pathol.*, *95*(1), 57–61.

50. Xu, D., Li. H., & Liu, J. P. Inhibition of telomerase by targeting MAP kinase signaling. *Telomerase Inhibition of the Series Methods in Molecular Biology™*, vol. *405*, pp. 147–165.

51. Kumar, M., Witt, B., Knippschild, U., Koch, S., Meena, J. K., Heinlein, C., Weise, J. M., Krepulat, F., Kuchenbauer, F., Iben, S., Rudolph, K. L., Deppert, W., & Günes, C., (2013). CEBP factors regulate telomerase reverse transcriptase promoter activity in whey acidic protein-T mice during mammary carcinogenesis. *Int. J. Cancer*, *132*(9), 2032–2043.

52. Van Doorslaer, K., & Burk, R. D., (2012). Association between hTERT activation by HPV E6 proteins and oncogenic risk. *Virology*, *433*(1), 216–219.

53. Wu, Y., Li, G., He, D., Yang, F., He, G., He, L., Zhang, H., Deng, Y., Fan, M., Shen, L., Zhou, D., & Zhang, Z., (2016). Telomerase reverse transcriptase methylation predicts lymph node metastasis and prognosis in patients with gastric cancer. *Onco Targets Ther.*, *9*, 279–286.

54. Zhu, J., Zhao, Y., & Wang, S., (2010). Chromatin and epigenetic regulation of the telomerase reverse transcriptase gene. *Protein Cell*, *1*(1), 22–32.

55. Sui, X., Kong, N., Wang, Z., & Pan, H., (2013). Epigenetic regulation of the human telomerase reverse transciptase gene: A potential therapeutic target for the treatment of leukemia (Review). *Oncol. Lett.*, *6*(2), 317–322.

56. Iliopoulos, D., Satra, M., Drakaki, A., Poultsides, G. A., & Tsezou, A., (2009). Epigenetic regulation of hTERT promoter in hepatocellular carcinomas. *Int. J. Oncol.*, *34*(2), 391–399.

57. Qing, H., Aono, J., Findeisen, H. M., Jones, K. L., Heywood, E. B., & Bruemmer, D., (2016). Differential regulation of telomerase reverse transcriptase promoter activation and protein degradation by histone deacetylase inhibition. *J. Cell Physiol.*, *231*(6), 1276–1282.

58. Xi, P., Zhou, L., Wang, M., Liu, J. P., & Cong, Y. S., (2013). Serine/threonine-protein phosphatase 2A physically interacts with human telomerase reverse transcriptase hTERT and regulates its subcellular distribution. *J. Cell Biochem.*, *114*(2), 409–417.

59. Chai, J. H., Zhang, Y., Tan, W. H., Chng, W. J., Li, B., & Wang, X., (2011). Regulation of hTERT by BCR-ABL at multiple levels in K562 cells. *BMC Cancer*, *11*, 512. doi: 10. 1186/1471-2407-11-512.

60. Lee, J. H., Khadka, P., Baek, S. H., & Chung, I. K., (2010). CHIP promotes human telomerase reverse transcriptase degradation and negatively regulates telomerase activity. *J. Biol. Chem.*, *285*, 42033–42045.

61. Mannoor, K., Liao, J., & Jiang, F., (2012). Small nucleolar RNAs in cancer. *Biochimica et Biophysica Acta*, *1826*(1), 10.

62. Egan, E. D., & Collins, K., (2012). An enhanced H/ACA RNP assembly mechanism for human telomerase RNA. *Molecular and Cellular Biology*, *32*(13), 2428–2439.

63. Kiss, T., Fayet-Lebaron, E., & Jády, B. E., (2010). Box H/ACA small ribonucleoproteins. *Mol Cell*, *37*(5), 597–606.

64. Cohen, S. B., Graham, M. E., Lovrecz, G. O., Bache, N., Robinson, P. J., & Reddel, R. R., (2007). Protein composition of catalytically active human telomerase from immortal cells. *Science*, *315*, 1850–1853.

65. Lewis, K. A., & Tollefsbol, T. O., (2016). Regulation of the telomerase reverse Transcriptase subunit through epigenetic mechanisms. *Frontiers in Genetics*, *7*, 83.

66. Kim, N. K., Theimer, C. A., Mitchell, J. R., Collins, K., & Feigon, J., (2010). Effect of pseudouridylation on the structure and activity of the catalytically essential P6. 1 hairpin in human telomerase RNA. *Nucleic Acids Res.*, *38*(19), 6746–6756.

67. Napier, C. E., Veas, L. A., Kan, C. Y., Taylor, L. M., et al., (2010). Mild hyperoxia limits hTR levels, telomerase activity, & telomere length maintenance in hTERT-transduced bone marrow endothelial cells. *Biochim Biophys Acta*, *1803*(10), 1142–1153.

68. Makhnevych, T., & Houry, W. A., (2012). The role of Hsp90 in protein complex assembly. *Biochim. Biophys. Acta*, *1823*(3), 674–682.

69. Jeong, S. A., Kim, K., Lee, J. H., Cha, J. S., Khadka, P., Cho, H. S., & Chung, I. K., (2015). Akt-mediated phosphorylation increases the binding affinity of hTERT for importin α to promote nuclear translocation. *J. Cell Sci.*, *128*(12), 2287–2301.

70. Frohnert, C., Hutten, S., Wälde, S., Nath, A., & Kehlenbach, R. H., (2014). Importin 7 and Nup358 promote nuclear import of the protein component of human telomerase. *PLoS One*, *9*(2), e88887.

71. Chen, Y., Deng, Z., Jiang, S., Hu, Q., et al., (2015). Human cells lacking coilin and Cajal bodies are proficient in telomerase assembly, trafficking and telomere maintenance. *Nucleic Acids Res.*, *43*(1), 385–395.

72. Vogan, J. M., Zhang, X., Youmans, D. T., et al., (2016). Minimized human telomerase maintains telomeres and resolves endogenous roles of H/ACA proteins, TCAB1, & Cajal bodies. Greider, C., ed. *eLife*, *5*, e18221.

73. Zhao, Y., Abreu, E., Kim, J., Stadler, G., Eskiocak, U., Terns, M. P., Terns, R. M., Shay, J. W., & Wright, W. E., (2011). Processive and distributive extension of human telomeres by telomerase under homeostatic and nonequilibrium conditions. *Mol Cell*, *42*(3), 297–307.

74. Shammas, M. A., (2011). Telomeres, lifestyle, cancer, & aging. *Curr. Opin. Clin. Nutr. Metab. Care*, *14*(1), 28–34.

75. Gire, V., & Dulic, V., (2015). Senescence from G2 arrest, revisited. *Cell Cycle*, *14*(3), 297–304.

76. Li, Y., & Tergaonkar, V., (2016). Telomerase reactivation in cancers: Mechanisms that govern transcriptional activation of the wild-type vs. mutant TERT promoters. *Transcription*, *7*(2), 44–49.

77. Bell, R. J., Rube, H. T., Xavier-Magalhães, A., Costa, B. M., Mancini, A., Song, J. S., & Costello, J. F., (2016). Understanding TERT promoter mutations: A common path to immortality. *Mol Cancer Res.*, *14*(4), 315–323.

78. Akincilar, S. C., Unal, B., & Tergaonkar, V., (2016). Reactivation of telomerase in cancer. *Cell Mol Life Sci.*, *73*(8), 1659–1670.

79. Vinothkumar, V., Arunkumar, G., Revathidevi, S., Arun, K., Manikandan, M., Rao, A. K., Rajkumar, K. S., Ajay, C., Rajaraman, R., Ramani, R., Murugan, A. K., & Munirajan, A. K., (2016). TERT promoter hot spot mutations are frequent in Indian cervical and oral squamous cell carcinomas. *Tumor. Biol.*, *37*(6), 7907–7913.

80. Jacob, S., Nayak, S., Kakar, R., Chaudhari, U. K., Joshi, D., Vundinti, B. R., Fernandes, G., Barai, R. S., Kholkute, S. D., & Sachdeva, G. A., (2016). Triad of telomerase, androgen receptor and early growth response 1 in prostate cancer cells. *Cancer Biol. Ther.*, *17*(4), 439–448.

81. Xu, Y., & Goldkorn, A., (2016). Telomere and telomerase therapeutics in cancer. *Genes*, *7*(6), pii: E22. doi: 10. 3390/genes7060022.

82. Zisuh, A. V., Han, T. Q., & Zhan, S. D., (2012). Expression of telomerase & its significance in the diagnosis of pancreatic cancer. *Indian J. Med. Res.*, *135*(1), 26–30.

83. Zuo, J., Wang, D. H., Zhang, Y. J., Liu, L., Liu, F. L., & Liu, W., (2013). Expression and mechanism of PinX1 and telomerase activity in the carcinogenesis of esophageal epithelial cells. *Oncol. Rep.*, *30*(4), 1823–1831.

84. Zheng, Y. L., Hu, N., Sun, Q., Wang, C., & Taylor, P. R., (2009). Telomere attrition in cancer cells and telomere length in stroma cells predict chromosome instability in esophageal squamous cell carcinoma: a genome-wide analysis. *Cancer Res.*, *69*(4), 1604–1614.

85. Heeg, S., Hirt, N., Queisser, A., Schmieg, H., Thaler, M., Kunert, H., Quante, M., Goessel, G., Von Werder, A., Harder, J., Beijersbergen, R., Blum, H. E., Nakagawa, H., & Opitz, O. G., (2011). EGFR overexpression induces activation of telomerase via PI3K/Akt-mediated phosphorylation and transcriptional regulation through Hif1-alpha in a cellular model of oral-esophageal carcinogenesis. *Cancer Sci.*, *102*(2), 351–360.

86. Merchant, N. B., Dutta, S. K., Girotra, M., Arora, M., & Meltzer, S. J., (2013). Evidence for enhanced telomerase activity in Barrett's esophagus with dysplasia and adenocarcinoma. *Asian Pac. J. Cancer Prev.*, *14*(2), 679–683.

87. Lu, R., Pal, J., Buon, L., Nanjappa, P., Shi, J., Fulciniti, M., Tai, Y. T., Guo, L., Yu, M., Gryaznov, S., Munshi, N. C., & Shammas, M. A., (2014). Targeting homologous recombination and telomerase in Barrett's adenocarcinoma: impact on telomere maintenance, genomic instability and growth. *Oncogene*, *33*(12), 1495–1505.

88. Hou, L., Savage, S. A., Blaser, M. J., Perez-Perez, G., Hoxha, M., Dioni, L., Pegoraro, V., Dong, L. M., Zatonski, W., Lissowska, J., Chow, W. H., & Baccarelli, A., (2009). Telomere length in peripheral leukocyte DNA and gastric cancer risk. *Cancer Epidemiol. Biomarkers Prev.*, *18*(11), 3103–3109.

89. Basu, N., Skinner, H. G., Litzelman, K., Vanderboom, R., Baichoo, E., & Boardman, L. A., (2013). Telomeres and telomere dynamics: relevance to cancers of the GI tract. *Expert Rev. Gastroenterol. Hepatol.*, *7*(8), 733–748.

90. Huang, D. S., Wang, Z., He, X. J., Diplas, B. H., Yang, R., Killela, P. J., Meng, Q., Ye, Z. Y., Wang, W., Jiang, X. T., Xu, L., He, X. L., Zhao, Z. S., Xu, W. J., Wang, H. J., Ma, Y. Y., Xia, Y. J., Li, L., Zhang, R. X., Jin, T., Zhao, Z. K., Xu, J., Yu, S., Wu, F., Liang, J., Wang, S., Jiao, Y., Yan, H., & Tao, H. Q., (2015). Recurrent TERT promoter mutations identified in a large-scale study of multiple tumor types are associated with increased TERT expression and telomerase activation. *Eur. J. Cancer*, *51*(8), 969–976.

91. Sasaki, T., Kuniyasu, H., Luo, Y., Kitayoshi, M., Tanabe, E., Kato, D., Shinya, S., Fujii, K., Ohmori, H., & Yamashita, Y., (2014). Akt activation and telomerase reverse

transcriptase expression are concurrently associated with prognosis of gastric cancer. *Pathobiology*, *81*(1), 36–41.

92. Bertorelle, R., Briarava, M., Rampazzo, E., et al., (2013). Telomerase is an independent prognostic marker of overall survival in patients with colorectal cancer. *British J. Cancer*, *108*(2), 278–284.

93. Qin, Y., Tang, B., Hu, C. J., Xiao, Y. F, Xie, R., Yong, X., Wu, Y. Y., Dong, H., & Yang, S. M., (2016). An hTERT/ZEB1 complex directly regulates E-cadherin to promote epithelial-to-mesenchymal transition (EMT) in colorectal cancer. *Oncotarget*, *7*(1), 351–361.

94. Ayiomamitis, G. D., Notas, G., Zaravinos, A., Zizi-Sermpetzoglou, A., Georgiadou, M., Sfakianaki, O., & Kouroumallis, E., (2014). Differences in telomerase activity between colon and rectal cancer. *Can. J. Surg.*, *57*(3), 199–208.

95. Bertorelle, R., Rampazzo, E., Pucciarelli, S., Nitti, D., & De Rossi, A., (2014). Telomeres, telomerase and colorectal cancer. *World J. Gastroenterol.*, *20*(8), 1940–1950.

96. Roger, L., Jones, R. E., Heppel, N. H., Williams, G. T., Sampson, J. R., & Baird, D. M., (2013). Extensive telomere erosion in the initiation of colorectal adenomas and its association with chromosomal instability. *J. Natl. Cancer Inst.*, *105*(16), 1202–1211.

97. Valls-Bautista, C., Bougel, S., Pinol-Felis, C., Vinas-Salas, J., & Benhattar, J., (2011). hTERT methylation is necessary but not sufficient for telomerase activity in colorectal cells. *Oncol Lett.*, *2*(6), 1257–1260.

98. El-Idrissi, M., Hervieu, V., Merle, P., Mortreux, F., & Wattel, E., (2013). Cause-specific telomere factors deregulation in hepatocellular carcinoma. *J. Exp. Clin. Cancer Res.*, *32*, 64.

99. Sunami, Y., Von Figura, G., Kleger, A., Strnad, P., et al., (2014). The role of telomeres in liver disease. *Prog. Mol Biol. Transl. Sci.*, *125*, 159–172.

100. Oh, B. K., Kim, Y. J., Park, Y. N., Choi, J., Kim, K. S., & Park, C., (2006). Quantitative assessment of hTERT mRNA expression in dysplastic nodules of HBV-related hepatocarcinogenesis. *Am. J. Gastroenterol.*, *101*(4), 831–838.

101. Nault, J. C., Mallet, M., Pilati, C., Calderaro, J., Bioulac-Sage, P., Laurent, C., Laurent, A., Cherqui, D., Balabaud, C., & Zucman-Rossi, J., (2013). High frequency of telomerase reverse-transcriptase promoter somatic mutations in hepatocellular carcinoma and preneoplastic lesions. *Nat. Commun.*, *4*, 2218.

102. Nault, J. C., Calderaro, J., Di Tommaso, L., Balabaud, C., Zafrani, E. S., Bioulac-Sage, P., Roncalli, M., & Zucman-Rossi, J., (2014). Telomerase reverse transcriptase promoter mutation is an early somatic genetic alteration in the transformation of premalignant nodules in hepatocellular carcinoma on cirrhosis. *Hepatology*, *60*(6), 1983–1992.

103. Quaas, A., Oldopp, T., Tharun, L., Klingenfeld, C., Krech, T., Sauter, G., & Grob, T. J., (2014). Frequency of TERT promoter mutations in primary s of the liver. *Virchows Arch.*, *465*(6), 673–677.

104. Heeg, S., (2015). Variations in telomere maintenance and the role of telomerase inhibition in gastrointestinal cancer. *Pharmgenomics Pers. Med.*, *8*, 171–180.

105. Weng, C. C., Kuo, K. K., Su, H. T., Hsiao, P. J., Chen, Y. W., Wu, D. C., Hung, W. C., & Cheng, K. H., (2016). Pancreatic progression associated with CD133 overexpression: Involvement of increased TERT expression and epidermal growth factor receptor-dependent Akt activation. *Pancreas*, *45*(3), 443–457.

106. Wang, L., Xiao, H., Zhang, X., Wang, C., & Huang, H., (2014). The role of telomeres and telomerase in hematologic malignancies and hematopoietic stem cell transplantation. *J. Hematol. Oncol.*, *7*, 61.

107. Gancarcikova, M., Zemanova, Z., Brezinova, J., Berkova, A., Vcelikova, S., Smigova, J., & Michalova, K., (2010). The role of telomeres and telomerase complex in haematological neoplasia: the length of telomeres as a marker of carcinogenesis and prognosis of disease. *Prague Med. Rep.*, *111*(2), 91–105.

108. Bruedigam, C., & Lane, S. W., (2016). Telomerase in hematologic malignancies. *Curr. Opin. Hematol.*, *23*(4), 346–353.

109. Capraro, V., Zane, L., Poncet, D., Perol, D., Galia, P., Preudhomme, C., Bonnefoy-Berard, N., Gilson, E., Thomas, X., El-Hamri, M., Chelghoun, Y., Michallet, M., Wattel, E., Mortreux, F., & Sibon, D., (2011). Telomere deregulations possess cytogenetic, phenotype, & prognostic specificities in acute leukemias. *Exp. Hematol.*, *39*(2), 195–202.

110. Wang, Y., Fang, M., Sun, X., & Sun, J., (2010). Telomerase activity and telomere length in acute leukemia: correlations with disease progression, subtypes and overall survival. *Int. J. Lab. Hematol.*, *32*, 230–238.

111. Braig, M., Pällmann, N., Preukschas, M., Steinemann, D., Hofmann, W., Gompf, A., Streichert, T., Braunschweig, T., Copland, M., Rudolph, K. L., Bokemeyer, C., Koschmieder, S., Schuppert, A., Balabanov, S., & Brümmendorf, T. H., (2014). A 'telomere-associated secretory phenotype' cooperates with BCR-ABL to drive malignant proliferation of leukemic cells. *Leukemia*, *28*(10), 2028–2039.

112. Samassekou, O., Li, H., Hebert, J., Ntwari, A., Wang, H., Cliche, C. G., Bouchard, E., Huang, S., & Yan, J., (2011). Chromosome arm-specific long telomeres: a new clonal event in primary chronic myelogenous leukemia cells. *Neoplasia*, *13*, 550–560.

113. Samassekou, O., Ntwari, A., Hebert, J., & Yan, J., (2009). Individual telomere lengths in chronic myeloid leukemia. *Neoplasia*, *11*, 1146–1154.

114. Samassekou, O., Malina, A., Hebert, J., & Yan, J., (2013). Presence of alternative lengthening of telomeres associated circular extrachromosome telomere repeats in primary leukemia cells of chronic myeloid leukemia. *J. Hematol. Oncol.*, *6*, 26. doi: 10. 1186/1756–8722–6–26.

115. Khosravi-Maharlooei, M., Jaberipour, M., Hosseini, K., Tashnizi, A., Attar, A., et al., (2015). Expression pattern of alternative splicing variants of human telomerase reverse transcriptase (hTERT) in cancer cell lines was not associated with the origin of the cells. *Int. J. Mol Cell Med.*, *4*(2), 109–119.

116. Ropio, J., Merlio, J. P., Soares, P., & Chevret, E., (2016). Telomerase activation in hematological malignancies. *Genes (Basel)*, *7*(9), 61.

117. Rollison, D. E., Epling-Burnette, P. K., Park, J. Y., Lee, J. H., Park, H., Jonathan, K., Cole, A. L., Painter, J. S., Guerrier, M., Melendez-Santiago, J., Fulp, W., Komrokji, R., Lancet, J., & List, A. F., (2011). Telomere length in myelodysplastic syndromes. *Leuk. Lymphoma*, *52*, 1528–1536.

118. Lange, K., Holm, L., Vang, N. K., Hahn, A., Hofmann, W., Kreipe, H., Schlegelberger, B., & Göhring, G., (2010). Telomere shortening and chromosomal instability in myelodysplastic syndromes. *Genes Chromosomes Cancer*, *49*(3), 260–269.

119. Bellon, M., & Nicot, C., (2015). Multiple pathways control the reactivation of telomerase in HTLV-I-associated leukemia. *Int. J. Cancer Oncol.*, *2*(2), pii: 215.

120. Hara, T., Matsumura-Arioka, Y., Ohtani, K., & Nakamura, M., (2008). Role of human T-cell leukemia virus type I Tax in expression of the human telomerase reverse transcriptase (hTERT) gene in human T-cells. *Cancer Sci.*, *99*, 1155–1163.

121. Jones, C. H., Pepper, C., & Baird, D. M., (2012). Telomere dysfunction and its role in haematological cancer. *British J. Haematol.*, *156*, 573–587.

122. Diaz de la Guardia, R., Catalina, P., Panero, J., Elosua, C., et al., (2012). Expression profile of telomere-associated genes in multiple myeloma. *J. Cell Mol Med.*, *16*(12), 3009–3021.
123. Brennan, S. K., Wang, Q., Tressler, R., Harley, C., Go, N., Bassett, E., Huff, C. A., Jones, R. J., & Matsui, W., (2010). Telomerase inhibition targets clonogenic multiple myeloma cells through telomere length-dependent and independent mechanisms. *PLoS One, 5*, e12487.
124. Rampazzo, E., Bonaldi, L., Trentin, L., Visco, C., Keppel, S., Giunco, S., Frezzato, F., Facco, M., Novella, E., Giaretta, I., Bianco, P. D., Semenzato, G., & De Rossi, A., (2012). Telomere length and telomerase levels delineate subgroups of B-cell chronic lymphocytic leukemia with different biological characteristics and clinical outcomes. *Haematologica, 97*(1), 56–63.
125. Hoxha, M., Fabris, S., Agnelli, L., Bollati, V., et al., (2014). Relevance of telomere/ telomerase system impairment in early stage chronic lymphocytic leukemia. *Genes Chromosomes Cancer*, *53*(7), 612–621.
126. Augereau, A., T'Kint de Roodenbeke, C., Simonet, T., Bauwens, S., Horard, B., Callanan, M., Leroux, D., Jallades, L., Salles, G., Gilson, E., & Poncet, D., (2011). Telomeric damage in early stage of chronic lymphocytic leukemia correlates with shelterin dysregulation. *Blood, 118*, 1316–1322.
127. Giunco, S., Celeghin, A., Gianesin, K., Dolcetti, R., Indraccolo, S., & De Rossi, A., (2015). Cross talk between EBV and telomerase: the role of TERT and NOTCH2 in the switch of latent/lytic cycle of the virus. *Cell Death Dis.*, *6*, e1774.
128. Dolcetti, R., Giunco, S., Dal Col, J., Celeghin, A., Mastorci, K., & De Rossi, A., (2014). Epstein-Barr virus and telomerase: from cell immortalization to therapy. *Infect Agent Cancer*, *9*(1), 8. doi: 10. 1186/1750-9378-9-8.
129. Wu, S., Huang, P., Li, C., Huang, Y., Li, X., Wang, Y., Chen, C., Lv, Z., Tang, A., Sun, X., Lu, J., Li, W., Zhou, J., Gui, Y., Zhou, F., Wang, D., & Cai, Z., (2014). Telomerase reverse transcriptase gene promoter mutations help discern the origin of urogenital s: a genomic and molecular study. *Eur. Urol.*, *65*(2), 274–277.
130. Prabhavathy, D., Subramanian, C. K., & Karunagaran, D., (2015). Re-expression of HPV16 E2 in SiHa (human cervical cancer) cells potentiates NF-κB activation induced by TNF-α concurrently increasing senescence and survival. *Biosci. Rep.*, *35*(1), pii: e00175. doi: 10. 1042/BSR20140160.
131. Liu, L., Liu, C., Lou, F., Zhang, G., Wang, X., Fan, Y., Yan, K., Wang, K., Xu, Z., Hu, S., Björkholm, M., & Xu, D., (2011). Activation of telomerase by seminal plasma in malignant and normal cervical epithelial cells. *J. Pathol.*, *225*(2), 203–211.
132. Petrenko, A. A., Korolenkova, L., Skvortsov, D. A., Fedorova, M. D., Skoblov, M. U., Baranova, A. V., Zvereva, M. E., Rubtsova, M. P., & Kisseljov, F. L., (2010). Cervical intraepithelial neoplasia: Telomerase activity and splice pattern of hTERT mRNA. *Biochimie, 92*(12), 1827–1831.
133. De-Wilde, J., Kooter, J. M., Overmeer, R. M., Classen-Kramer, D., Meijer, C. J. L. M., Snijders, P. J. F., & Steenbergen, R. D. M., (2010). hTERT promoter activity and CpG methylation in HPV-induced carcinogenesis. *BMC Cancer, 10*(271), http://www. biomedcentral.com/1471–2407/10/271.
134. Raghunandan, B. N., Sanjai, K., Kumaraswamy, J., Papaiah, L., Pandey, B., & Jyothi, B. M., (2016). Expression of human telomerase reverse transcriptase protein in oral epithelial dysplasia and oral squamous cell carcinoma: An immunohistochemical study. *J. Oral Maxillofac. Pathol.*, *20*(1), 96–101.

135. Gupta, O. P., Suhail, S., Kumar, D., Kumar, V., Patil, R., & Gupta, S., (2015). Telomerase- a biomarker in oral cancer cell proliferation. *World J. Pharmaceu. Res.*, *4*(6), 531–540.

136. Shigeishi, H., Sugiyama, M., Tahara, H., Ono, S., Kumar, B. U., Okura, M., Kogo, M., Shinohara, M., Shindoh, M., Shintani, S., Hamakawa, H., Takata, T., & Kamata, N., (2011). Increased telomerase activity and hTERT expression in human salivary gland carcinomas. *Oncol Lett.*, *2*(5), 845–850.

137. Zhao, T., Hu, F., Qiao, B., Chen, Z., & Tao, Q., (2015). Telomerase reverse transcriptase potentially promotes the progression of oral squamous cell carcinoma through induction of epithelial-mesenchymal transition. *Int. J. Oncol.*, *46*(5), 2205–2215.

138. Qiao, B., Chen, Z., Hu, F., Tao, Q., & Lam, A. K., (2013). BMI-1 activation is crucial in hTERT-induced epithelial-mesenchymal transition of oral epithelial cells. *Exp. Mol Pathol.*, *95*(1), 57–61.

139. Holysz, H., Lipinska, N., Paszel-Jaworska, A., & Rubis, B., (2013). Telomerase as a useful target in cancer fighting-the breast cancer case. *Tumor Biol.*, *34*(3), 1371–1380.

140. Vageli, D., Ioannou, M. G., & Koukoulis, G. K., (2009). Transcriptional activation of hTERT in breast carcinomas by the Her2-ER81-related pathway. *Oncol Res.*, *17*(9), 413–423.

141. Piscuoglio, S., Ng, C. K., Murray, M., Burke, K. A., et al., (2016). Massively parallel sequencing of phyllodes tumours of the breast reveals actionable mutations, & TERT promoter hotspot mutations and TERT gene amplification as likely drivers of progression. *J. Pathol.*, *238*(4), 508–518.

142. Lu, L., Zhang, C., Zhu, G., et al., (2011). Telomerase expression and telomere length in breast cancer and their associations with adjuvant treatment and disease outcome. *Breast Cancer Research: BCR*, *13*(3), R56.

143. Zhang, Y., Toh, L., Lau, P., & Wang, X., (2012). Human telomerase reverse transcriptase (hTERT) is a novel target of the Wnt/beta-catenin pathway in human cancer. *J. Biol. Chem.*, *287*, 32494–32511.

144. Tamakawa, R. A., Fleisig, H. B., & Wong, J. M., (2010). Telomerase inhibition potentiates the effects of genotoxic agents in breast and colorectal cancer cells in a cell cycle-specific manner. *Cancer Res.*, *70*(21), 8684–8694.

145. Gansner, J. M., & Rosas, I. O., (2013). Telomeres in lung disease. *Transl. Res.*, *162*(6), 343–352.

146. Jeon, H. S., Choi, J. E., Jung, D. K., Choi, Y. Y., Kang, H. G., Lee, W. K., Yoo, S. S., Lim, J. O., & Park, J. Y., (2012). Telomerase activity and the risk of lung cancer. *J. Korean Med Sci.*, *27*(2), 141–145.

147. Dobija-Kubica, K., Zalewska-Ziob, M., Brulinski, K., Rogozinski, P., Wiczkowski, A., Gawrychowska, A., & Gawrychowski, J., (2016). Telomerase activity in non-small cell lung cancer. *Kardiochir. Torakochirurgia Pol.*, *13*(1), 15–20.

148. Liu, W., Yin, Y., Wang, J., Shi, B., Zhang, L., Qian, D., Li, C., Zhang, H., Wang, S., Zhu, J., Gao, L., Zhang, Q., Jia, B., Hao, L., Wang, C., & Zhang, B., (2016). Kras mutations increase telomerase activity and targeting telomerase is a promising therapeutic strategy for Kras-mutant NSCLC. *Oncotarget*, doi: 10. 18632/oncotarget. 10162. [Epub ahead of print].

149. Shen, C., Liu, Y., Wen, Z., Yang, K., Li, G., Zhang, S., & Zhang, X., (2015). Influence and mechanism of PinX1 gene on the chemotherapy sensitivity of nasopharyngeal carcinoma cells in response to Cisplatin. *Zhonghua Yi Xue Za Zhi*, *95*(24), 1951–1956.

150. Hu, W., Jia, Y., Yu, Z., Lv, K., Chen, Y., Wang, L., Luo, X., Liu, T., Li, W., Li, Y., Zhang, C., Shi, D., Huang, W., Sun, B., & Deng, W. G., (2016). KLF4 downregulates hTERT expression and telomerase activity to inhibit lung carcinoma growth. *Oncotarget*, doi: 10. 18632/oncotarget. 9141. [Epub ahead of print].

151. Guo, W., Lu, J., Dai, M., Wu, T., Yu, Z., Wang, J., Chen, W., Shi, D., Yu, W., Xiao, Y., Yi, C., Tang, Z., Xu, T., Xiao, X., Yuan, Y., Liu, Q., Du, G., & Deng, W., (2014). Transcriptional coactivator CBP upregulates hTERT expression and growth and predicts poor prognosis in human lung cancers. *Oncotarget*, 5(19), 9349–9361.

152. Chen, W., Lu, J., Qin, Y., Wang, J., Tian, Y., Shi, D., Wang, S., Xiao, Y., Dai, M., Liu, L., Wei, G., Wu, T., Jin, B., Xiao, X., Kang, T. B., Huang, W., & Deng, W., (2014). Ret finger protein-like 3 promotes cell growth by activating telomerase reverse transcriptase expression in human lung cancer cells. *Oncotarget*, 5(23), 11909–11923.

153. Wei, R., Cao, L., Pu, H., Wang, H., Zheng, Y., Niu, X., Weng, X., Zhang, H., Favus, M. J., Zhang, L., Jia, W., Zeng, Y., Amos, C. I., Lu, S., Wang, H. Y., Liu, Y., & Liu, W., (2015). TERT polymorphism rs2736100-C is associated with EGFR mutation-positive non-small cell lung cancer. *Clin Cancer Res.*, 21(22), 5173–5180.

154. Wang, F., Fu, P., Pang, Y., Liu, C., Shao, Z., Zhu, J., Li, J., Wang, T., Zhang, X., & Liu, J., (2014). TERT rs2736100T/G polymorphism upregulates interleukin 6 expression in non-small cell lung cancer especially in adenocarcinoma. *Tumor Biol.*, 35(5), 4667–4672.

155. Hsu, C. P., Lee, L. W., Tang, S. C., Hsin, I. L., Lin, Y. W., & Ko, J. L., (2015). Epidermal growth factor activates telomerase activity by direct binding of Ets-2 to hTERT promoter in lung cancer cells. *Tumor Biol.*, 36(7), 5389–5398.

156. Tallet, A., Nault, J. C., Renier, A., Hysi, I., Galateau-Salle, F., Cazes, A., Copin, M. C., Hofman, P., Andujar, P., Le Pimpec-Barthes, F., Zucman-Rossi, J., Jaurand, M. C., & Jean, D., (2014). Overexpression and promoter mutation of the TERT gene in malignant pleural mesothelioma. *Oncogene*, 33(28), 3748–3752.

157. Rane, J. K., Greener, S., Frame, F. M., Mann, V. M., Simms, M. S., Collins, A. T., Berney, D. M., & Maitland, N. J., (2016). Telomerase activity and telomere length in human benign prostatic hyperplasia stem-like cells and their progeny implies the existence of distinct basal and luminal cell lineages. *Eur. Urol.*, 69(4), 551–554.

158. Wu, S., Huang, P., Li, C., Huang, Y., Li, X., Wang, Y., Chen, C., Lv, Z., Tang, A., Sun, X., Lu, J., Li, W., Zhou, J., Gui, Y., Zhou, F., Wang, D., & Cai, Z., (2014). Telomerase reverse transcriptase gene promoter mutations help discern the origin of urogenital s: a genomic and molecular study. *Eur. Urol.*, 65(2), 274–277.

159. Marion, R. M., & Blasco, M. A., (2010). Telomere rejuvenation during nuclear reprogramming. *Adv. Exp. Med. Biol.*, 695, 118–131.

160. Zanetti, M., (2016). A second chance for telomerase reverse transcriptase in anticancer immunotherapy. *Nat. Rev. Clin. Oncol.*, doi: 10. 1038/nrclinonc. 67.

161. Teichroeb, J. H., Kim, J., & Betts, D. H., (2016). The role of telomeres and telomerase reverse transcriptase isoforms in pluripotency induction and maintenance. *RNA Biol.*, 19, 1–13.

162. Shay, J. W., & Wright, W. E., (2010). Telomeres and telomerase in normal and cancer stem cells. *FEBS Lett.*, 584(17), 3819–3825.

163. De Bonis, M. L., Ortega, S., & Blasco, M. A., (2014). SIRT1 is necessary for proficient telomere elongation and genomic stability of induced pluripotent stem cells. *Stem Cell Reports*, 2(5), 690–706.

164. Terali, K., & Yilmazer, A., (2016). New surprises from an old favourite: The emergence of telomerase as a key player in the regulation of cancer stemness. *Biochimie, 121,* 170–178.

165. Sprouse, A. A., Steding, C. E., & Herbert, B. S., (2012). Pharmaceutical regulation of telomerase and its clinical potential. *J. Cell Mol Med., 16*(1), 1–7.

166. Cosan, D. T., & Soyocak, A., (2012). Inhibiting telomerase activity and inducing apoptosis in cancer cells by several natural food compounds. Reviews on selected topics of telomere biology, edited by Bibo, L. pp. 123–148,

167. Alibakhshi, A., Ranjbari, J., Pilehvar-Soltanahmadi, Y., Nasiri, M., Mollazade, M., & Zarghami, N., (2016). An update on phytochemicals substances in molecular target therapy of cancer: Potential inhibitory effect on telomerase activity. *Curr. Med. Chem.,* [Epub ahead of print].

168. Roy, M., Mukherjee, S., & Biswas J., (2012). Inhibition of an epigenetic modulator, histone deacetylase by PEITC in breast cancer- a detailed mechanistic approach. *Int. J. Ther. Applicn., 5,* 1–13.

169. Mukherjee, S., Dey, S., Bhattacharya, R. K., & Roy, M., (2009). Isothicyanates sensitize the effect of chemotherapeutic drugs via modulation of protein kinase C and telomerase in cervical cancer cells. *Mol Cell Biochem., 330,* 9–22.

170. Mukherjee, S., Bhattacharya, R. K., & Roy, M., (2009). Targeting PKC and telomerase by PEITC sensitizes PC-3 cells towards chemotherapeutic drug induced apoptosis. *J. Env. Pathol. Toxicol. Oncol., 28*(4), 269–282.

171. Roy, M., Mukherjee, S., Sarkar, R., & Biswas, J., (2011). Curcumin sensitizes chemotherapeutic drugs via modulation of PKC, telomerase, NF-κB and HDAC in breast cancer. *Ther. Deliv., 2*(10), 1275–1293.

CHAPTER 3

CELL CYCLE CHECKPOINTS IN CANCER

SREEPARNA CHAKRABORTY[1] and ABHIK SEN[2]

[1]*West Virginia University, USA, E-mail: sree.chakraborty@gmail.com*

[2]*Centre For Neurodegenerative Diseases, Blanchette Rockefeller Neurosciences Institute West Virginia University, USA, E-mail: abhiksen78@gmail.com*

CONTENTS

ABSTRACT

The cell cycle is an exceptionally structured physiological mechanism governing the duplication and transmission of hereditary genetic material from one cell generation to the next and therefore requires control. Accurate control of this cyclical progression at different "checkpoints" is fundamental for deciding when a cell ought to focus on deoxyribonucleic acid (DNA) synthesis and division versus proliferation arrest, DNA repair, or apoptosis. Ideally, checkpoints delay transition from one cell cycle phase to another by a complex system of positive and negative regulatory mechanisms, until the specific endogenous or exogenous condition has been satisfied. Inappropriate cell proliferation that bypasses normal cell checkpoints is the hallmark of cancer cells. The gain-of-function mutations in oncogenes and loss-of-functions in tumor suppressor genes were initially shown to contribute to cancer development. Recent studies have focused on the signaling pathways of cell cycle regulatory genes in the hope of modulating cancer progression. However, it is not clearly understood, exactly how does single (or even multiple) gene sequence modifications, translational upregulation, or obliterated regulatory domains influence the mechanism of cell cycle. Therefore, understanding the underlying regulatory signaling networks may give us knowledge on the parity of a typical cell cycle and carcinogenic cell expansion and recommend techniques for disease treatment.

3.1   INTRODUCTION

The sequence of growth and division of a eukaryotic cell into daughter cells can be described as a series of coordinated events that compose a "cell division cycle." The process starts with the cell triggered to enter the cell cycle, followed by genetic material synthesis, equal partitioning, and cleavage of the cell during cytokinesis. In 1950–1960s, Alma Howard's and Stephen Pelc's pioneering work in broad bean, *Vicia faba*, further revealed that during this cyclical division, a cell goes through discrete phases that can be broadly identified as follows: the interphase [consisting of gap 1 (G1), DNA synthesis (S), and gap 2 (G2)] and mitosis (M) phases [1]. Entry into the cycle from a previous mitotic cycle is made during G1, followed in sequence by DNA synthesis in the S phase; time lapse between synthesis and division is the G2 phase, and subsequently, genetic material division occurs during the M phase. To maintain this cell cycle integrity, cells are governed by a complex network of control system popularly known as "checkpoints." Both intracellular and extracellular signals control cyclical progression by modulating these checkpoints. Thus, depending upon the signals received, when a cell fails to complete a crucial stage of cell cycle or experiences unfavorable conditions, the cell cycle progression can either be arrested or be diverged at the start of G1 into a quiescent nondividing phase called G0 (gap zero). These molecular checkpoints are functionally classified as follows: first, a cascade of protein kinases that modulate cell cycle progression and second, an arrangement of flagging checkpoints that screen finishing of critical stages and even defer movement to the following stage if necessary.

Principal among the cell cycle control mechanisms are a group of serine/threonine kinases, known as cyclin-dependent kinases (CDKs) and their modulator cyclin subunits. These kinases are in turn regulated further regulated by binding of cyclin-dependent kinase inhibitors (CKIs) as well as by a host of post-translational modifications. Moreover, transcriptional control by intrinsic and extrinsic factors limits cyclin production to specific phases of the cell cycle. The ubiquitin-mediated proteolysis of cyclin further guarantees irreversible inactivation of the related CDK. This periodicity of the cyclins, regulated by their synthesis and proteolytic degradation, gives the cell unique control over advancement from one cycle to the next [2]. Considering that aberrant entry into the cell cycle and uncontrolled cell proliferation are hallmarks of cancer development, it is not surprising that dysregulation of the CDKs plays a central role in tumorigenesis.

A more supervisory role is played by a complex network of signaling pathways, known as checkpoint control. These checkpoints are essential for maintaining genetic integrity of a dividing cell. The cell cycle checkpoints are not limited to a particular phase of the cycle and therefore continuously monitor to sense flaws in critical events such as DNA replication and chromosome segregation [3]. For instance, when cells have DNA damages that need to be repaired, they can activate DNA damage checkpoints at G1/S, intra-S phase, and also DNA replication checkpoint at G2/M transition. When these checkpoints are activated, signals are relayed to the cell cycle progression machinery. These signals then can delay cycle progression, until normal DNA replication is restored. Similarly, checkpoints such as the spindle checkpoint arrests cell cycle at the M phase until all chromosomes are aligned on the spindle and are equally distributed.

One of the fundamental aspects of cancer is dysregulation of these cell cycle regulatory mechanisms for inappropriate cell proliferation. Unlike typical cells that multiply upon specific developmental or mitogenic signals in light of tissue growth needs, the proliferation of cancer cells proceeds essentially uncontrolled. Moreover, this cell number excess is linked in a vicious cycle with a reduction in sensitivity to signals that normally tell a cell to adhere, differentiate, or die by negating cell cycle progression controls in the presence of damaged DNA or other physiological insults.

3.2   PROGRESSION OF CELL CYCLE

As discussed earlier, cell cycle transitions are controlled by cyclin-dependent kinases (CDK) that are dependent on a cyclin regulatory subunit for activity. The cyclins are unstable proteins that are transcribed and synthesized periodically during the cell cycle. Regulatory phosphorylation and dephosphorylation in the activities of various cyclin-CDK complexes lead to the initiation and progression of various cell cycle events and are described below in a phase specific manner.

3.2.1   G1 PHASE

The human cell cycle starts at the G1 phase, when dormant cells at the G0 phase are stimulated to enter the cycle under influence of mitogenic growth factors via the Ras-myc signaling pathway. This phase is marked by an increased expression of the D cyclins encoded by *CCND1* (11q13) and *CCND2* (12p13), especially during mid-G1. The D cyclins actively associate with CDK4 and/or CDK6, resulting in their phosphorylation and subsequent activation [4]. Full activation of cyclin D-CDK4/6 complexes requires dephosphorylation of inhibitory sites (threonine-14 and tyrosine-15) by the dual-specific phosphatase Cdc25 and phosphorylation by the CDK-activating kinase (CAK) (Figure 3.1). Negative regulation of the cyclin-dependent kinase inhibitors (CKIs), the INK4 family proteins (p15^{INK4b}, p16^{INK4a}, p18^{INK4c}, and p19^{INK4d}) and the CIP/KIP family proteins (p21^{Cip1} and p57^{Kip2}) is further removed by proteolysis prior to CDK4/6 activity [5]. In addition to their inhibitory role, the CIP/KIP family proteins especially p21^{Cip1} and p27^{Kip1} also helps in stabilizing cyclin D-CDK4/6 complexes promoting their activation and nuclear accumulation [6]. The activated CDKs then phosphorylates a family of nuclear phosphoproteins (Rb/p105, p107 and Rb2/p130), encoded by a tumor suppressor retinoblastoma gene (*RB*). In the dephosphorylated or hypophosphorylated state, the retinoblastoma proteins bind to members of the E2F family of transcription factors and inhibit their transcription [7]. Thus, by modulating E2F and other co-repressors, these

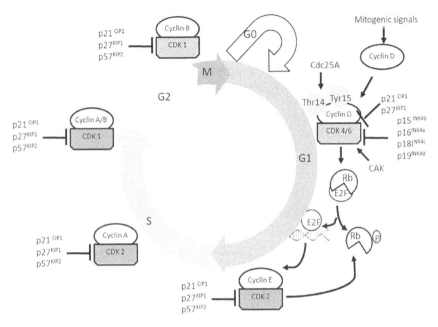

FIGURE 3.1 Phase-specific expression of various cyclins and corresponding cyclin-dependent kinases during cell cycle progression. Cyclin-CDK complexes are further activated by Cdc25 and CAK and inhibited by the INK4 and CIP/KIP family of cyclin-dependent kinase inhibitors.

"pocket proteins" functions as the gatekeeper of the cell cycle, halting cell cycle progression at G1.

3.2.2 G1/S TRANSITION

After successive phosphorylation of pRb by cyclin D-CDK4/6 complexes, phosphorylated RB dissociates from E2F, allowing E2F to transcribe a number of genes, including cyclin E at *CCNE* (19q12) [7, 8]. This in turn enables activation of cyclin E-CDK2 complex by removal of negative cyclin kinase inhibitors (p21^{Cip1}, p27^{Kip1} and p57^{Kip2}). Activated cyclin E-CDK2 complex further hyperphosphorylates pRb, inducing maximal activation of E2F factors in a feedback regulatory loop and facilitates cell cycle progression through G1/S transition (Figure 3.1) [9, 10]. Cyclin E-CDK2 also regulates multiple cellular processes by phosphorylating and activating numerous downstream proteins like Smad3 (a key mediator of the TGF-β pathway)

[11], CBP/p300, and E2F-5 [12]. The retinoblastoma protein (pRb) is maintained in its hyperphosphorylated state throughout the remainder of the
cycle. Thereafter, in preparation of DNA synthesis in the following S phase,
cyclin E initiates the assembly of a pre-replication complex by modulating
activities of nucleophosmin (NPM) and CP110 in the centrosome and cen-
triole, respectively [13, 14].

3.2.3 S PHASE

Just prior to the G1/S transition, S phase cyclin (cyclin A) synthesis increases
gradually by active transcription of *CCNA* at chromosome 4 (q25–q31), and
its expression persists through the entire S phase. Cyclin A associates with
CDK2 and plays a key role in S phase entry and initiation of DNA synthesis (3.1). Premature activity of cyclin A-CDK2 complexes prior to the S
phase is repressed by phosphorylation at tyrosine-15 site of CDK2 and by
the association of the CKIs, p27[Kip1] and p21[Cip1]. The entry into the S phase is
therefore initiated by dephosphorylation of inhibitory phosphates by Cdc25
phosphatases and by SCF ubiquitin ligase complex-mediated degradation
of p27[Kip1] and p21[Cip1] [15]. Cyclin A-CDK2 complex is further activated by
phosphorylation at threonine-160 located in the "T-loop" of CDK2 by CAK
[16]. Activated cyclin A-CDK2 subsequently initiates and ensures completion of DNA synthesis in the S phase. In addition, this cyclin-CDK complex
modulates activity of other cyclin complexes, chiefly the cyclin B-CDK1
during G2 phase primarily at the centrosome and in the nucleus [17]. At
a later stage of the S phase, cyclin A partners with CDK1 and is then subsequently substituted by cyclin B prior to mitosis [18]. Although CDK2
assumes the essential part in controlling entry into the S phase, numerous
studies show that due to cyclin-dependent kinase redundancy, CDK1 too
may initiate G1/S transition [19].

3.2.4 G2/M TRANSITION

In contrast to the role of cyclins and their respective kinases at G1/S checkpoint, the corresponding G2/M events are still poorly understood. Recent
studies reveal that both cyclin A-CDK2 and cyclin B-CDK1 complexes are
crucial for G2/M transition and M phase progression [20]. Although cyclin
A-CDK2 activity is primarily noted at the onset of the S phase, a significant

upregulation occurs in the early G2 phase. Translation control of accumulated cyclin A along with the removal of the inhibitory tyrosine-15 phosphorylation on CDK2 by the dual-specific phosphatase Cdc25A in the S phase and Cdc25B in the G2 phase modulates the activity of cyclin A [21]. Once activated by cyclin A, CDK2 regulates several transcription factors, chief among them being FoxM1 (member of the fork-head box superfamily of transcription factors) [22]. This transcription factor is essential for its role in downstream activation of a set of target genes that regulate mitosis and spindle assembly checkpoint [23, 24]. To prevent untimely activity of FoxM1, its N-terminal repressor domain (RD) binds to and represses C-terminal transactivation domain (TAD). Cyclin A-CDK2 hyperphosphorylates TAD, displacing RD, and relieving this autoinhibition. Histone deacetylase p300/CREB binding protein (Ep300/Crebbp), a transcriptional co-activator, now can bind to FoxM1. The resultant complex modulates downstream genes, thereby promoting their expression during mitotic entry [23]. As an additional precautionary measure against any premature activation, the phosphorylation of FoxM1 can also be reversed by protein phosphatase 2A (PP2A) and its regulatory subunit B55α [25]. These consolidated activities of phosphorylation by cyclin A-CDK2 and dephosphorylation by PP2A/B55α limit the transcriptional activity of FoxM1 within the mitotic window. Cyclin A may further complex with CDK1 and modulate cyclin B synthesis via transcription factors NF-Y, FoxM1, and B-Myb. Therefore, with increased transcription of the cyclin B gene *CCNB* (5q12), the cell undergoes a dramatic upheaval for the M phase. Consequent increase in cyclin B therefore leads to activation of CDK1 and formation of cyclin B-CDK1 complexes for entry into mitosis. Because the upregulation of cyclin B precedes the formation of the cyclin B-CDK1 complex at G2/M transition, it is in an ideal position to regulate G2 phase progression (Figure 3.1). Further phosphoryation by CAK at threonine-161 completes the activation of cyclin B-CDK1 complex. To forestall premature mitosis, this complex is inactivated by phosphorylation of CDK1 on tyrosine-15 and threonine-14 residues by Wee1 and Myt1 kinases [26].

3.2.5 M PHASE

During late G2, as the cell approaches mitosis, combined events promote the activation of cyclin B-CDK1 complex. These include phosphorylation of Cdc25C and Cdc25B by Polo-like kinase 1 (PLK1) promoting their nuclear localization [27]. However, prior to M phase, PLK1 itself is activated by Aurora A-dependent phosphorylation at threonine-210 in association with Bora protein [28]. Activated by PLK1, Cdc25C phosphorylates and removes inhibitory kinase Myt1 and Wee1 suppression at tyrosine-15 and threonine-14 residues, leading to the activation of the cyclin B-CDK1 complex (also known as maturation promoting factor). Cyclin B-CDK1 feedback loops further simultaneously activate Cdc25C and inactivate Wee1/Myt1 [29], resulting in a critical proportion of activated cyclin B1-CDK1 complexes, allowing a rapid entry into mitosis [30, 31]. Active cyclin B-CDK1 contributes to chromosome condensation and nuclear envelope breakdown and interacts with a variety of other key proteins and pathways that regulate cell growth and progression of mitosis. Finally, when the chromosomes are properly aligned during anaphase, rapid inactivation of CDK1 occurs. This loss of function of CDK1 at the end of mitosis is mediated by ubiquitin-mediated degradation of cyclin B by anaphase-promoting complex/cyclosome (APC/C) [32]. Cyclin B-CDK1 complexes can also negatively regulate its degradation by phosphorylating and activating APC/C and its subunit Cdc20, thus initiating mitotic exit and completion of the cell cycle [33].

3.3   CONCERTED ROLE OF CDK, CYCLIN, AND CKI IN CELL CYCLE REGULATION

As described before, cell cycle progression is regulated at the G1–S and the G2–M transitions as well as in the S phase and mitosis. At the molecular level, a normal cell cycle can be seen as an intricate network of cyclins and CDKs that are further modified and controlled by phosphorylations and dephosphorylations with inhibitors and assembly factors. Precise transcriptional activity and proteosomal degradation for maintaining critical levels of cyclins, along with subcellular and nuclear localization and transport indicate a complex control that can halt cell cycle progression at different stages on sensing genomic damage or failure of completion previous activity. A detailed understanding of cyclin-dependent kinases along with their activators and repressor molecules will provide tremendous insight into how these key components modulate cell cycle progression.

3.3.1   CYCLINS AND THEIR ASSOCIATED CANCERS

Cyclins belong to a family of proteins that are principally involved in cell division regulation and are structurally identified by conserved "cyclin box" regions. The cyclin boxes are composed of about 100 amino acid residues, arranged in 5 helical regions, and are critical for binding partner proteins like cyclin-dependent kinases (CDKs). Cyclins were discovered as proteins that oscillate in synchrony with the cell cycle, accumulate progressively through interphase and disappear abruptly at mitosis, in marine invertebrates [34]. In humans, cyclins A and B were the first mitotic cyclins to be identified, followed by other cell cycle progression cyclins (C, D, E). Subsequently, on the basis of sequence similarity and their timing of appearance during the cell cycle, several cyclin families (F-L, O, T and Y), each including more subfamilies were isolated [35]. Since then, mammalian cyclins can be broadly grouped as G1 cyclins (D1-D3 and E1-E2), S phase cyclins (A1-A2), and mitotic cyclins (B1-B3). As their names suggest, the G1-S cyclins are essential for the control of the cell cycle at G1 and S phases, while the M cyclins accumulate steadily during G2 and are abruptly destroyed as cells exit mitosis. Cyclins are also the first example of accessory subunits that are activating rather than being inhibited by protein kinases. Each cyclin is known to interact with one or two cyclin-dependent kinases, and most cyclin-dependent kinases associate with one or two cyclins in a redundant manner to control cell cycle transcription and differentiation.

3.3.1.1   Cyclin D

Cyclin D family consists of D1, D2, and D3 subtypes that are differentially expressed in the nucleus, nuclear membrane, and cytoplasm in a cell lineage-specific manner. It is one of the foremost cyclins that are synthesized when quiescent (G0) cells are stimulated by extracellular signaling cues to enter the cell cycle. These are therefore the principle rate-limiting cyclins of the G1 phase and are vital for cell cycle progression. The D cyclins, especially D1 subtype, in different combinations allosterically regulate and bind with either CDK4 or CDK6 proteins to form a serine/threonine kinase holoenzyme complex [4]. As described previously, the cyclin D-CDK4 complex plays an important role in the mid-G1 phase by phosphorylating Rb family proteins to disable their function as transcriptional suppressor and allowing activation of the E2F-dependent transcription of several cell cycle progression genes. Moreover, in support of the notion that the retinoblastoma protein pRb is a critical downstream target of D cyclins, cells lacking functional pRb do not require cyclin-dependent kinases for passage from G1 into the S phase. The three D cyclins subtypes, however, have different affinities for Rb, with cyclin D1 playing a principle role. In addition, D1 cyclins are also shown to interact with SMAD3, breast cancer 1 (BRCA1), and cyclin-dependent kinase inhibitors (CDKN1A, and CDKN1B), thus indicating a wider range of cellular activities [36]. Quite similar to its other subtypes, cyclin D1 located at 11q13, comprises cyclin-like terminal, cyclin-N terminal, and cyclin-C terminal domain along with specific sequences for serine/threonine dual-specificity protein kinase (catalytic domain). The expression level of cyclin D1 is highly responsive to the action of proliferative signals including growth factor receptors of the mitogen-activated protein kinase Ras-Raf-MEK-ERK pathways [37]. Moreover, unlike other cyclins, cyclin D1 levels do not oscillate during the cell cycle. Its expression is controlled chiefly by growth factors and can shuttle in and out of the nucleus of cycling cells. On receiving adequate mitogenic signals, cyclin D1 expression, activation, and nuclear accumulation occur during the mid-G1 phase. Activated cyclin D1-CDK 4 complex then modulates G1 sequences by targeting its primary substrate, the retinoblastoma family of proteins [38]. Cyclin D1 is also capable of interfering with DNA synthesis in the following S phase by binding with proliferating cell nuclear antigen (PCNA), a critical regulator of DNA synthesis. Therefore, a precise and regulated proteolysis of cyclin D1 at late G1 is vital to maintain efficient cell cycle progression. Thus, during the S phase, cyclin D1 activation is negated by glycogen synthase kinase 3β (GSK3β) in proline-287-directed phosphorylation at threonine-286 [39]. This phosphorylation triggers cyclin D1 nuclear export and ubiquitination-mediated proteolysis [40].

Altered activity of cyclin D1, and to a lesser extent, cyclins D2 and D3 are expressed in several solid tumors [41]. An increased transcription of cyclin D1 mRNA is observed in parathyroid adenoma and is probably due to translocation t(11;11)(q13;p15) with the parathyroid hormone (PTH) enhancer [42]. Overexpression is also observed in mantle cell (centrocytic) lymphoma, breast, esophageal, and squamous cell carcinomas [43]. Moreover, chromosomal aberration involving translocation of cyclin D1 with the IgH locus t(11;14)(q13;q32) is found in multiple myeloma [42]. Furthermore, it can be noted that more than half of reported breast cancers had increased expression of cyclin D1 protein. This elevated cyclin D1 level is best observed in early breast cancer pathogenesis such as ductal carcinoma *in situ* (DCIS). Once cyclin D1 overexpression is acquired by the tumor cells, it is maintained at the same level throughout breast cancer progression from DCIS to invasive carcinoma and is preserved even in metastatic lesions [44]. Thus, an increase in cyclin D1 expression serves to identify mammary epithelial cell malignancies. Other than its role in tumor development, the overexpression of cyclin D1 (via activation of E2F-1 positive feedback loop) is known to promote cancer cell metastasis by modulating fibroblast growth factor receptor 1 (FGFR-1) activity [45]. Upregulation of FGFR-1 is frequently observed in several cancers including brain, breast, prostate, thyroid, skin, and salivary gland tumors and is correlated with increased invasiveness and poor prognosis. Moreover, deregulated cyclin D1 levels may initiate angiogenesis and tumor metastasis by altering mitochondrial integrity, thereby leading to increased production of reactive oxygen species [46]. In the case of cyclin D2, an elevated mRNA expression is most frequently noted in Ewing's sarcomas [47]. Increased protein levels of cyclin D2 is also observed during pathogenesis of cancers like B-cell lymphocytic leukemia and lymphoplasmacytic lymphomas and in early male germ cell tumors [48]. Higher than normal levels of cyclin D3 is often detected in cancers like glioblastomas, renal cell carcinomas, pancreatic adenocarcinomas, and several B-cell malignancies such as diffuse large B-cell lymphomas or multiple myelomas [48, 49]. The altered expression of cyclin D and its subtypes in various tumors, conclusively suggests that dysregulation of these cell regulators may promote malignant transformation.

3.3.1.2 Cyclin E

Cyclin E is transcribed from the chromosomal region 19q12→q13 along with a host of 39- to 52-kDa polypeptides during the G1 phase. Further posttranslational modifications lead to several cyclin E isoforms, of which two subtypes (E1 and E2) principally govern the activity of the catalytic subunit, CDK2. The nuclear protein cyclin E1 transcribed from *CCNE1* at 19q12 was first identified by screening for genes that could complement G1 cyclin mutations in *Saccharomyces cerevisiae*. The second member of cyclin E family, termed cyclin E2 (*CCNE2* at 8q22.1), is nearly 70% homologous with cyclin E1 and is thus largely regarded as functionally redundant with cyclin E1 [50]. Highest activity of cyclin E-CDK2 is observed during the G1-S phase following phosphorylation of retinoblastoma (Rb) by cyclin D-CDK4/6. Cyclin E has an unique role in being a component of the Rb-E2F pathway as well as a downstream target gene with defined E2F binding sites [51]. Therefore, not only cyclin E-CDK2 hyperphosphorylates (and inactivates) Rb, cyclin E may promote its own expression via a positive feedback loop. Binding and modulation of CDK2 activity by inhibitory and activating phosphorylations along with transcriptional and posttranscriptional modifications maintain cyclin E levels in normal cells. To prevent untimely activity and normal cell cycle progression, cyclin E is degraded either by the Cul-3 protein ubiquitin-proteasome system (monomeric cyclin E1) or by SCF-Fbw7 ubiquitin ligase (targets cyclin E1-CDK2 complexes) [50, 52]. These numerous layers of control guarantee that the cyclin E level is precisely modulated during cell cycle as any alterations may lead to generation of malignant cells.

Cyclin E and its low-molecular-weight isoforms have been isolated and extensively studied in human breast, endometrium, cervix, uterus, and ovarian cancers. Increased transcriptional activity is often correlated with ovarian cancer, the fourth leading cause of cancer deaths in women of United States of America [53]. Elevated levels are also detected in the early stages of gastrointestinal tract cancers, promoting transformation from adenoma to adenocarcinoma principally in the stomach and the colorectal region. Cyclin E expression was increased in nearly 50% of reported stomach cancers, leading to its use as a prognostic marker [46, 54]. Moreover, tissue microarrays techniques have frequently isolated cyclin E gene amplifications in rhabdomyosarcoma and pheochromocytoma [55]. Several studies have also implicated cyclin E in pathogenesis of lung cancers and adrenocortical tumors [50]. Low-molecular-weight isoforms of cyclin E are also quite prominent in metastatic melanomas. These biologically hyperactive molecules are thought to be a principle factor promoting perineural invasion and metastasis when compared to the full-length cyclin E [56].

3.3.1.3   Cyclin A

Cyclin A is especially intriguing among the cyclin family as it can regulate two distinctive CDKs in two different phases: S stage and mitosis. Since its isolation from sea urchin embryos during 1973, several homologues of cyclin A have been identified in *Drosophila, Xenopus*, mice, and humans. In humans, an embryonic form of cyclin A (cyclin A1, *CCNA1* at chromosome 13q12.3-q13) is observed only during meiosis and early embryogenesis, while, all somatic cells express subtype cyclin A2 (*CCNA2* at chromosome 4q27). As described earlier, peak cyclin A accumulation precedes DNA synthesis phase, and along with CDK2 complexes, it targets downstream phosphorylation of DNA replication machinery [57]. However, the precise role of cyclin A-CDK1 complexes during mitosis is still debatable, and probably confers stability to cyclin B-CDK1 units. Following its activity, cyclin A is abruptly degraded by ubiquitin-dependent proteolysis prior to mitotic metaphase.

Owing to its pivotal role in cell cycle regulation, altered expression of cyclin A2 is often associated with proliferation markers such as PCNA, Ki67, and altered p53 tumor suppressor activities. Cyclin A increase is shown to promote dysregulated proliferation of malignant cells in leukemia, lymphoma, liver, colorectal, and gastric cancer [57, 58]. Moreover, increase in cyclin A is also noted in melanoma, esophageal cancer, lung cancers, osteosarcoma, soft-tissue sarcoma, and smooth muscle cancers [59, 60]. Overexpression of cyclin A is also frequently noticed in astrocytoma [61]. Increased expression of cyclin A can be used to determine tumor stages and is positively correlated with poor prognosis in breast cancer and that of the reproductive tract including ovary, cervical and testicular cancers [62, 63].

3.3.1.4   Cyclin B

Cyclin B is a member of the highly conserved cyclin family required during G2/M transition and consists of B1 (*CCNB1*; 5q12), B2 (CCNB2; 15q22.2), and B3 (*CCNB3*; Xp11) subtypes. Rapid accumulation of cyclin B1 during the G2 phase is essential for mitotic entry of the dividing cell. Following which, this protein accumulates in the nucleus and is shuttled to kinetochores, spindle microtubules, and centrosomes during the prometaphase [64]. Thereafter, cyclin B1 interacts with CDK1-forming maturation-promoting factor (MPF) and helps in chromosome condensation and alignment and nuclear envelope dissolution by acting upon nuclear lamins, microtubules, and downstream chromatin-associated proteins [65]. Finally, mitotic exit is facilitated by rapid proteolytic degradation of cyclin B1 by APC/C prior to anaphase onset. Cyclin B3 is also known to interact with CDK2 during meiosis [66].

Overexpression of cyclin B (especially B1 isoform) has been reported in various human tumors, such as in both small cell (SCLC) and nonsmall cell lung cancer (NSCLC) and in head and neck squamous cell carcinoma [67, 68]. This upregulation is closely associated with poor prognosis in NSCLC patients, particularly those with nonsquamous cell carcinoma [69, 70]. In patients with squamous cell carcinoma subtype (SCC) of NSCLC, cyclin B1 expression is often regarded as a stage-specific prognostic marker [71]. Consistent with this finding, increased cyclin B1 level can also be correlated with aggressive disease progression in SCC of the tongue [68]. In addition, altered expression of cyclin B1 is related to aneuploidy and high proliferation rate of human mammary and cervical carcinomas [72, 73]. Furthermore, elevated cyclin B1 in prostate cancer cells promoted increased expression of the proto-oncogenic serine/threonine kinase (Pim1) leading to polyploidy [74]. Pharmaceutical interventions leading to lowered cyclin B1 levels improved sensitivity of DNA mismatch repair-deficient prostate cancer cells to alkylating agents [75] and apoptosis of prostate cancer cells in vitro [74]. Increased cyclin B1 synthesis and cellular localizations are also positively correlated with stage and progression of renal cell carcinoma [76]. Cyclin B expression is also increased in several colorectal cancers, indicating dysregulation of cell proliferation mechanism [77]. Moreover, suppression of E-cadherin via Cyclin B1 may lead to lymph node metastasis and subsequent invasion of colorectal cancer cells [78]. In vitro studies have revealed that cyclin B1-CDK is increased in astrocytoma [79] and glioblastoma of brain tissues [80], the expression rate which can be correlated with pathologic grades of disease progression [81]. Moreover, owing to its differential gene expression, cyclin B1 along with MYC (v-myc, myelocytomatosis viral oncogene) and lactate dehydrogenase B (LDHB) is considered a strong and independent survival marker in patients with medulloblastoma [82]. Upregulation of this cyclin kinase activity is also implicated in the genesis and/or progression of malignant lymphomas as evident during Hodgkin's lymphoma, diffuse large B-cell lymphoma [83], and follicular lymphoma [84]. In contrast, less aggressive, well-differentiated adenocarcinomas and noninvasive tumors of gastric cancer showed low endogenous levels of this cyclin [85, 86].

3.3.2 CYCLIN-DEPENDENT KINASES AND THEIR ROLE IN CARCINOGENESIS

Cyclin-dependent kinases (CDKs) are a group of proline-directed serine/ threonine kinases that serve as the catalytic unit in CDK-cyclin heterodimers during cell cycle progression [18]. Along with cyclins, altered expression of CDKs have been implicated in the genesis of several cancers. These kinases belong to the CMGC family named after its members as CDKs, mitogen-activated protein kinases (MAPKs), glycogen synthase kinases (GSKs), and CDK-like kinases (CLKs) [87, 88]. CDKs were first implicated in cell cycle control in concurrence with different cyclins, based on pioneering work in budding yeast *S. cerevisiae* (Cdc28) and fission yeast *Schizosaccharomyces pombe* (Cdc2). Since then, CDKs have been identified and cloned independently as cell cycle-regulating gene products in starfish, *Xenopus*, and humans [34]. Albeit reasonably like the framework in yeast, mammalian cells, however, vary both CDKs and cyclins (rather than simply the cyclin) during cell cycle to guarantee successive movement through the cell cycle stages in a precise manner. Therefore, while several CDKs are encoded from almost 12 gene loci, only five have known cell cycle regulatory functions (CDK1, CDK2, CDK3, CDK4, and CDK6). Other CDKs show varied role in basal gene transcription by RNA polymerase II (CDK7-CDK9), RNA modifications (CDK11, CDK12) and neuronal differentiation (CDK5, CDK10). This mammalian CDK diversity in addition to their role in cell cycle probably confers a unique control on cell proliferation during transition from unicellular to complex multicellular organisms [18, 34].

Similar to other kinases, CDKs are characterized by a smaller amino-terminal lobe composed primarily of β-sheets and a PSTAIRE-like cyclin-binding domain. The larger carboxy terminal lobe comprises α-helices along with a T-loop (also known as activation loop). The ATP active site is located deep in-between the two lobes and is obstructed by the T-loop in cyclin free monomers. Inhibitory kinases Wee1 and Myt1 further phosphorylates the active site at threonine-13 and tyrosine-15 respectively, thereby preventing ATP transfer. Cyclins and several noncyclin CDK activators such as viral cyclins and RINGO/Speedy functionally activate CDKS [89, 90]. Phosphorylation of T-loop at threonine-161 by CDK-activating kinases (CAKs) further facilitates cyclin binding [91]. The CDKs are unique in their substrate specificity and require binding with cyclin via the PSTAIRE helix for further reconfiguration of critical residues and subsequent activation [92]. However, in spite of this specificity, detailed studies have deduced a functional redundancy in CDKs and their cyclin-regulating units. Knockout mice lacking functional CDKs showed that CDK1 is capable of binding with several cyclins sequentially, thereby compensating for nearly all interphase CDKs during cell cycle progression [93]. This is best observed under pathological conditions, when nearly all CDKs or cyclins (except for cyclins B1 and A2) are bypassed and replaced with altered complexes of diverse functions [93, 94]. Deregulation of these key cell cycle components by altered cyclin levels or INK4, Cip/Kip inhibitors-mediated suppression is probably one of the primary causes of carcinogenesis and has often been targeted for therapeutic interventions [95].

3.3.2.1 Cyclin-Dependent Kinase 1

Cyclin-dependent kinase 1 (*CDK1*; 10q21.1), a key kinase known for its role during mitosis, is the human homologue of Cdc2 isolated from fission yeast (*S. pombe*). Activity of CDK1 requires binding to its regulating partner (cyclin B1) along with phosphorylation of threonine-161 residue on the T-loop. Cyclin B1-CDK1 heterodimer, popularly known as the "maturation-promoting factor," determines precise moment for the onset of mitosis [96]. The cyclin B-CDK1 complex induces mitosis by phosphorylating and activating enzymes regulating chromatin condensation, nuclear membrane breakdown, mitosis-specific microtubule reorganization, and actin cytoskeleton, thereby allowing for mitotic rounding up of the cell. Subsequent entry into the anaphase critically relies on the sudden destruction of the cyclin B-CDK1 activity by the ubiquitin ligase APC/C [30].

The transcription control of mitotic kinase cyclin B-CDK1 is very stable throughout the cell cycle. This is vital in mammalian cells, as CDK1 is unique in its ability to independently perform the essential functions of all other cell cycle-regulating CDKs. It is, therefore, one of the least mutated kinases in human cancers. However, an increase in CDK1 expression is noted in several cancers like pancreatic adenocarcinoma [97], lymphoma [98], and advanced melanoma [99]. Decreased levels of CDK1 has also been correlated with poor prognosis and chemotherapeutic resistance in lung cancer [100].

3.3.2.2 Cyclin-Dependent Kinase 2

In humans, the *CDK2* gene is located on chromosome 12q13, and its translated product is actively involved in control of the cell cycle; it is essential for meiosis, but dispensable for mitosis. As described earlier, this serine/threonine protein kinase performs dual activity by binding cyclin E during the S phase and cyclin A during G2 for progressing from the S phase to mitosis [17]. Cyclin-dependent kinase 2 (CDK2) is also known to control cell cycle by phosphorylating downstream cyclin B-CDK1 in the centrosome and nucleus, therefore playing a crucial part in DNA duplication. It can interact with a host of cyclins, namely cyclins A, B1, B3, D, or E, and can actively phosphorylate p53/TP53 [101], CDK7 [102], Rb1, BRCA2 [103], and MYC [104]. The CDK2 is also actively involved in G1/S phase DNA damage checkpoint, where it controls DNA damaged cells from dividing and initiates homologous recombination-dependent repair by phosphorylating BRCA2 [103].

Deregulation of this CDK therefore may promote carcinogenesis as observed in several cancers including laryngeal squamous cell cancer [105], advanced melanoma [99], and breast cancer [106]. However, frequent hyperactivation of CDK2 is mostly due to an increased transcription or translational alteration in its regulating cyclin units (cyclin A/E). As discussed earlier, such increased expression of CDK2-cyclin A/E complexes are observed in malignancies of breast, endometrium, ovary, lung and thyroid [106].

3.3.2.3 Cyclin-Dependent Kinase 3

Encoded by the gene located on chromosome 17q25.1, this cyclin-dependent kinase has a high sequence identity with CDK1 and CDK2 [107]. The activity of cyclin-dependent kinase 3 (CDK3) was first observed in the early G1 phase where it associates with cyclin C to phosphorylate pRb1, thereby promoting exit from G0 [108, 109]. CDK3 principally enhances progression through G1 into the S phase in the mammalian cell cycle, and its expression reaches its peak in mid G1. Thereafter, CDK3 binds to E2F family of transcription factors and increases their transcriptional activities, thus playing an essential role at the G1/S transition.

Transcriptional activity of CDK3 has also been found to be dysregulated in numerous human tumors. Viral components (DNA tumor virus proteins EIA, SV40 large T, E7, and herpes simplex virus) frequently modulate CDK3 activity via the RB-E2F pathway leading to malignant modifications [110, 111]. Increased CDK3 expression is noted in glioblastoma and neuroblastoma cell lines and play an important role in cell proliferation and malignant alterations [112, 113]. Aberrant CDK3 activity is also noted in nasopharyngeal cancer and can be associated with the degree of infiltration, lymph node metastasis, and clinical staging [114].

3.3.2.4 Cyclin-Dependent Kinase 4

Cyclin-dependent kinase 4 (*CDK4*; 12q14) in association with its activating partner, cyclin D, are the central regulators of the G1 phase and G1/S transition during cell cycle. CDK4 phosphorylates and inhibit members of the retinoblastoma protein family allowing subsequent transcription of E2F target genes that are responsible for progression through the G1 phase, control transcriptional processes, and regulate cell proliferation components. Considering the pivotal role of CDK4 in cell cycle, it is not surprising that dysregulation of this CDK plays a central role in tumorigenesis.

The significance of CDK4 in human cancers were first noted during a germ line CDK4-Arg24Cys (R24C) mutation that led to constitutive activation of the kinase by preventing CDK4 and its inhibitor p16^{INK4a} binding [115]. This resulted in a predisposition to familial melanomas [116], lymphomas, and lung cancers [117, 118]. In fact, inactivation of the p16^{INK4a} gene by deletion, silencing, or mutation is one of the most recurrent tumor suppressor mutations in human malignancies that results in imperfect inhibition of CDK4 and consequent hyperactivity [119]. Transcriptional and translational alteration in CDK4 expression has also been noted in a variety of cancers including refractory rhabdomyosarcoma [120], osteosarcoma [121], liposarcoma [122], glioblastoma multiforme [123], neuroblastoma [124], and sporadic melanoma [125]. This increase in CDK4 activity during malignancies can be further associated either with cyclin D gene overexpression, amplification, polymorphism, and/or translocation. Cyclin-dependent kinase 4 in conjunction with cyclin D1 is also extensively used in clinical staging of human primary lung cancers and is an attractive pharmacological target for lung cancer therapeutics [117, 126].

3.3.2.5   Cyclin-Dependent Kinase 5

Although cyclin-dependent kinase 5 (*CDK5*; 7q36) has nearly 60% structural identity with cyclin-dependent kinase family members, unlike them, it does not associate with regulator cyclins for kinase activity [127]. Instead, CDK5 is activated by association with CDK5-specific activator proteins, p35 (CDK5R1) or p39 (CDK5R2) and p67, principally in postmitotic neurons [128]. This neuronal-specific expression is vital for proper development and function of human brain via signal transduction "cross-talk" governing neuronal migration, axon guidance, and synaptic transmission [129].

Owing to its vital role in nervous tissues, altered expression of CDK5 is often associated with the development of neurodegenerative diseases. Neurotoxicity of CDK5/p25 units developed from cleavage of CDK5/p35 is shown to have increased proteolytic and apoptotic functions in inducing neuronal cell death, Alzheimer's disease, amyotrophic lateral sclerosis (ALS), and Parkinson's disease [130, 131]. Aside from its contribution to neurodegenerative diseases, CDK5 activity has been correlated with the development of neuronal cancers including glioblastoma and neuroblastoma [132]. CDK5 is also considered a marker of poor prognosis in lung cancer [133]. Owing to its ability to regulate cell motility and migration, CDK5 plays a vital role in metastatic progression of pancreatic ductal adenocarcinoma cells [134]. Aberrant CDK5 activity has been reported during multiple myeloma, lymphoma, colorectal, head, neck, breast, ovarian, lymphoma, prostate, sarcoma, and bladder cancers in humans [106, 134].

3.3.2.6   Cyclin-Dependent Kinase 6

Cyclin-dependent kinase 6 (CDK6, also known as serine/threonine-protein kinase PLSTIRE), encoded in the 7q21-22 chromosomal region, is the catalytic regulatory component of the Cyclin D-CDK complex formed during the G1 phase of the cell cycle. As described previously, CDK6 along with other G1 phase CDKs (CDK2 and CDK4) modulates the inhibiting activity of retinoblastoma protein (pRb). The cyclin D-CDK6 complex is vital for phosphorylating pRb, leading to downstream activation of E2F transcription factors that further regulates S phase genes. Other than its regulatory cyclin unit, CDK6 is simultaneously activated by the CAK complex. Conversely, CDK inhibitors of the INK4 and Cip/Kip families represses untimely activation of CDK6. In spite of these unique controlling mechanisms, dysregulation of CDK6 is often manifested as unregulated proliferation as well as genomic and chromosomal instability in malignant cells.

CDK6 is preferentially expressed in almost all hematopoietic cell types and subsequently upregulated in different cancers such as leukemia and lymphomas. Altered CDK6 levels have been observed in T-cell lymphoblastic lymphoma/leukemia (T-LBL/ALL) and in cancers of pancreas and urinary bladder [2, 135, 136]. Furthermore, a CDK6 mutation that disables p16^{INK4a}-mediated CDK suppression leads to uncontrolled CDK6 protein kinase activity and consequent deregulated cell proliferation in human neuroblastoma via the pRb1-E2F pathway [137].

3.3.2.7   Cyclin-Dependent Kinase 7

The cyclin-dependent kinase 7 (CDK7) gene is located on chromosome 5q12.1, and its encoded protein forms a trimeric complex with cyclin H and MAT1 (menage a trois 1). This CDK7-cyclin H and MAT1 complex is unique in its role as it functions as a CDK-activating kinase (CAK) [138]. Moreover, it is a vital part of the transcription factor II human (TFIIH), which can phosphorylate the C-terminal domain (CTD) of the large subunit of RNA polymerase II (RNA pol II), and is actively involved in transcription initiation and DNA repair mechanisms [91]. This protein is thought to serve as a direct link between transcription regulation and cell cycle progression by phosphorylating and activating several essential kinases, including CDK1, CDK2, CDK3, CDK4, and CDK6 [91, 138]. CDK-activating kinase can also phosphorylate the retinoic acid receptor-alpha, octamer transcription factors (Oct-1), and p53 [139, 140]. Consistent with its multidimensional role in cell cycle regulation, aberrant CDK7 expression is frequently noted in association with cyclin H during cancer cell metastasis. This increased expression of CDK7 is thought to be the driving factor promoting ovarian cancer cell migration and endometrium lymphovascular space invasion [141, 142].

3.3.2.8   Cyclin-Dependent Kinase 8

Encoded by chromosome region 13q12, cyclin-dependent kinase 8 (CDK8) is a critical negative regulator of transcription. The "CDK8 complex" (comprising CDK8, cyclin C, Med12, and Med13) can inhibit the activity of Mediator multiunit subcomplex and RNA polymerase II (RNA pol II) through several mechanisms, thereby preventing initiation and re-initiation of transcription. For example, CDK8 and its regulatory subunit cyclin C negatively regulates the larger subunit of RNA polymerase II through phosphorylation of its C-terminal domain (CTD), thereby disrupting its association with Mediator–polymerase II. This kinase has also been shown to regulate transcription by targeting cyclin H-CDK7 subunits of TFIIH, thereby connecting functions of Mediator-like protein complexes and basal transcription machinery of the cells [143].

Owing to its important role in transcription regulation, aberrant expression of CDK8 has been frequently reported in several human cancers. The oncogenic property of this kinase is best elucidated in its ability to regulate β-catenin-induced malignant transformation and expression of various downstream β-catenin transcriptional targets. The altered levels of both CDK8 and β-catenin can be associated with carcinogenesis, tumor staging, and increased colon cancer-related deaths [144, 145]. Moreover, in gastric adenocarcinomas, a higher levels of CDK8 activities along with delocalization of β-catenin may be one of the determining factors for initiation and clinical progression of the disease [146]. Upregulation of CDK8 expression is further elucidated in the highly proliferative malignant melanoma cells that are depleted of tumor suppressive properties of the histone variant macroH2A (mH2A) chromatin region [147]. Likewise, lowering endogenous of CDK8 levels through gene silencing in breast cancer cell lines leads to a decrease in cellular proliferation potential [148]. Therefore, it is safe to conclude that, in humans, CDK8 kinase activities are plausibly exploited by cancer cells for promoting growth and maintaining a dedifferentiating state.

3.3.2.9   Cyclin-Dependent Kinase 9

Cyclin-dependent kinase 9 (CDK9), encoded in the chromosomal region 9q34.1, is a major component of the multiprotein complex TAK/P-TEFb. In association with cyclins T1, T2a, T2b, or K, this complex functions as an elongation factor for RNA polymerase II-directed transcription by phosphorylating the C-terminal domain of the largest subunit of RNA polymerase II [149]. Moreover, by binding with its regulatory cyclin K subunit and not cyclin T, CDK9 functions principally as a DNA repair complex. It maintains genomic integrity by promoting replication arrest, suppressing DNA:RNA hybrids, and limiting single-stranded DNA (ssDNA) in response to replication stress [149].

Owing to its significant role in DNA repair and transcription control, dysregulation of CDK9-mediated signal transduction pathways is frequently observed during tumorigenesis in several human cancers [150]. Increased cyclin T1-CDK9 activity is essentially associated with different grades of neuroblastoma, primary neuroectodermal tumor, rhabdomyosarcoma, and prostate cancer [106, 151, 152]. Hyperactivity of CDK9 and cyclin T1 has also been reported in myeloid leukemia and several lymphomas, including B- and T-cell precursor-derived lymphomas, anaplastic large T-cell lymphoma, follicular lymphomas, and Hodgkin's lymphoma [152]. Moreover, aberrant amplification of CDK9 and cyclin T1 mRNA is frequently observed in Burkitt's lymphoma and diffuse large B-cell lymphoma [152].

3.3.2.10   Cyclin-Dependent Kinase 10

Cyclin-dependent kinase 10 (CDK10) is unique among other CDKs owing to its ability to interact directly with transcription factors like Ets2 (v-ets, erythroblastosis virus E26 oncogene homolog 2) repressing its activity in normal cells [153]. Although in vitro breast cancer cell lines have shown a regulating role of cyclin M, despite having a PSTAIRE-like cyclin binding motif and all the structural features of a functional catalytic domain, a cyclin partner for CDK10 leaves scope for further elucidation [154]. However, owing to its ability to interact with Ets2, CDK10 is an important determinant of resistance to breast cancer treatment [155]. In normal cells, it is thought to function as a tumor suppressor protein and its subsequent downregulation is noted in biliary tract tumors and hepatocarcinoma [156, 157]. Overexpression of CDK10 has also been linked to chemotherapeutic resistance in malignant cells [156].

Although initially thought to represent a family of protein kinases that are crucial cell cycle regulators, newer research has identified several CDKs with little known cell progression kinase activity. Instead, kinases such as CDK11, CDK12, and CDK13 [158] in association with their activator cyclin L are essential during transcription control and splicing regulation [159, 160]. Furthermore, CDK12 when activated by cyclin K acts as a vital component in DNA repair mechanisms of the cell [161]. These low-molecular-weight molecules also serve as signal molecules that intricately connect cell cycle with transcription regulation and RNA splicing. This is particularly highlighted by the role of CDK14-cyclin Y during Wnt/β-catenin signaling [162]. Diverse roles of CDK16 and cyclin Y complex have been recognized during presynaptic protein trafficking [163] as well as during spermatogenesis [164].

3.3.3   CYCLIN-DEPENDENT KINASE INHIBITORS AND CANCER

As described in the previous sections, human cell cycle is precisely regulated by the sequential activation of CDKs by their cyclin partners. To prevent any aberrant CDK expression that may lead to future malignancies, a deactivation mechanism is equally important during the cell cycle. Cyclin-dependent kinase inhibitors (CKIs), serve as brakes that modulate CDK activities, thus restricting their expression in a phase-specific manner. Thus, while most cyclins initiate CDK activation, CKIs limits the kinase activity. CKIs are subdivided into two classes based on their structure and CDK specificity. The INK4 family of proteins [p16^{INK4a} (*CDKN2A*), p15^{INK4b} (*CDKN2B*), p18^{INK4c} (*CDKN2C*), and p19^{INK4d} (*CDKN2D*)] composed of multiple ankyrin repeats primarily target monomeric CDK4/6 or heteromeric CDK4/6 and cyclin D complexes [165]. Conversely, the Cip/Kip family members [p21^{Cip1} (*CDKN1A*), p27^{Kip1} (*CDKN1B*) and p57^{Kip2} (*CDKN1C*)] have a broader range and interfere with cyclin A, B, D, and E-dependent kinase complex activities [166]. Owing to their inhibitory activity, CKIs promote lowered proliferation potential and aberrant growth suppression (notably via pRb-regulated pathways) thus possessing unique tumor suppressor properties in human cells.

3.3.3.1   Cip/Kip Family of Cyclin-Dependent Inhibitors

Relative binding of Cip/Kip family of CKIs (p21^{Cip1}, p27^{Kip1}, and p57^{Kip2}) directly to components of the transcriptional machinery aid in cell cycle regulation. Although their interaction is analogous with CDK/cyclin complexes, this association is usually inhibitory. Among this family of inhibitors, the cyclin-dependent kinase inhibitor p21^{Cip1} is best known to interact with G1 cyclin-CDK complexes and also with several transcription factors. It has a vital role in inhibition of E2F-transcribed proteins, thereby enhancing the repression of downstream E2F-responsive genes and inducing efficient cell cycle arrest [166]. In addition to p21, the other Cip/Kip proteins p27 and p57 also participate in the assembly of catalytically active cyclin D-CDK4/6 complexes [167]. p21^{Cip1} is also known to disrupt the interaction between CDK and retinoblastoma family of proteins such as Rb1/pRb, Rbl1 (p107), and Rbl2 (p130), thereby halting cell cycle progression [166]. p21^{Cip1} effectively modulates the different phases of cell cycle by p53-dependent gene repression of downstream targets like *CDC25C*, *CDK1*, *CHEK1*, *CCNB1* (which encodes cyclin B1), *TERT* (which encodes telomerase reverse transcriptase), and the antiapoptotic gene *BIRC5* (survivin) [168, 169]. Moreover, p21^{Cip1} levels are regulated by posttranslational means via its degradation by E3 ubiquitin ligases, thereby promoting cyclin-mediated CDK activation [170]. Quite surprisingly, Cip/Kip proteins are capable of modulating cell cycle independently of cyclins and CDKs by inhibiting components of the DNA replication machinery during unfavorable conditions. This low-molecular-weight protein, p21^{Cip1}, has the unique ability to bind to PCNA, a DNA polymerase δ unit, via its carboxyl terminus (C-terminus amino acids 143–160) and suppress DNA synthesis [170]. In contrast to p21^{Cip1}, p27^{Kip1} functions primarily to restrict the entry of cells into the cell division cycle and is therefore expressed chiefly in mitogen-deprived and quiescent cells [171]. Other than its classical role as cyclin-CDK inhibitor, p27^{Kip1} can modulate normal cell motility by modifying cellular cytoskeleton. Thus, deficiency in endogenous p27^{Kip1} levels is often implicated in increased tumor aggressiveness and poor prognosis [172]. p27^{Kip1} in association with p130/E2F4 also functions as a transcription regulator by binding at the promoter regions of genes involved in vital cellular functions such as mitochondrial units, cellular respiration, and splicing and processing of RNA. This localization further enhances the binding of transcriptional co-repressors such as mSIN3A and histone deacetylases (HDACs [172]. Unlike ubiquitously expressed p21^{Cip1} and p27^{Kip1}, p57^{Kip1} has a tissue-restricted expression pattern as observed in regulation of cell cycle during embryogenesis [173].

Originally described as inhibitors of CDK-cyclin complexes, these molecules owing to their conformational flexibility are able sequester a wide diversity of proteins in a multitude of pathways and therefore are often aberrantly expressed in cancer cells [174]. Several viral proteins like the human papilloma virus (HPV) E6 protein, hepatitis C virus core protein, and adeno-associated virus type 2 preferentially downregulates the p21^{Cip1} protein in infected cells along with an increase in CDK2, thus promoting tumorigenesis [175]. Furthermore, in infected cells, human papillomavirus-16 E7 protein may bind to both p21^{Cip1} and p27^{Kip1}, thereby suppressing their inhibitory activity toward CDK2-cyclin complexes [176]. Moreover, increased cytoplasmic expression of p21^{Cip1} is a poor prognostic and aggressive tumor marker in human carcinomas of pancreas, breast, prostate, ovary, and cervix, and in glioblastomas [177, 178]. Lowered endogenous p27^{Cip1} expression levels have also been successfully correlated with increased tumor aggressiveness of several malignancies, including colon, prostate, stomach, lung, brain, breast, and ovarian carcinoma, thus highlighting the role of p27^{Kip1} as a prognosis marker [179, 180]. Similar to the other members of the Cip/Kip family, the role of p57^{Kip1} is essentially that of tumor suppression, and its inactivation is documented in carcinomas of the lung, gastrointestinal tract, liver, pancreas, breast, and head and neck and acute myeloid leukemia [181, 182].

3.3.3.2 INK4 Family of Cyclin-Dependent Kinase Inhibitor

The INK4 *family of proteins are structurally related* inhibitors of CDK4 and/ or CDK6 encoded in a 35-kb human *INK4a/ARF/INK4b (CDKN2A* and *CDKN2B)* genome locus. Principal among them is *CDKN2A,* located at 9p21, which encodes two different proteins, p16^{INK4a} and p14^{ARF} (p19^{ARF} in mouse) using an alternative reading frame. Although the tumor suppressor properties of p14^{ARF} is extensively studied, little is known about its role in cell cycle regulation. Other members of this family are *CDKN2B* at 9p21 (encoding p15^{INK4b}), *CDKN2C* at 1p32 (encoding p18^{INK4c}), and *CDKN2D* at 19q13 (encoding p19^{INK4d}). Among themselves, these 15 to 19 kDa polypeptides share about 40% homology and can bind both monomeric CDK4/6 and cyclin D-bound CDK4/6 [165, 183]. The binding of p16^{INK4a} with CDK4/6 induces allosteric modifications, repressing their activation by cyclin D. This in turn prevents CDK4/6-mediated pRb phosphorylation, continuing its suppression of E2F transcription factors, and leading to G1 arrest. In addition, to their role in cell cycle G1/S transition, these low-molecular-weight proteins (p14^{ARF}, p15^{INK4b}, and p16^{INK4a}) also show tumor suppressor properties. This is best elucidated through p53-mediated tumor suppressor activities of p14^{ARF}. Unlike other INK4 members, p14^{ARF} does not bind to any cyclin-CDK complexes, but rather suppresses Mouse double minute 2 homolog (Mdm2), a p53 E3-ubiquitin ligase, following genotoxic stress. p14^{ARF} Mdm2 association leads to relocalization of the ligase from the nucleus to the cell nucleolus, thus promoting p53 nuclear stabilization. Stabilized p53 further upregulates its transcriptional activity, leading to increased synthesis of downstream targets like Mdm2 and p21^{Cip1} and finally prompting a p53-dependent cell cycle arrest [184].

The shared genomic sequences, close loci proximity, and interconnected activities of p16^{INK4a} and p14^{ARF} family members controlling several essential cell cycle signaling pathways make them a vulnerable target for oncogenic onslaught. Therefore, mutations in the INK4 family, specially CDKN2A and CDKN2B tumor suppressor genes, have been found frequently in several human tumors. Alterations of the *CDKN2C* gene has also been reported in human tumors, albeit at much lower frequency. Moreover, due to p16^{INK4a} and p14^{ARF} role in tumor suppression and modulating activities of Rb and p53 pathways, it is not surprising that genetic and epigenetic changes in this locus are frequently detected in the majority of tumor types. Thus, homozygous deletion or mutations of the p16^{INK4a} gene is frequently observed in anaplastic meningiomas [185]. Promoter silencing of this gene through methylation leads to loss of control of the restriction point in the G1 phase of the cell cycle and is observed in NSCLC [186]. Epigenetic modulation by hypermethylation of p15^{INK4b} gene is noted in glial tumors, leukemia, and myelodysplasia and is frequently deleted in multiple myeloma [187, 188]. Furthermore, selective inactivation of the tumor suppressor gene p19^{ARF} has also been reported in cancers like familial melanoma [189, 190].

3.4   SIGNALING PATHWAYS REGULATING THE CELL CYCLE

Cycling cells are constantly subjected to chemical, radiation, or biological stresses that can potentially induce aberrant DNA alterations. Genomic damage may result from endogenous agents such as reactive oxygen species generated as a byproduct of cellular metabolism, through spontaneous depurination of DNA, and by collapse of the replicating fork. Exogenous sources of DNA damage include viral infective agents, chemicals such as cisplatin, and ionizing and ultraviolet radiation [191]. To prevent transmitting these aberrant genomic changes, it is vital that the cell cycle progression is halted, and DNA alterations are repaired prior to DNA duplication and segregation, thereby ensuring that each daughter cell receives a full complement of undamaged DNA.

3.4.1 DNA DAMAGE AND REPLICATION CHECKPOINT

Concurrently with cyclin-CDK mediated cell cycle regulation, eukaryotic genomic integrity is maintained at the DNA damage checkpoints by synchronized actions of several signaling pathways that can sense genotoxic damage and DNA replication interference and effectively transduce this signal to downstream effector molecules [192]. In contrast to popular belief, these checkpoint activities are not restricted to a particular point in the cell cycle. Instead, these surveillance mechanisms constantly monitor the integrity of the cell cycle and may generate distinct DNA damage response (DDR) via kinase-mediated phosphorylations to slow and/or halt cell cycle progression, thereby allowing time for repair of DNA lesions and disrupted DNA forks that gives rise to strand breaks [193]. This is of vital importance as deficiencies in DNA damage responses may result in faulty repair, damaged or improperly segregated DNA leading to poor cellular viability, genetic instability, and even carcinogenesis. Conceptually, the term "checkpoint" is described based on the cell cycle transition phase that is being inhibited by DNA damage. Thus, while DNA damage checkpoints monitors total structural genomic integrity at G1/S, S, and G2/M phases, the DNA replication checkpoint screens for proper synthesis of DNA at the intra-S checkpoint. Although seemingly diverse in functions, these checkpoints share several decisive pathways and are functionally interlinked. Therefore, just like other signal transduction pathways, the genes involved in DNA damage checkpoint can be functionally classified into four categories, namely sensors, mediators, transducers, and effectors [193]. This classification is purely for better understanding the complex response system, as there is no clear demarcation between the various proteins involved in DNA damage sensing, signal transduction, and effector steps of the DNA damage checkpoints. For instance, several DNA damage sensor proteins may also function as signal transducer molecules. Additionally, mediator proteins that are thought to have intermediate functioning between sensors and signal transducers seem to partake in more than one stage of the checkpoint response.

Principally, two protein kinases of the phosphatidylinositol-3 (PI-3) kinase-like kinase family (PIKK), ATM (ataxia telangiectasia mutated) and ATR (AT and Rad3-related), and four gene products (RAD17, RAD1, RAD9, and HUS1) that are homologous to replication proteins are involved in DNA damage recognition and signal initiation of these checkpoints, forming an integral part of the DNA damage response (DDR) [194]. The ataxia telangiectasia mutated kinase activity is immediately activated in the presence of DNA double-stranded breaks (DSBs) generated by ionizing radiation or radiomimetic drugs. In response to this type of DNA damage characterized particularly by double-stranded DNA (dsDNA), inactive dimeric or oligomeric ATM is autophosphorylated at serine-1981 into activated monomer units [195]. The MRN complex [Mre11 (Meiotic recombination protein), NBS1 (Nimegen breakage syndrome) and Rad50 (Radiation sensitive 50)] associates with ATM, further enhancing its activity and rapidly directing its localization to damaged DNA sites [196]. Whereas ATR, in concert with ATM, responds broadly to replication blockage due to ssDNA and damage from UV and ionizing radiation [193, 197]. In the case of ATR, its activation is preceded by recognition and binding of ssDNA by replication protein A (RPA). The regulatory unit of ATR, known as ATR-interacting protein (ATRIP), recognizes these RPA-coated ssDNA and helps in localizing ATR-ATRIP complex to DNA damage sites [198]. Along with ATRIP, ATR forms a heterodimer with two additional protein complexes, the Rad17 and 9-1-1 complex, for complete functional activation. The 9-1-1 trimeric complex has a sliding clamp-like configuration comprising Rad9, Rad1, and Hus1 proteins and is structurally similar to PCNA, a processivity factor for DNA polymerase-δ [199]. The Rad17 protein, resembling the subunits of the replication factor C (RFC1) forms a RFC-like complex with the four small RFC subunits (RFC2-RFC5). Similar to eukaryotic DNA replication mechanisms involving RFC-mediated recognition of primer template junction and consequent recruitment of PCNA onto DNA, during DDR, RAD17 acts as a DNA damage-activated loader of the 9-1-1 clamp onto damaged DNA [200, 201]. Although the activity of ATR kinase is vital for initiating ssDNA repair, its functioning during dsDNA breaks is dependent on ATM. In contrast to rapid activation of ATM during DSB resection, ATR is activated slowly, predominantly in the later phases of cell cycle. This differential expression can be attributed to the role of several exo- and endo nucleases like the MRN complex (an exo- and endonuclease), CtIP (an endonuclease activator of MRN) and EXO1 (an exonuclease) that form long stretches of ssDNA adjacent to the DSBs. These long stretches of ssDNA are required for ATR activation during ATM-mediated DSB resection [202]. Further modulation of DNA replication origin firing sites occur sequentially through phosphorylation of downstream ATR-interacting protein (ATRIP) and checkpoint kinase 1 (Chk1) [198, 201]. DNA-dependent protein kinase (DNA-PK) belonging to the PIKK family is another important DDR kinase that is activated by DNA damage and plays a prominent role in non-homologous end joining (NHEJ) of dsDNA breaks [201]. It is composed of a catalytic subunit (DNA-PKcs) and DNA-binding Ku heterodimer consisting of Ku70/ 80 subunits [203]. In response to various genotoxic stresses, DNA-PKs are rapidly phosphorylated at several serine and threonine residues. Phosphorylation at the threonine-2609 cluster region is particularly important during DSB repair and is regulated by both ATM and ATR. Moreover, once activated and recruited to the DNA break sites, the PIKKs phosphorylate several mediator and transducer downstream genes. In the case of ATM, the mediator molecules upregulated are NBS1, tumor suppressor p53-binding protein (53BP1), structural maintenance of chromosome 1 (SMC1), and breast cancer 1 (BRCA1). This leads to activation of transducers like ATM itself along with checkpoint kinase 2 (Chk2) and finally effector proteins like Cdc25A, B, C phosphatases; CDKs; and p53 [193, 204]. During ssDNA breaks, ATR effectively phosphorylates p53 along with sensors like Rad17 and transducers such as ATRIP and Chk1 to control cell cycle progression [198, 205]. In view of their complexity, a detailed understanding of how these intricate signaling pathways detect DNA damage and subsequently prevent cell cycle progression at G1/S, intra-S, and G2/M phases is warranted.

3.4.1.1   The G1/S DNA Damage Checkpoint

During favorable cell cycle conditions, eukaryotic cells in the G1 phase become committed to enter the S phase at a stage known as the restriction point. In humans, this restriction point is at least 2 h prior to DNA synthesis. Regardless of whether cells have or have not progressed through the restriction point, in presence of DNA damage, G1/S checkpoint prevents the progression of cells from G1 to the S phase by several mechanisms. Although transcription factor p53 was primarily thought to be the key molecule for this effect, various studies have highlighted a rapid p53-independent signal transduction response prior to p53 synthesis, activation, and further posttranslational modifications. Thus, depending on the source, DNA damage may trigger a rapid cascade of phosphorylation response events involving kinases like ATM (upon IR) or ATR (during UV radiation). These phosphorylations result in the activation of two types of biochemical pathways: firstly to initiate the G1/S arrest and secondly to maintain it. The phosphorylation that initiates rapid G1/S arrest begins with ATM- or ATR-mediated phosphorylation of Chk2 or Chk1 kinases, respectively. Being phosphorylated by Chk1/Chk2 kinase, Cdc25A phosphatase is subjected to nuclear exclusion and Skp1-Cul1-F-box protein ubiquitin ligase-mediated proteosomal degradation. The Cdc25A phosphatase is essential for removing inhibitory control at threonine-14 and tyrosine-15 residues of CDK2, allowing its activation by cyclin E during the G1 cell cycle phase. Consequently, inactive (phosphorylated) CDK2 is unable of loading Cdc45, a binding molecule for several DNA polymerases, onto DNA pre-replication complexes, thereby promoting a DNA-damaged induced G1 block. This ATM/ATR–Chk2/Chk1–Cdc25A–CDK2-Cdc45 pathway(s) aptly explains a p53-independent initiation of the G1/S checkpoint and rapidly executes cell cycle arrest by a cascade of protein–protein interactions, phosphorylations, ubiquitination, and proteolysis of the key target, the Cdc25A phosphatase (Figure 3.2).

Tumor suppressor protein and an important transcription factor, p53, plays the vital role in maintaining G1/S arrest. Under normal conditions, the cellular level of the p53 protein is low due to its relatively short half-life and through targeted ubiquitin-dependent degradation by Mdm2, a p53-E3 ubiquitin ligase that restricts p53 activity [206]. Depending on the nature of DNA damage incurred, p53 is phosphorylated by ATM/ATR directly at serine-15 or by downstream Chk2 kinases at serine-20. This deters p53 interaction with Mdm2, inhibiting its degradation and ensuring its stability [207, 208]. In addition, ATM may promote p53 stabilization, accumulation and nuclear retention in DNA damaged cells by phosphorylating its negative regulator Mdm2 at serine-395 [206]. As a consequence of p53 activation, transcriptional upregulation of the cyclin-dependent kinase inhibitor p21[Cip1] occurs. Direct binding of p21[Cip1] to S phase-promoting cyclin E-CDK2 complexes leads to G1/S transition inhibition [20]. Moreover, by binding with CDK4/6-cyclinD complex, p21[Cip1] prevents it from phosphorylating Rb (Figure 3.2). As described previously, the phosphorylation of Rb is essential for the activation of E2F transcription factor that controls transcription of downstream target genes required to proceed to the S phase. In addition to p53, several novel members of p53 family have been identified for their possible role in DNA damage. These include tumor suppressor, p33[ING], which co-precipitates with p53, and is required for p53-mediated p21[Cip1] induction in response to IR [209]. Two other members of p53 transcription family, p63 and p73, with significant sequential similarity in their DNA binding (DBD), oligomerization domain (OD), and transactivation domains (TA), are capable of similar functions, including modulation of several common

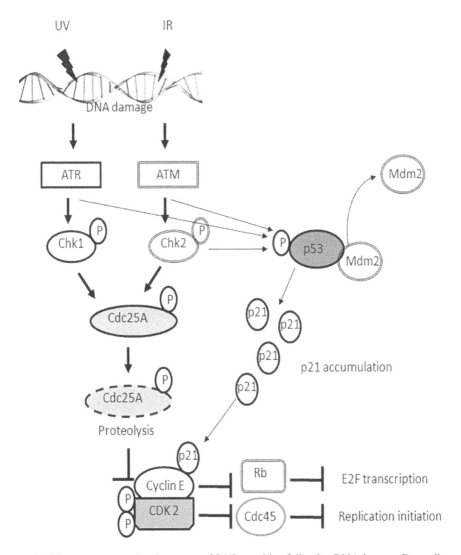

FIGURE 3.2   Arrest and maintenance of G1/S transition following DNA damage. Depending on the source, DNA damage rapidly upregulates ATM/Chk2 (ionizing radiation) or ATR/Chk1 (UV radiation) kinases that phosphorylates Cdc25A and primes it for proteosomal degradation. Absence of Cdc25A inhibits cyclin E-CDK2 activation, blocking replication initiation and inducing G1/S arrest. Once initiated G1/S arrest is maintained by ATR/ATM/Chk2-mediated p53 upregulation and by suppressing the activities of its inhibitor Mdm2 ligase, thereby ensuring stable p53 transcription. Consequently, p53 upregulates cyclin-dependent kinase inhibitor p21 that prevents activation of G1 cyclin complexes (cyclin E-CDK2 and cyclin D-CDK4/6) leading to DNA damage-induced G1/S arrest. The arrow head indicates transcriptional activation. The line ending with a bar indicates inhibition of cell cycle transcription.

downstream targets and even induction of cell cycle arrest upon DNA damage. This role of the isoforms in regulation of cell cycle is extremely complex involving several posttranslational modifications in response to various stimuli including stress [210]. Similar to p53, both p63 and p73 can induce G1 block via upregulation of p21^{Cip1}. Likewise, p73 may also upregulate Mdm2 ligase expression. However, unlike p53, Mdm2 do not target p73 for ubiquitin-dependent degradation. Instead, Mdm2 regulates p73 transcription activator functions by preventing its binding with p300/CBP, a component of the eukaryotic transcription complex. During DNA damage, activated ATM further phosphorylates and activates c-Abl kinase, a nonreceptor tyrosine kinase which in turn can activate p73 and potentially result in the transactivation of p21^{Cip1} and GADD45 (growth arrest and DNA damage) genes. Thus, ATM may mediate G1/S checkpoint through direct phosphorylation of p53 or indirectly through phosphorylation of c-Abl which in turn can upregulate p21^{Cip1} via p73 activation [211]. Another mechanism by which p53 plausibly induces a G1 arrest is by interacting with cyclin H of the CDK-activating complex (CAK; CDK7/cyclin H/Mat1) [91]. This nontranscriptional mechanism inhibits CAK from phosphorylating CDK2, thereby preventing its activation during G1.

3.4.1.2   S Phase (Replication) Checkpoint

Cells are increasingly vulnerable to DNA damage during its synthesis and replication phase. In order to negate this DNA damage, cells activate a complex network of signal transduction pathways collectively referred to as the intra-S replication checkpoint. Checkpoint control of the S phase is of particular importance because "replication stress" induced by stalled replication forks, mis-incorporated bases, secondary DNA structures, DNA–RNA hybrids, fragile DNA sites, constitutive activation of oncogenes like C-Myc, and DNA lesions incurred by exogenous agents constantly hinder the replication process. Repair in the S phase also may be the final step of defense to eliminate DNA damage before they are converted into inheritable mutation. As previously described, the principal components of DNA damage response, ATR [212] and ATM [213] play the pivotal role in replication distress through two distinct pathways, namely *ATM/ATR–Chk1/Chk2–CDC25A* and *ATM–NBS1–SMC1* [214]. ATR is probably the key kinase as it can localize and initiate signaling pathways in the presence of ssDNA structures involved in replication stress induced by stalled replication forks. Consequently, in the presence of ssDNA, the ssDNA-binding protein RPA binds to the ATRIP-ATR complex, thereby helping in localizing the kinase to the DNA lesion site. This leads to further recruitment of Rad17 multimer, which helps to load the Rad9–Hus1–Rad1 (9-1-1) complex for DNA repair initiation. Thereafter, in the presence of allosteric activator TopBP1, the activated ATR modulates the transcription of essential downstream targets chiefly Chk1. Upregulated Chk1 phosphorylates Cdc25A phosphatase and inhibits it from activating the critical serine/threonine kinase CDK2, thereby effectively attenuating the initiation of S phase replication origin firings [215]. Moreover, another mechanism by which ATR-dependent checkpoints inhibits replication initiation is by lowering Cdc7-Dbf4 protein kinase activity, which is required for Cdc45 binding to chromatin. Therefore, the down-regulation of either cyclin E-CDK2 or Cdc7/Dbf4 complexes may result in the inhibition of late replication origins during the intra-S checkpoint [216]. Similar to the ATM-induced damage responses, ATR-mediated signaling also results in phosphorylation of mediators like BRCA1 and NBS1, which promotes repair of collapsed replication forks [216]. Despite the fact that ATR is thought to be the actual kinase intervening the reaction to replication stress, mostly because of its capacity to act during the intra-S stage checkpoint, evidence exists to support a role for ATM activation in response to replication stress. This alternate intra-S checkpoint signal transduction pathway is induced following ionizing radiation and is initiated by phosphorylation of Nbs1 by ATM and its recruitment to DNA damaged sites. The Mre11–Rad50-Nbs1 (MRN) complex further activates and upregulates ATM on sensing dsDNA lesions [204]. Phosphorylated Nbs1 also modulates one of the components of the cohesion complex, SMC1 (structure maintenance of chromosome) protein, by phosphorylating at serine-957 and serine-966 [217]. This signal transduction pathway is critical not only for arresting cell cycle but also because it activates the DNA repair process mediated by these various effector proteins. However, several studies have questioned the probability of ATR activation and not that of ATM during recruitment of the MRN complex and Mre11 and Nbs1 interaction at stalled fork sites [218, 219]. Moreover, another study showed both ATR and ATM are essential for Mre11-dependent regulation of stalled forks [220]. In case of a DSB resulting from replication of a nicked DNA, ATM along with the MRN complex and mediator protein BRCA1 can also initiate the standard checkpoint response following the ATM-Chk2-Cdc25A-Cdk2 pathway.

ATM activity may plausibly resolve replication forks by directly upregulating downstream RecQ family of DNA helicases such as Werner syndrome protein (WRN) and Bloom syndrome protein (BLM) [221]. Furthermore, in the absence of Nbs1, mediator-adaptor proteins such as 53BP1 can initiate ATM-MRN complex interaction, resulting in the phosphorylation of downstream proteins such as Chk1, Chk2, and Nbs1. The pivotal role of ATM is further elucidated when a lack of functional ATM kinase renders the intra-S phase checkpoint defective, causing radio-resistant DNA synthesis (RDS), a hallmark of A-T cells [222].

3.4.1.3   G2/M Checkpoint in DNA Damage

Active during the late G2 phase, this G2/M checkpoint principally prevent cells with DNA damage from mitotic entry, thereby preventing the damaged DNA from being segregated into daughter cells. Similar to other checkpoints, at the G2/M transition checkpoint, both ATM-Chk2 and/or ATR-Chk1 signaling initiates and maintains cell cycle arrest during IR- or UV-mediated DNA damage, respectively. In any case, checkpoint kinases prevent entry into mitosis by inhibiting cyclin B-CDK1 activity and upregulating inhibitory Wee1 transcription. This is done through several mechanisms including the inhibition of cyclin B-CDK1 kinase by Chk1/Chk2, degradation, and inhibition of the Cdc25 family of phosphatases. Phosphorylated by ATM/ATR-induced responses via *ATM–Chk2–Cdc25A* and/or the *ATR– Chk1– Cdc25A* pathways, the mediator proteins such as 53BP1 and MDC1 (mediator of DNA damage checkpoint protein 1) play critical roles in the activation of Chk1 and Chk2. These kinases further phosphorylate Cdc25A leading to its degradation and subsequent inactivation of CDK1. Cdc25A phosphatase activity is essential for the removal of inhibitory phosphorylations at theronin-14 and tyrosine-15 residues from CDK1. Further phosphorylation of Cdc25C on serine-216 by Chk1 or Chk2 creates a binding site for 14-3-3 proteins and results in export to and retention in the cytoplasm, resulting in loss of function [223]. The initiation of G2/M arrest is also achieved via p53-regulated pathways. The critical transcription targets of p53 are the CDK inhibitor p21[Cip1] and GADD45 that cause the dissociation of the cyclinB-CDK1 kinase complex. Adaptor protein 14-3-3σ then sequesters the cyclin B-CDK1 kinase in the cytoplasm, thus allowing time for DNA repair [224]. The transcription factor p53 can also decrease the promoter activity of cyclin

B1, thereby lowering intracellular cyclin B1 and leading to cell cycle arrest [225]. Moreover, p73 isoform of p53 has been shown to modulate several key G2/M regulator genes such as *Cdc25B, Cdc25C,* and *Cyclin B1* and *B2,* thus highlighting its importance in cell cycle progression [226]. Cells lacking these genes exhibit a G2/M checkpoint defect and may promote genomic instability and cancer.

3.4.1.4 DNA Damage Checkpoint and Cancer

DNA damage mechanisms involved in cellular DNA damage response pathways are frequently altered in human cancer susceptibility syndromes, leading to aberrant cellular transformation. Several cancer susceptible syndromes arise due to inheritance of one or more different mutated genes involved in repair of DNA DSBs, including nonpolyposis colon cancer syndrome, Fanconi's anemia, Li-Fraumeni syndrome, ataxia-telangiectasia, and xeroderma pigmentosum. Inheritance of a single mutated copy of either the *BRCA1* or *BRCA2* genes, both of which participate in DNA damage signaling, markedly increases the risk of women for developing breast or ovarian cancers. Translational activation of RAD51, BRCA1, ERCC1 (Excision Repair Cross-Complementation Group 1), and PARP1 (Poly-ADP-Ribose Polymerase 1) is also observed in various chemotherapeutic-resistant cancers [227]. The tumor suppressor role of p53 is best elucidated during DNA damage checkpoint activation. This damage-inducible p53 checkpoint pathway effectively prevents tumorigenesis by inducing either growth arrest or apoptosis [168]. Cancer cells thus frequently initiate modifications like missense mutations or loss of the p53 gene; inactivation of wild-type p53 protein function by interaction with the proto-oncogenic cellular protein mdm2, or the inability to induce downstream effector molecules such as p21^{Cip1} leading to uncontrolled growth [228]. Furthermore, an increased autophosphorylation of ATM and ATM-dependent phosphorylation of Chk2 are reported in both early-stage and late-stage tumors, suggesting that DDRs not only serve as a barrier to malignant progression of tumor but may also promote tumor metastasis regardless of cancer stage [229, 230]. Increased expression of DNA damage checkpoint genes like *NBS1, RAD50, Chk1, Chk2, Cdc25A, Cdc25B*, and *Cdc25C* are also frequently reported in several malignancies [227, 231]. Furthermore, DNA-PK catalytic subunit is reported to be overexpressed in radiation-resistant tumors of the prostate and in glioblastoma multiforme malignancies associated with poor survival [232, 233].

3.4.2 SPINDLE ASSEMBLY CHECKPOINT

The spindle assembly checkpoint (SAC) is a highly conserved cell cycle supervision mechanism that is active during the prometaphase and comprises several genes and their products that are involved in pathways responsible for preventing precocious separation of sister chromatids [234, 235]. This cell cycle checkpoints screens chromosomal kinetochore for proper spindle microtubular attachment during mitosis. Therefore, in the presence of unattached or improperly attached kinetochores, SAC is activated. One of the first responses of SAC activation is the assembly of mitotic checkpoint complex (MCC), an inhibitory signal of metaphase to anaphase transition by preventing proteolysis of cyclin-dependent kinase, blocks sister-chromatid separation and cell entrance into the anaphase. The MCC comprises highly conserved proteins Mad2 (mitotic arrest deficient 2) and mitotic checkpoint serine/threonine-protein kinase BubR1 and Bub3 along with the Cdc20 protein. Plausible initiation of MCC response occurs by autoactivation and accumulation of Mps1 (monopolar spindle 1), a serine/threonine kinase at unattached kinetochores. This results in recruitment of several checkpoint associated proteins such as Mad1-Mad2 and Bub3-BubR1 complexes, motor protein CENP-E and proteins of the Zeste White 10 (ZW10), and ROD and zwilch complex, which act simultaneously with Cdc20, thus promoting and amplifying SAC activity [236, 237]. For example, Mad2 and Cdc20 found in a complex with BubR1 and Bub3 (mitotic checkpoint complex) are a more potent inhibitor of the APC/C than Mad2-Cdc20 alone [236]. Moreover, within the kinetochore, Mps1 also phosphorylates an array of Met-Glu-Leu-Thr (MELT) motifs of kinetochore associated protein KNL-1, which acts as the recruitment site for Bub3:Bub1 and Bub3:BubR1 complex [238, 239]. The Cdc20 protein of the MCC, is one of the two identified co-activators of the APC/C. This E3 ubiquitin ligase degrades two vital regulators of mitosis, namely securin and cyclin B, by 26S proteasome leading to anaphase onset [236]. The MCC generated on unattached kinetochores prevents Cdc20 activation of APC/C, thereby prolonging expression of cyclin B. As discussed previously, cyclin B is the key regulatory factor of CDK1 and its expression is vital for maintaining normal cell cycle progression during mitosis. Spindle assembly checkpoint also prevents ubiquitination of securin by inhibiting Cdc20 activity. Securin binds to and stochiometrically inhibits a protease known as separase. Separase is required to cleave cohesin, the molecular glue that holds sister chromatids together, thus allowing chromatids to be pulled to opposite poles [240]. Hence by repressing Cdc20 activity, the SAC postpones prometaphase until all chromosomes are accurately oriented on the metaphase plate between separate spindle poles. The chromosome bi-orientation finally switches off the checkpoint, relieving mitotic arrest. Mad1/Mad2 and BubR1 are transported away from the kinetochore along microtubules by dynein, thereby preventing further inhibitory signaling [241]. In mammalian cells, the binding of microtubules to centrosome-associated protein E downregulates BubR1 kinase activity, resulting in checkpoint silencing, and finally, phosphorylation of Mad2 disrupts MCC formation [242, 243]. Degraded MCC results in an upregulation of Cdc20 activities, which becomes free to activate the APC/C complex. This ligase complex now targets securin and cyclin B for further degradation, thus leading to sister-chromatid separation and promoting mitotic exit.

3.4.2.1   Spindle Assembly Checkpoint: Aneuploidy and Cancer

A dysregulated spindle assembly checkpoint is the key source of aneuploidy-related tumorigenesis. Improper mitosis promotes chromosomal instability (CIN) by gain or loss of chromosomes. This gives rise to an aneuploid progeny, a common feature of solid tumor and becomes the precursor cells of tumors [244]. In primary head and neck squamous cell cancer tissues, a significant higher expression of Cdc20 is observed at the transcription level [245]. The expression of another essential mitotic complex gene, MAD1, has been identified as a cellular target of the human T-cell leukemia virus type 1 oncoprotein Tax [246]. Mitotic checkpoint defects have also been found frequently in human colorectal and lung carcinomas [247]. Although MAD2 gene mutations are quite rare in human cancers, lowered expression of the Mad2 protein has been correlated with defective spindle checkpoint function and CIN in breast cancer [248, 249]. Moreover, silencing of the MAD2 promoter activity has been implicated in human liver carcinogenesis [250].

3.5 CONCLUSION

Cell cycle is thus a highly complex process, which requires a tight coordination of various mechanisms that control different stages of DNA synthesis, replication, and segregation into daughter cells. This chapter has detailed the concerted and sequential activities of cyclins, CDKs, and various interdependent signal transduction pathways in maintaining the integrity and progression of cell cycle in normal cells. Concurrently, it highlights the susceptibility of cells to DNA damage by alteration in any component of cell division machinery.

3.6 SUMMARY

- Normal cell cycle progression is maintained and continuously monitored by an intricate network of signal transduction pathways comprising cyclins, CDKs, CKIs, and several checkpoint gene products.
- Deregulation associated with synthesis, amplification, or mutation of cell cycle regulator proteins, tumor suppressors, and transcription factors is reported in a wide variety of human cancers. Therefore, loss of cell cycle checkpoint control is one of the principle causes of genetic instability that lead to malignancies.
- Thus, elucidating novel molecular mechanisms in cell cycle progression and checkpoint control can not only help in early detection of cancers and serve as prognostic markers but may also aid in predicting cancer susceptibility.
- Better characterization of known defects of pivotal checkpoint genes may help to reconstruct altered DNA damage responses aiding in designing targeted cancer therapeutic strategies. One such example is the cyclin-dependent kinase inhibitors. These low-molecular-weight units constitute attractive pharmacological targets for silencing or disrupting kinase hyperactivity in human cancers.
- Finally, because most of the components of human cell progression and control pathways play an equally essential role in other physiological processes like transcription, differentiation, neuronal, immunological response, and senescence, effective therapeutic strategies involving these pathways would promote better health outcomes.

KEYWORDS

- **cancer**
- **cell cycle**
- **cell cycle checkpoints**
- **cyclin**
- **DNA damage**

REFERENCES

1. Dubrovsky, J. G., & Ivanov, V. B., (2003). Celebrating 50 years of the cell cycle. *Nature, 426*(6968), 759.
2. Malumbres, M., & Barbacid, M., (2009). Cell cycle, CDKs and cancer: a changing paradigm. *Nat. Rev. Cancer, 9*(3), 153–166.
3. Barnum, K. J., & O'Connell, M. J., (2014). Cell cycle regulation by checkpoints. *Methods Mol Biol., 1170,* 29–40.
4. Alao, J. P., (2007). The regulation of cyclin D1 degradation: roles in cancer development and the potential for therapeutic invention. *Mol Cancer, 6,* 24.
5. Nishitani, H., Shiomi, Y., Iida, H., Michishita, M., Takami, T., & Tsurimoto, T., (2008). CDK inhibitor p21 is degraded by a proliferating cell nuclear antigen-coupled Cul4-DDB1Cdt2 pathway during S phase and after UV irradiation. *J. Biol. Chem., 283*(43), 29045–29052.
6. Sherr, C. J., Beach, D., & Shapiro, G. I., (2016). Targeting CDK4 and CDK6: From discovery to therapy. *Cancer Disco., 6*(4), 353–367.
7. Sengupta, S., & Henry, R. W., (2015). Regulation of the retinoblastoma-E2F pathway by the ubiquitin-proteasome system. *Biochim. Biophys. Acta., 1849*(10), 1289–1297.
8. Trimarchi, J. M., & Lees, J. A., (2002). Sibling rivalry in the E2F family. *Nat. Rev. Mol Cell Biol., 3*(1), 11–20.
9. Boonstra, J., (2003). Progression through the G1-phase of the on-going cell cycle. *J. Cell Biochem., 90*(2), 244–252.
10. Giacinti, C., & Giordano, A., (2006). RB and cell cycle progression. *Oncogene, 25*(38), 5220–5227.
11. Cooley, A., Zelivianski, S., & Jeruss, J. S., (2010). Impact of cyclin E overexpression on Smad3 activity in breast cancer cell lines. *Cell Cycle, 9*(24), 4900–4907.
12. Morris, L., Allen, K. E., & La Thangue, N. B., (2000). Regulation of E2F transcription by cyclin E-Cdk2 kinase mediated through p300/CBP co-activators. *Nat. Cell Biol., 2*(4), 232–239.
13. Chen, Z., Indjeian, V. B., McManus, M., Wang, L., & Dynlacht, B. D., (2002). CP110, a cell cycle-dependent CDK substrate, regulates centrosome duplication in human cells. *Dev. Cell, 3*(3), 339–350.

14. Huang, H., Regan, K. M., Lou, Z., Chen, J., & Tindall, D. J., (2006). CDK2-dependent phosphorylation of FOXO1 as an apoptotic response to DNA damage. *Science*, *314*(5797), 294–297.

15. Hitomi, M., Yang, K., Guo, Y., Fretthold, J., Harwalkar, J., & Stacey, D. W., (2006). p27Kip1 and cyclin dependent kinase 2 regulate passage through the restriction point. *Cell Cycle*, *5*(19), 2281–2289.

16. Morris, M. C., Gondeau, C., Tainer, J. A., & Divita, G., (2002). Kinetic mechanism of activation of the Cdk2/cyclin A complex. Key role of the C-lobe of the Cdk. *J. Biol. Chem.*, *277*(26), 23847–23853.

17. De Boer, L., Oakes, V., Beamish, H., Giles, N., Stevens, F., Somodevilla-Torres, M., Desouza, C., & Gabrielli, B., (2008). Cyclin A/cdk2 coordinates centrosomal and nuclear mitotic events. *Oncogene*, *27*(31), 4261–4268.

18. Doree, M., & Hunt, T., (2002). From Cdc2 to Cdk1: when did the cell cycle kinase join its cyclin partner? *J. Cell Sci.*, *115*(12), 2461–2464.

19. Bashir, T., & Pagano, M., (2005). Cdk1: the dominant sibling of Cdk2. *Nat. Cell Biol.*, *7*(8), 779–781.

20. Baus, F., Gire, V., Fisher, D., Piette, J., & Dulic, V., (2003). Permanent cell cycle exit in G2 phase after DNA damage in normal human fibroblasts. *EMBO J.*, *22*(15), 3992–4002.

21. Goldstone, S., Pavey, S., Forrest, A., Sinnamon, J., & Gabrielli, B., (2001). Cdc25-dependent activation of cyclin A/cdk2 is blocked in G2 phase arrested cells independently of ATM/ATR. *Oncogene*, *20*(8), 921–932.

22. Hannenhalli, S., & Kaestner, K. H., (2009). The evolution of fox genes and their role in development and disease. *Nat. Rev. Genet.*, *10*(4), 233–240.

23. Laoukili, J., Kooistra, M. R., Bras, A., Kauw, J., Kerkhoven, R. M., Morrison, A., Clevers, H., & Medema, R. H., (2005). FoxM1 is required for execution of the mitotic programme and chromosome stability. *Nat. Cell Biol.*, *7*(2), 126–136.

24. Sadasivam, S., Duan, S., & De Caprio, J. A., (2012). The MuvB complex sequentially recruits B-Myb and FoxM1 to promote mitotic gene expression. *Genes Dev.*, *26*(5), 474–489.

25. Alvarez-Fernandez, M., Halim, V. A., Aprelia, M., Laoukili, J., Mohammed, S., & Medema, R. H., (2011). Protein phosphatase 2A (B55alpha) prevents premature activation of forkhead transcription factor FoxM1 by antagonizing cyclin A/cyclin-dependent kinase-mediated phosphorylation. *J. Biol. Chem.*, *286*(38), 33029–33036.

26. Mitra, J., & Enders, G. H., (2004). Cyclin A/Cdk2 complexes regulate activation of Cdk1 and Cdc25 phosphatases in human cells. *Oncogene*, *23*(19), 3361–3367.

27. Roshak, A. K., Capper, E. A., Imburgia, C., Fornwald, J., Scott, G., & Marshall, L. A., (2000). The human polo-like kinase, PLK, regulates cdc2/cyclin B through phosphorylation and activation of the cdc25C phosphatase. *Cell Signal*, *12*(6), 405–411.

28. Seki, A., Coppinger, J. A., Jang, C. Y., Yates, J. R., & Fang, G., (2008). Bora and the kinase Aurora a cooperatively activate the kinase Plk1 and control mitotic entry. *Science*, *320*(5883), 1655–1658.

29. Lindqvist, A., Rodriguez-Bravo, V., & Medema, R. H., (2009). The decision to enter mitosis: feedback and redundancy in the mitotic entry network. *J. Cell Biol.*, *185*(2), 193–202.

30. Nigg, E. A., (2001). Mitotic kinases as regulators of cell division and its checkpoints. *Nat. Rev. Mol Cell Biol.*, *2*(1), 21–32.

31. Takizawa, C. G., & Morgan, D. O., (2000). Control of mitosis by changes in the subcellular location of cyclin-B1-Cdk1 and Cdc25C. *Curr. Opin. Cell Biol., 12*(6), 658–665.

32. Fung, T. K., & Poon, R. Y., (2005). A roller coaster ride with the mitotic cyclins. *Semin. Cell Dev. Biol., 16*(3), 335–342.

33. Yu, H., (2007). Cdc20: a WD40 activator for a cell cycle degradation machine. *Mol Cell., 27*(1), 3–16.

34. Lim, S., & Kaldis, P., (2013). Cdks, cyclins and CKIs: roles beyond cell cycle regulation. *Development, 140*(15), 3079–3093.

35. Satyanarayana, A., & Kaldis, P., (2009). Mammalian cell-cycle regulation: several Cdks, numerous cyclins and diverse compensatory mechanisms. *Oncogene, 28*(33), 2925–2939.

36. Zelivianski, S., Cooley, A., Kall, R., & Jeruss, J. S., (2010). Cyclin-dependent kinase 4-mediated phosphorylation inhibits Smad3 activity in cyclin D-overexpressing breast cancer cells. *Mol Cancer Res., 8*(10), 1375–1387.

37. Chambard, J. C., Lefloch, R., Pouyssegur, J., & Lenormand, P., (2007). ERK implication in cell cycle regulation. *Biochim. Biophys. Acta, 1773*(8), 1299–1310.

38. Fu, M., Wang, C., Li, Z., Sakamaki, T., & Pestell, R. G., (2004). Minireview: Cyclin D1: normal and abnormal functions. *Endocrinology, 145*(12), 5439–5447.

39. Takahashi-Yanaga, F., & Sasaguri, T., (2008). GSK-3beta regulates cyclin D1 expression: a new target for chemotherapy. *Cell Signal, 20*(4), 581–589.

40. Alt, J. R., Cleveland, J. L., Hannink, M., & Diehl, J. A., (2000). Phosphorylation-dependent regulation of cyclin D1 nuclear export and cyclin D1-dependent cellular transformation. *Genes Dev., 14*(24), 3102–3114.

41. Bahnassy, A. A., Zekri, A. R., El-Houssini, S., El-Shehaby, A. M., Mahmoud, M. R., Abdallah, S., & El-Serafi, M., (2004). Cyclin A and cyclin D1 as significant prognostic markers in colorectal cancer patients. *BMC Gastroenterol, 4*, 22.

42. Diehl, J. A., (2002). Cycling to cancer with cyclin D1. *Cancer Biol. Ther., 1*(3), 226–231.

43. Aquino, G., Franco, R., Ronconi, F., Anniciello, A., Russo, L., De Chiara, A., & Panico, L., (2012). Peripheral T-cell lymphoma with cyclin D1 overexpression: A case report. *Diagn. Pathol., 7*, 79.

44. Mohammadizadeh, F., Hani, M., Ranaee, M., & Bagheri, M., (2013). Role of cyclin D1 in breast carcinoma. *J. Res. Med. Sci., 18*(12), 1021–1025.

45. Tashiro, E., Tsuchiya, A., & Imoto, M., (2007). Functions of cyclin D1 as an oncogene and regulation of cyclin D1 expression. *Cancer Sci., 98*(5), 629–635.

46. Stamatakos, M., Palla, V., Karaiskos, I., Xiromeritis, K., Alexiou, I., Pateras, I., & Kontzoglou, K., (2010). Cell cyclins: triggering elements of cancer or not? *World J. Surg. Oncol., 8*, 111.

47. Kawano, M., Tanaka, K., Itonaga, I., Iwasaki, T., & Tsumura, H., (2015). c-Myc represses tumor-suppressive microRNAs, let-7a, miR-16 and miR-29b, & induces cyclin D2-mediated cell proliferation in ewing's sarcoma cell line. *PLoS One, 10*(9), e0138560.

48. Deshpande, A., Sicinski, P., & Hinds, P. W., (2005). Cyclins and cdks in development and cancer: A perspective. *Oncogene, 24*(17), 2909–2915.

49. Sawai, C. M., Freund, J., Oh, P., Ndiaye-Lobry, D., Bretz, J. C., Strikoudis, A., Genesca, L., Trimarchi, T., Kelliher, M. A., Clark, M., Soulier, J., Chen-Kiang, S., & Aifantis, I., (2012). Therapeutic targeting of the cyclin D3:CDK4/6 complex in T cell leukemia. *Cancer Cell, 22*(4), 452–465.

50. Hwang, H. C., & Clurman, B. E., (2005). Cyclin E in normal and neoplastic cell cycles. *Oncogene, 24*(17), 2776–2786.
51. Sherr, C. J., & Mc-Cormick, F., (2002). The RB and p53 pathways in cancer. *Cancer Cell, 2*(2), 103–112.
52. Siu, K. T., Rosner, M. R., & Minella, A. C., (2012). An integrated view of cyclin E function and regulation. *Cell Cycle, 11*(1), 57–64.
53. Bedrosian, I., Lu, K. H., Verschraegen, C., & Keyomarsi, K., (2004). Cyclin E deregulation alters the biologic properties of ovarian cancer cells. *Oncogene, 23*(15), 2648–2657.
54. Li, J. Q., Miki, H., Ohmori, M., Wu, F., & Funamoto, Y., (2001). Expression of cyclin E and cyclin-dependent kinase 2 correlates with metastasis and prognosis in colorectal carcinoma. *Hum. Pathol., 32*(9), 945–953.
55. Schraml, P., Schwerdtfeger, G., Burkhalter, F., Raggi, A., Schmidt, D., Ruffalo, T., King, W., Wilber, K., Mihatsch, M. J., & Moch, H., (2003). Combined array comparative genomic hybridization and tissue microarray analysis suggest PAK1 at 11q13. 5-q14 as a critical oncogene target in ovarian carcinoma. *Am. J. Pathol., 163*(3), 985–992.
56. Bales, E., Mills, L., Milam, N., McGahren-Murray, M., Bandyopadhyay, D., Chen, D., Reed, J. A., Timchenko, N., Van den Oord, J. J., Bar-Eli, M., Keyomarsi, K., & Medrano, E. E., (2005). The low molecular weight cyclin E isoforms augment angiogenesis and metastasis of human melanoma cells in vivo. *Cancer Res., 65*(3), 692–697.
57. Yam, C. H., Fung, T. K., & Poon, R. Y., (2002). Cyclin A in cell cycle control and cancer. *Cell Mol Life Sci., 59*(8), 1317–1326.
58. Ohashi, R., Gao, C., Miyazaki, M., Hamazaki, K., Tsuji, T., Inoue, Y., Uemura, T., Hirai, R., Shimizu, N., & Namba, M., (2001). Enhanced expression of cyclin E and cyclin A in human hepatocellular carcinomas. *Anticancer Res., 21*(1B), 657–662.
59. Florenes, V. A., Maelandsmo, G. M., Faye, R., Nesland, J. M., & Holm, R., (2001). Cyclin A expression in superficial spreading malignant melanomas correlates with clinical outcome. *J. Pathol., 195*(5), 530–536.
60. Sherr, C. J., (2000). Cell cycle control and cancer. *Harvey Lect., 96*, 73–92.
61. Allan, K., Jordan, R. C., Ang, L. C., Taylor, M., & Young, B., (2000). Overexpression of cyclin A and cyclin B1 proteins in astrocytomas. *Arch. Pathol. Lab. Med., 124*(2), 216–220.
62. Bukholm, I. R., Bukholm, G., & Nesland, J. M., (2001). Over-expression of cyclin A is highly associated with early relapse and reduced survival in patients with primary breast carcinomas. *Int. J. Cancer, 93*(2), 283–287.
63. Bukholm, I. R., Bukholm, G., & Nesland, J. M., (2001). Coexpression of cyclin A and beta-catenin and survival in breast cancer patients. *Int. J. Cancer, 94*(1), 148–149.
64. Chen, Q., Zhang, X., Jiang, Q., Clarke, P. R., & Zhang, C., (2008). Cyclin B1 is localized to unattached kinetochores and contributes to efficient microtubule attachment and proper chromosome alignment during mitosis. *Cell Res., 18*(2), 268–280.
65. Bentley, A. M., Normand, G., Hoyt, J., & King, R. W., (2007). Distinct sequence elements of cyclin B1 promote localization to chromatin, centrosomes, & kinetochores during mitosis. *Mol Biol. Cell., 18*(12), 4847–4858.
66. Nguyen, T. B., Manova, K., Capodieci, P., Lindon, C., Bottega, S., Wang, X. Y., Refik-Rogers, J., Pines, J., Wolgemuth, D. J., & Koff, A., (2002). Characterization and expression of mammalian cyclin b3, a prepachytene meiotic cyclin. *J. Biol. Chem., 277*(44), 41960–41969.

67. Igarashi, T., Jiang, S. X., Kameya, T., Asamura, H., Sato, Y., Nagai, K., & Okayasu, I., (2004). Divergent cyclin B1 expression and Rb/p16/cyclin D1 pathway aberrations among pulmonary neuroendocrine tumors. *Mod. Pathol., 17*(10), 1259–1267.

68. Hassan, K. A., Ang, K. K., El-Naggar, A. K., Story, M. D., Lee, J. I., Liu, D., Hong, W. K., & Mao, L., (2002). Cyclin B1 overexpression and resistance to radiotherapy in head and neck squamous cell carcinoma. *Cancer Res., 62*(22), 6414–6417.

69. Singhal, S., Vachani, A., Antin-Ozerkis, D., Kaiser, L. R., & Albelda, S. M., (2005). Prognostic implications of cell cycle, apoptosis, & angiogenesis biomarkers in non-small cell lung cancer: A review. *Clin. Cancer Res., 11*(11), 3974–3986.

70. Arinaga, M., Noguchi, T., Takeno, S., Chujo, M., Miura, T., Kimura, Y., & Uchida, Y., (2003). Clinical implication of cyclin B1 in non-small cell lung cancer. *Oncol. Rep., 10*(5), 1381–1386.

71. Soria, J. C., Jang, S. J., Khuri, F. R., Hassan, K., Liu, D., Hong, W. K., & Mao, L., (2000). Overexpression of cyclin B1 in early-stage non-small cell lung cancer and its clinical implication. *Cancer Res., 60*(15), 4000–4004.

72. Suzuki, T., Urano, T., Miki, Y., Moriya, T., Akahira, J., Ishida, T., Horie, K., Inoue, S., & Sasano, H., (2007). Nuclear cyclin B1 in human breast carcinoma as a potent prognostic factor. *Cancer Sci., 98*(5), 644–651.

73. Zhao, M., Kim, Y. T., Yoon, B. S., Kim, S. W., Kang, M. H., Kim, S. H., Kim, J. H., Kim, J. W., & Park, Y. W., (2006). Expression profiling of cyclin B1 and D1 in cervical carcinoma. *Exp. Oncol., 28*(1), 44–48.

74. Roh, M., Song, C., Kim, J., & Abdulkadir, S. A., (2005). Chromosomal instability induced by Pim-1 is passage-dependent and associated with dysregulation of cyclin B1. *J. Biol. Chem., 280*(49), 40568–40577.

75. Rasmussen, L. J., Rasmussen, M., Lutzen, A., Bisgaard, H. C., & Singh, K. K., (2000). The human cyclin B1 protein modulates sensitivity of DNA mismatch repair deficient prostate cancer cell lines to alkylating agents. *Exp. Cell Res., 257*(1), 127–134.

76. Ikuerowo, S. O., Kuczyk, M. A., Mengel, M., Van der Heyde, E., Shittu, O. B., Vaske, B., Jonas, U., Machtens, S., & Serth, J., (2006). Alteration of subcellular and cellular expression patterns of cyclin B1 in renal cell carcinoma is significantly related to clinical progression and survival of patients. *Int. J. Cancer, 119*(4), 867–874.

77. Fang, Y., Yu, H., Liang, X., Xu, J., & Cai, X., (2014). Chk1-induced CCNB1 overexpression promotes cell proliferation and tumor growth in human colorectal cancer. *Cancer Biol. Ther., 15*(9), 1268–1279.

78. Fang, Y., Liang, X., Jiang, W., Li, J., Xu, J., & Cai, X., (2015). Cyclin b1 suppresses colorectal cancer invasion and metastasis by regulating e-cadherin. *PLoS One, 10*(5), e0126875.

79. Scott, I. S., Morris, L. S., Rushbrook, S. M., Bird, K., Vowler, S. L., Burnet, N. G., & Coleman, N., (2005). Immunohistochemical estimation of cell cycle entry and phase distribution in astrocytomas: applications in diagnostic neuropathology. *Neuropathol. Appl. Neurobiol., 31*(5), 455–466.

80. Holtkamp, N., Afanasieva, A., Elstner, A., Van Landeghem, F. K., Konneker, M., Kuhn, S. A., Kettenmann, H., & Von Deimling, A., (2005). Brain slice invasion model reveals genes differentially regulated in glioma invasion. *Biochem. Biophys. Res. Commun., 336*(4), 1227–1233.

81. Chen, H., Huang, Q., Dong, J., Zhai, D. Z., Wang, A. D., & Lan, Q., (2008). Overexpression of CDC2/CyclinB1 in gliomas, & CDC2 depletion inhibits proliferation of human glioma cells in vitro and in vivo. *BMC Cancer, 8*, 29.

82. De Haas, T., Hasselt, N., Troost, D., Caron, H., Popovic, M., Zadravec-Zaletel, L., Grajkowska, W., Perek, M., Osterheld, M. C., Ellison, D., Baas, F., Versteeg, R., & Kool, M., (2008). Molecular risk stratification of medulloblastoma patients based on immunohistochemical analysis of MYC, LDHB, & CCNB1 expression. *Clin. Cancer Res.*, *14*(13), 4154–4160.

83. Obermann, E. C., Went, P., Pehrs, A. C., Tzankov, A., Wild, P. J., Pileri, S., Hofstaedter, F., & Dirnhofer, S., (2005). Cyclin B1 expression is an independent prognostic marker for poor outcome in diffuse large B-cell lymphoma. *Oncol Rep.*, *14*(6), 1461–1467.

84. Bjorck, E., Ek, S., Landgren, O., Jerkeman, M., Ehinger, M., Bjorkholm, M., Borrebaeck, C. A., Porwit-MacDonald, A., & Nordenskjold, M., (2005). High expression of cyclin B1 predicts a favorable outcome in patients with follicular lymphoma. *Blood*, *105*(7), 2908–2915.

85. Yasuda, M., Takesue, F., Inutsuka, S., Honda, M., Nozoe, T., & Korenaga, D., (2002). Overexpression of cyclin B1 in gastric cancer and its clinicopathological significance: An immunohistological study. *J. Cancer Res. Clin. Oncol.*, *128*(8), 412–416.

86. Kim, D. H., (2007). Prognostic implications of cyclin B1, p34cdc2, p27(Kip1) and p53 expression in gastric cancer. *Yonsei Med. J.*, *48*(4), 694–700.

87. Hartwell, L. H., (2002). Nobel Lecture. Yeast and cancer. *Biosci. Rep.*, *22*(3–4), 373–394.

88. Hunt, T., (2002). Nobel Lecture. Protein synthesis, proteolysis, & cell cycle transitions. *Biosci Rep.*, *22* (5–6), 465–486.

89. Nebreda, A. R., (2006). CDK activation by non-cyclin proteins. *Curr. Opin. Cell Biol.*, *18*(2), 192–198.

90. Mouron, S., De Carcer, G., Seco, E., Fernandez-Miranda, G., Malumbres, M., & Nebreda, A. R., (2010). RINGO C is required to sustain the spindle-assembly checkpoint. *J. Cell Sci.*, *123*(15), 2586–2595.

91. Lolli, G., & Johnson, L. N., (2005). CAK-Cyclin-dependent Activating Kinase: a key kinase in cell cycle control and a target for drugs? *Cell Cycle*, *4*(4), 572–577.

92. Malumbres, M., Harlow, E., Hunt, T., Hunter, T., Lahti, J. M., Manning, G., Morgan, D. O., Tsai, L. H., & Wolgemuth, D. J., (2009). Cyclin-dependent kinases: a family portrait. *Nat. Cell Biol.*, *11*(11), 1275–1276.

93. Santamaria, D., Barriere, C., Cerqueira, A., Hunt, S., Tardy, C., Newton, K., Caceres, J. F., Dubus, P., Malumbres, M., & Barbacid, M., (2007). Cdk1 is sufficient to drive the mammalian cell cycle. *Nature*, *448*(7155), 811–815.

94. Bendris, N., Lemmers, B., & Blanchard, J. M., (2015). Cell cycle, cytoskeleton dynamics and beyond: the many functions of cyclins and CDK inhibitors. *Cell Cycle*, *14*(12), 1786–1798.

95. Knockaert, M., Greengard, P., & Meijer, L., (2002). Pharmacological inhibitors of cyclin-dependent kinases. *Trends Pharmacol. Sci.*, *23*(9), 417–425.

96. Brown, N. R., Korolchuk, S., Martin, M. P., Stanley, W. A., Moukhametzianov, R., Noble, M. E., & Endicott, J. A., (2015). CDK1 structures reveal conserved and unique features of the essential cell cycle CDK. *Nat. Commun.*, *6*, 6769.

97. Ito, Y., Takeda, T., Wakasa, K., Tsujimoto, M., Okada, M., & Matsuura, N., (2002). Expression of the G2-M modulators in pancreatic adenocarcinoma. *Pancreatology*, *2*(2), 138–145.

98. Zhao, M. Y., Auerbach, A., D'Costa, A. M., Rapoport, A. P., Burger, A. M., Sausville, E. A., Stass, S. A., Jiang, F., Sands, A. M., Aguilera, N., & Zhao, X. F., (2009). Phospho-

p70S6K/p85S6K and cdc2/cdk1 are novel targets for diffuse large B-cell lymphoma combination therapy. *Clin. Cancer Res.*, *15*(5), 1708–1720.

99. Abdullah, C., Wang, X., & Becker, D., (2011). Expression analysis and molecular targeting of cyclin-dependent kinases in advanced melanoma. *Cell Cycle*, *10*(6), 977–988.

100. Zhang, C., Elkahloun, A. G., Robertson, M., Gills, J. J., Tsurutani, J., Shih, J. H., Fukuoka, J., Hollander, M. C., Harris, C. C., Travis, W. D., Jen, J., & Dennis, P. A., (2011). Loss of cytoplasmic CDK1 predicts poor survival in human lung cancer and confers chemotherapeutic resistance. *PLoS One*, *6*(8), e23849.

101. Luciani, M. G., Hutchins, J. R., Zheleva, D., & Hupp, T. R., (2000). The C-terminal regulatory domain of p53 contains a functional docking site for cyclin A. *J. Mol Biol.*, *300*(3), 503–518.

102. Garrett, S., Barton, W. A., Knights, R., Jin, P., Morgan, D. O., & Fisher, R. P., (2001). Reciprocal activation by cyclin-dependent kinases 2 and 7 is directed by substrate specificity determinants outside the T loop. *Mol Cell Biol.*, *21*(1), 88–99.

103. Neganova, I., Vilella, F., Atkinson, S. P., Lloret, M., Passos, J. F., Von Zglinicki, T., O'Connor, J. E., Burks, D., Jones, R., Armstrong, L., & Lako, M., (2011). An important role for CDK2 in G1 to S checkpoint activation and DNA damage response in human embryonic stem cells. *Stem Cells*, *29*(4), 651–659.

104. Hydbring, P., & Larsson, L. G., (2010). Tipping the balance: Cdk2 enables Myc to suppress senescence. *Cancer Res.*, *70*(17), 6687–6691.

105. Liu, J. L., Ma, H. P., Lu, X. L., Sun, S. H., Guo, X., & Li, F. C., (2011). NF-kappaB induces abnormal centrosome amplification by upregulation of CDK2 in laryngeal squamous cell cancer. *Int. J. Oncol.*, *39*(4), 915–924.

106. Peyressatre, M., Prevel, C., Pellerano, M., & Morris, M. C., (2015). Targeting cyclin-dependent kinases in human cancers: from small molecules to Peptide inhibitors. *Cancers (Basel)*, *7*(1), 179–237.

107. Malumbres, M., & Barbacid, M., (2005). Mammalian cyclin-dependent kinases. *Trends Biochem Sci.*, *30*(11), 630–641.

108. Ren, S., & Rollins, B. J., (2004). Cyclin C/cdk3 promotes Rb-dependent G0 exit. *Cell*, *117*(2), 239–251.

109. Keezer, S. M., & Gilbert, D. M., (2002). Evidence for a pre-restriction point Cdk3 activity. *J. Cell Biochem.*, *85*(3), 545–552.

110. Lu, J., Zhang, Z. L., Huang, D., Tang, N., Li, Y., Peng, Z., Lu, C., Dong, Z., & Tang, F., (2016). Cdk3-promoted epithelial-mesenchymal transition through activating AP-1 is involved in colorectal cancer metastasis. *Oncotarget*, *7*(6), 7012–7028.

111. Schang, L. M., Bantly, A., & Schaffer, P. A., (2002). Explant-induced reactivation of herpes simplex virus occurs in neurons expressing nuclear cdk2 and cdk4. *J. Virol*, *76*(15), 7724–7735.

112. Zheng, D., Cho, Y. Y., Lau, A. T., Zhang, J., Ma, W. Y., Bode, A. M., & Dong, Z., (2008). Cyclin-dependent kinase 3-mediated activating transcription factor 1 phosphorylation enhances cell transformation. *Cancer Res.*, *68*(18), 7650–7660.

113. Du, J., Widlund, H. R., Horstmann, M. A., Ramaswamy, S., Ross, K., Huber, W. E., Nishimura, E. K., Golub, T. R., & Fisher, D. E., (2004). Critical role of CDK2 for melanoma growth linked to its melanocyte-specific transcriptional regulation by MITF. *Cancer Cell*, *6*(6), 565–576.

114. Wang, L., Hu, H. Y., Lin, Y. L., Zhao, Z. X., Tan, L., Yu, P., Wan, H. J., Jin, Z., & Zheng, D., (2014). CDK3 expression and its clinical significance in human nasopharyngeal carcinoma. *Mol Med. Rep.*, *9*(6), 2582–2586.

115. Rane, S. G., Cosenza, S. C., Mettus, R. V., & Reddy, E. P., (2002). Germ line transmission of the Cdk4(R24C) mutation facilitates tumorigenesis and escape from cellular senescence. *Mol Cell Biol.*, *22*(2), 644–656.

116. Chawla, R., Procknow, J. A., Tantravahi, R. V., Khurana, J. S., Litvin, J., & Reddy, E. P., (2010). Cooperativity of Cdk4R24C and Ras in melanoma development. *Cell Cycle*, *9*(16), 3305–3314.

117. Puyol, M., Martin, A., Dubus, P., Mulero, F., Pizcueta, P., Khan, G., Guerra, C., Santamaria, D., & Barbacid, M., (2010). A synthetic lethal interaction between K-Ras oncogenes and Cdk4 unveils a therapeutic strategy for non-small cell lung carcinoma. *Cancer Cell*, *18*(1), 63–73.

118. Sotillo, R., Renner, O., Dubus, P., Ruiz-Cabello, J., Martin-Caballero, J., Barbacid, M., Carnero, A., & Malumbres, M., (2005). Cooperation between Cdk4 and p27kip1 in tumor development: a preclinical model to evaluate cell cycle inhibitors with therapeutic activity. *Cancer Res.*, *65*(9), 3846–3852.

119. Borg, A., Sandberg, T., Nilsson, K., Johannsson, O., Klinker, M., Masback, A., Westerdahl, J., Olsson, H., & Ingvar, C., (2000). High frequency of multiple melanomas and breast and pancreas carcinomas in CDKN2A mutation-positive melanoma families. *J. Natl. Cancer Inst.*, *92*(15), 1260–1266.

120. Park, S., Lee, J., Do, I. G., Jang, J., Rho, K., Ahn, S., Maruja, L., Kim, S. J., Kim, K. M., Mao, M., Oh, E., Kim, Y. J., Kim, J., & Choi, Y. L., (2014). Aberrant CDK4 amplification in refractory rhabdomyosarcoma as identified by genomic profiling. *Sci. Rep.*, *4*, 3623.

121. Yoshida, A., Ushiku, T., Motoi, T., Beppu, Y., Fukayama, M., Tsuda, H., & Shibata, T., (2012). MDM2 and CDK4 immunohistochemical coexpression in high-grade osteosarcoma: correlation with a dedifferentiated subtype. *Am. J. Surg. Pathol.*, *36*(3), 423–431.

122. Dei Tos, A. P., Doglioni, C., Piccinin, S., Sciot, R., Furlanetto, A., Boiocchi, M., Dal Cin, P., Maestro, R., Fletcher, C. D., & Tallini, G., (2000). Coordinated expression and amplification of the MDM2, CDK4, & HMGI-C genes in atypical lipomatous tumours. *J. Pathol.*, *190*(5), 531–536.

123. Michaud, K., Solomon, D. A., Oermann, E., Kim, J. S., Zhong, W. Z., Prados, M. D., Ozawa, T., James, C. D., & Waldman, T., (2010). Pharmacologic inhibition of cyclin-dependent kinases 4 and 6 arrests the growth of glioblastoma multiforme intracranial xenografts. *Cancer Res.*, *70*(8), 3228–3238.

124. Su, W. T., Alaminos, M., Mora, J., Cheung, N. K., La Quaglia, M. P., & Gerald, W. L., (2004). Positional gene expression analysis identifies 12q overexpression and amplification in a subset of neuroblastomas. *Cancer Genet. Cytogenet.*, *154*(2), 131–137.

125. Sheppard, K. E., & McArthur, G. A., (2013). The cell-cycle regulator CDK4: an emerging therapeutic target in melanoma. *Clin. Cancer Res.*, *19*(19), 5320–5328.

126. Dobashi, Y., Goto, A., Fukayama, M., Abe, A., & Ooi, A., (2004). Overexpression of cdk4/cyclin D1, a possible mediator of apoptosis and an indicator of prognosis in human primary lung carcinoma. *Int. J. Cancer*, *110*(4), 532–541.

127. Dhavan, R., & Tsai, L. H., (2001). A decade of CDK5. *Nat. Rev. Mol Cell Biol.*, *2*(10), 749–759.

128. Shah, K., & Lahiri, D. K., (2014). Cdk5 activity in the brain - multiple paths of regulation. *J. Cell Sci.*, *127*(11), 2391–2400.

129. Su, S. C., & Tsai, L. H., (2011). Cyclin-dependent kinases in brain development and disease. *Annu. Rev. Cell Dev. Biol.*, *27*, 465–491.

130. Cheung, Z. H., & Ip, N. Y., (2012). Cdk5: a multifaceted kinase in neurodegenerative diseases. *Trends Cell Biol.*, *22*(3), 169–175.
131. Smith, P. D., Crocker, S. J., Jackson-Lewis, V., Jordan-Sciutto, K. L., Hayley, S., Mount, M. P., O'Hare, M. J., Callaghan, S., Slack, R. S., Przedborski, S., Anisman, H., & Park, D. S., (2003). Cyclin-dependent kinase 5 is a mediator of dopaminergic neuron loss in a mouse model of Parkinson's disease. *Proc. Natl. Acad. Sci. USA.*, *100*(23), 13650–13655.
132. Catania, A., Urban, S., Yan, E., Hao, C., Barron, G., & Allalunis-Turner, J., (2001). Expression and localization of cyclin-dependent kinase 5 in apoptotic human glioma cells. *Neuro Oncol.*, *3*(2), 89–98.
133. Liu, J. L., Wang, X. Y., Huang, B. X., Zhu, F., Zhang, R. G., & Wu, G., (2011). Expression of CDK5/p35 in resected patients with non-small cell lung cancer: Relation to prognosis. *Med. Oncol.*, *28*(3), 673–678.
134. Eggers, J. P., Grandgenett, P. M., Collisson, E. C., Lewallen, M. E., Tremayne, J., Singh, P. K., Swanson, B. J., Andersen, J. M., Caffrey, T. C., High, R. R., Ouellette, M., & Hollingsworth, M. A., (2011). Cyclin-dependent kinase 5 is amplified and overexpressed in pancreatic cancer and activated by mutant K-Ras. *Clin. Cancer Res.*, *17*(19), 6140–6150.
135. Lee, K. H., Lotterman, C., Karikari, C., Omura, N., Feldmann, G., Habbe, N., Goggins, M. G., Mendell, J. T., & Maitra, A., (2009). Epigenetic silencing of MicroRNA miR-107 regulates cyclin-dependent kinase 6 expression in pancreatic cancer. *Pancreatology*, *9*(3), 293–301.
136. Wang, G., Zheng, L., Yu, Z., Liao, G., Lu, L., Xu, R., Zhao, Z., & Chen, G., (2012). Increased cyclin-dependent kinase 6 expression in bladder cancer. *Oncol. Lett.*, *4*(1), 43–46.
137. Tadesse, S., Yu, M., Kumarasiri, M., Le, B. T., & Wang, S., (2015). Targeting CDK6 in cancer: State of the art and new insights. *Cell Cycle*, *14*(20), 3220–3230.
138. Schachter, M. M., & Fisher, R. P., (2013). The CDK-activating kinase Cdk7: taking yes for an answer. *Cell Cycle*, *12*(20), 3239–3240.
139. Chebaro, Y., Amal, I., Rochel, N., Rochette-Egly, C., Stote, R. H., & Dejaegere, A., (2013). Phosphorylation of the retinoic acid receptor alpha induces a mechanical allosteric regulation and changes in internal dynamics. *PLoS Comput. Biol.*, *9*(4), e1003012.
140. Fisher, R. P., (2005). Secrets of a double agent: CDK7 in cell-cycle control and transcription. *J. Cell Sci.*, *118*(22), 5171–5180.
141. Collins, C. S., Hong, J., Sapinoso, L., Zhou, Y., Liu, Z., Micklash, K., Schultz, P. G., & Hampton, G. M., (2006). A small interfering RNA screen for modulators of tumor cell motility identifies MAP4K4 as a promigratory kinase. *Proc. Natl. Acad. Sci. USA*, *103*(10), 3775–3780.
142. Kayaselcuk, F., Erkanli, S., Bolat, F., Seydaoglu, G., Kuscu, E., & Demirhan, B., (2006). Expression of cyclin H in normal and cancerous endometrium, its correlation with other cyclins, & association with clinicopathologic parameters. *Int. J. Gynecol. Cancer*, *16*(1), 402–408.
143. Akoulitchev, S., Chuikov, S., & Reinberg, D., (2000). TFIIH is negatively regulated by cdk8-containing mediator complexes. *Nature*, *407*(6800), 102–106.
144. Firestein, R., Shima, K., Nosho, K., Irahara, N., Baba, Y., Bojarski, E., Giovannucci, E. L., Hahn, W. C., Fuchs, C. S., & Ogino, S., (2010). CDK8 expression in *470* colorectal cancers in relation to beta-catenin activation, other molecular alterations and patient survival. *Int. J. Cancer*, *126*(12), 2863–2873.

145. Seo, J. O., Han, S. I., & Lim, S. C., (2010). Role of CDK8 and beta-catenin in colorectal adenocarcinoma. *Oncol. Rep., 24*(1), 285–291.

146. Kim, M. Y., Han, S. I., & Lim, S. C., (2011). Roles of cyclin-dependent kinase 8 and beta-catenin in the oncogenesis and progression of gastric adenocarcinoma. *Int. J. Oncol., 38*(5), 1375–1383.

147. Kapoor, A., Goldberg, M. S., Cumberland, L. K., Ratnakumar, K., Segura, M. F., Emanuel, P. O., Menendez, S., Vardabasso, C., Leroy, G., Vidal, C. I., Polsky, D., Osman, I., Garcia, B. A., Hernando, E., & Bernstein, E., (2010). The histone variant macroH2A suppresses melanoma progression through regulation of CDK8. *Nature, 468*(7327), 1105–1109.

148. Li, X. Y., Luo, Q. F., Wei, C. K., Li, D. F., & Fang, L., (2014). siRNA-mediated silencing of CDK8 inhibits proliferation and growth in breast cancer cells. *Int. J. Clin. Exp. Pathol., 7*(1), 92–100.

149. Yu, D. S., & Cortez, D., (2011). A role for CDK9-cyclin K in maintaining genome integrity. *Cell Cycle, 10*(1), 28–32.

150. Romano, G., (2013). Deregulations in the cyclin-dependent kinase-9-related pathway in cancer: implications for drug discovery and development. *ISRN Oncol., 2013.* 305371.

151. De Falco, G., Bellan, C., D'Amuri, A., Angeloni, G., Leucci, E., Giordano, A., & Leoncini, L., (2005). Cdk9 regulates neural differentiation and its expression correlates with the differentiation grade of neuroblastoma and PNET tumors. *Cancer Biol. Ther., 4*(3), 277–281.

152. Bellan, C., De Falco, G., Lazzi, S., Micheli, P., Vicidomini, S., Schurfeld, K., Amato, T., Palumbo, A., Bagella, L., Sabattini, E., Bartolommei, S., Hummel, M., Pileri, S., Tosi, P., Leoncini, L., & Giordano, A., (2004). CDK9/CYCLIN T1 expression during normal lymphoid differentiation and malignant transformation. *J. Pathol., 203*(4), 946–952.

153. Kasten, M., & Giordano, A., (2001). Cdk10, a Cdc2-related kinase, associates with the Ets2 transcription factor and modulates its transactivation activity. *Oncogene, 20*(15), 1832–1838.

154. Guen, V. J., Gamble, C., Flajolet, M., Unger, S., Thollet, A., Ferandin, Y., Superti-Furga, A., Cohen, P. A., Meijer, L., & Colas, P., (2013). CDK10/cyclin M is a protein kinase that controls ETS2 degradation and is deficient in STAR syndrome. *Proc. Natl. Acad. Sci. USA., 110*(48), 19525–19530.

155. Iorns, E., Turner, N. C., Elliott, R., Syed, N., Garrone, O., Gasco, M., Tutt, A. N., Crook, T., Lord, C. J., & Ashworth, A., (2008). Identification of CDK10 as an important determinant of resistance to endocrine therapy for breast cancer. *Cancer Cell, 13*(2), 91–104.

156. Yu, J. H., Zhong, X. Y., Zhang, W. G., Wang, Z. D., Dong, Q., Tai, S., Li, H., & Cui, Y. F., (2012). CDK10 functions as a tumor suppressor gene and regulates survivability of biliary tract cancer cells. *Oncol. Rep., 27*(4), 1266–1276.

157. Zhong, X. Y., Xu, X. X., Yu, J. H., Jiang, G. X., Yu, Y., Tai, S., Wang, Z. D., & Cui, Y. F., (2012). Clinical and biological significance of Cdk10 in hepatocellular carcinoma. *Gene, 498*(1), 68–74.

158. Chen, H. H., Wong, Y. H., Geneviere, A. M., & Fann, M. J., (2007). CDK13/CDC2L5 interacts with L-type cyclins and regulates alternative splicing. *Biochem. Biophys. Res. Commun., 354*(3), 735–740.

159. Hu, D., Mayeda, A., Trembley, J. H., Lahti, J. M., & Kidd, V. J., (2003). CDK11 complexes promote pre-mRNA splicing. *J. Biol. Chem., 278*(10), 8623–8629.

160. Chen, H. H., Wang, Y. C., & Fann, M. J., (2006). Identification and characterization of the CDK12/cyclin L1 complex involved in alternative splicing regulation. *Mol Cell Biol.*, *26*(7), 2736–2745.

161. Blazek, D., Kohoutek, J., Bartholomeeusen, K., Johansen, E., Hulinkova, P., Luo, Z., Cimermancic, P., Ule, J., & Peterlin, B. M., (2011). The Cyclin K/Cdk12 complex maintains genomic stability via regulation of expression of DNA damage response genes. *Genes Dev.*, *25*(20), 2158–2172.

162. Davidson, G., Shen, J., Huang, Y. L., Su, Y., Karaulanov, E., Bartscherer, K., Hassler, C., Stannek, P., Boutros, M., & Niehrs, C., (2009). Cell cycle control of wnt receptor activation. *Dev. Cell*, *17*(6), 788–799.

163. Ou, C. Y., Poon, V. Y., Maeder, C. I., Watanabe, S., Lehrman, E. K., Fu, A. K., Park, M., Fu, W. Y., Jorgensen, E. M., Ip, N. Y., & Shen, K., (2010). Two cyclin-dependent kinase pathways are essential for polarized trafficking of presynaptic components. *Cell*, *141*(5), 846–858.

164. Mikolcevic, P., Sigl, R., Rauch, V., Hess, M. W., Pfaller, K., Barisic, M., Pelliniemi, L. J., Boesl, M., & Geley, S., (2012). Cyclin-dependent kinase 16/PCTAIRE kinase 1 is activated by cyclin Y and is essential for spermatogenesis. *Mol Cell Biol.*, *32*(4), 868–879.

165. Jeffrey, P. D., Tong, L., & Pavletich, N. P., (2000). Structural basis of inhibition of CDK-cyclin complexes by INK4 inhibitors. *Genes Dev.*, *14*(24), 3115–3125.

166. Bonelli, P., Tuccillo, F. M., Borrelli, A., Schiattarella, A., & Buonaguro, F. M., (2014). CDK/CCN and CDKI alterations for cancer prognosis and therapeutic predictivity. *Biomed. Res. Int.*, 361020.

167. Larrea, M. D., Liang, J., Da Silva, T., Hong, F., Shao, S. H., Han, K., Dumont, D., & Slingerland, J. M., (2008). Phosphorylation of p27Kip1 regulates assembly and activation of cyclin D1-Cdk4. *Mol Cell Biol.*, *28*(20), 6462–6472.

168. Taylor, W. R., & Stark, G. R., (2001). Regulation of the G2/M transition by p53. *Oncogene*, *20*(15), 1803–1815.

169. Lohr, K., Moritz, C., Contente, A., & Dobbelstein, M., (2003). p21/CDKN1A mediates negative regulation of transcription by p53. *J. Biol. Chem.*, *278*(35), 32507–32516.

170. Soria, G., & Gottifredi, V., (2010). PCNA-coupled p21 degradation after DNA damage: The exception that confirms the rule? *DNA Repair (Amst)*, *9*(4), 358–364.

171. Besson, A., Gurian-West, M., Chen, X., Kelly-Spratt, K. S., Kemp, C. J., & Roberts, J. M., (2006). A pathway in quiescent cells that controls p27Kip1 stability, subcellular localization, & tumor suppression. *Genes Dev.*, *20*(1), 47–64.

172. Pippa, R., Espinosa, L., Gundem, G., Garcia-Escudero, R., Dominguez, A., Orlando, S., Gallastegui, E., Saiz, C., Besson, A., Pujol, M. J., Lopez-Bigas, N., Paramio, J. M., Bigas, A., & Bachs, O., (2012). p27Kip1 represses transcription by direct interaction with p130/E2F4 at the promoters of target genes. *Oncogene*, *31*(38), 4207–4220.

173. Rossi, M. N., & Antonangeli, F., (2015). Cellular response upon stress: p57 contribution to the final outcome. *Mediators Inflamm.*, *2015*, 259325.

174. Lacy, E. R., Filippov, I., Lewis, W. S., Otieno, S., Xiao, L., Weiss, S., Hengst, L., & Kriwacki, R. W., (2004). p27 binds cyclin-CDK complexes through a sequential mechanism involving binding-induced protein folding. *Nat. Struct. Mol Biol.*, *11*(4), 358–364.

175. Abbas, T., & Dutta, A., (2009). p21 in cancer: intricate networks and multiple activities. *Nat. Rev. Cancer*, *9*(6), 400–414.

176. Jones, R. W., Coughlan, E. P., Reid, J. S., Sykes, P., Watson, P. D., & Cook, C., (2007). Human papilloma virus vaccines and their role in cancer prevention. *New Zealand Med. J., 120*(1266), U2829.

177. Biankin, A. V., Kench, J. G., Morey, A. L., Lee, C. S., Biankin, S. A., Head, D. R., Hugh, T. B., Henshall, S. M., & Sutherland, R. L., (2001). Overexpression of p21(WAF1/CIP1) is an early event in the development of pancreatic intraepithelial neoplasia. *Cancer Res., 61*(24), 8830–8837.

178. Roninson, I. B., (2002). Oncogenic functions of tumour suppressor p21(Waf1/Cip1/Sdi1): association with cell senescence and tumour-promoting activities of stromal fibroblasts. *Cancer Lett., 179*(1), 1–14.

179. Besson, A., Gurian-West, M., Schmidt, A., Hall, A., & Roberts, J. M., (2004). p27Kip1 modulates cell migration through the regulation of RhoA activation. *Genes Dev., 18*(8), 862–876.

180. Blain, S. W., Scher, H. I., Cordon-Cardo, C., & Koff, A., (2003). p27 as a target for cancer therapeutics. *Cancer Cell, 3*(2), 111–115.

181. Besson, A., Dowdy, S. F., & Roberts, J. M., (2008). CDK inhibitors: cell cycle regulators and beyond. *Dev. Cell, 14*(2), 159–169.

182. Lai, S., Goepfert, H., Gillenwater, A. M., Luna, M. A., & El-Naggar, A. K., (2000). Loss of imprinting and genetic alterations of the cyclin-dependent kinase inhibitor p57KIP2 gene in head and neck squamous cell carcinoma. *Clin. Cancer Res., 6*(8), 3172–3176.

183. Canepa, E. T., Scassa, M. E., Ceruti, J. M., Marazita, M. C., Carcagno, A. L., Sirkin, P. F., & Ogara, M. F., (2007). INK4 proteins, a family of mammalian CDK inhibitors with novel biological functions. *IUBMB Life, 59*(7), 419–426.

184. Kim, W. Y., & Sharpless, N. E., (2006). The regulation of INK4/ARF in cancer and aging. *Cell, 127*(2), 265–275.

185. Bostrom, J., Meyer-Puttlitz, B., Wolter, M., Blaschke, B., Weber, R. G., Lichter, P., Ichimura, K., Collins, V. P., & Reifenberger, G., (2001). Alterations of the tumor suppressor genes CDKN2A (p16(INK4a)), p14(ARF), CDKN2B (p15(INK4b)), & CDKN2C (p18(INK4c)) in atypical and anaplastic meningiomas. *Am. J. Pathol., 159*(2), 661–669.

186. Voorhoeve, P. M., & Agami, R., (2003). The tumor-suppressive functions of the human INK4A locus. *Cancer Cell, 4*(4), 311–319.

187. Esteller, M., Cordon-Cardo, C., Corn, P. G., Meltzer, S. J., Pohar, K. S., Watkins, D. N., Capella, G., Peinado, M. A., Matias-Guiu, X., Prat, J., Baylin, S. B., & Herman, J. G., (2001). p14ARF silencing by promoter hypermethylation mediates abnormal intracellular localization of MDM2. *Cancer Res., 61*(7), 2816–2821.

188. Li, J., Bi, L., Lin, Y., Lu, Z., & Hou, G., (2014). Clinicopathological significance and potential drug target of p15INK4B in multiple myeloma. *Drug Des. Devel. Ther., 8*, 2129–2136.

189. Hewitt, C., Lee Wu, C., Evans, G., Howell, A., Elles, R. G., Jordan, R., Sloan, P., Read, A. P., & Thakker, N., (2002). Germline mutation of ARF in a melanoma kindred. *Hum. Mol Genet., 11*(11), 1273–1279.

190. Randerson-Moor, J. A., Harland, M., Williams, S., Cuthbert-Heavens, D., Sheridan, E., Aveyard, J., Sibley, K., Whitaker, L., Knowles, M., Bishop, J. N., & Bishop, D. T., (2001). A germline deletion of p14(ARF) but not CDKN2A in a melanoma-neural system tumour syndrome family. *Hum. Mol Genet., 10*(1), 55–62.

191. Hartwell, L. H., & Kastan, M. B., (1994). Cell cycle control and cancer. *Science, 266*(5192), 1821–1828.

192. Houtgraaf, J. H., Versmissen, J., & Van der Giessen, W. J., (2006). A concise review of DNA damage checkpoints and repair in mammalian cells. *Cardiovasc. Revasc. Med.*, *7*(3), 165–172.

193. Niida, H., & Nakanishi, M., (2006). DNA damage checkpoints in mammals. *Mutagenesis*, *21*(1), 3–9.

194. O'Connell, M. J., Walworth, N. C., & Carr, A. M., (2000). The G2-phase DNA-damage checkpoint. *Trends Cell Biol.*, *10*(7), 296–303.

195. Bakkenist, C. J., & Kastan, M. B., (2003). DNA damage activates ATM through intermolecular autophosphorylation and dimer dissociation. *Nature*, *421*(6922), 499–506.

196. Lee, J. H., & Paull, T. T., (2004). Direct activation of the ATM protein kinase by the Mre11/Rad50/Nbs1 complex. *Science*, *304*(5667), 93–96.

197. Abraham, R. T., (2001). Cell cycle checkpoint signaling through the ATM and ATR kinases. *Genes Dev.*, *15*(17), 2177–2196.

198. Cortez, D., Guntuku, S., Qin, J., & Elledge, S. J., (2001). ATR and ATRIP: partners in checkpoint signaling. *Science*, *294*(5547), 1713–1716.

199. Venclovas, C., & Thelen, M. P., (2000). Structure-based predictions of Rad1, Rad9, Hus1 and Rad17 participation in sliding clamp and clamp-loading complexes. *Nucleic Acids Res.*, *28*(13), 2481–2493.

200. Majka, J., & Burgers, P. M., (2004). The PCNA-RFC families of DNA clamps and clamp loaders. *Prog. Nucleic Acid Res. Mol Biol.*, *78*, 227–260.

201. Marechal, A., & Zou, L., (2013). DNA damage sensing by the ATM and ATR kinases. *Cold Spring Harb Perspect Biol.*, *5*(9).

202. Shiotani, B., & Zou, L., (2009). ATR signaling at a glance. *J. Cell Sci.*, *122*(3), 301–304.

203. Lee, S. H., & Kim, C. H., (2002). DNA-dependent protein kinase complex: a multifunctional protein in DNA repair and damage checkpoint. *Mol Cells.*, *13*(2), 159–166.

204. Lim, D. S., Kim, S. T., Xu, B., Maser, R. S., Lin, J., Petrini, J. H., & Kastan, M. B., (2000). ATM phosphorylates p95/nbs1 in an S-phase checkpoint pathway. *Nature*, *404*(6778), 613–617.

205. Zou, L., Cortez, D., & Elledge, S. J., (2002). Regulation of ATR substrate selection by Rad17-dependent loading of Rad9 complexes onto chromatin. *Genes Dev.*, *16*(2), 198–208.

206. Maya, R., Balass, M., Kim, S. T., Shkedy, D., Leal, J. F., Shifman, O., Moas, M., Buschmann, T., Ronai, Z., Shiloh, Y., Kastan, M. B., Katzir, E., & Oren, M., (2001). ATM-dependent phosphorylation of Mdm2 on serine 395: role in p53 activation by DNA damage. *Genes Dev.*, *15*(9), 1067–1077.

207. Moll, U. M., & Petrenko, O., (2003). The MDM2-p53 interaction. *Mol Cancer Res.*, *1*(14), 1001–1008.

208. Bartek, J., & Lukas, J., (2001). Mammalian G1- and S-phase checkpoints in response to DNA damage. *Curr. Opin. Cell Biol.*, *13*(6), 738–747.

209. Guo, R., Chen, J., Mitchell, D. L., & Johnson, D. G., (2011). GCN5 and E2F1 stimulate nucleotide excision repair by promoting H3K9 acetylation at sites of damage. *Nucleic Acids Res.*, *39*(4), 1390–1397.

210. Murray-Zmijewski, F., Lane, D. P., & Bourdon, J. C., (2006). p53/p63/p73 isoforms: an orchestra of isoforms to harmonise cell differentiation and response to stress. *Cell Death Differ.*, *13*(6), 962–972.

211. Li, L. S., Morales, J. C., Hwang, A., Wagner, M. W., & Boothman, D. A., (2008). DNA mismatch repair-dependent activation of c-Abl/p73alpha/GADD45alpha-mediated apoptosis. *J. Biol. Chem.*, *283*(31), 21394–1403.

212. Lopez-Contreras, A. J., & Fernandez-Capetillo, O., (2010). The ATR barrier to replication-born DNA damage. *DNA Repair (Amst.)*, *9*(12), 1249–1255.

213. Derheimer, F. A., & Kastan, M. B., (2010). Multiple roles of ATM in monitoring and maintaining DNA integrity. *FEBS Lett.*, *584*(17), 3675–3681.

214. Falck, J., Petrini, J. H., Williams, B. R., Lukas, J., & Bartek, J., (2002). The DNA damage-dependent intra-S phase checkpoint is regulated by parallel pathways. *Nat. Genet.*, *30*(3), 290–294.

215. Costanzo, V., Robertson, K., Ying, C. Y., Kim, E., Avvedimento, E., Gottesman, M., Grieco, D., & Gautier, J., (2000). Reconstitution of an ATM-dependent checkpoint that inhibits chromosomal DNA replication following DNA damage. *Mol Cell.*, *6*(3), 649–659.

216. Sancar, A., Lindsey-Boltz, L. A., Unsal-Kacmaz, K., & Linn, S., (2004). Molecular mechanisms of mammalian DNA repair and the DNA damage checkpoints. *Annu. Rev. Biochem.*, *73*, 39–85.

217. Kim, S. T., Xu, B., & Kastan, M. B., (2002). Involvement of the cohesin protein, Smc1, in Atm-dependent and independent responses to DNA damage. *Genes Dev.*, *16*(5), 560–570.

218. Duursma, A. M., Driscoll, R., Elias, J. E., & Cimprich, K. A., (2013). A role for the MRN complex in ATR activation via TOPBP1 recruitment. *Mol Cell.*, *50*(1), 116–122.

219. Shiotani, B., Nguyen, H. D., Hakansson, P., Marechal, A., Tse, A., Tahara, H., & Zou, L., (2013). Two distinct modes of ATR activation orchestrated by Rad17 and Nbs1. *Cell Rep.*, *3*(5), 1651–1662.

220. Trenz, K., Smith, E., Smith, S., & Costanzo, V., (2006). ATM and ATR promote Mre11 dependent restart of collapsed replication forks and prevent accumulation of DNA breaks. *EMBO J.*, *25*(8), 1764–1774.

221. Mazouzi, A., Velimezi, G., & Loizou, J. I., (2014). DNA replication stress: causes, resolution and disease. *Exp. Cell Res.*, *329*(1), 85–93.

222. Gamper, A. M., Choi, S., Matsumoto, Y., Banerjee, D., Tomkinson, A. E., & Bakkenist, C. J., (2012). ATM protein physically and functionally interacts with proliferating cell nuclear antigen to regulate DNA synthesis. *J. Biol. Chem.*, *287*(15), 12445–12454.

223. Mailand, N., Podtelejnikov, A. V., Groth, A., Mann, M., Bartek, J., & Lukas, J., (2002). Regulation of G(2)/M events by Cdc25A through phosphorylation-dependent modulation of its stability. *EMBO J.*, *21*(21), 5911–5920.

224. Mhawech, P., (2005). 14–3–3 proteins-an update. *Cell Res.*, *15*(4), 228–236.

225. Krause, K., Wasner, M., Reinhard, W., Haugwitz, U., Dohna, C. L., Mossner, J., & Engeland, K., (2000). The tumour suppressor protein p53 can repress transcription of cyclin B. *Nucleic Acids Res.*, *28*(22), 4410–4418.

226. Allocati, N., Di Ilio, C., & De Laurenzi, V., (2012). p63/p73 in the control of cell cycle and cell death. *Exp. Cell Res.*, *318*(11), 1285–1290.

227. Hosoya, N., & Miyagawa, K., (2014). Targeting DNA damage response in cancer therapy. *Cancer Sci.*, *105*(4), 370–388.

228. Kruiswijk, F., Labuschagne, C. F., & Vousden, K. H., (2015). p53 in survival, death and metabolic health: a lifeguard with a licence to kill. *Nat. Rev. Mol Cell Biol.*, *16*(7), 393–405.

229. Bartkova, J., Horejsi, Z., Koed, K., Kramer, A., Tort, F., Zieger, K., Guldberg, P., Seh-ested, M., Nesland, J. M., Lukas, C., Orntoft, T., Lukas, J., & Bartek, J., (2005). DNA damage response as a candidate anti-cancer barrier in early human tumorigenesis. *Nature*, *434*(7035), 864–870.

230. Sun, M., Guo, X., Qian, X., Wang, H., Yang, C., Brinkman, K. L., Serrano-Gonzalez, M., Jope, R. S., Zhou, B., Engler, D. A., Zhan, M., Wong, S. T., Fu, L., & Xu, B., (2012). Activation of the ATM-Snail pathway promotes breast cancer metastasis. *J. Mol Cell Biol.*, *4*(5), 304–315.

231. Dzikiewicz-Krawczyk, A., (2008). The importance of making ends meet: mutations in genes and altered expression of proteins of the MRN complex and cancer. *Mutat. Res.*, *659*(3), 262–273.

232. Kase, M., Vardja, M., Lipping, A., Asser, T., & Jaal, J., (2011). Impact of PARP-1 and DNA-PK expression on survival in patients with glioblastoma multiforme. *Radiother. Oncol.*, *101*(1), 127–131.

233. Bouchaert, P., Guerif, S., Debiais, C., Irani, J., & Fromont, G., (2012). DNA-PKcs ex-pression predicts response to radiotherapy in prostate cancer. *Int. J. Radiat. Oncol. Biol. Phys.*, *84*(5), 1179–1185.

234. Musacchio, A., & Salmon, E. D., (2007). The spindle-assembly checkpoint in space and time. *Nat. Rev. Mol Cell Biol.*, *8*(5), 379–393.

235. Taylor, S. S., Scott, M. I., & Holland, A. J., (2004). The spindle checkpoint: a qual-ity control mechanism which ensures accurate chromosome segregation. *Chromosome Res.*, *12*(6), 599–616.

236. Sudakin, V., Chan, G. K., & Yen, T. J., (2001). Checkpoint inhibition of the APC/C in HeLa cells is mediated by a complex of BUBR1, BUB3, CDC20, & MAD2. *J. Cell Biol.*, *154*(5), 925–936.

237. Morrow, C. J., Tighe, A., Johnson, V. L., Scott, M. I., Ditchfield, C., & Taylor, S. S., (2005). Bub1 and aurora B cooperate to maintain BubR1-mediated inhibition of APC/CCdc20. *J. Cell Sc.*, *118*(16), 3639–3652.

238. Krenn, V., Overlack, K., Primorac, I., Van Gerwen, S., & Musacchio, A., (2014). KI motifs of human Knl1 enhance assembly of comprehensive spindle checkpoint com-plexes around MELT repeats. *Curr. Biol.*, *24*(1), 29–39.

239. De Antoni, A., Pearson, C. G., Cimini, D., Canman, J. C., Sala, V., Nezi, L., Mapelli, M., Sironi, L., Faretta, M., Salmon, E. D., & Musacchio, A., (2005). The Mad1/Mad2 complex as a template for Mad2 activation in the spindle assembly checkpoint. *Curr. Biol*, *15*(3), 214–225.

240. Peters, J. M., (2006). The anaphase promoting complex/cyclosome: a machine designed to destroy. *Nat. Rev. Mol Cell Biol.*, *7*(9), 644–656.

241. Howell, B. J., McEwen, B. F., Canman, J. C., Hoffman, D. B., Farrar, E. M., Rieder, C. L., & Salmon, E. D., (2001). Cytoplasmic dynein/dynactin drives kinetochore protein transport to the spindle poles and has a role in mitotic spindle checkpoint inactivation. *J. Cell Biol.*, *155*(7), 1159–1172.

242. Mao, Y., Abrieu, A., & Cleveland, D. W., (2003). Activating and silencing the mitotic checkpoint through CENP-E-dependent activation/inactivation of BubR1. *Cell*, *114*(1), 87–98.

243. Wassmann, K., Liberal, V., & Benezra, R., (2003). Mad2 phosphorylation regulates its association with Mad1 and the APC/C. *EMBO J.*, *22*(4), 797–806.

244. Kops, G. J., Weaver, B. A., & Cleveland, D. W., (2005). On the road to cancer: aneu-ploidy and the mitotic checkpoint. *Nat. Rev. Cancer*, *5*(10), 773–785.

245. Mondal, G., Sengupta, S., Panda, C. K., Gollin, S. M., Saunders, W. S., & Roychoud-hury, S., (2007). Overexpression of Cdc20 leads to impairment of the spindle assembly checkpoint and aneuploidization in oral cancer. *Carcinogenesis*, *28*(1), 81–92.

246. Jin, D. Y., Spencer, F., & Jeang, K. T., (1998). Human T cell leukemia virus type 1 on-coprotein Tax targets the human mitotic checkpoint protein MAD1. *Cell*, *93*(1), 81–91.

247. Wang, X., Jin, D. Y., Ng, R. W., Feng, H., Wong, Y. C., Cheung, A. L., & Tsao, S. W., (2002). Significance of MAD2 expression to mitotic checkpoint control in ovarian can-cer cells. *Cancer Res.*, *62*(6), 1662–1668.

248. Fung, M. K., Cheung, H. W., Wong, H. L., Yuen, H. F., Ling, M. T., Chan, K. W., Wong, Y. C., Cheung, A. L., & Wang, X., (2007). MAD2 expression and its significance in mitotic checkpoint control in testicular germ cell tumour. *Biochim. Biophys. Acta*, *1773*(6), 821–832.

249. Yoon, D. S., Wersto, R. P., Zhou, W., Chrest, F. J., Garrett, E. S., Kwon, T. K., & Gabrielson, E., (2002). Variable levels of chromosomal instability and mitotic spindle checkpoint defects in breast cancer. *Am. J. Pathol.*, *161*(2), 391–397.

250. Jeong, S. J., Shin, H. J., Kim, S. J., Ha, G. H., Cho, B. I., Baek, K. H., Kim, C. M., & Lee, C. W., (2004). Transcriptional abnormality of the hsMAD2 mitotic checkpoint gene is a potential link to hepatocellular carcinogenesis. *Cancer Res.*, *64*(23), 8666–8673.

CHAPTER 4

ANGIOGENESIS, ITS IMPORTANCE, AND IMPLICATION IN TUMOR GROWTH AND PROGRESSION, AND IN ANTICANCER THERAPY: AN UPDATE

CHANDRANI SARKAR and DEBANJAN CHAKROBORTY

Department of Pathology, The Ohio State University, 1645 Neil Avenue, Columbus, OH 43210, USA, E-mail: Chandrani Sarkar: Chandrani.Sarkar@osumc.edu, Debanjan Chakroborty: Debanjan. Chakroborty@osumc.edu

CONTENTS

ABSTRACT

Angiogenesis is the process of formation of new blood vessels from preexisting vasculature. Blood vessels deliver nutrients and oxygen to the tissues and subsequently remove waste products from them and are thus important for tissue growth and survival. Apart from their role in normal physiology, blood vessels also play a critical role in the initiation, growth, progression, and metastasis of tumors. Decades of research has identified multiple steps and various check points in the growth of tumor vasculature. Moreover, a multitude of factors that either promote or inhibit angiogenesis have also been identified. Key regulatory molecules of angiogenesis have been considered as potential therapeutic targets in the treatment of cancer, and numerous therapeutic possibilities have been envisaged through successful inhibition of the process. Over the years, many inhibitors of angiogenesis have been identified and tested in clinical trials, some of which have received approval and are being used in treatment of patients with different types of cancer. In this chapter, we will discuss about the development in the field of tumor angiogenesis, the essential steps involved, the factors that control the angiogenic process, the antiangiogenic drugs that have been approved for the treatment of cancer, and finally, their advantages and disadvantages.

4.1   INTRODUCTION

The term "angiogenesis" ("angêion" meaning vase and genesis meaning "birth" in Greek) was first used by John Hunter, a British Surgeon, in 1794 to describe the growth of blood vessels in reindeer antlers [1, 2]. During embryonic development, blood vessels are formed from angioblasts or endothelial precursor cells originating in the bone marrow by a process termed as vasculogenesis [3, 4]. Thereafter, new blood vessels in adults are mostly formed by sprouting or branching of these existing blood vessels through the process of angiogenesis [5]. Blood vessels are formed mainly from two types of cells, endothelial cells and the surrounding mural cells (pericytes in small vessels and smooth muscle cells in larger vessels). The newly sprouted vessels are stabilized by mural cells that cover them through a process known as arteriogenesis [6-8]. Because blood vessels are the key route for supply of nutrients and oxygen to different tissues within the body, the process of angiogenesis occurs to meet tissue demands in both physiological and pathological conditions. In the adult, continued angiogenesis is required for functioning of the female reproductive system, oocyte development, and for tissue repair during healing of wounds. Here, the process is strictly regulated by maintaining a balance between the endogenous promoters and inhibitors of angiogenesis. The loss of this balance may lead to many pathological disorders. An excess of promoters leading to excessive angiogenesis may contribute to the growth of tumors, psoriasis, inflammatory bowel diseases, and atherosclerosis. Similarly, an excess of inhibitors leading to reduced and improper vessel growth may result in diseases like ischemia, pre-eclampsia, neurodegeneration, and osteoporosis [9–13].

4.2   IMPORTANCE OF ANGIOGENESIS DURING TUMOR GROWTH

Long back in 1865, Virchow, the founder of pathological anatomy, first drew attention to the fact that the tumor mass consists of numerous blood vessels [14]. In 1907, Goldman was the first to study tumor vascularization systematically [15]. Later, Algire and colleagues mentioned the importance of new blood vessels or neovascularization in tumor growth [16]. However, the first concrete proof of this concept was provided by Judah Folkman in 1971, when he and colleagues provided evidence that to grow beyond a size of 2 mm^3, tumors require new blood vessels to be formed to supply the rapidly multiplying cells with nutrients and oxygen [17, 18]. This finding led to an entirely new concept in the treatment of cancer: the antiangiogenic strategy, where the endothelial cells were targeted instead of tumor cells to restrict the growth of tumors [17, 19-24]. The search for effective anti-angiogenic targets/strategies has thus governed cancer research for decades, and over the years, numerous promoters and inhibitors of angiogenesis have been identified and tested and some have been successful in clinical trials.

Blood vessels form an integral component of tissue growth and maintenance within the body [11, 23]. Tumors are composed of rapidly proliferating host-derived cells that have lost control over cell division and are in constant need for adequate supply of nutrients and oxygen and effective removal of waste products. When tumor growth exceeds a specific size, the existing blood supply is not sufficient to meet their nutritional requirements. The tumor cells then cleverly hijack and manipulate the very basic process of blood vessel formation in the tissues to meet their own excessive need of nutrients and oxygen for rapid growth. Tumors liberate a variety of growth factors that augment the process of angiogenesis. The newly formed vessels in turn support further growth and progression of tumor cells [25–27]. Angiogenesis plays a crucial role not only in the growth of primary tumors but also helps in the metastatic spread of the tumor cells to distant sites in the body [26–28]. To get disseminated into other sites, tumor cells have to break the physiological barriers imposed by primary tissue structure. Blood vessels provide the routes through which the tumor cells get dispersed to other sites within the body. The tumor cells first need to gain access into the blood vessels. Newly formed vessels within the tumor are nascent and fragile and do not have enough basement membrane coverage that enhances the chances of tumor cells to penetrate the blood vessels as the cells then require lesser invasive potential than that required to invade normal intact blood vessels. Eventually, the tumor cells that are shed into the nearest blood vessel get carried away with the circulation, escape from vasculature, and get seeded to other organs where they can start a fresh secondary growth [29–31]. Even at the secondary sites, these cells require new vessels to grow beyond the size of 1–2 mm in diameter. Hence, the same process of neovessel formation, tumor growth, and tumor cell dissemination is repeated, leading to the metastatic cascade in the body. Thus, angiogenesis plays a pivotal role in the growth of both primary and secondary tumors [32–35]. Research work over the last few decades has provided sufficient evidence to support this idea. Both in vivo and in vitro studies have proved that for successful growth, tumors rely on the formation of new blood vessels, and inhibition of angiogenic processes result in stunted or diminished tumor growth [18, 19, 21]. Direct relevance of the importance of angiogenesis in the growth of tumors comes from studies where it has been shown that agents or molecules that specifically act on endothelial cells and not on tumor cells have inhibitory effect on overall tumor growth and progression [35–37]. Indirect evidences come from the fact that endothelial cells, which are otherwise quiescent in the normal state, are extremely active and highly proliferating within the tumor microenvironment [38, 39]. Reports further show that the interaction between tumor cells and endothelial cells occurs in both direction; endothelial cells are stimulated by paracrine signals from tumor cells and endothelial cells also secret cytokines and other growth factors that promote tumor cell growth and metastases [40–42]. Numerous studies so far have also shown that the degree of vascularization (determined by intratumoral microvessel density) directly correlates with the aggressiveness of the tumors and the metastasizing potential of tumor cells [43–45]. Consequently, inhibition of angiogenesis has emerged as a novel and rational approach to inhibit metastasis as targeting the blood vessels appeared to be easier and specific compared to targeting the heterogeneous, unstable, and resistant tumor cells [46, 47].

4.3 PROCESS OF NEOVASCULARIZATION

The "angiogenic switch" that helps tumors to proceed from the avascular (approximately 1–2 mm^3) to a vascular state depends largely on *sprouting angiogenesis* where new capillaries are formed from existing vasculature [48, 49]. This process is initiated when the basement membrane and extracellular matrix are degraded, leading to migration and invasion of endothelial cells into the surrounding matrix. These migrated endothelial cells then proliferate and organize themselves to create a lumen and thus form an immature new vessel that is stabilized when mural cells surround the endothelial cells to form a sheath and an extracellular matrix is laid onto it. This newly formed vessel then anastomoses into a preexisting vessel to establish blood flow. The entire process is controlled by a number of regulators, both pro- and antiangiogenic, and their balance determines the efficiency of the process [48, 50–52]. In addition to sprouting angiogenesis, several other mechanisms of tumor neovascularization have also been identified [48]. *Intussusceptive tumor angiogenesis* where a preexisting vessel splits into two vessels through extension of the capillary wall into the lumen forming interstitial tissue pillars has also been reported in tumors. The process of intussusception is a fast and energy efficient process that relies on endothelial cell expansion and subsequent thinning of cellular structure as opposed to proliferation as in sprouting angiogenesis. Here, at first, the adjacent capillary walls come in contact with each other and form a transluminal bridge. Then, restructuring of the endothelial cell junctions leads to formation of gaps in the vessel bilayer; this allows growth factors and cells to enter the lumen to form a core at the contact region, which is then surrounded by pericytes and myofibroblasts followed by retraction of endothelial cells and formation of two separate vessels [48, 53–55]. Another mechanism of tumor neovessel formation, *vasculogenesis* was first reported by Ashahara et al. [56, 57] where endothelial progenitor cells (EPC) from bone marrow migrate and incorporate themselves into the tumor vasculature to promote new vessel formation [58]. However, the extent to which EPC control the process of new vessel formation greatly varies with the type of tumor. Tumors in tissues rich in blood vessels like brain can grow without eliciting an angiogenic response by a mechanism known as *vessel co-option* where the tumor cells line up along the existing blood vessels and derive nutrients from them [48, 55, 59]. In rapidly growing tumors, to meet the nutrient needs of the tumor cells, it has also been observed that tumor cells themselves dedifferentiate into an endothelial cell-like phenotype and form tubular structures, thereby creating a secondary circulatory system within the tumors. This process is known as *vasculogenic mimicry* [48, 55, 60]. Regardless of the mechanism or mechanisms involved in promoting angiogenesis in tumors, it is now well accepted that the onset of angiogenesis is a crucial factor that determines the fate of tumors; this establishes angiogenesis as a potential target for anticancer treatment.

4.4   HOW IS TUMOR VASCULATURE DIFFERENT FROM NORMAL VASCULATURE?

Unlike normal cells and tissues that satisfy their metabolic needs from physiological angiogenesis and vasculogenesis, tumor cells build their own supply of blood vessels. However, the tumor blood vessels differ from normal vessels in both structure and function [61]. Normal vessels maintain a hierarchy of arterioles, capillaries, and venules and are evenly distributed, whereas tumor vessels lack any hierarchy, are irregularly distributed, chaotic in organization, form tortuous networks with irregular branching patterns, and are dilated [24,27, 62]. The tight endothelial monolayer that is required for normal barrier function of blood vessels is lacking in tumor vessels. Many tumor vessels lack functional pericytes, and their basement membrane is defective in structure and composition; they are also extremely leaky or permeable due to the presence of fenestrae and transcellular gaps [63-65]. Chromosomal abnormalities in endothelial cell nuclei like aneuploidy with abnormal centrosomes have also been reported in tumor blood vessels [66]. Some tumor vessels are "mosaic" in which both endothelial cells and tumor cells form the luminal surface [67,68]. Abnormal tumor vessels also exhibit bidirectional blood flow [69].

Functional abnormality of tumor vessels is manifested by the fact that they are hyperpermeable, thereby allowing large macromolecules to escape into the surrounding tissue. They are also inefficient in oxygen supply and clearing of wastes. The fluid that extravasates from the tumor blood vessels is similar in composition to plasma. This protein-rich fluid after leakage interacts with tissue factor in the stroma, which then activates the clotting system and deposits fibrin. The fibrin gel clots formed helps in tumor growth by absorbing water and inhibiting fluid clearance, leading to edema and creating a pressure gradient that aids diffusion from the interstitial fluid to the vessel lumen. In addition, fibrin deposition supplies a stroma that activates the growth of new blood vessels and fibroblasts and formation of fibrovascular stroma. It also helps in the migration of tumor cells, endothelial cells, pericytes, fibroblasts, and inflammatory cells (neutrophils, monocytes). Many growth factors get trapped in the fibrin gel and are rescued from degradation and hence can continue with secretion of proangiogenic factors, leading to more angiogenesis. Also fibrin is broken down by matrix metalloproteinases (MMPs) to form Fragment E, which promotes angiogenesis directly. Thus, abnormal tumor blood vessels are inefficient in function but are successful in creating an environment that promotes the growth and development of tumors [70, 71].

4.5 KEY REGULATORS OF ANGIOGENESIS

The process of angiogenesis is controlled by a number of conditions, cytokines, and growth factors that are prevalent in the tumor microenvironment. We will next discuss the key regulators controlling this process during tumor growth and progression (see Table 4.1)

4.5.1 VASCULAR ENDOTHELIAL GROWTH FACTOR (VEGF) FAMILY

Among the growth factors that regulate the process of angiogenesis, the VEGF family has drawn the maximum attention and has been most widely studied. This family includes the growth factors VEGF-A/VEGF or vascular permeability factor (VPF), VEGF-B, VEGF-C, VEGF-D, and placental growth factor (PlGF) [51, 72–74]. Of these, VEGF-A or VPF is the most important cytokine that regulates the process of both normal angiogenesis and tumor neovascularization and was the first member of the VEGF family to be isolated and studied. VEGF-A/VPF was initially identified as an

TABLE 4.1 Endogenous Regulators of Angiogenesis

Name	Mode of action	Effect on angiogenesis (Stimulation =Angiogenesis ↑ and Inhibition =Angiogenesis↓)	References
Vascular endothelial growth factor (VEGF) (VEGF-A. VEGF-B, VEGF-C, VEGF-D, VEGF-E and Placental growth factor (PlGF))	Promotes endothelial cell proliferation, migration, tube formation, sprouting, extracellular matrix degradation, endothelial progenitor cell mobilization, lymphatic endothelial cell proliferation and mobilization	Angiogenesis ↑ Vasculogenesis ↑ Lymphangiogenesis ↑	51, 72–77, 91
Fibroblast Growth Factor (FGF)	Promotes endothelial cell proliferation, migration, tube formation, degradation of extra cellular matrix proteins, alteration of intra cellular adhesion proteins, endothelial progenitor cell mobilization and enhances VEGF production by tumor cells	Angiogenesis ↑ Vasculogenesis ↑	31, 102, 103
Angiopoietin	Vessel maintenance, vessel stabilization; promotes mural cell recruitment to newly formed vessels, endothelial sprouting and tube formation.	Angiogenesis ↑	92, 95, 98
Epidermal Growth Factor (EGF)	Enhances proliferation of endothelial cells, promotes endothelial cell migration, increases angiogenic cytokines production by tumor cells.	Angiogenesis ↑	105, 106
Platelet-Derived Growth Factor(PDGF)	Increases endothelial cell sprouting, maintains pericyte homeostasis, stimulates pericye mobilization and recruitment, and controls endothelial-pericyte interaction.	Angiogenesis ↑	31, 74, 112

Matrix Metalloproteinases (MMPs)	Promotes endothelial cell proliferation, mobilization, tube formation and helps in the process of vasculogenic mimicry, matrix degradation, extracellular matrix remodeling, endothelial progenitor cell mobilization and pericyte recruitment.	Angiogenesis ↑ Vasculogenesis ↑	114, 115, 120–124
Endostatin	Endothelial cell apoptosis, cell cycle arrest, prevents endothelial cell matrix degradation, inhibits functions of VEGF activities MMPs	Angiogenesis ↓	177–179, 181
Thrombospondin	Inhibits endothelial cell proliferation, migration and tube formation and induces apoptosis of endothelial cells	Angiogenesis ↓	183–186
Tumstatin	Inhibits endothelial cell proliferation and promotes endothelial cell apoptosis	Angiogenesis ↓	190, 191
Arresten	Inhibits endothelial cell proliferation and promotes endothelial cell apoptosis and also inhibits the actions of VEGF and FGF.	Angiogenesis ↓	196, 197
Canstatin	Inhibits endothelial cell proliferation and promotes endothelial cell apoptosis.	Angiogenesis ↓	194, 195
Endorepellin	Inhibits endothelial cell proliferation, migration and tube formation.	Angiogenesis ↓	198, 199
Interleukins	Suppress FGF induced angiogenesis.	Angiogenesis ↓	210–212
Interferons	Inhibit FGF induced angiogenesis, production and activity of MMP9, M2 polarization of macrophages.	Angiogenesis ↓	201–209
Platelet factor 4(PF4)	Inhibits proliferation and migration of endothelial cells.	Angiogenesis ↓	214, 215

TABLE 4.1 (Continued)

Name	Mode of action	Effect on angiogenesis (Stimulation =Angiogenesis ↑ and Inhibition =Angiogenesis↓)	References
Angiostatin	Inhibits proliferation, migration of endothelial cells, induces apoptosis.	Angiogenesis ↓	127, 221
Pigment epithelium derived factor (PEDF)	Inhibits proliferation, migration of endothelial cells, promotes FasL dependent endothelial cell death.	Angiogenesis ↓	224, 225
Prolactin fragments (PRLs)	Inhibits VEGF mediated angiogenesis.	Angiogenesis ↓	229
Vasostatin	Inhibits growth factor induced angiogenesis, effective against bFGF, inhibits endothelial cell attachment to basement membrane.	Angiogenesis ↓	226, 227, 229
Troponin1	Inhibits endothelial cell proliferation and migration.	Angiogenesis ↓	230, 231
2 methoxyestradiol (2-ME)	Inhibits VEGF production, HIF1α production and accumulation.	Angiogenesis ↓	232–234
Soluble Fms like tyrosine kinase1 (sFlt1)	Binds to VEGF and inhibits VEGF mediated angiogenesis.	Angiogenesis ↓	236
Chondromodulin I(ChM-I)	Inhibits endothelial cell migration.	Angiogenesis ↓	237, 238
Isthmin 1 (ISM1)	Inhibits VEGF and FGF induced endothelial cell proliferation, capillary network formation and induces endothelial cell apoptosis.	Angiogenesis ↓	240
Carboxy-terminus of Hsc70 interacting protein (CHIP)	Inhibits endothelial cell growth and tubule formation.	Angiogenesis ↓	240

Rho GTPase activating protein 18 (ARHGAP18)	Induces premature senescence in endothelial cells, inhibits endothelial cell migration, inhibits endothelial cell sprouting.	Angiogenesis ↓	240
G-protein-coupled receptor 56 (GPR56)	Inhibits VEGF secretion and synthesis.	Angiogenesis ↓	240
Zinc finger protein 24 (ZNF24)	Suppresses expression of VEGF and PDGFRβ.	Angiogenesis ↓	240
Multimerin2 (MMRN2)	Inhibits endothelial cell migration, vessel sprouting and VEGF-VEGFR interaction.	Angiogenesis ↓	240
Suppressor of cytokine signaling-3 (SOCS3)	Inhibits inflammation and growth factor mediated angiogenesis, regulates growth factor mediated endothelial cell proliferation.	Angiogenesis ↓	240
FK506 binding protein like (FKBPL)	Inhibits migration and tube formation of endothelial cells, increases vessel diameter and induces vessel normalization and improves drug delivery.	Angiogenesis ↓	240

inducer of vascular hyperpermeability in vivo [75–77]. It promotes vascular endothelial cell proliferation, sprouting, and tubule formation; helps in extracellular matrix degradation by activating enzymes thereby increasing vascular permeability; helps in mobilization of endothelial precursor cells from bone marrow; and protects endothelial cells from apoptosis [51]. It is expressed in almost all solid tumors studied (lung, breast, gastrointestinal tract, kidney, bladder, and ovary) as well as in certain hematological malignancies [51]. VEGF-A acts as a survival factor for endothelial cells in both in vivo and in vitro conditions [78]. The human *vegf* gene is located on chromosome 6 and consists of 8 exons separated by 7 introns. Alternative splicing of mRNA results in four mature isoforms of VEGF (VEGF121, VEGF165, VEGF189, and VEGF206), of which VEGF165, which lacks the amino acid residues encoded by exon 6, is most common and is overexpressed in a large number of solid tumors [79]. VEGF145 and VEGF183 are other lesser known isoforms of VEGF [80]. Mouse VEGF gene is located on chromosome 17 and has 8 exons. In mouse, each VEGF isoform is one amino acid less than their corresponding human isoform. VEGF-A executes its functions mainly through two transmembrane tyrosine kinase receptors, VEGF receptor-1 (VEGFR-1) or fms like tyrosine kinase-1 (Flt-1) and VEGFR-2 or kinase insert domain containing receptor/fetal liver kinase -1 (KDR/Flk-1) that are expressed on endothelial cells. VEGFR-2 is considered as the main receptor through which the proangiogenic functions of VEGF-A are executed. In addition, VEGF-A also acts through the neuropilin receptors (NP-1 and NP-2) that are expressed on neurons and vascular endothelium [81]. Binding of VEGF-A to NP-1 has been reported to increase the interaction between VEGF-A and VEGFR-2. Two polypeptide forms of VEGF-B, VEGF-B167 and VEGF-B186, have been reported in humans [82]. VEGF-B, a VEGF A homologue, specifically binds to VEGFR-1 but does not interact with other VEGF receptors, i.e., VEGFR-2 or VEGFR-3 [83]. The exact role of VEGF-B, expressed in the heart, skeletal muscles, and vascular cells, in angiogenesis is debatable with some studies reporting its role in the promotion of pathological angiogenesis, and other showing that it lacks any such property. A recent study has shown that VEGF-B can promote cancer metastasis through an angiogenesis-independent mechanism [84]. VEGF-C and VEGF-D bind and activate VEGFR-2 and VEGFR-3 [85, 86]. Both these growth factors promote angiogenesis as well as lymphangiogenesis or the growth of new lymphatic vessels [87, 88]. VEGF-E is proangiogenic and stimulates VEGFR-2 to promote endothelial cell growth [89]. Another important growth factor of VEGF family is placental growth factor (PlGF). It is a dimeric protein that has more than 50% similarity with the platelet-derived growth factor region of VEGF. High expression of PlGF is seen in the placenta throughout all the stages of gestation. The four isoforms of human PlGF, PlGF-1, PlGF-2, PlGF-3 and PlGF-4 bind to VEGFR-1. PlGF can alternatively activate VEGFR-2 as it competes with VEGF-A for VEGFR-1 and displaces VEGF-A from VEGFR-1 which eventually leaves more VEGF-A to bind and activate VEGFR-2 [90]. The human *plgf* gene is located on chromosome 14q24. In mice, the gene is located on chromosome 12 [72]. At first, its role in promotion of angiogenesis was controversial, but subsequent studies supported its inclusion as a proangiogenic growth factor. PlGF can promote angiogenesis in both direct and indirect manner [13]. Although the role of PlGF in physiological angiogenesis is not very prominent, it has been reported to play an important role in pathological angiogenesis like tumor growth and ocular and limb ischemia. Studies using *plgf* knockout mice show that PlGF is not required for normal vessel development as the newborns are found healthy and fertile and are born at Mendelian frequency [91].

4.5.2 ANGIOPOIETINS AND TIE RECEPTORS

Tie receptors (Tie 1 and Tie 2) are tyrosine kinase receptors that are expressed on endothelial cells. The Tie 2 gene is located on chromosome 9. Angiopoietins, mainly Ang-1 and Ang-2, are secretory oligomeric glycoprotein growth factors that act as ligands for Tie receptors, and together they play a key role in blood vessel maintenance, growth, and stabilization [92]. Apart from these two factors, other members of the Angiopoietin family are Ang-3 and Ang-4. Ang-1 is widely distributed throughout the normal adult vasculature and is mainly secreted by mural cells or pericytes [93]. Secretion of Ang-2 occurs only when cells are stimulated. In resting or normal circumstances, the molecules are stored in endothelial Weibel-Palade bodies [94]. Ang-1 by acting through Tie2 receptor, a 150-kDa transmembrane receptor tyrosine kinase, helps to recruit pericytes to newly formed vessels and thus plays a major role in vessel stabilization and reduces vessel permeability [95]. Mice lacking either Ang-1 or Tie-2

die before birth as a result of incomplete vascular development characterized by abnormal vasculature that is leaky and devoid of branching and
sprouting vessels. Tie1-deficient mice also die either perinatally [96] or
between days 13.5 and 14.5 of gestation due to inefficient vascular integrity, which proves that Tie1 is necessary for the vessel integrity and survival of endothelial cells during angiogenesis [97]. The role of Ang-2 in
angiogenesis is kind of complicated. Unlike Ang-1, Ang-2 acts as a partial
agonist or as an antagonist of Tie-2 receptor, blocking Ang-1-Tie-2 interaction and therefore antagonizes Tie 2 response to Ang-1 and helps in the
loss of pericytes and destabilization of vessels. Such vessels are characterized by increased endothelial cell sprouting and tubule formation. The
balance between Ang-1 and Ang-2 is therefore crucial in the maintenance
of healthy blood vessels. Ang-1 is an anti-inflammatory molecule that is
needed for vessel stabilization whereas Ang-2 is highly inflammatory in
nature and activates endothelial cells and destabilizes the endothelial barrier function and thereby promotes vascular inflammation and angiogenesis. Studies have shown that blocking Ang-2 inhibits tumor angiogenesis
and therefore retards tumor growth [92, 98].

4.5.3   FIBROBLAST GROWTH FACTOR (FGF)

Another important growth factor family that mediates angiogenic response
is the fibroblast family of growth factors or FGF growth factor family. The
two prototypical types of FGF are acidic or aFGF and basic or bFGF [31].
Unlike VEGF, which is a more specific mitogen for endothelial cells, FGF
can elicit mitotic actions to nearly all kinds of cells of neuroectodermal or
embryonic mesodermal origin [99]. The action of FGF is mediated through
the FGF receptor (FGFR) [100, 101]. Studies attribute a less significant role
of FGF in normal generalized angiogenesis but indicate that FGF plays a
major role in remodeling and maintenance of damaged vessels both in case
of tumor angiogenesis as well as during healing of wounds [102]. The role
played by FGF in tumor angiogenesis includes stimulation of endothelial
cell proliferation, degradation of extracellular matrix proteins, alteration of
intercellular adhesion and junction by affecting cadherins [31]. Studies also
indicate the role of FGF in mobilization and subsequent recruitment of endothelial progenitor cells to the tumor beds [103]. There is also evidence of
substantial crosstalk between FGFR and VEGFR signaling in angiogenesis,

and the FGFR system might mediate resistance to VEGFR targeting in some situations [104].

4.5.4   EPIDERMAL GROWTH FACTOR (EGF)

The epidermal growth factor (EGF) family is another family of growth factors that plays a very important role in angiogenesis during tumor growth. EGF is a low-molecular-weight polypeptide with a molecular weight of 6 kDa. It binds with epidermal growth factor receptor (EGFR), which is a member of the Her/erb family of receptor tyrosine kinases, with maximum affinity. The EGF-EGFR pathway is a well-established pathway that induces angiogenesis during tumor growth [105]. EGF increases the production of angiogenic cytokines from tumor cells through activation of the EGFR pathway. Multiple studies have shown that the addition of EGF to cultures of gastric, pancreatic, and glioblastoma cancer cell lines can induce the production of angiogenic factors such as VEGF, bFGF, and IL-8 in these cells. In vivo studies have also shown that treatment with EGFR inhibitors decreases intratumoral expression of angiogenic factors like VEGF and IL-8 that leads to reduction of angiogenesis [106].

4.5.5   PLATELET-DERIVED GROWTH FACTOR (PDGF)

The platelet-derived growth factors (PDGF) are a family of dimeric disulfide-bound growth factors with molecular weight of 30 kDa that regulates the process of angiogenesis in many ways. Though initially purified from platelets, many other cell types like fibroblasts, astrocytes, keratinocytes, and endothelial cells were subsequently identified to secret PDGF [107]. Heterodimers (PDGF-AB) as well as homodimers (PDGF-AA or PDGF-BB) of PDGF composed of polypeptide chains A and B have been identified. Recently, 2 new members, PDGF-CC and PDGF-DD were also identified. They act through cell membrane tyrosine kinase PDGF receptors (PDGF-$\alpha\alpha$, PDGF-$\alpha\beta$, and PDGF-$\beta\beta$) [108]. PDGF through PDGF-beta receptor in capillary endothelial cells increases DNA synthesis and forms angiogenic sprouts in vitro [109, 110]. The main role played by PDGF in regulating endothelial cell functions seems to be the regulation of pericytes that are required for stability of the microvessels. PDGF has been reported to play a role in pericyte homeostasis, proliferation, migration, and recruitment to growing capillaries in tumors [31, 74]. Mouse models with deficient pericytes show a wide range of abnormalities in the blood vessels [74]. Targeted deletion of PDGF-B or the PDGF-β receptor leads to ablation of the microvascular pericytes from the capillary walls. Furthermore, mice bred without PDGF-BB or its receptor dies prenatally due to leaky blood vessels [31, 111]. PDGF through its receptors in pericytes stimulates the expression of Ang-1, which helps the pericytes to interact with the endothelial cells to maintain the stability of the newly formed vessels [112]. Also, PDGF-D also increases the interstitial fluid pressure by recruiting macrophages to expression sites and inhibits the vascular leakage caused due to growth factor-induced angiogenesis. Furthermore, PDGF-D also induces macrophage recruitment, increases interstitial pressure, and promotes blood vessel maturation during angiogenesis [113].

4.5.6   MATRIX METALLOPROTEINASES (MMPS)

The matrix metalloproteinases or metrixins are the family of enzymes that plays a critical role in the angiogenic process. These are zinc-containing enzymes or endopeptidases. There are over 20 or more members that have been identified till date that are part of the MMP family [114, 115]. MMPs are found in soluble or in cell membrane-associated forms, membrane type-MMP or MT-MMPs [74]. Although MMPs play a significant role during the angiogenic process, the role played by MMPs are not specific to tumor angiogenesis alone. Low levels of constitutive expression of MMPs is seen in normal physiological states such as placental growth, embryogenesis, and during wound healing, but overexpression of MMPs is associated virtually with all human cancers [114, 116]. Normally, MMPs remain in inactive form, i.e., as zymogen or proenzyme, and upon activation, they become functional and participate in subsequent cellular and molecular events [114, 115]. In tumor bed, the major contributors that synthesize and secret MMPs are tumor cells, tumor infiltrating inflammatory cells, tumor-associated macrophages or TAM, tumor-associated neutrophils or TAN, and the endothelial cells [117]. Additionally, stromal cells and mural cells/pericytes also secret MMPs in the tumor microenvironment [118]. The angiogenic factors like VEGF and FGF can induce synthesis and production of MMPs in endothelial cells. MMPs identified so far can be divided into 5 sub-categories: matrilysins, stromelysins, gelatinases, collagenases, and MT-MMPs [114, 115,

119]. Together, they perform numerous functions to promote angiogenesis. MMPs, both soluble and membrane type, are capable of degrading the components of vascular basement membrane and the extracellular matrix (ECM) components. ECM remodeling by MMPs helps in the degradation of proteins and growth factors that often remain in an inactive state in the matrix, and release of their active forms make them suitable for participation in blood vessel formation [114, 115]. Apart from these functions, MMPs also show a number of effects on endothelial cells; mainly endothelial cell proliferation, mobilization, sprouting, and can also influence tube formation capabilities [120]. Among the MMPs, exogenous addition of MMP9 has been shown to directly control the process of angiogenesis in vitro. MMP2 and MMP13 have also been shown to induce neovessel formations [121]. MMPs also play a prominent role in the process of vasculogenic mimicry. MMP-2 and MT1-MMP have been shown to play this role in melanoma where they confer the endothelial property to tumor cells [122]. MMPs also play a role in vasculogenesis where they help in mobilization of endothelial progenitor cells (EPCs) from bone marrow to circulation [123]. MMPs also have influence on mural cells or pericytes. Studies have shown that MMP9-knockout animals have defects in recruiting pericytes and their blood vessels have reduced coverage [124].

However, the role played by MMPs in regulation of angiogenesis is not that simple as was initially thought. Besides the role in angiogenesis promotion, a significant number of studies have also demonstrated that several members of the MMP family can play negative roles during neovessel formation, thus leading to further confusion. However, antiangiogenic properties of MMPs are mostly attributed to their proteolytic functions. They degrade ECM components via proteolytic processes to generate fragments that inhibit neovessel formation through suppression of processes like endothelial cell proliferation, migration, and invasion. Among MMPs, MMP9, MMP2, MMP7, and MMP12 have been shown to have antiangiogenic properties [121, 125]. It has been shown that MMP-7 and MMP-9 have the capabilities to hydrolyze plasminogen, a matrix component, to generate angiostatin, a natural endogenous inhibitor of angiogenesis [125]. Furthermore, forced overexpression of MMP9 within tumor cells results in reduced angiogenesis and tumor growth inhibition [126]. MMPs derived from macrophages, especially MMP12 has been shown to inhibit neovessel formation through the generation of angiostatin [127, 128]. Endostatin, tumstatin, and canstatin are among the other inhibitors that are generated through proteolytic cleavage of ECM by different MMPs [121, 129]

In physiological conditions, MMPs, both soluble and membrane type, are kept in check by tissue inhibitors of matrix metalloproteinases (TIMPs). They usually form inhibitory complexes with MMPs, thereby prohibiting the later from taking part in the neovascularization process. The balance between TIMPs and MMPs is crucial and depending on which either stimulation or inhibition of vessel growth takes place. Based on the type of MMPs, TIMPs also participate in both stimulation and inhibition of angiogenic processes and hence the tumor growth [130, 131]

4.5.7 HYPOXIA

Hypoxia or hypoxic conditions, i.e., less availability of oxygen to cells or tissues, dictate the necessity of formation of new blood vessels within the tumor mass [132]. In solid tumors, as the tumor grows in size, the proliferating cells adjacent to the supplying blood vessels push their neighboring cells outwards, thus creating the distance between these cells and existing blood supply, which makes it difficult for nutrients and oxygen to reach these cells. As further growth requires constant supply of oxygen and metabolites, this temporary deficit of nutrients and oxygen within tumor mass thus emerges as a key driver of further vessel growth or angiogenesis [17, 132]. Hypoxia has been shown to regulate both physiological angiogenesis as in follicular development and pathological conditions like in tumor growth by both direct and indirect ways [75, 133] Hypoxia inducible factor (HIF), a transcription factor, is the key regulatory protein in hypoxia-driven angiogenesis. HIF complex consists of the α and β subunits and co-activators. There are three HIFα subunits, namely HIF1α, HIF2α, and HIF3α, that have been reported to take part in angiogenic regulation during tumor growth. Upon hydroxylation by propyl hydroxylases (PHDs), these subunits are recognized by von Hippel-Lindau (VHL) ubiquitin-ligase complex resulting in degradation. During low oxygen conditions, PHDs are less active, which allows these subunits to escape recognition and hence VHL- mediated degradation. These HIFα subunits then form heterodimers with the β subunits and activate the transcription of important genes in the nucleus [134]. HIF1 is the master regulator of many angiogenic events and is most ubiquitously present and accordingly has been regarded as a promising therapeutic target.

Both HIF1α and HIF1β are constitutively expressed in normoxic conditions. However, HIF1α in the normoxic state has a shorter half-life than that in the hypoxic state. In hypoxic conditions, as the stability of HIF 1α increases, it forms a stable heterodimer with HIF1β which then binds to hypoxia responsive element binding region and regulates the transcription of VEGF mRNA and its expression [135]. It also indirectly increases the secretion of MMP-2 and MMP-9 and therefore regulates angiogenesis and metastases [136]. In addition to VEGF, HIF1 also regulates a number of other cytokines like stromal cell derived factor 1 (SDF1) and placental growth factor (PLGF) that take part in the process of angiogenesis [91, 137, 138]. Using forced expression of HIF1, studies have shown that HIF1 is associated with more angiogenic phenotype of the tumor characterized by increase in the angiogenic and vasculogenic potential of endothelial cells and promotes hyperaggressiveness in tumor cells [139–142]. Similarly, transfection of dominant negative form of HIF1 to tumor cells resulted in a less angiogenic tumor and hence reduction in the growth [142]. In addition to manipulating the expression of VEGF and other angiogenic growth factors [143, 144], HIF1 also has autoregulatory effects on endothelial cells and can directly control proliferation and migration of these cells [145, 146].

4.5.8   NEURAL REGULATION OF VESSEL GROWTH AND ANGIOGENESIS

Several years ago, it was observed that the majority of growing tumors lack innervation. However, sporadic presence of nerve fibers was reported in some tumors [147–149]. It has been further reported that perineural invasion is directly associated with poor prognosis in certain types of malignant tumors [150–152]. Normal blood vessels are innervated by sympathetic nerves, and the neuromediators released from these nerve endings regulate vessel growth, structure, and functions [153–156]. Observations from several clinical and animal studies prove that behavioral conditions like stress can modulate the progression of different types of cancers [157–159]. Chronic stress activates the sympathetic nervous system (SNS) which in turn releases neurotransmitters such as norepinephrine, epinephrine, and dopamine. Stress-induced immune suppression was previously thought to be the reason for enhanced tumor growth [160]. However, stress has also been shown to promote the angiogenic phenotype of primary tumors and also their metastatic dissemination [161]. Increased sympathetic activity has been reported to mediate cancer progression [159]. Also, loss of sympathetic innervation has been shown to favor dysregulated vessel growth and increase vessel permeability and vessel tortuosity, which are the characteristics of angiogenic or intratumoral blood vessels [156]. The catecholamine neurotransmitters epinephrine and norepinephrine have been shown to promote angiogenesis during tumor growth [12] whereas the other catecholamine neurotransmitter dopamine has been shown to inhibit the process of angiogenesis [159, 162–166]. Epinephrine and norepinephrine augment the production of proangiogenic factors like VEGFA and IL6 in tumor tissues [167–168]. This aids in promotion of angiogenesis and tumor growth. However, and interestingly, dopamine acts differently as it inhibits VEGFA-VEGFR2 interaction resulting in the inhibition of VEGFA-induced angiogenesis and tumor growth [162, 163, 165, 166, 169]. In addition, dopamine also plays a major role in regulating the process of vasculogenesis [170]. Dopamine present in the bone marrow has been shown to regulate mobilization of EPCs from the bone marrow to the circulation. Loss of dopamine in the bone marrow during tumor growth results in the egress of EPC from bone marrow to circulation [170]. Dopamine also plays a major role in restructuring of aberrant tumor blood vessels or in "normalizing" of abnormal vessels. This is particularly important because normalization of tumor blood vessels is essential for increased delivery of anticancer drugs and radiation to the tumor cells [159, 171]. In addition, the co-neurotransmitters or molecules such as serotonin, neuropeptide Y, acetylcholine, or nitric oxide or small peptides like somatostatin and substance P have been reported to play roles in tumor angiogenesis, affecting the process either directly or through regulation of other angiogenic factors [161, 172–176].

4.5.9   ENDOGENOUS INHIBITORS OF ANGIOGENESIS

Numerous naturally present endogenous inhibitors of angiogenesis are also found in the body. These are mainly protein components or fragments of proteins generated during proteolytic processing of compounds found in the ECM. Under normal physiological circumstances, these inhibitors maintain a balance with the endogenous proangiogenic growth factors and stringently regulate the process of angiogenesis. Depending on the pathological circumstances, the balance is tipped toward inhibitors or stimulators, depending on which angiogenesis is either suppressed or stimulated. Additionally, partially digested ECM components, hormones or hormone metabolite fragments, clotting factors, and proteins of the immune system may also act as inhibitors of angiogenic processes.

4.5.9.1 Inhibitors Derived from Matrix or ECM Breakdown

Endostatin, discovered in 1997, is a 20- to 22-kDa carboxy terminal fragment of collagen VIII [177] that inhibits proliferation, migration, and tube formation of endothelial cells [177], which results in reduced growth of tumors [178]. The other direct effects of endostatin on endothelial cells include induction of apoptosis and cell cycle arrest [179]. Endostatin stabilizes endothelial cell-matrix junctions preventing cell detachment that is required during neovessel formation. It also interferes with VEGF binding to VEGF receptors and inhibits activities of MMPs [181].

Thrombospondin, another natural inhibitor of neovascularization, is a multidomain, heparin-binding matrix glycoprotein [182]. There are two members of the thrombospondin family, namely thrombospondin 1 (TSP-1) and thrombospondin 2 (TSP-2). Both TSP-1 and TSP-2 have been shown to inhibit proliferation, migration, and tubule-forming capabilities of endothelial cells and induce apoptosis [183–186]. Although TSPs are recognized as molecules that inhibit the process of angiogenesis, studies have also shown that they might also show proangiogenic activities, which indicate their biphasic role [187]. TSP-1 depletion in mice results in manifold increase in tumor growth [188]. Moreover, antiangiogenic therapy has been shown to increase circulating TSP-1 in mice supporting its role as an inhibitor of angiogenesis [189].

Tumstatin is a derivative of collagen IV. It is a small 28-kDa protein fragment specifically shown to inhibit proliferation of endothelial cells and promote cell apoptosis [190, 191]. The domain named Tum-5 located within aa 54–132 of this fragment has been attributed with antiangiogenic functions and has been widely studied both in vitro and in vivo [192]. Preclinical studies have shown that Tumstatin is effective as an antiangiogenic agent alone and in combination with anticancer drugs [193].

Canstatin is a 24-kDa, matrix-derived fragment of N terminal α2 chain of collagen IV that also has the capability to inhibit proliferation, migration and tubule-forming properties of endothelial cells. Canstatin can promote apoptosis of endothelial cells through downregulation of end antiapoptotic proteins. It specifically acts on endothelial cells and does not have any inhibitory action on cells other than the endothelial origin [194]. Canstatin has been shown to suppress tumor growth in vivo by inhibition of endothelial cell proliferation [195].

Arresten is a 26-kDa protein fragment derived from the carboxy terminal of the α chain of collagen IV. It has inhibitory action on VEGF- and FGF-induced endothelial cell proliferation, migration, and tube formation [196, 197]. It has also been shown to inhibit expression of VEGF and HIF1α in tumors [197].

Endorepellin is an 85-kDa protein fragment derived from the carboxy terminal angiostatic module of perlecan, a well-known heparin sulfate proteoglycan. It inhibits tumor growth by inhibition of angiogenic processes. Using mouse tumor models, it has been shown that endorepellin can inhibit proliferation, migration, and tubule formation of endothelial cells [198, 199]. Recent reports have shown that endorepellin modulates the expression of autophagic markers via suppression of VEGFR2 in endothelial cells and thereby induces autophagy in these cells [200]. Apart from matrix-derived endogenous fragments there are other growth factors and cytokines that function as inhibitors of angiogenic processes in vivo.

4.5.9.2   Inhibitors Derived from Blood or Other Cells

Interferons (IFNs) are a family of secreted glycoproteins produced by cells of the immune system. They play a prominent role in the regulation of angiogenic processes ranging from controlling endothelial cell behavior to production of angiogenic cytokines both in vivo and in vitro [201, 202]. IFN α was the first IFN to be identified. Later, IFNβ and IFNγ have also been reported to inhibit angiogenic functions. IFNs are most effective against tumors that secrete high amounts of FGF2, like brain hemangiomas, angioblastomas, and pulmonary hemangiomatosis [203–205]. IFN α also suppresses IL-8 [206] secreted by tumor cells and IFN-γ and IFN-β inhibit expression and enzymatic activity of MMP-9 [207]. Furthermore, IFN γ also inhibits the differentiation of monocytes to M2 macrophages in the tumor microenvironment [208]. M2 macrophages secret VEGF and help in angiogenesis [209]. Inhibition of M2 polarization by IFN γ thus prevents further angiogenesis.

Interleukins(ILs) are leukocyte-derived protein factors and cytokines that have a variety of physiological roles. Among the ILs, IL-1β, IL-4, IL-12, and IL-18 have been reported to have antiangiogenic functions [210]. IL-4 directly effects the migration and proliferation of endothelial cells. It also inhibits bFGF-induced vessel sprouting [211]. IL-1β and IL-18 were shown to suppress FGF-induced tumor angiogenesis. IL-12 and IL-18 also induce IFNγ and prevent angiogenesis [212].

Platelet factor 4 (PF4) is a bloodborne secretory angiostatic cytokine derived from platelet α granules. It binds to and neutralizes heparin [212, 213]. Using in vitro assays, it has been shown that PF4 specifically and directly can inhibit the proliferation and migration of endothelial cells [214]. It inhibits endothelial cell migration by blocking MMP1 and MMP3 [215]. In vivo antiangiogenic properties have been tested in multiple myeloma, murine melanoma, and human colon cancer xenografts, where it has been found that PF4 specifically inhibits endothelial cells [216–218].

Angiostatin derived from plasminogen via hydrolysis by MMPs is a naturally occurring 38-kDa fragment known to inhibit angiogenesis [219]. It contains triple disulfide-bonded kringle domains. Different kringle domains confer different angiogenic properties to the angiostatin molecule [127, 220]. Angiostatin is very specific to proliferating or growing endothelial cells and does not have any effect on resting endothelial cells [127]. It inhibits proliferation, migration, and tubule formation and induces proapoptotic behavior in endothelial cells [221].

Pigment epithelium-derived factor (PEDF) is a serpin family member and a very potent and selective antiangiogenic agent [222]. It only targets the newly formed blood vessels and is therefore very successful in inhibiting tumor growth via suppression of angiogenesis [223]. PEDF can inhibit proliferation, migration, and specifically induce FasL-dependent cell death of endothelial cells. It can also disrupt the balance between pro- and antiangiogenic factors in vivo [224]. Even in the presence of proangiogenic factors like VEGF, IL-8, and FGF, PEDF can inhibit endothelial cell migration [225]. Antiangiogenic properties of PEDF have been explored in many mouse and human tumor xenografts including glioma, melanoma and in Wilm's tumor. The antiangiogenic therapeutic efficacies of PEDF or PEDF gene delivery have also been well documented in several mouse tumors [212].

Vasostatin, the amino terminal domain of calreticulin, is a potent inhibitor of endothelial cell proliferation and angiogenesis. It is particularly effective against tumor angiogenesis stimulated by several growth factors

[226, 227]. It inhibits growth of colon and ovarian tumors in mice through inhibition of angiogenesis [226]. The delivery of recombinant vasostatin DNA to mouse tumor also successfully reduces the growth [228]. It is particularly shown to be effective against bFGF-induced angiogenesis and to prohibit endothelial cell attachment to basement membrane component laminin in vitro [229].

Troponin I is an endogenously produced cartilage-derived angiogenesis inhibitor that inhibits angiogenesis both in vitro and in vivo. It can inhibit FGF-induced endothelial cell proliferation, migration as well as EC proliferation in unstimulated conditions [230, 231].

2-Methoxyestradiol (2-ME) is an endogenous metabolite produced from estradiol-17β and is an inhibitor of angiogenesis [232, 233]. It interferes with VEGF synthesis as it inhibits HIF1α production and accumulation within the nucleus [234]. 2-ME is a potent inhibitor of endothelial cell proliferation and can also inhibit migration of these cells. 2-ME can induce apoptosis of endothelial cells by upregulating Fas and Bcl-2 [232]. Although the compound is orally available and well tolerated, its fast pass metabolism and low solubility restricts its use in therapy [235].

Soluble Fms-like tyrosine kinase 1 (sFlt1) is soluble VEGFR1 and has strong binding affinity for VEGF and PlGF. It binds to circulating VEGF, rendering it less available to endothelial cells and thereby indirectly inhibits VEGF-induced angiogenesis in vivo [236].

Chondromodulin-I (ChM-I) is a 25-kDa glycoprotein angiogenesis inhibitor that was initially isolated from fetal bovine epiphyseal cartilage [237]. It inhibits invasive potential of endothelial cells in vivo. Studies show its efficacy as an antiangiogenic agent in tumors [238].

Prolactin fragments (PRLs) 16 kDa and 8kDa, enzymatically and endogenously derived from proangiogenic prolactin, are antiangiogenic in nature. They interfere with VEGF- and FGF-mediated angiogenesis [239].

Apart from these endogenous angiogenic inhibitors, in recent years, several other endogenously produced antiangiogenic molecules have been identified, like isthmin1 (ISM1), suppressor of cytokine signaling-3 (SOCS-3), tumor protein 73-alpha (TAp73), FK506-binding protein-like (FKBPL), carboxy-terminus of Hsc70 interacting protein (CHIP), multimerin-2 (MMRN2), Rho GTPase activating protein 18 (ARHGAP18), zinc finger protein 24 (ZNF24), G-protein coupled receptor 56 (GPR56), and JWA. These proteins have the potential to be developed into antiangiogenic drugs for cancer or other diseases that involve excessive angiogenesis [240]. They are superior to artificially designed synthetic angiogenesis inhibitors as they are expected to be better tolerated by the patients and be less toxic. It is also expected that patients will not develop resistance to these compounds. In the last two decades, we have seen that several of these antiangiogenic molecules have entered the clinical trials for cancer and other diseases where angiogenesis plays a crucial role and some have received approval (endostatin and angiostatin) [241–244].

4.6   ANTIANGIOGENIC THERAPY

Angiogenesis is a complex multistep process regulated by a number of pro- and antiangiogenic factors involving many signaling pathways that offer numerous potential targets for therapy. Based on the current understanding of this process, a number of antiangiogenic therapeutic strategies have been approved for the treatment of a broad range of cancers (Table 4.2), and several other antiangiogenic agents are in the process of being approved.

The first antiangiogenic agent to be approved for treatment by US Food and Drug Administration (FDA) was bevacizumab (Avastin ™, Genentech) in 2004 for the treatment of metastatic colorectal cancer (mCRC) as a first line treatment after phase III trial in patients showed improved overall survival, progression-free survival, and response rate. Bevacizumab is a humanized monoclonal antibody that targets VEGFA and prevents it from binding to its receptors to initiate signaling cascades leading to angiogenesis. Later, it has been used as the second-line treatment for mCRC and in treatment of nonsmall cell lung cancer (NSCLC), ovarian cancer, and metastatic renal cell carcinoma (mRCC) [245–250]. Other monoclonal antibodies approved for treatment include cetuximab (Erbitux, Bristol-Myers Squibb) for the treatment of mCRC and head and neck cancer and panitumumab (Vectibix, Amgen) for the treatment of mCRC. Both these agents target the epidermal growth factor receptor (EGFR) [251–256]. Monoclonal antibodies targeting EGFR in the last stages of development are nimotuzumab in glioma and head and neck cancer, zalutumumab in head and neck cancer, and necitumumab in NSCLC [257–259]. Ramucirumab (Cyramza, Eli Lilly), a monoclonal antibody targeting VEGFR2 has shown significant overall and progression-free survival in randomized placebo-controlled clinical trial and improved survival in a chemoresistant setting when added with paclitaxel in patients with refractory gastro-esophageal cancer. It has been

TABLE 4.2 List of Approved Anti-Angiogenic Agents in Cancer Treatment

Antiangiogenic agent	Type of cancer treated	Mechanism of action	Treatment	Major complications	References
Bevacizumab	Colorectal cancer (metastatic)(mCRC), Ovarian cancer, Non-small cell lung cancer (NSCLC), Renal cell carcinoma (RCC)	Acts against VEGF, inhibits VEGF-VEGFR2 interaction	First and second line with chemotherapeutic agents for mCRC, first line with chemotherapy for NSCLC, with Interferon for RCC, first line with chemotherapy for ovarian cancer	Hypertension, bowel perforation, fistulas, thrombotic microangiopathy, hemorrhage	245–250, 263
Sorafenib	Thyroid cancer, Renal cell carcinoma (RCC), Hepatocellular carcinoma (HCC)	Tyrosine kinase inhibitor of Raf/MEK/ERK and VEGFR and PDGFR signaling	Single drug, first line for RCC and HCC, refractory to radioactive iodine for thyroid cancer	Hemorrhage, hypertension, neutropenia, myocardial ischemia and myocardial infarction.	248, 263, 272–274, 277
Sunitinib	Pancreatic neuroendocrine tumors, Renal cell carcinoma (RCC), Gastrointestinal stromal Tumor (GIST)	Tyrosine kinase inhibitor of VEGFR, PDGFR, FLT-3, c-KIT, RET and CSF-1R	Single drug,first line for RCC and pancreatic neuroendocrine tumors,GIST after disease progression with or intolerance to imatinib mesylate	Hypertension, diarrhea, fatigue, hypothyroidism.	248, 263, 274–276, 278
Vandetanib	Medullary Thyroid cancer	Inhibitor of VEGFR-1, VEGFR-2, VEGFR-3 and EGFR	Single drug to unresectable, locally advanced or metastatic disease	Hypertension, diarrhea, Headache, abdominal pain	248, 263, 285, 286

Axitinib	Renal cell carcinoma (RCC)	Tyrosine kinase inhibitor of VEGFR1, VEGFR2 and VEGFR3	Single drug, second line	Weight gain, nausea, diarrhea, dysphonia, fatigue, hypertension,	248, 263, 287, 288
Aflibercept	Colorectal cancer	Binds to VEGF-A, VEGF-B and PlGF	Second line	Neutropenia, leukopenia, fistula, diarrhea, hypertension, compromised wound healing	248, 263, 268–271
Pazopanib	Soft tissue carcinoma, Renal cell carcinoma (RCC)	Multi targeted tyrosine kinase inhibitor	Single drug for soft tissue carcinoma, single drug /first line for RCC	Electrolyte imbalance, myelosuppression, hypertension, hypo and hyper glycemia, neutropenia, thrombocytopenia	248, 263
Regorafenib	Refractory metastatic colorectal cancer, Gastrointestinal stromal Tumor (GIST)	Multi kinase inhibitor	Single drug, refractory mCRC, surgically non removable GIST, non-responsive to imatinib and sunitinib	Hand foot syndrome, loss of appetite, intestine perforation, severe bleeding, liver damage	263, 268, 279, 280
Ramucirumab	Metastatic colorectal cancer Non-small cell lung cancer, (NSCLC), Gastric and gastro-esophageal cancer	Blocks the binding of VEGF to VEGFR2	Refractory with or without chemotherapy	Anemia, headache, diarrhea, hypertension, arterial thromboembolic events, GI perforation, neutropenia	258, 260–263

TABLE 4.2 (Continued)

Antiangiogenic agent	Type of cancer treated	Mechanism of action	Treatment	Major Complications	References
Lenvatenib	Thyroid cancer	Inhibits VEGFR2 and VEGFR3	Radioactive iodine refractory, recurrent or metastatic cancer	High blood pressure, common fatigue, nausea, diarrhea, muscle ache, mouth sores	263
Trastuzumab	Metastatic breast cancer; metastatic Non-small cell lung cancer (NSCLC)	Humanized monoclonal antibody against HER2	Single-agent, second-line therapy for metastatic breast cancer that over-express HER2, combination with doxorubicin, cyclophosphamide, and paclitaxel for HER2-overexpressing, node-positive breast cancer, second line for NSCLC	Cardiac toxicity, congestive heart failure	258, 265–267
Thalidomide	Multiple Myeloma	Multitarget drug	In combination with dexamethasone	Myelosuppression, edema, hypotension, myalgia, drowsiness, hematuria	296
Gefitinib	Advanced and metastatic non-small cell lung cancer (NSCLC)	Inhibits EGFR tyrosine kinase	Second line, locally advanced or metastatic NSCLC	Elevation of liver enzymes, vomiting, nausea, diarrhea, asthenia	281, 282

Erlotinib	Non-small cell lung cancer (NSCLC), pancreatic cancer	EGFR/HER1 receptor tyrosine kinase inhibitor	Monotherapy for NSCLC, locally advanced, unresectable, metastatic pancreatic cancer in combination with gemcitabine as first line treatment	Rash, diarrhea, fatigue, loss of appetite.	283, 284
Temsirolimus	Renal cell carcinoma (RCC)	mTOR kinase inhibitor	For advanced RCC	Fatigue, skin rash, decrease of hemoglobin, lymphocytes	293–295
Everolimus	Renal cell carcinoma (RCC), progressive neuroendocrine tumors of pancreatic origin	mTOR kinase inhibitor	Advanced RCC after failure of treatment with sunitinib and sorafenib, for unresectable, locally advanced, metastatic neuroendocrine tumors of pancreatic origin	Stomatitis, diarrhea, peripheral edema, fatigue, neutropenia	293–295

approved by FDA for the treatment of gastric cancer and NSCLC in 2014 [258, 260–263]. Trastuzumab (Herceptin, Genentech), humanized mono-clonal antibody against HER2 [264], is approved as single-agent, second-line therapy for metastatic breast cancer that overexpresses HER2 and as adjuvant treatment in combination with doxorubicin, cyclophosphamide, and paclitaxel for HER2-overexpressing, node-positive breast cancer [258, 265, 266]. It has also been approved for the treatment of metastatic NSCLC after failure of chemotherapy regimen [258, 267]. Aflibercept (VEGF-trap, Regeneron), a novel recombinant soluble fusion protein that binds to VEGF-A, VEGF-B, and PlGF, was recently approved for the treatment of mCRC in combination with chemotherapeutic drugs [263, 268–271].

The second group of antiangiogenic agents includes the tyrosine kinase inhibitors (TKIs) that target different signaling pathways in angiogenesis. TKIs targeting the VEGF pathway have proved to be very successful in the treatment of mRCC. Sorafenib (Nexavar, Bayer/Onyx Pharmaceuticals), an inhibitor of Raf/MEK/ERK and the VEGFR and PDGFR signaling path-ways, was the first to be identified and approved by FDA for RCC in 2005 [272–274]. Sorafenib was followed by sunitinib (Sutent, Pfizer), an oral inhibitor of VEGFR-2, PDGFR, FLT-3, c-KIT, RET, and CSF-1R, in 2006 for gastrointestinal stromal tumor (GIST) and advanced mRCC [274–276]. Sorafinib is also used in the treatment of metastatic hepatocellular carcinoma (mHCC) and thyroid cancer [263, 277], and Sunitinib in the treatment of pancreatic neuroendocrine tumors [263, 278]. Rogarafenib (Stivarga, Bayer HealthCare), another TKI, was reported recently to increase the overall survival of mCRC patients whose disease had progressed upon receiving standard therapy, i.e., for those who have been previously treated with fluo-ropyrimidine-, oxaliplatin-, and irinotecan-based chemotherapy [279, 280]. Gefitinib (Iressa, AstraZeneca and Teva) is a first-generation TKI targeting EGFR that received approval from the FDA as a second-line treatment for advanced NSCLC after two phase II trials showed an overall survival of 6 to 8 months [281, 282]. Erlotinib (Tarceva, Genentech), an oral inhibi-tor of EGFR/HER1 receptor tyrosine kinase, was approved in 2004 after a phase III trial showed that erlotinib monotherapy provided a 2-month sur-vival benefit over best supportive care in patients with chemotherapy-refrac-tory advanced NSCLC [283, 284]. Vandetanib (Caprelsa, Astrazeneca), orally available, small molecule TKI that acts as an inhibitor of VEGFR-1, VEGFR-2, VEGFR-3, and EGFR has been approved for the treatment of symptomatic or progressive medullary thyroid cancer in patients showing unresectable, locally advanced, or metastatic forms of the disease [263, 285, 286]. Axitinib (Inlyta, Pfizer), a second generation inhibitor of VEGFR1, VEGFR2, and VEGFR3, was approved for the treatment of RCC in 2012 [287, 288]. Imatinib (Gleevec, Novartis) selectively inhibits Bcr/Abl and is approved for the treatment of gastrointestinal stromal tumors (GIST), chronic myelogenous leukemia (CML), and acute lymphoblastic leukemia [248, 289]. Lapatinib (Tykerb, GlaxoSmithKline), an oral TKI targeting EGFR and ErbB/Her2 was approved for the treatment of metastatic breast cancer in 2007 [290, 291]. Lenvatinib (Lenvima, Eisai Co), a VEGFR-2 and VEGFR-3 inhibitor, has been approved in 2015 for the treatment of progressive radioactive iodine refractory-differentiated thyroid cancer [263, 292]. Several other TKIs are in the final stages of clinical development for the treatment of ovarian cancer, breast cancer, medullary thyroid cancer, glioblastoma, and biliary tract cancer.

Inhibitors of mTOR, a serine threonine kinase, phosphorylation of which is a key downstream signaling event in the PI3K/Akt signaling cascade that regulates several cellular processes including angiogenesis, form the third class of antiangiogenic agents in therapy. Two mTOR inhibitors, Temsirolimus (Torisel, Wyeth) and Everolimus (Afinitor, Novartis), have also been approved for the treatment of RCC [293–295].

In 2006, thalidomide (Thalomid, Celgene Corporation) in combination with dexamethasone received approval from FDA for the treatment of newly diagnosed multiple myeloma (MM) patients. Thalidomide is a potent teratogen that inhibits angiogenesis by decreasing expression of bFGF, VEGF, COX-2, IL-6, and tumor necrosis factor (TNF-α). Lenalidomide (Revlimid), a synthetic analog of thalidomide with potent immunomodulatory and antiangiogenic properties and lower adverse effects was also approved by FDA for the second-line treatment of MM in combination with dexamethasone [296].

4.7   ADVANTAGES OF ANTIANGIOGENIC THERAPY AND COMPLICATIONS

Conventional chemotherapy targets the tumor cells by interfering with the processes of DNA replication, cell division, or metabolism. However, such chemotherapeutic drugs have their limitations as they lack specificity, as a result of which not only cancer cells but also normal dividing cells are damaged. Standard chemotherapy therefore comes with a number of serious side effects like hair loss, bone marrow suppression, low blood counts, gastrointestinal symptoms, and infections. In an attempt to avoid/lessen these undesired effects, suboptimal doses of the drugs are administered, which results in partial response to chemotherapy and early relapse of disease. Problems like resistance to drugs due to genomic instability of cancer cells and impaired delivery of drugs to tumor sites due to abnormal blood vessels also exist [9, 297–302]. Antiangiogenic inhibitors target the blood vessels rather than directly targeting the tumor cells. Their success in specifically restricting tumor cells from growing was guaranteed for different reasons. These drugs target endothelial cells that unlike tumor cells are genetically stable, and hence, it was assumed that there would be no resistance to these drugs. Further, as in normal physiological state, endothelial cells remain mostly quiescent; thus, antiangiogenic drugs would specifically target only the actively proliferating endothelial cells in blood vessels that supply to tumors. In addition, the process of physiological angiogenesis is distinct from tumor angiogenesis. Specific targeting of tumor blood vessels would result in no/less side effects than standard chemotherapy [303–305]. Success of antiangiogenic therapy in preclinical studies also led to impractical expectations. Recent conducted clinical trials have proved some of these expectations to be wrong and have revealed a number of adverse side effects associated with these agents. Very commons effects include hypertension, proteinuria, thromboembolism (cardiac ischemia, cerebral vascular accident, peripheral arterial thrombosis) cardiomyopathy, hemorrhage, delayed or impaired wound healing, gastrointestinal perforation, fistulas, reversible posterior leukoenkephalopathy syndrome, hypothyroidism, and myelosuppression [263, 306, 307]. Some of these adverse effects can be monitored and treated in a routine fashion. Excessive toxicity of some may require interruptions in treatment, reduction in dosage, or even total stoppage of treatment, which may limit the therapeutic efficacy. Interestingly, it has also been proposed that certain side effects of these drugs can be used as a predictive biomarker for their therapeutic efficacy. Here, we will discuss some of the commonly observed side effects associated with antiangiogenic treatments.

Hypertension, which is relatively easier to control, is the best reported cardiovascular adverse effect of VEGF/VEGFR inhibitors that occurs in approximately 25% of the patients. This may result in temporary interruption of anti-VEGF therapy if the patient is symptomatic or if there are chances that the rise in blood pressure may lead to other acute complications. These patients are treated with standard medications for hypertension, like calcium channel inhibitors or angiotensin-converting enzyme (ACE) inhibitors or with both. Anti-VEGF therapy at the same or lower dose is resumed once the blood pressure level is controlled. Rarely patients suffer from uncontrolled hypertension or hypertensive crisis (grade 4), with deadly complications. Such cases would require permanent discontinuation of anti-VEGF therapy. VEGF inhibitors cause vasoconstriction as signaling through VEGFR2 is essential for the synthesis of nitric oxide and prostaglandin I_2, which are required for endothelial cell-dependent vasodilation of blood vessels. This might be the reason for hypertension induced by anti-VEGF inhibitors. Another cause of hypertension may be rarefaction or the decrease in the number and density of arterioles and capillaries by anti-VEGF agents [245, 308–311].

VEGF inhibitors increase the risk of *thromboembolism*, mainly arterial thrombosis (about 5%). Cardiac and cerebral ischemia are most commonly seen in the treated patients. Patients with a history of arterial thromboembolism and elderly patients are at increased risk of developing aggravated form of this disease, which indicates the need for careful risk–benefit assessment before the start of antiangiogenic therapy. VEGF plays a major role in endothelial cell-platelet homeostasis. VEGF secreted by these cells prevent blood cells from adhering to the vasculature. In addition, VEGF also helps in the survival, proliferation and migration of endothelial cells. It also controls tissue factor-mediated coagulation cascade. Inhibition of VEGF signaling therefore might induce apoptosis of endothelial cells, disrupt the endothelial cell lining, and promote aggregation of platelets [245, 310, 312].

Proteinuria with significantly increased protein concentration in urine (more than 3.5 g protein loss in 24 hours) has been reported in 3% of patients in most of the clinical trials and in 7–8% of patients with RCC. VEGF is important in the homeostasis of kidney glomerulus, and it thus regulates the renal function. Inhibition of VEGF leads to improper glomerular function, decreased protein reabsorption from urine, or increase in filtration. Proteinuria rarely might lead to the development of nephrotic syndrome or result in renal failure. Thrombotic microangiopathy in the kidney possibly due to the direct targeting of VEGF has also been reported with the use of bevacizumab, VEGF-trap, and sunitinib [263, 311, 313, 314].

Hemorrhage or bleeding is increased in patients treated with anti-VEGF or anti-VEGFR agents and was a big concern in clinical trials. Bleeding has been reported in all clinical trials of bevacizumab (about 40%). Sunitinib and other VEGF/VEGFR inhibitors such as axitinib and VEGF-trap also cause bleeding. The risk of bleeding also varies with the tumor type, with tumors in the lungs and gastrointestinal tract showing the highest risk of excessive bleeding following anti-VEGF therapies. In patients with metastatic NSCLC, treatment with bevacizumab led to life-threatening hemoptysis. Sorafenib, sunitinib, axitinib, and motesanib also caused fatal pulmonary hemorrhage in patients with NSCLC. Targeting VEGF most likely results in the disruption of the endothelial cell-platelet interaction leading to loss of vascular integrity, which results in bleeding [306, 315–320].

Antiangiogenic inhibitors disturb the process of *wound healing* primarily because the process requires active angiogenesis at the wound site and is regulated by interactions between endothelial cells, platelets, and the coagulation cascade. VEGF is a major regulator of the process and blocking VEGF signaling results in disruption of the process. Impaired wound healing at the site of surgery caused by anti-VEGF/VEGFR agents may be due to dehiscence of wounds in patients who had undergone surgery prior to treatment with these agents or delay or lack of proper healing in patients who underwent surgery after the start of treatment. The problems in wound healing were reported to increase from 0.5% to 1.3% in CRC patients who underwent surgery before treatment with a combination of bevacizumab and chemotherapy in contrast to patients receiving chemotherapy alone. In CRC patients who underwent surgery while being treated with a combination of bevacizumab and chemotherapy compared to those who underwent surgery while being treated with chemotherapy alone, wound complications increased from 3.4% to 13% [306, 321–323].

Increased hypoxia and impaired wound healing due to inhibition of VEGF might increase the risk of *bowel perforation or formation of fistulas.* Patients with intra-abdominal tumors like ovarian, colorectal, gastric, and pancreatic are at even more risk of developing gastrointestinal fistulas or bowel perforations. In metastatic ovarian cancer patients, the risk of bowel perforation upon receiving bevacizumab ranged from 0% to 11.4%, with patients in more advanced stages of the disease or patients who had pelvic diseases and had undergone bowel surgery before, being at a higher risk. An increase in bowel perforation was also reported in metastatic CRC patients who received bevacizumab. Other drugs like sunitinib and sorafinib might also cause gastrointestinal perforation and fistulas [306, 324, 325].

As the thyroid gland is heavily fenestrated, VEGF blockage also results in reduction of blood capillaries and affects the proper functioning of the thyroid. *Hypothyroidism* has been reported in 36% of patients treated with TKIs [326, 327].

Hematopoietic cells and endothelial precursor cells express VEGFRs. Therefore, targeting VEGF or VEGFR might lead to *myelosuppression*. TKIs like sunitinib and sorafenib cause neutropenia and thrombocytopenia [317, 328, 329]. Apart from the above mentioned side effects, other adverse effects of antiangiogenic drugs include malaise, hand-foot syndrome, diarrhea, mucositis, skin reactions, hair loss, and hypophosphatemia [248, 330, 331].

4.8   RESISTANCE TO ANTIANGIOGENIC DRUGS

It was believed that resistance to antiangiogenic drugs would not develop as these drugs target genetically stable endothelial cells rather than the unstable tumor cells. However, clinical results have not supported this view and both intrinsic (when tumors do not respond from the beginning of treatment) and acquired (when tumors elicit initial response and then progress to unresponsive stage) resistance to antiangiogenic therapy is a challenging issue in the treatment course that has led to variable results and also failure of these drugs in many cases. Most of the antiangiogenic therapies are based on targeting the VEGF/VEGFR axis [24]. Several possible reasons and mechanisms have been cited for the development of resistance to these therapies. Endothelial cells of tumor blood vessels contain aberrant genomes that are not seen in the normal vasculature and are not as stable as was previously assumed to be [303, 304, 332, 333]. Furthermore, vascular regression caused due to antiangiogenic agents creates tissue hypoxia in the tumor microenvironment, which elevates the expression of HIF1α, which in turn promotes the upregulation of multiple alternate angiogenic factors that are not targeted by the antiangiogenic/anti-VEGF agents being used. Moreover, the hypoxic environment caused due to antiangiogenic treatment leads to the selection of tumor cells that are more invasive and hence drug resistant [24, 324–326]. Reports have further shown that targeting the VEGF pathway leads to the upregulation of other proangiogenic factors like ANG1-2, EGF, PDGF, FGF2 and interleukin 8 that induce the new pathways to restore angiogenesis in growing tumors. Thus, anti-VEGF drugs develop resistance by this alternate compensatory mechanism [327, 328]. Further, anti-VEGF agents create a major shift in cellular composition, increasing the number of cells like inflammatory cells and stromal fibroblasts, which are major sources of cytokines and non-VEGF angiogenic factors [329, 330]. In addition, recruitment of proangiogenic cells from the bone marrow, increased pericyte recruitment to form mature vessels (studies have also shown that VEGF-targeted therapies inhibit the growth of neo vessels but not that of established mature tumor vessels), or increased ability of tumor cells to utilize the established normal vessels may also be the different VEGF-independent ways of promoting angiogenesis [324, 326, 331]. The heterogeneous nature of the tumor vessels consisting of some vessels that are more responsive to these drugs while others that are relatively less responsive might be a reason for intrinsic resistance. Six blood vessel sub-types (mother vessels, capillaries, glomeruloid microvascular proliferations, vascular malformations, feeder arteries, and draining veins) have been identified in tumors. Among these, only the early vessels, mother vessels, and glomeruloid microvascular proliferations are dependent on the VEGF/VEGFR interaction and are therefore responsive to anti-VEGF-VEGFR treatment. The other four subtypes or the late vessels that arise from these early vessels are not dependent on VEGF/VEGFR interaction. Treatment might result in change in proportions of the sensitive and independent vessels, thus leading to acquired resistance [27]. Mechanisms of tumor neovascularization other than VEGF-dependent sprouting angiogenesis, which are not targeted by antiangiogenic drugs, like vessel cooption, vascular mimicry, intussusception, and vasculogenesis, also continue to support tumor angiogenesis and hence also contribute to antiangiogenic drug resistance and support further growth of the tumors [60, 332].

4.9   CONCLUSION

It is now well established that the process of angiogenesis plays an important role in cancer progression [17–21]. The various pro- and antiangiogenic factors and conditions that control this complex and multistep process have also been identified. Research in this field has also improved our understanding of the molecular pathways that dictate angiogenesis. Angiogenesis is now considered as a promising target for cancer therapy. The first generation of antiangiogenic drugs that were approved after successful phase III clinical trials, have been able to prolong the progression-free survival and, in some cases, the overall survival of patients suffering from different types of cancer. Unanticipated adverse effects of these antiangiogenic drugs have emerged with the extended use of the drugs. However, with the exceptions of some complications that might be life-threatening or fatal, the majority of these side effects are manageable [263, 306]. Because there are varied results following the use of antiangiogenic agents in the clinics, there is an urgent need to identify patients who are most likely to be benefitted from these drugs and patients who will present with adverse effects. Hence, the development of predictive markers for toxicity or efficacy of antiangiogenic drugs is needed for successful treatment using these angiogenesis inhibitors [306]. Studies are also being undertaken to determine the mechanisms of resistance to angiogenic inhibitors. Because late stages of the disease may not only depend on the VEGF pathway, the identification of other angiogenic pathways and proangiogenic molecules that control this process, such as PDGF, Ang2, and bFGF, will help in the development of newer therapeutic targets and agents that will act on more than one factor/pathway concurrently and thereby will be more effective. In addition, continued research and identification of novel targets that contribute to tumor angiogenesis and progression will further improve treatment using these inhibitors to achieve the goal of curing cancer.

4.10 SUMMARY

- Angiogenesis is necessary for tumor growth and progression.
- Multiple endogenous regulators (pro- and antiangiogenic) control the process of angiogenesis.
- Tumor blood vessels differ from normal blood vessels in structure and function.
- The multiple steps in the process of angiogenesis and pathways governing the process provide potential therapeutic targets.
- Targeting the tumor vasculature instead of directly targeting the genetically unstable tumor cells to treat cancer is advantageous.
- Over the years, numerous antiangiogenic agents have been identified and tested in clinical trials. Some of these agents have been approved for the treatment of different cancers.
- The antiangiogenic drugs alone or in combination with standard therapy have been successful in prolonging the progression-free survival

of patients. In some cases, the overall survival of patients has also improved.

- Expanded use of antiangiogenic agents has revealed some adverse effects.
- Intrinsic and acquired resistance to antiangiogenic therapy is a challenging issue.
- Development of predictive markers for toxicity or efficacy of antiangiogenic drugs is required for successful treatment using angiogenesis inhibitors.
- Identification of therapeutic targets that control more than one factors/pathways in angiogenesis will increase the efficacy of treatment.

ACKNOWLEDGMENTS

The authors thank Sujit Basu, MD, PhD, Professor, Department of Pathology, Division of Medical Oncology, Department of Internal Medicine and Comprehensive Cancer Center, The Ohio State University, for his insightful comments and suggestions.

KEYWORDS

- **angiogenesis**
- **anti angiogenic treatment**
- **tumor growth**

REFERENCES

1. Hunter, J., (2007). A treatise on the blood, inflammation, & gun-shot wounds 1794. *Clin. Orthop. Relat. Res., 458*, 27–34.
2. Mariotti, M., & Maier, J. A., (2006). Angiogenesis: an overview. In: *New Frontiers in Angiogenesis*, Forough, R., Springer, Netherlands, pp. 1–29.
3. Risau, W., (1997). Mechanisms of angiogenesis. *Nature, 386*, 671–674.
4. Flamme, I., Frölich, T., & Risau, W., (1997). Molecular mechanisms of vasculogenesis and embryonic angiogenesis. *J. Cell Physiol., 173*, 206–210.
5. Folkman, J., (1995). Angiogenesis in cancer, vascular, rheumatoid and other disease. *Nat. Med., 1*, 27–31.

6. Bergers, G., & Song, S., (2005). The role of pericytes in blood-vessel formation and maintenance. *Neuro. Oncol., 7*, 452–464.

7. Zhang, J., Cao, R., Zhang, Y., Jia, T., Cao, Y., & Wahlberg, E., (2009). Differential roles of PDGFR-alpha and PDGFR-beta in angiogenesis and vessel stability. *FASEB J., 23*, 153–163.

8. Armulik, A., Genové, G., & Betsholtz, C., (2011). Pericytes: developmental, physiological, & pathological perspectives, problems, & promises. *Dev. Cell., 21*, 193–215.

9. Hanahan, D., & Folkman, J., (1996). Patterns and emerging mechanisms of the angiogenic switch during tumorigenesis. *Cell, 86*, 353–364.

10. Carmeliet, P., & Jain, R. K., (2000). Angiogenesis in cancer and other diseases. *Nature, 407*, 249–257.

11. Carmeliet, P., (2003). Angiogenesis in health and disease. *Nat. Med., 9*, 653–660.

12. Dvorak, H. F., (2005). Angiogenesis: update 2005. *J. Thromb. Haemost., 3*, 1835–1842.

13. Carmeliet, P., & Jain, R. K., (2011). Molecular mechanisms and clinical applications of angiogenesis. *Nature, 473*, 298–307.

14. Ribatti, D., Vacca, A., & Dammacco, F., (1999). The role of the vascular phase in solid tumor growth: a historical review. *Neoplasia., 1*, 293–302.

15. Goldman, E., (1907). The growth of malignant disease in man and the lower animals with special reference to the vascular system. *Lancet., II*, 1236–1240.

16. Algire, G. H., Chalkley, H. W., Legallais, F. Y., & Park, H. D., (1945). Vascular reactions of normal and malignant tissues in vivo. I. Vascular reactions of mice to wounds and to normal and neoplastic transplants. *J. Natl. Cancer Inst., 6*, 73–85.

17. Folkman, J., (1971). Tumor angiogenesis: therapeutic implications. *N. Engl. J. Med., 285*, 1182–1186.

18. Gimbrone, M. A. Jr., Leapman, S. B., Cotran, R. S., & Folkman, J., (1972). Tumor dormancy in vivo by prevention of neovascularization. *J. Exp. Med., 136*, 261–276.

19. Langer, R., Conn, H., Vacanti, J., Haudenschild, C., & Folkman, J., (1980). Control of tumor growth in animals by infusion of an angiogenesis inhibitor. *Proc. Natl. Acad. Sci. USA, 77*, 4331–4335.

20. Kerbel, R. S., (1991). Inhibition of tumor angiogenesis as a strategy to circumvent acquired resistance to anti-cancer therapeutic agents. *Bioessays., 3*, 31–36.

21. Kim, K. J., Li, B., Winer, J., Armanini, M., Gillett, N., Phillips, H. S., & Ferrara, N., (1993). Inhibition of vascular endothelial growth factor-induced angiogenesis suppresses tumour growth in vivo. *Nature, 362*, 841–844.

22. Gasparini, G. 1., Longo, R., Toi, M., & Ferrara, N., (2005). Angiogenic inhibitors: a new therapeutic strategy in oncology. *Nat. Clin. Pract. Oncol., 2*, 562–577.

23. Potente, M., Gerhardt, H., & Carmeliet, P., (2011). Basic and therapeutic aspects of angiogenesis. *Cell, 146*, 873–887.

24. Dvorak, H. F., (2015). Tumor Stroma, Tumor Blood Vessels, & Antiangiogenesis Therapy. *Cancer J., 21*, 237–243.

25. Folkman, J., (1990). What is the evidence that tumors are angiogenesis dependent? *J. Natl. Cancer Inst., 82*, 4–6.

26. Folkman, J., (2002). Role of angiogenesis in tumor growth and metastasis. *Semin. Oncol., 29*, 15–18.

27. Nagy, J. A., Chang, S. H., Dvorak, A. M., & Dvorak, H. F., (2009). Why are tumour blood vessels abnormal and why is it important to know? *Br. J. Cancer, 100*, 865–869.

28. Lee, H. T., Xue, J., Chou, P. C., Zhou, A., Yang, P., Conrad, C. A., Aldape, K. D., Priebe, W., Patterson, C., Sawaya, R., Xie, K., & Huang, S., (2015). Stat3 orchestrates

interaction between endothelial and tumor cells and inhibition of Stat3 suppresses brain metastasis of breast cancer cells. *Oncotarget, 6,* 10016–10029.

29. Bockhorn, M., Jain, R. K., & Munn, L. L., (2007). Active versus passive mechanisms in metastasis: do cancer cells crawl into vessels, or are they pushed? *Lancet. Oncol., 8,* 444–448.

30. Bielenberg, D. R., & Zetter, B. R., (2015). The Contribution of Angiogenesis to the Process of Metastasis. *Cancer, J., 2,* 1267–1273.

31. Papetti, M., Herman I. M., (2002). Mechanisms of normal and tumor-derived angiogenesis. *Am. J. Physiol. Cell Physiol., 282,* 947–970.

32. Blood, C. H., & Zetter, B. R., (1990). Tumor interactions with the vasculature: angiogenesis and tumor metastasis. *Biochim. Biophys. Acta., (1032),* 89–118.

33. Li, C. Y., Shan, S., Huang, Q., Braun, R. D., Lanzen, J., Hu, K., Lin, P., & Dewhirst, M. W., (2000). Initial stages of tumor cell-induced angiogenesis: evaluation via skin window chambers in rodent models. *J. Natl. Cancer Inst., 92,* 143–147.

34. Van Zijl, F., Krupitza, G., & Mikulits, W., (2011). Initial steps of metastasis: cell invasion and endothelial transmigration. *Mutat. Res., 728,* 23–34.

35. Millauer, B., Longhi, M. P., Plate, K. H., Shawver, L. K., Risau, W., Ullrich, A., & Strawn, L. M., (1996). Dominant-negative inhibition of Flk-1 suppresses the growth of many tumor types in vivo. *Cancer Res., 56,* 1615–1620.

36. Kumar, C. C., Malkowski, M., Yin, Z., Tanghetti, E., Yaremko, B., Nechuta, T., Varner, J., Liu, M., & Smith, E. M., (2001). Inhibition of angiogenesis and tumor growth by SCH221153, a dual alpha(v)beta3 and alpha(v)beta5 integrin receptor antagonist. *Cancer Res., 61,* 2232–2238.

37. Kudo, S., Konda, R., Obara, W., Kudo, D., Tani, K., Nakamura, Y., & Fujioka, T., (2007). Inhibition of tumor growth through suppression of angiogenesis by brain-specific angiogenesis inhibitor 1 gene transfer in murine renal cell carcinoma. *Oncol. Rep., 18,* 785–791.

38. Vartanian, R. K., & Weidner, N., (1994). Correlation of intratumoral endothelial cell proliferation with microvessel density (tumor angiogenesis) and tumor cell proliferation in breast carcinoma. *Am. J. Pathol., 144,* 1188–1194.

39. Imura, S., Miyake, H., Izumi, K., Tashiro, S., & Uehara, H., (2004). Correlation of vascular endothelial cell proliferation with microvessel density and expression of vascular endothelial growth factor and basic fibroblast growth factor in hepatocellular carcinoma. *J. Med. Invest., 51,* 202–209.

40. Rak, J. W., St Croix, B. D., & Kerbel, R. S., (1995). Consequences of angiogenesis for tumor progression, metastasis and cancer therapy. *Anticancer Drugs, 6,* 3–18.

41. Indraccolo, S., Minuzzo, S., Masiero, M., Pusceddu, I., Persano, L., Moserle, L., Reboldi, A., Favaro, E., Mecarozzi, M., Di Mario, G., Screpanti, I., Ponzoni, M., Doglioni, C., & Amadori, A., (2009). Cross-talk between tumor and endothelial cells involving the Notch3-Dll4 interaction marks escape from tumor dormancy. *Cancer Res., 69,* 1314–1323.

42. Zeng, Q., Li, S., Chepeha, D. B., Giordano, T. J., Li, J., Zhang, H., Polverini, P. J., Nor, J., Kitajewski, J., & Wang, C. Y., (2005). Crosstalk between tumor and endothelial cells promotes tumor angiogenesis by MAPK activation of Notch signaling. *Cancer Cell, 8,* 13–23.

43. Brem, S., Cotran, R., & Folkman, J., (1972). Tumor angiogenesis: a quantitative method for histologic grading. *J. Natl. Cancer Inst., 48,* 347–356.

44. Weidner, N., Carroll, P. R., Flax, J., Blumenfeld, W., & Folkman, J., (1993). Tumor angiogenesis correlates with metastasis in invasive prostate carcinoma. *Am. J. Pathol., 143*, 401–409.

45. Labiche, A., Elie, N., Herlin, P., Denoux, Y., Crouet, H., Heutte, N., Joly, F., Héron, J. F., Gauduchon, P., & Henry-Amar, M., (2009). Prognostic significance of tumour vascularisation on survival of patients with advanced ovarian carcinoma. *Histol. Histopathol., 24*, 425–435.

46. Fidler, I. J., & Ellis, L. M., (1994). The implications of angiogenesis for the biology and therapy of cancer metastasis. *Cell, 79*, 185–188.

47. Welti, J., Loges, S., Dimmeler, S., & Carmeliet, P., (2013). Recent molecular discoveries in angiogenesis and antiangiogenic therapies in cancer. *J. Clin. Invest., 123*, 3190–3200.

48. Hillen, F., & Griffioen, A. W., (2007). Tumour vascularization: sprouting angiogenesis and beyond. *Cancer Metastasis Rev., 26*, 489–502.

49. Ribatti, D., & Crivellato, E., (2012). "Sprouting angiogenesis", a reappraisal. *Dev. Biol., 372*, 157–165.

50. Bergers, G., & Benjamin, L. E., (2003). Tumorigenesis and the angiogenic switch. *Nat. Rev. Cancer, 3*, 401–410.

51. Ferrara, N., Gerber, H. P., & Le Couter, J., (2003). The biology of VEGF and its receptors. *Nature Medicine, 9*, 669–676.

52. Jain, R. K., (2003). Molecular regulation of vessel maturation. *Nature Medicine, 9*, 685–693.

53. Patan, S., Haenni, B., & Burri, P. H., (1993). Evidence for intussusceptive capillary growth in the chicken chorio-allantoic membrane (CAM). *Anatomy and Embryology (Berl), 187*, 121–130.

54. Patan, S., Munn, L. L., & Jain, R. K., (1996). Intussusceptive microvascular growth in a human colon adenocarcinoma xenograft: A novel mechanism of tumor angiogenesis. *Microvascular Research, 51*, 260–272.

55. Döme, B., Hendrix, M. J., Paku, S., Tóvári, J., & Tímár, J., (2007). Alternative vascularization mechanisms in cancer: Pathology and therapeutic implications. *Am. J. Pathol., 170*, 1–15.

56. Asahara, T., Murohara, T., Sullivan, A., Silver, M., van der Zee, R., Li, T., Witzenbichler, B., Schatteman, G., & Isner, J. M., (1997). Isolation of putative progenitor endothelial cells for angiogenesis. *Science, 275*, 964–967.

57. Kalka, C., Masuda, H., Takahashi, T., Kalka-Moll, W. M., Silver, M., Kearney, M., Li, T., Isner, J. M., & Asahara, T., (2000). Transplantation of ex vivo expanded endothelial progenitor cells for therapeutic neovascularization. *Proc. Natl. Acad. Sci. USA, 97*, 3422–3427.

58. Kopp, H. G., Ramos, C. A., & Rafii, S., (2006). Contribution of endothelial progenitors and proangiogenic hematopoietic cells to vascularization of tumor and ischemic tissue. *Curr. Opin. Hematol., 13*, 175–181.

59. Holash, J., Maisonpierre, P. C., Compton, D., Boland, P., Alexander, C. R., Zagzag, D., Yancopoulos, G. D., & Wiegand, S. J., (1999). Vessel cooption, regression, & growth in tumors mediated by angiopoietins and VEGF. *Science, 284*, 1994–1998.

60. Maniotis, A. J., Folberg, R., Hess, A., Seftor, E. A., Gardner, L. M., Pe'er, J., Trent, J. M., Meltzer, P. S., & Hendrix, M. J., (1999). Vascular channel formation by human melanoma cells in vivo and in vitro: vasculogenic mimicry. *Am. J. Pathol., 155*, 739–752.

61. Nagy, J. A., Dvorak, A. M., & Dvorak, H. F., (2012). Vascular hyperpermeability, angiogenesis, & stroma generation. *Cold Spring Harb. Perspect. Med., 2*, a006544.

62. Fu, Y., Nagy, J., Dvorak, A., & Dvorak, H., (2007). Tumor blood vessels: structure and function. In *Cancer Drug Discovery and Function. Antiangiogenic Agents in Cancer Therapy,* Teicher, B., Ellis, L. Eds., Humana Press Inc: Totowa, NJ, pp. 205–224.

63. Morikawa, S., Baluk, P., Kaidoh, T., Haskell, A., Jain, R. K., & McDonald, D. M., (2002). Abnormalities in pericytes on blood vessels and endothelial sprouts in tumors. *Am. J. Pathol., 160*, 985–1000.

64. McDonald, D. M., & Baluk, P., (2002). Significance of blood vessel leakiness in cancer. *Cancer Res., 62*, 5381–5385.

65. Hosaka, K., Yang, Y., Seki, T., Nakamura, M., Andersson, P., Rouhi, P., Yang, X., Jensen, L., Lim, S., Feng, N., Xue, Y., Li, X., Larsson, O., Ohhashi, T., & Cao, Y., (2013). Tumour PDGF-BB expression levels determine dual effects of anti-PDGF drugs on vascular remodelling and metastasis. *Nat. Commun., 4*, 2129.

66. Akino, T., Hida, K., Hida, Y., Tsuchiya, K., Freedman, D., Muraki, C., Ohga, N., Matsuda, K., Akiyama, K., Harabayashi, T., Shinohara, N., Nonomura, K., Klagsbrun, M., & Shindoh, M., (2009). Cytogenetic abnormalities of tumor-associated endothelial cells in human malignant tumors. *Am. J. Pathol., 175*, 2657–2667.

67. Chang, Y. S., di Tomaso, E., McDonald, D. M., Jones, R., Jain, R. K., & Munn, L. L., (2000). Mosaic blood vessels in tumors: frequency of cancer cells in contact with flowing blood. *Proc. Natl. Acad. Sci. USA, 97*, 14608–14613.

68. Sood, A. K., Seftor, E. A., Fletcher, M. S., Gardner, L. M., Heidger, P. M., Buller, R. E., Seftor, R. E., & Hendrix, M. J., (2001). Molecular determinants of ovarian cancer plasticity. *Am. J. Pathol., 158*, 1279–1288.

69. Ziyad, S., & Iruela-Arispe, M. L., (2011). Molecular mechanisms of tumor angiogenesis. *Genes Cancer, 2*, 1085–1096.

70. Nagy, J. A., Benjamin, L., Zeng, H., Dvorak, A. M., & Dvorak, H. F., (2008). Vascular permeability, vascular hyperpermeability and angiogenesis. *Angiogenesis, 11*, 109–119.

71. Thompson, W. D., Smith, E. B., Stirk, C. M., Marshall, F. I., Stout, A. J., & Kocchar, A., (1992). Angiogenic activity of fibrin degradation products is located in fibrin fragment E. *J. Pathol., 168*, 47–53.

72. Maglione, D., Guerriero, V., Viglietto, G., Delli-Bovi, P., & Persico, M. G., (1991). Isolation of a human placenta cDNA coding for a protein related to the vascular permeability factor. *Proc. Natl. Acad. Sci. USA, 88*, 9267–9271.

73. Ellis, L. M., & Hicklin, D. J., (2008). VEGF-targeted therapy: mechanisms of antitumour activity. *Nat. Rev. Cancer, 8*, 579–591.

74. Otrock, Z. K., Mahfouz, R. A., Makarem, J. A., & Shamseddine, A. I., (2007). Understanding the biology of angiogenesis: review of the most important molecular mechanisms. *Blood Cells Mol. Dis., 39*, 212–220.

75. Brown, L. F., Detmar, M., Claffey, K., Nagy, J. A., Feng, D., Dvorak, A. M., & Dvorak, H. F., (1997). Vascular permeability factor/vascular endothelial growth factor: a multifunctional angiogenic cytokine. *EXS, 79*, 233–269.

76. Dvorak, H. F., Nagy, J. A., Feng, D., Brown, L. F., & Dvorak, A. M., (1999). Vascular permeability factor/vascular endothelial growth factor and the significance of microvascular hyperpermeability in angiogenesis. *Curr. Top. Microbiol. Immunol., 237*, 97–132.

77. Ferrara, N., (2004). Vascular endothelial growth factor as a target for anticancer therapy. *Oncologist., 9*, 2–10.

78. Nör, J. E., Christensen, J., Mooney, D. J., & Polverini, P. J., (1999). Vascular endothelial growth factor (VEGF)-mediated angiogenesis is associated with enhanced endothelial cell survival and induction of Bcl-2 expression. *Am. J. Pathol., 154*, 375–384.

79. Tischer, E., Mitchell, R., Hartman, T., Silva, M., Gospodarowicz, D., Fiddes, J. C., & Abraham, J. A., (1991). The human gene for vascular endothelial growth factor. Multiple protein forms are encoded through alternative exon splicing. *J. Biol. Chem., 266*, 11947–11954.

80. Neufeld, G., Cohen, T., Gengrinovitch, S., & Poltorak, Z., (1999). Vascular endothelial growth factor (VEGF) and its receptors. *FASEB J., 13*, 9–22.

81. Dvorak, H. F., (2002). Vascular permeability factor/vascular endothelial growth factor: a critical cytokine in tumor angiogenesis and a potential target for diagnosis and therapy. *J. Clin. Oncol., 20*, 4368–4380.

82. Silins, G., Grimmond, S., Egerton, M., & Hayward, N., (1997). Analysis of the promoter region of the human VEGF-related factor gene. *Biochem. Biophys. Res. Commun., 230*, 413–418.

83. Nash, A. D., Baca, M., Wright, C., & Scotney, P. D., (2006). The biology of vascular endothelial growth factor-B (VEGF-B). *Pulm. Pharmacol. Ther., 19*, 61–69.

84. Yang, X., Zhang, Y., Hosaka, K., Andersson, P., Wang, J., Tholander, F., Cao, Z., Morikawa, H., Tegnér, J., Yang, Y., Iwamoto, H., Lim. S., & Cao, Y., (2015). VEGF-B promotes cancer metastasis through a VEGF-A-independent mechanism and serves as a marker of poor prognosis for cancer patients. *Proc. Natl. Acad. Sci. USA, 112*, E2900-E2909.

85. Achen, M. G., Jeltsch, M., Kukk, E., Mäkinen, T., Vitali, A., Wilks, A. F., Alitalo, K., & Stacker, S. A., (1998). Vascular endothelial growth factor D (VEGF-D) is a ligand for the tyrosine kinases VEGF receptor 2 (Flk1) and VEGF receptor 3 (Flt4). *Proc. Natl. Acad. Sci. USA., 95*, 548–553.

86. Lee, J., Gray, A., Yuan, J., Luoh, S. M., Avraham, H., & Wood, W. I., (1996). Vascular endothelial growth factor-related protein: a ligand and specific activator of the tyrosine kinase receptor Flt4 . *Proc. Natl. Acad. Sci. USA, 93*, 1988–1992.

87. Cao, Y., Linden, P., Farnebo, J., Cao, R., Eriksson, A., Kumar, V., Qi, J. H., Claesson-Welsh, L., & Alitalo, K., (1998). Vascular endothelial growth factor C induces angiogenesis in vivo. *Proc. Natl. Acad. Sci. USA, 95*, 14389–14394.

88. Marconcini, L., Marchio, S., Morbidelli, L., Cartocci, E., Albini, A., Ziche, M., Bussolino, F., & Oliviero, S., (1999). c-fos-induced growth factor/vascular endothelial growth factor D induces angiogenesis in vivo and in vitro. *Proc. Natl. Acad. Sci. USA., 96*, 9671–9676.

89. Shibuya, M., (2011). Vascular endothelial growth factor (VEGF) and its receptor (VEGFR) signaling in angiogenesis: A crucial target for anti- and pro-angiogenic therapies. *Genes Cancer, 2*, 1097–1105.

90. De Falco, S., (2012). The discovery of placenta growth factor and its biological activity. *Exp. Mol. Med., 44*, 1–9.

91. Carmeliet, P., Moons, L., Luttun, A., Vincenti, V., Compernolle, V., De Mol, M., Wu, Y., Bono, F., Devy, L., Beck, H., Scholz, D., Acker, T., DiPalma, T., Dewerchin, M., Noel, A., Stalmans, I., Barra, A., Blacher, S., VandenDriessche, T., Ponten, A., Eriksson, U., Plate, K. H., Foidart, J. M., Schaper, W., Charnock-Jones, D. S., Hicklin, D. J., Herbert, J. M., Collen, D., & Persico, M. G., (2001). Synergism between vascular endothelial growth factor and placental growth factor contributes to angiogenesis and plasma extravasation in pathological conditions. *Nat. Med., 7*, 575–583.

92. Augustin, H. G., Koh, G. Y., Thurston, G., & Alitalo, K., (2009). Control of vascular morphogenesis and homeostasis through the angiopoietin-Tie system. *Nat. Rev. Mol. Cell Biol., 10*, 165–177.

93. Armulik, A., Abramsson, A., & Betsholtz, C., (2005). Endothelial/pericyte interactions. *Circ. Res., 97*, 512–523.

94. Fiedler, U., Scharpfenecker, M., Koidl, S., Hegen, A., Grunow, V., Schmidt, J. M., Kriz, W., Thurston, G., & Augustin, H. G., (2004). The Tie-2 ligand angiopoietin-2 is stored in and rapidly released upon stimulation from endothelial cell Weibel-Palade bodies. *Blood, 103*, 4150–4156.

95. Schubert, S. Y., Benarroch, A., Monter-Solans, J., & Edelman, E. R., (2011). Primary monocytes regulate endothelial cell survival through secretion of angiopoietin-1 and activation of endothelial Tie2. *Arterioscler. Thromb. Vasc. Biol., 31*, 870–875.

96. Saharinen, P., Kerkelä, K., Ekman, N., Marron, M., Brindle, N., Lee, G. M., Augustin, H., Koh, G. Y., & Alitalo, K., (2005). Multiple angiopoietin recombinant proteins activate the Tie1 receptor tyrosine kinase and promote its interaction with Tie2. *J. Cell Biol., 169*, 239–243.

97. Puri, M. C., Rossant, J., Alitalo, K., Bernstein, A., & Partanen, J., (1995). The receptor tyrosine kinase TIE is required for integrity and survival of vascular endothelial cells. *EMBO J., 14*, 5884–5891.

98. Thomas, M., & Augustin, H. G., (2009). The role of the Angiopoietins in vascular morphogenesis. *Angiogenesis, 12*, 125–137.

99. Thomas, K. A., (1987). Fibroblast growth factors. *FASEB J., 1*, 434–440.

100. Cross, M. J., & Claesson-Welsh, L., (2001). FGF and VEGF function in angiogenesis: signalling pathways, biological responses and therapeutic inhibition. *Trends Pharmacol. Sci., 22*, 201–207.

101. Beenken, A., & Mohammadi, M., (2009). The FGF family: biology, pathophysiology and therapy. *Nat. Rev. Drug Discov., 8*, 235–253.

102. Miller, D. L., Ortega, S., Bashayan, O., Basch, R., & Basilico, C., (2000). Compensation by fibroblast growth factor 1 (FGF1) does not account for the mild phenotypic defects observed in FGF2 null mice. *Mol Cell Biol., 20*, 2260–2268.

103. Fons, P., Gueguen-Dorbes, G., Herault, J. P., Geronimi, F., Tuyaret, J., Frédérique, D., Schaeffer, P., Volle-Challier, C., Herbert, J. M., & Bono, F., (2015). Tumor vasculature is regulated by FGF/FGFR signaling-mediated angiogenesis and bone marrow-derived cell recruitment: this mechanism is inhibited by SSR128129E, the first allosteric antagonist of FGFRs. *J. Cell Physiol., 230*, 43–51.

104. Turner, N., & Grose, R., (2010). Fibroblast growth factor signalling: from development to cancer. *Nat. Rev. Cancer, 10*, 116–129.

105. Gullick, W. J., (2009). The epidermal growth factor system of ligands and receptors in cancer. *Eur. J. Cancer, 45*, 205–210.

106. Van Cruijsen, H., Giaccone, G., & Hoekman, K., (2005). Epidermal growth factor receptor and angiogenesis: Opportunities for combined anticancer strategies. *Int. J. Cancer, 117*, 883–888.

107. Heldin, C. H., & Westermark, B., (1999). Mechanism of action and in vivo role of platelet-derived growth factor. *Physiol. Rev., 79*, 1283–1316.

108. Cao, Y., Cao, R., & Hedlund, E. M., (2008). Regulation of tumor angiogenesis and metastasis by FGF and PDGF signaling pathways. *J. Mol. Med. (Berl), 86*, 785–789.

109. Battegay, E. J., Rupp, J., Iruela-Arispe, L., Sage, E. H., & Pech, M., (1994). PDGF-BB modulates endothelial proliferation and angiogenesis in vitro via PDGF beta-receptors. *J. Cell Biol., 125*, 917–928.

110. Nicosia, R. F., Nicosia, S. V., & Smith, M., (1994). Vascular endothelial growth factor, platelet-derived growth factor, & insulin-like growth factor-1 promote rat aortic angiogenesis in vitro. *Am. J. Pathol., 145*, 1023–1029.

111. Levéen, P., Pekny, M., Gebre-Medhin, S., Swolin, B., Larsson, E., & Betsholtz, C., (1994). Mice deficient for PDGF B show renal, cardiovascular, & hematological abnormalities. *Genes Dev., 8*, 1875–1887.

112. Nishishita, T., & Lin, P. C., (2004). Angiopoietin 1, PDGF-B, & TGF-beta gene regulation in endothelial cell and smooth muscle cell interaction. *J. Cell Biochem, 91*, 584–593.

113. Uutela, M., Wirzenius, M., Paavonen, K., Rajantie, I., He, Y., Karpanen, T., Lohela, M., Wiig, H., Salven, P., Pajusola, K., Eriksson, U., & Alitalo, K., (2004). PDGF-D induces macrophage recruitment, increased interstitial pressure, & blood vessel maturation during angiogenesis. *Blood, 104*, 3198–3204.

114. Nagase, H., & Woessner, J. F., (1999). Jr. Matrix metalloproteinases, *J. Biol. Chem., 274*, 21491–21494.

115. McCawley, L. J., & Matrisian, L. M., (2001). Matrix metalloproteinases: They're not just for matrix anymore! *Curr. Opin. Cell Biol., 13*, 534–540.

116. Löffek, S., Schilling, O., & Franzke, C. W., (2011). Series "matrix metalloproteinases in lung health and disease": Biological role of matrix metalloproteinases: a critical balance. *Eur. Respir. J., 38*, 191–208.

117. Deryugina, E. I., Zajac, E., Juncker-Jensen, A., Kupriyanova, T. A., Welter, L., & Quigley, J. P., (2014). Tissue-infiltrating neutrophils constitute the major in vivo source of angiogenesis-inducing MMP-9 in the tumor microenvironment. *Neoplasia., 16*, 771–788.

118. Takata, F., Dohgu, S., Matsumoto, J., Takahashi, H., Machida, T., Wakigawa, T., Harada, E., Miyaji, H., Koga, M., Nishioka, T., Yamauchi, A., & Kataoka, Y., (2011). Brain pericytes among cells constituting the blood-brain barrier are highly sensitive to tumor necrosis factor-α, releasing matrix metalloproteinase-9 and migrating in vitro. *J. Neuroinflammation., 26*, 8, 106.

119. Stamenkovic, I., (2003). Extracellular matrix remodelling: the role of matrix metalloproteinases. *J. Pathol., 200*, 448–464.

120. Van Hinsbergh, V. W., & Koolwijk, P., (2008). Endothelial sprouting and angiogenesis: matrix metalloproteinases in the lead. *Cardiovasc. Res., 78*, 203–212.

121. Rundhaug, J. E., (2005). Matrix metalloproteinases and angiogenesis. *J. Cell Mol. Med., 9*, 267–285.

122. Hess, A. R., Seftor, E. A., Seftor, R. E., & Hendrix, M. J., (2003). Phosphoinositide 3-kinase regulates membrane Type 1-matrix metalloproteinase (MMP) and MMP-2 activity during melanoma cell vasculogenic mimicry. *Cancer Res., 63*, 4757–4762.

123. Heissig, B., Hattori, K., Dias, S., Friedrich, M., Ferris, B., Hackett, N. R., Crystal, R. G., Besmer, P., Lyden, D., Moore, M. A., Werb, Z., & Rafii, S., (2002). Recruitment of stem and progenitor cells from the bone marrow niche requires MMP-9 mediated release of kit-ligand. *Cell, 109*, 625–637.

124. Chantrain, C. F., Shimada, H., Jodele, S., Groshen, S., Ye, W., Shalinsky, D. R., Werb, Z., Coussens, L. M., & DeClerck, Y. A., (2004). Stromal matrix metalloproteinase-9

regulates the vascular architecture in neuroblastoma by promoting pericyte recruitment. *Cancer Res., 64*, 1675–1686.

125. Patterson, B. C., & Sang, Q. A., (1997). Angiostatin-converting enzyme activities of human matrilysin (MMP-7) and gelatinase B/type IV collagenase (MMP-9). *J. Biol. Chem., 272*, 28823–28825.

126. Pozzi, A., LeVine, W. F., & Gardner, H. A., (2002). Low plasma levels of matrix metalloproteinase 9 permit increased tumor angiogenesis. *Oncogene., 21*, 272–281.

127. O'Reilly, M. S., Holmgren, L., Shing, Y., Chen, C., Rosenthal, R. A., Moses, M., Lane, W. S., Cao, Y., Sage, E. H., & Folkman, J., (1994). Angiostatin: a novel angiogenesis inhibitor that mediates the suppression of metastases by a Lewis lung carcinoma. *Cell, 79*, 315–328.

128. Dong, Z., Kumar, R., Yang, X., & Fidler, I. J., (1997). Macrophage-derived metalloelastase is responsible for the generation of angiostatin in Lewis lung carcinoma. *Cell, 88*, 801–810.

129. Kalluri, R., (2003). Basement membranes: structure, assembly and role in tumour angiogenesis. *Nat. Rev. Cancer, 3*, 422–433.

130. Sang, Q. X., (1998). Complex role of matrix metalloproteinases in angiogenesis. *Cell Res., 8*, 171–177.

131. Moses, M. A., (1997). The regulation of neovascularization of matrix metalloproteinases and their inhibitors. *Stem Cells, 15*, 180–189.

132. Liao, D., & Johnson, R. S., (2007). Hypoxia: a key regulator of angiogenesis in cancer. *Cancer Metastasis Rev., 26*, 281–290.

133. Neeman, M., Abramovitch, R., Schiffenbauer, Y. S., & Tempel, C., (1997). Regulation of angiogenesis by hypoxic stress: from solid tumours to the ovarian follicle. *Int. J. Exp. Pathol., 78*, 57–70.

134. Wang, Z., Dabrosin, C., Yin, X., Fuster, M. M., Arreola, A., Rathmell, W. K., Generali, D., Nagaraju, G. P., El-Rayes, B., Ribatti, D., Chen, Y. C., Honoki, K., Fujii, H., Georgakilas, A. G., Nowsheen, S., Amedei, A., Niccolai, E., Amin, A., Ashraf, S. S., Helferich, B., Yang, X., Guha, G., Bhakta, D., Ciriolo, M. R., Aquilano, K., Chen, S., Halicka, D., Mohammed, S. I., Azmi, A. S., Bilsland, A., Keith, W. N., & Jensen, L. D., (2015). Broad targeting of angiogenesis for cancer prevention and therapy. *Semin. Cancer Biol., 35*, 224–243.

135. Masoud, G. N., & Li, W., (2015). HIF-1α pathway: role, regulation and intervention for cancer therapy. *Acta. Pharm. Sin. B., 5*, 378–389.

136. Mori, H., Yao, Y., Learman, B. S., Kurozumi, K., Ishida, J., Ramakrishnan, S. K., Overmyer, K. A., Xue, X., Cawthorn, W. P., Reid, M. A., Taylor, M., Ning, X., Shah, Y. M., & MacDougald, O. A., (2016). Induction of WNT11 by hypoxia and hypoxia-inducible factor-1α regulates cell proliferation, migration and invasion. *Sci. Rep., 10*(6), 21520.

137. Kelly, B. D., Hackett, S. F., Hirota, K., Oshima, Y., Cai, Z., Berg-Dixon, S., Rowan, A., Yan, Z., Campochiaro, P. A., & Semenza, G. L., (2003). Cell type-specific regulation of angiogenic growth factor gene expression and induction of angiogenesis in nonischemic tissue by a constitutively active form of hypoxia-inducible factor 1. *Circ. Res., 28*(93), 1074–1081.

138. Ceradini, D. J., Kulkarni, A. R., Callaghan, M. J., Tepper, O. M., Bastidas, N., Kleinman, M. E., Capla, J. M., Galiano, R. D., Levine, J. P., & Gurtner, G. C., (2004). Progenitor cell trafficking is regulated by hypoxic gradients through HIF-1 induction of SDF-1. *Nat. Med., 10*, 858–864.

139. Jensen, R. L., Ragel, B. T., Whang, K., & Gillespie, D., (2006). Inhibition of hypoxia inducible factor-1alpha (HIF-1alpha) decreases vascular endothelial growth factor (VEGF) secretion and tumor growth in malignant gliomas. *J. Neurooncol., 78*, 233–247.

140. Bos, R., Zhong, H., Hanrahan, C. F., Mommers, E. C., Semenza, G. L., Pinedo, H. M., Abeloff, M. D., Simons, J. W., van Diest, P. J., van der Wall, E., (2001). Levels of hypoxia-inducible factor-1 alpha during breast carcinogenesis. Levels of hypoxia-inducible factor-1 alpha during breast carcinogenesis. *J. Natl. Cancer Inst., 93*, 309–314.

141. Ravi, R., Mookerjee, B., Bhujwalla, Z. M., Sutter, C. H., Artemov, D., Zeng, Q., Dillehay, L. E., Madan, A., Semenza, G. L., & Bedi, A., (2000). Regulation of tumor angiogenesis by p53-induced degradation of hypoxia-inducible factor 1alpha. *Genes Dev. Jan. 1, 14*(1), 34–44.

142. Gillespie, D. L., Flynn, J. R., Ragel, B. T., Arce-Larreta, M., Kelly, D. A., Tripp, S. R., & Jensen, R. L., (2009). Silencing of HIF-1alpha by RNA interference in human glioma cells in vitro and in vivo. *Methods Mol. Biol., 487*, 283–301.

143. Park, Y. S., Kim, G., Jin, Y. M., Lee, J. Y., Shin, J. W., & Jo, I., (2016). Expression of angiopoietin-1 in hypoxic pericytes: Regulation by hypoxia-inducible factor-2α and participation in endothelial cell migration and tube formation. *Biochem. Biophys. Res. Commun., 469*, 263–269.

144. Hu, K., Babapoor-Farrokhran, S., Rodrigues, M., Deshpande, M., Puchner, B., Kashiwabuchi, F., Hassan, S. J., Asnaghi, L., Handa, J. T., Merbs, S., Eberhart, C. G., Semenza, G. L., Montaner, S., & Sodhi, A., (2016). Hypoxia-inducible factor 1 upregulation of both VEGF and ANGPTL4 is required to promote the angiogenic phenotype in uveal melanoma. *Oncotarget*, doi: 10. 18632/oncotarget. 6868. [Epub ahead of print].

145. Kütscher, C., Lampert, F. M., Kunze, M., Markfeld-Erol, F., Stark, G. B., & Finkenzeller, G., (2016). Overexpression of hypoxia-inducible factor-1 alpha improves vasculogenesis-related functions of endothelial progenitor cells. *Microvasc Res., 105*, 85–92.

146. Pichiule, P., Chavez, J. C., & LaManna, J. C., (2004). Hypoxic regulation of angiopoietin-2 expression in endothelial cells. *J. Biol. Chem., 279*, 12171–12180.

147. Willis, R. A., (1973). *The Spread of Tumors in the Human Body*, 3rd edition., Butterworths: London,.

148. Li, S., Sun, Y., & Gao, D., (2013). Role of the nervous system in cancer metastasis. *Oncol. Lett., 5*, 1101–1111.

149. Seifert, P., & Spitznas, M., (2001). Tumours may be innervated. *Virchows. Arch., 438*, 228–231.

150. Poeschl, E. M., Pollheimer, M. J., Kornprat, P., Lindtner, R. A., Schlemmer, A., Rehak, P., Vieth, M., & Langner, C., (2010). Perineural invasion: correlation with aggressive phenotype and independent prognostic variable in both colon and rectum cancer. *J. Clin. Oncol., 28*, e358-e360.

151. Hibi, T., Mori, T., Fukuma, M., Yamazaki, K., Hashiguchi, A., Yamada, T., Tanabe, M., Aiura, K., Kawakami, T., Ogiwara, A., Kosuge, T., Kitajima, M., Kitagawa, Y., & Sakamoto, M., (2009). Synuclein-gamma is closely involved in perineural invasion and distant metastasis in mouse models and is a novel prognostic factor in pancreatic cancer. *Clin. Cancer Res., 15*, 2864–2871.

152. Karak, S. G., Quatrano, N., Buckley, J., & Ricci, A., (2010). Jr. Prevalence and significance of perineural invasion in invasive breast carcinoma. *Conn. Med., 74*, 17–21.

153. Tsuru, H., Tanimitsu, N., & Hirai, T., (2002). Role of perivascular sympathetic nerves and regional differences in the features of sympathetic innervation of the vascular system. *Jpn. J. Pharmacol., 88*, 9–13.

154. Carmeliet, P., (2003). Blood vessels and nerves: Common signals, pathways and diseases. *Nat. Rev. Genet., 4*, 710–720.

155. Krimer, L. S, Muly, E. C. 3rd., Williams, G. V., & Goldman-Rakic, P. S., (1998). Dopaminergic regulation of cerebral cortical microcirculation. *Nat. Neurosci., 1*, 286–289.

156. Chakroborty, D., Sarkar, C., Yu, H., Wang, J., Liu, Z., Dasgupta, P. S., & Basu, S., (2011). Dopamine stabilizes tumor blood vessels by up-regulating angiopoietin 1 expression in pericytes and Kruppel-like factor-2 expression in tumor endothelial cells. *Proc. Natl. Acad. Sci. USA, 108*, 20730–20735.

157. Antoni, M. H., Lutgendorf, S. K., Cole, S. W., Dhabhar, F. S., Sephton, S. E., McDonald, P. G., Stefanek, M., & Sood, A. K., (2006). The influence of bio-behavioural factors on tumour biology: pathways and mechanisms. *Nat. Rev. Cancer, 6*, 240–248.

158. Lee, J. W., Shahzad, M. M., Lin, Y. G., Armaiz-Pena, G., Mangala, L. S., Han, H. D., Kim, H. S., Nam, E. J., Jennings, N. B., Halder, J., Nick, A. M., Stone, R. L., Lu, C., Lutgendorf, S. K., Cole, S. W., Lokshin, A. E., & Sood, A. K., (2009). Surgical stress promotes tumor growth in ovarian carcinoma. *Clin. Cancer Res., 15*, 2695–2702.

159. Thaker, P. H., Han, L. Y., Kamat, A. A., Arevalo, J. M., Takahashi, R., Lu, C., Jennings, N. B., Armaiz-Pena, G., Bankson, J. A., Ravoori, M., Merritt, W. M., Lin, Y. G., Mangala, L. S., Kim, T. J., Coleman, R. L., Landen, C. N., Li, Y., Felix, E., Sanguino, A. M., Newman, R. A., Lloyd, M., Gershenson, D. M., Kundra, V., Lopez-Berestein, G., Lutgendorf, S. K., Cole, S. W., & Sood, A. K., (2006). Chronic stress promotes tumor growth and angiogenesis in a mouse model of ovarian carcinoma. *Nat. Med., 12*, 939–944.

160. Godbout, J. P., & Glaser, R., (2006). Stress-induced immune dysregulation: implications for wound healing, infectious disease and cancer. *J. Neuroimmune. Pharmacol., 1*, 421–427.

161. Mancino, M., Ametller, E., Gascón, P., & Almendro, V., (2011). The neuronal influence on tumor progression. *Biochim. Biophys. Acta., 1816*, 105–118.

162. Basu, S., Nagy, J. A., Pal, S., Vasile, E., Eckelhoefer, I. A., Bliss, V. S., Manseau, E. J., Dasgupta, P. S., Dvorak, H. F., & Mukhopadhyay, D., (2001). The neurotransmitter dopamine inhibits angiogenesis induced by vascular permeability factor/vascular endothelial growth factor. *Nat Med., 7*, 569–574.

163. Chakroborty, D., Sarkar, C., Mitra, R. B., Banerjee, S., Dasgupta, P. S., & Basu, S., (2004). Depleted dopamine in gastric cancer tissues: dopamine treatment retards growth of gastric cancer by inhibiting angiogenesis. *Clin. Cancer Res., 10*, 4349–4356.

164. Basu, S., Sarkar, C., Chakroborty, D., Nagy, J., Mitra, R. B., Dasgupta, P. S., & Mukhopadhyay, D., (2004). Ablation of peripheral dopaminergic nerves stimulates malignant tumor growth by inducing vascular permeability factor/vascular endothelial growth factor-mediated angiogenesis. *Cancer Res., 64*, 5551–5555.

165. Chakroborty, D., Sarkar, C., Basu, B., Dasgupta, P. S., & Basu, S., (2009). Catecholamine's regulate tumor angiogenesis. *Cancer Res., 69*, 3727–3730.

166. Sarkar, C., Chakroborty, D., & Basu, S., (2013). Neurotransmitters as regulators of tumor angiogenesis and immunity: the role of catecholamines. *J. Neuroimmune. Pharmacol., 8*, 7–14.

167. Moreno-Smith, M., Lutgendorf, S. K., & Sood, A. K., (2010). Impact of stress on cancer metastasis. *Future Oncol., 6*, 1863–1881.

168. Madden, K. S., Szpunar, M. J., & Brown, E. B., (2011). β-Adrenergic receptors (β-AR) regulate VEGF and IL-6 production by divergent pathways in high β-AR-expressing breast cancer cell lines. *Breast Cancer Res. Treat., 130,* 747–758.

169. Sarkar, C., Chakroborty, D., Mitra, R. B., Banerjee, S., Dasgupta, P. S., & Basu, S., (2004). Dopamine in vivo inhibits VEGF-induced phosphorylation of VEGFR-2, MAPK, & focal adhesion kinase in endothelial cells. *Am. J. Physiol. Heart Circ. Physiol., 287,* 1554–1560.

170. Chakroborty, D., Chowdhury, U. R., Sarkar, C., Baral, R., Dasgupta, P. S., & Basu, S., (2008). Dopamine regulates endothelial progenitor cell mobilization from mouse bone marrow in tumor vascularization. *J. Clin. Invest., 118,* 1380–1389.

171. Sarkar, C., Chakroborty, D., Chowdhury, U. R., Dasgupta, P. S., & Basu, S., (2008). Dopamine increases the efficacy of anticancer drugs in breast and colon cancer preclinical models. *Clin. Cancer Res., 14,* 2502–2510.

172. Peters, M. A., Walenkamp, A. M., Kema, I. P., Meijer, C., de Vries, E. G., & Oosting, S. F., (2014). Dopamine and serotonin regulate tumor behavior by affecting angiogenesis. *Drug Resist. Updat., 17,* 96–104.

173. Muñoz, M., & Coveñas, R., (2013). Involvement of substance P and the NK-1 receptor in cancer progression. *Peptides, 48,* 1–9.

174. Gallo, O., Masini, E., Morbidelli, L., Franchi, A., Fini-Storchi, I., Vergari, W. A., & Ziche, M., (1998). Role of nitric oxide in angiogenesis and tumor progression in head and neck cancer. *J. Natl. Cancer Inst., 90,* 587–596.

175. Tilan, J., & Kitlinska, J., (2010). Sympathetic neurotransmitters and tumor angiogenesis-Link between stress and cancer progression. *J. Oncol., 2010,* 539706.

176. Florio, T., Morini, M., Villa, V., Arena, S., Corsaro, A., Thellung, S., Culler, M. D., Pfeffer, U., Noonan, D. M., Schettini, G., & Albini, A., (2003). Somatostatin inhibits tumor angiogenesis and growth via somatostatin receptor-3-mediated regulation of endothelial nitric oxide synthase and mitogen-activated protein kinase activities. *Endocrinology, 144,* 1574–1584.

177. O'Reilly, M. S., Boehm, T., Shing, Y., Fukai, N., Vasios, G., Lane, W. S., Flynn, E., Birkhead, J. R., Olsen, B. R., & Folkman, J., (1997). Endostatin: an endogenous inhibitor of angiogenesis and tumor growth. *Cell, 88,* 277–285.

178. Dhanabal, M., Ramchandran, R., Volk, R., Stillman, I. E., Lombardo, M., Iruela-Arispe, M. L., Simons, M., & Sukhatme, V. P., (1999). Endostatin: yeast production, mutants, & antitumor effect in renal cell carcinoma. *Cancer Res., 59,* 189–197.

179. Dhanabal, M., Ramchandran, R., Waterman, M. J., Lu, H., Knebelmann, B., Segal, M., & Sukhatme, V. P., (1999). Endostatin induces endothelial cell apoptosis. *J. Biol. Chem., 274,* 11721–11726.

180. Dixelius, J., Cross, M., Matsumoto, T., Sasaki, T., Timpl, R., & Claesson-Welsh, L., (2002). Endostatin regulates endothelial cell adhesion and cytoskeletal organization. *Cancer Res., 62,* 1944–1947.

181. Kim, Y. M., Hwang, S., Kim, Y. M., Pyun, B. J., Kim, T. Y., Lee, S. T., Gho, Y. S., & Kwon, Y. G., (2002). Endostatin blocks vascular endothelial growth factor-mediated signaling via direct interaction with KDR/Flk-1. *J. Biol. Chem., 277,* 27872–27879.

182. Good, D. J., Polverini, P. J., Rastinejad, F., Le Beau, M. M., Lemons, R. S., Frazier, W. A., & Bouck, N. P., (1990). A tumor suppressor-dependent inhibitor of angiogenesis is immunologically and functionally indistinguishable from a fragment of thrombospondin. *Proc. Natl. Acad. Sci. USA, 87,* 6624–6628.

183. Taraboletti, G., Roberts, D., Liotta, L. A., & Giavazzi, R., (1990). Platelet thrombos-pondin modulates endothelial cell adhesion, motility, & growth: a potential angiogen-esis regulatory factor. *J. Cell Biol., 111*, 765–772.

184. Iruela-Arispe, M. L., Bornstein, P., & Sage, H., (1991). Thrombospondin exerts an anti-angiogenic effect on cord formation by endothelial cells in vitro. *Proc. Natl. Acad. Sci. USA*, 88, 5026–5030.

185. Jiménez, B., Volpert, O. V., Crawford, S. E., Febbraio, M., Silverstein, R. L., & Bouck, N., (2000). Signals leading to apoptosis-dependent inhibition of neovascularization by thrombospondin-1. *Nat. Med., 6*, 41–48.

186. Noh, Y. H., Matsuda, K., Hong, Y. K., Kunstfeld, R., Riccardi, L., Koch, M., Oura, H., Dadras, S. S., Streit, M., & Detmar, M., (2003). An N-terminal 80 kDa recombinant fragment of human thrombospondin-2 inhibits vascular endothelial growth factor in-duced endothelial cell migration in vitro and tumor growth and angiogenesis in vivo. *J. Invest. Dermatol., 121*, 1536–1543.

187. Nicosia, R. F., & Tuszynski, G. P., (1994). Matrix-bound thrombospondin promotes angiogenesis in vitro. *J. Cell Biol., 124*, 183–193.

188. Rodriguez-Manzaneque, J. C., Lane, T. F., Ortega, M. A., Hynes, R. O., Lawler, J., & Iruela-Arispe, M. L., (2001). Thrombospondin-1 suppresses spontaneous tumor growth and inhibits activation of matrix metalloproteinase-9 and mobilization of vascular en-dothelial growth factor. *Proc. Natl. Acad. Sci. USA, 98*, 12485–12490.

189. Bocci, G., Francia, G., Man, S., Lawler, J., & Kerbel, R. S., (2003). Thrombospondin 1, a mediator of the antiangiogenic effects of low-dose metronomic chemotherapy. *Proc. Natl. Acad. Sci. USA, 100*, 12917–12922.

190. Hamano, Y., & Kalluri, R., (2005). Tumstatin, the NC1 domain of alpha3 chain of type IV collagen, is an endogenous inhibitor of pathological angiogenesis and suppresses tumor growth. *Biochem. Biophys. Res. Commun., 333*, 292–298.

191. Maeshima, Y., Colorado, P. C., & Kalluri, R., (2000). Two RGD-independent alpha v beta 3 integrin binding sites on tumstatin regulate distinct anti-tumor properties. *J. Biol. Chem., 275*, 23745–23750.

192. Maeshima, Y., Manfredi, M., Reimer, C., Holthaus, K. A., Hopfer, H., Chandamuri, B. R., Kharbanda, S., & Kalluri, R., (2001). Identification of the anti-angiogenic site with-in vascular basement membrane-derived tumstatin. *J. Biol. Chem., 276*, 15240–15248.

193. Eikesdal, H. P., Sugimoto, H., Birrane, G., Maeshima, Y., Cooke, V. G., Kieran, M., & Kalluri, R., (2008). Identification of amino acids essential for the antiangiogenic activ-ity of tumstatin and its use in combination antitumor activity. *Proc. Natl. Acad. Sci. USA, 105*, 15040–15045.

194. Kamphaus, G. D., Colorado, P. C., Panka, D. J., Hopfer, H., Ramchandran, R., Torre, A., Maeshima, Y., Mier, J. W., Sukhatme, V. P., & Kalluri, R., (2000). Canstatin, a novel ma-trix-derived inhibitor of angiogenesis and tumor growth. *J. Biol. Chem., 275*, 1209–1215.

195. He, G. A., Luo, J. X., Zhang, T. Y., Wang, F. Y., & Li, R. F., (2003). Canstatin-N frag-ment inhibits in vitro endothelial cell proliferation and suppresses in vivo tumor growth. *Biochem. Biophys. Res. Commun., 312*, 801–805.

196. Colorado, P. C., Torre, A., Kamphaus, G., Maeshima, Y., Hopfer, H., Takahashi, K., Volk, R., Zamborsky, E. D., Herman, S., Sarkar, P. K., Ericksen, M. B., Dhanabal, M., Simons, M., Post, M., Kufe, D. W., Weichselbaum, R. R., Sukhatme, V. P., & Kalluri, R., (2000). Anti-angiogenic cues from vascular basement membrane collagen. *Cancer Res., 60*, 2520–2526.

197. Sudhakar, A., Nyberg, P., Keshamouni, V. G., Mannam, A. P., Li, J., Sugimoto, H., Cosgrove, D., & Kalluri, R., (2005). Human alpha1 type IV collagen NC1 domain exhibits distinct antiangiogenic activity mediated by alpha1beta1 integrin. *J. Clin. Invest., 115,* 2801–2810.

198. Mongiat, M., Sweeney, S. M., San Antonio, J. D., Fu, J., & Iozzo, R. V., (2003). Endorepellin, a novel inhibitor of angiogenesis derived from the C terminus of perlecan. *J. Biol. Chem., 278,* 4238–4249.

199. Bix, G., Castello, R., Burrows, M., Zoeller, J. J., Weech, M., Iozzo, R. A., Cardi, C., Thakur, M. L., Barker, C. A., Camphausen, K., & Iozzo, R. V., (2006). Endorepellin in vivo: targeting the tumor vasculature and retarding cancer growth and metabolism. *J. Natl. Cancer Inst., 98,* 1634–1646.

200. Poluzzi, C., Casulli, J., Goyal, A., Mercer, T. J., Neill, T., & Iozzo, R. V., (2014). Endorepellin evokes autophagy in endothelial cells. *J. Biol. Chem., 289,* 16114–16128.

201. Brouty-Boyé, D., & Zetter, B. R., (1980). Inhibition of cell motility by interferon. *Science, 208,* 516–518.

202. Ribatti, D., Vacca, A., Iurlaro, M., Ria, R., Roncali, L., & Dammacco, F., (1996). Human recombinant interferon alpha-2a inhibits angiogenesis of chick area vasculosa in shell-less culture. *Int. J. Microcirc. Clin. Exp., 16,* 165–169.

203. Ezekowitz, R. A., Mulliken, J. B., & Folkman, J., (1992). Interferon alfa-2a therapy for life-threatening hemangiomas of infancy. *N. Engl. J. Med., 326,* 1456–1463.

204. Kaban, L. B., Troulis, M. J., Ebb, D., August, M., Hornicek, F. J., & Dodson, T. B., (2002). Antiangiogenic therapy with interferon alpha for giant cell lesions of the jaws. *J. Oral. Maxillofac. Surg., 60,* 1103–1111.

205. Ginns, L. C., Roberts, D. H., Mark, E. J., Brusch, J. L., & Marler, J. J., (2003). Pulmonary capillary hemangiomatosis with atypical endotheliomatosis: successful antiangiogenic therapy with doxycycline. *Chest, 124,* 2017–2022.

206. Indraccolo, S., (2010). Interferon-alpha as angiogenesis inhibitor: learning from tumor models. *Autoimmunity, 43,* 244–247.

207. Ma, Z., Qin, H., & Benveniste, E. N., (2001). Transcriptional suppression of matrix metalloproteinase-9 gene expression by IFN-gamma and IFN-beta: critical role of STAT-1alpha. *J. Immunol., 167,* 5150–5159.

208. Sun, T., Yang, Y., Luo, X., Cheng, Y., Zhang, M., Wang, K., & Ge, C., (2014). Inhibition of tumor angiogenesis by interferon-γ by suppression of tumor-associated macrophage differentiation. *Oncol. Res., 21,* 227–235.

209. Lamagna, C., Aurrand-Lions, M., & Imhof, B. A., (2006). Dual role of macrophages in tumor growth and angiogenesis. *J. Leukoc. Biol., 80,* 705–713.

210. Nyberg, P., Xie, L., & Kalluri, R., (2005). Endogenous inhibitors of angiogenesis. *Cancer Res., 65,* 3967–3979.

211. Volpert, O. V., Fong, T., Koch, A. E., Peterson, J. D., Waltenbaugh, C., Tepper, R. I., & Bouck, N. P., (1998). Inhibition of angiogenesis by interleukin 4. *J. Exp. Med., 188,* 1039–1046.

212. Ribatti, D., (2009). Endogenous inhibitors of angiogenesis: a historical review. *Leuk. Res., 33,* 638–644.

213. Taylor, S., Folkman J., (1982). Protamine is an inhibitor of angiogenesis. *Nature, 297*(5864), 307–312.

214. Sharpe, R. J., Byers, H. R., Scott, C. F., Bauer, S. I., & Maione, T. E., (1990). Growth inhibition of murine melanoma and human colon carcinoma by recombinant human platelet factor 4. *J. Natl. Cancer Inst., 82,* 848–853.

215. Bikfalvi, A., (2004). Platelet factor 4: an inhibitor of angiogenesis. *Semin. Thromb. Hemost., 30*, 379–385.

216. Yang, L., Du, J., Hou, J., Jiang, H., & Zou, J., (2011). Platelet factor-4 and its p17–70 peptide inhibit myeloma proliferation and angiogenesis in vivo. *BMC Cancer, 11*, 261.

217. Fang, S., Liu, B., Sun, Q., Zhao, J., Qi, H., & Li, Q., (2014). Platelet factor 4 inhibits IL-17/Stat3 pathway via upregulation of SOCS3 expression in melanoma. *Inflammation, 37*, 1744–1750.

218. Maione, T. E., Gray, G. S., Hunt, A. J., & Sharpe, R. J., (1991). Inhibition of tumor growth in mice by an analogue of platelet factor 4 that lacks affinity for heparin and retains potent angiostatic activity. *Cancer Res., 51*, 2077–2083.

219. Wahl, M. L., Kenan, D. J., Gonzalez-Gronow, M., & Pizzo, S. V., (2005). Angiostatin's molecular mechanism: aspects of specificity and regulation elucidated. *J. Cell Biochem., 96*, 242–261.

220. Cao, Y., Ji, R. W., Davidson, D., Schaller, J., Marti, D., Söhndel, S., McCance, S. G., O'Reilly, M. S., Llinás, M., & Folkman, J., (1996). Kringle domains of human angiostatin. Characterization of the anti-proliferative activity on endothelial cells. *J. Biol. Chem., 271*, 29461–29467.

221. Claesson-Welsh, L., Welsh, M., Ito, N., Anand-Apte, B., Soker, S., Zetter, B., O'Reilly, M., & Folkman, J., (1998). Angiostatin induces endothelial cell apoptosis and activation of focal adhesion kinase independently of the integrin-binding motif RGD. *Proc. Natl. Acad. Sci. USA, 95*, 5579–5583.

222. Dawson, D. W., Volpert, O. V., Gillis, P., Crawford, S. E., Xu, H., Benedict, W., & Bouck, N. P., (1999). Pigment epithelium-derived factor: a potent inhibitor of angiogenesis. *Science, 285*, 245–248.

223. Bouck, N., (2002). PEDF: anti-angiogenic guardian of ocular function. *Trends. Mol. Med., 8*, 330–334.

224. Ek, E. T., Dass, C. R., & Choong, P. F., (2006). Pigment epithelium-derived factor: a multimodal tumor inhibitor. *Mol. Cancer Ther., 5*, 1641–1646.

225. Tombran-Tink, J., & Barnstable, C. J., (2003). PEDF: a multifaceted neurotrophic factor. *Nat. Rev. Neurosci., 4*, 628–636.

226. Pike, S. E., Yao, L., Jones, K. D., Cherney, B., Appella, E., Sakaguchi, K., Nakhasi, H., Teruya-Feldstein, J., Wirth, P., Gupta, G., & Tosato, G., (1998). Vasostatin, a calreticulin fragment, inhibits angiogenesis and suppresses tumor growth. *J. Exp. Med., 188*, 2349–2356.

227. Pike, S. E., Yao, L., Setsuda, J., Jones, K. D., Cherney, B., Appella, E., Sakaguchi, K., Nakhasi, H., Atreya, C. D., Teruya-Feldstein, J., Wirth, P., Gupta, G., & Tosato, G., (1999). Calreticulin and calreticulin fragments are endothelial cell inhibitors that suppress tumor growth. *Blood, 94*, 2461–2468.

228. Xiao, F., Wei, Y., Yang, L., Zhao, X., Tian, L., Ding, Z., Yuan, S., Lou, Y., Liu, F., Wen, Y., Li, J., Deng, H., Kang, B., Mao, Y., Lei, S., He, Q., Su, J., Lu, Y., Niu, T., Hou, J., & Huang, M. J., (2002). A gene therapy for cancer based on the angiogenesis inhibitor, vasostatin. *Gene Ther., 9*, 1207–1213.

229. Yao, L., Pike, S. E., & Tosato, G., (2002). Laminin binding to the calreticulin fragment vasostatin regulates endothelial cell function. *J. Leukoc. Biol., 71*, 47–53.

230. Moses, M. A., Wiederschain, D., Wu, I., Fernandez, C. A., Ghazizadeh, V., Lane, W. S., Flynn, E., Sytkowski, A., Tao, T., & Langer, R., (1999). Troponin I is present in human cartilage and inhibits angiogenesis. *Proc. Natl. Acad. Sci. USA, 96*, 2645–2650.

231. Feldman, L., & Rouleau, C., (2002). Troponin I inhibits capillary endothelial cell proliferation by interaction with the cell's bFGF receptor. *Microvasc. Res., 63*, 41–49.

232. Yue, T. L., Wang, X., Louden, C. S., Gupta, S., Pillarisetti, K., Gu, J. L., Hart, T. K., Lysko, P. G., & Feuerstein, G. Z., (1997). 2-Methoxyestradiol, an endogenous estrogen metabolite, induces apoptosis in endothelial cells and inhibits angiogenesis: possible role for stress-activated protein kinase signaling pathway and Fas expression. *Mol. Pharmacol., 51*, 951–962.

233. Fotsis, T., Zhang, Y., Pepper, M. S., Adlercreutz, H., Montesano, R., Nawroth, P. P., & Schweigerer, L., (1994). The endogenous oestrogen metabolite 2-methoxyoestradiol inhibits angiogenesis and suppresses tumour growth. *Nature, 368*, 237–239.

234. Mabjeesh, N. J., Escuin, D., LaVallee, T. M., Pribluda, V. S., Swartz, G. M., Johnson, M. S., Willard, M. T., Zhong, H., Simons, J. W., & Giannakakou, P., (2003). 2ME2 inhibits tumor growth and angiogenesis by disrupting microtubules and dysregulating HIF. *Cancer Cell, 3*, 363–375.

235. Verenich, S., & Gerk, P. M., (2010). Therapeutic promises of 2-methoxyestradiol and its drug disposition challenges. *Mol. Pharm., 7*, 2030–2039.

236. Zhu, H., Li, Z., Mao, S., Ma, B., Zhou, S., Deng, L., Liu, T., Cui, D., Zhao, Y., He, J., Yi, C., & Huang, Y., (2011). Antitumor effect of sFlt-1 gene therapy system mediated by Bifidobacterium Infantis on Lewis lung cancer in mice. *Cancer Gene Ther., 18*, 884–896.

237. Hiraki, Y., Tanaka, H., Inoue, H., Kondo, J., Kamizono, A., & Suzuki, F., (1991). Molecular cloning of a new class of cartilage-specific matrix, chondromodulin-I, which stimulates growth of cultured chondrocytes. *Biochem. Biophys. Res. Commun., 175*, 971–977.

238. Hayami, T., Shukunami, C., Mitsui, K., Endo, N., Tokunaga, K., Kondo, J., Takahashi, H. E., & Hiraki, Y., (1999). Specific loss of chondromodulin-I gene expression in chondrosarcoma and the suppression of tumor angiogenesis and growth by its recombinant protein in vivo. *FEBS Lett., 458*, 436–440.

239. D'Angelo, G., Struman, I., Martial, J., & Weiner, R. I., (1995). Activation of mitogen-activated protein kinases by vascular endothelial growth factor and basic fibroblast growth factor in capillary endothelial cells is inhibited by the antiangiogenic factor 16-kDa N-terminal fragment of prolactin. *Proc. Natl. Acad. Sci. USA, 92*, 6374–6378.

240. Rao, N., Lee, Y. F., & Ge, R., (2015). Novel endogenous angiogenesis inhibitors and their therapeutic potential. *Acta. Pharmacol. Sin., 36*, 1177–1190.

241. Ryan, D. P., Penson, R. T., Ahmed, S., Chabner, B. A., & Lynch, T. J., (1999). Jr. Reality testing in cancer treatment: the phase I trial of endostatin. *Oncologist, 4*, 501–508.

242. Thomas, J. P., Arzoomanian, R. Z., Alberti, D., Marnocha, R., Lee, F., Friedl, A., Tutsch, K., Dresen, A., Geiger, P., Pluda, J., Fogler, W., Schiller, J. H., & Wilding, G., (2003). Phase I pharmacokinetic and pharmacodynamic study of recombinant human endostatin in patients with advanced solid tumors. *J. Clin. Oncol., 21*, 223–231.

243. Rong, B., Yang, S., Li, W., Zhang, W., & Ming, Z., (2012). Systematic review and meta-analysis of Endostar (rh-endostatin) combined with chemotherapy versus chemotherapy alone for treating advanced non-small cell lung cancer. *World J. Surg. Oncol., 10*, 170.

244. Ge, W., Cao, D. D., Wang, H. M., Jie, F. F., Zheng, Y. F., & Chen, Y., (2011). Endostar combined with chemotherapy versus chemotherapy alone for advanced NSCLCs: a meta-analysis. *Asian Pac. J. Cancer Prev., 12*, 2705–2711.

245. Hurwitz, H., Fehrenbacher, L., Novotny, W., Cartwright, T., Hainsworth, J., Heim, W., Berlin, J., Baron, A., Griffing, S., Holmgren, E., Ferrara, N., Fyfe, G., Rogers, B., Ross, R., & Kabbinavar, F., (2004). Bevacizumab plus irinotecan, fluorouracil, & leucovorin for metastatic colorectal cancer. *N. Engl. J. Med., 350*, 2335–2342.

246. Herbst, R. S., Johnson, D. H., Mininberg, E., Carbone, D. P., Henderson, T., Kim, E. S., Blumenschein, G. Jr., Lee, J. J., Liu, D. D., Truong, M. T., Hong, W. K., Tran, H., Tsao, A., Xie, D., Ramies, D. A., Mass, R., Seshagiri, S., Eberhard, D. A., Kelley, S. K., & Sandler, A., (2005). Phase I/II trial evaluating the anti-vascular endothelial growth factor monoclonal antibody bevacizumab in combination with the HER-1/epidermal growth factor receptor tyrosine kinase inhibitor erlotinib for patients with recurrent non-small-cell lung cancer. *J. Clin. Oncol., 23*, 2544–2555.

247. Shih, T., & Lindley, C., (2006). Bevacizumab: an angiogenesis inhibitor for the treatment of solid malignancies. *Clin. Ther., 28*, 1779–1802.

248. Al-Husein, B., Abdalla, M., Trepte, M., Deremer, D. L., & Somanath, P. R., (2012). Antiangiogenic therapy for cancer: an update. *Pharmacotherapy, 32*, 1095–1111.

249. Rini, B. I., (2007). Vascular endothelial growth factor-targeted therapy in renal cell carcinoma: current status and future directions. *Clin. Cancer Res., 13*, 1098–1106.

250. Gerber, H. P., & Ferrara, N., (2005). Pharmacology and pharmacodynamics of bevacizumab as monotherapy or in combination with cytotoxic therapy in preclinical studies. *Cancer Res., 65*, 671–680.

251. Song, J. Y., Lee, S. W., Hong, J. P., Chang, S. E., Choe, H., & Choi, J., (2009). Epidermal growth factor competes with EGF receptor inhibitors to induce cell death in EGFR-overexpressing tumor cells. *Cancer Lett., 283*, 135–142.

252. Humblet, Y., (2004). Cetuximab: an IgG(1) monoclonal antibody for the treatment of epidermal growth factor receptor-expressing tumours. *Expert Opin. Pharmacother., 5*, 1621–1633.

253. Cunningham, D., Humblet, Y., Siena, S., Khayat, D., Bleiberg, H., Santoro, A., Bets, D., Mueser, M., Harstrick, A., Verslype, C., Chau, I., Van Cutsem, E., (2004). Cetuximab monotherapy and cetuximab plus irinotecan in irinotecan-refractory metastatic colorectal cancer. *N. Engl. J. Med., 351*, 337–345.

254. Burtness, B., (2005). Cetuximab and cisplatin for chemotherapy-refractory squamous cell cancer of the head and neck. *J. Clin. Oncol., 23*, 5440–5442.

255. Giusti, R. M., Shastri, K. A., Cohen, M. H., Keegan, P., & Pazdur, R., (2007). FDA drug approval summary: panitumumab (Vectibix). *Oncologist, 12*(5), 577–583.

256. Giusti, R. M., Shastri, K., Pilaro, A. M., Fuchs, C., Cordoba-Rodriguez, R., Koti, K., Rothmann, M., Men, A. Y., Zhao, H., Hughes, M., Keegan, P., Weiss, K. D., & Pazdur, R. U. S., (2008). Food and Drug Administration approval: panitumumab for epidermal growth factor receptor-expressing metastatic colorectal carcinoma with progression following fluoropyrimidine-, oxaliplatin-, & irinotecan-containing chemotherapy regimens. *Clin. Cancer Res., 14*, 1296–1302.

257. Shuptrine, C. W., Surana, R., & Weiner, L. M., (2012). Monoclonal antibodies for the treatment of cancer. *Semin. Cancer Biol., 22*, 3–13.

258. Vacchelli, E., Aranda, F., Eggermont, A., Galon, J., Sautès-Fridman, C., Zitvogel, L., Kroemer, G., & Galluzzi, L., (2014). Trial Watch: Tumor-targeting monoclonal antibodies in cancer therapy. *Oncoimmunology, 3*, e27048.

259. Kuenen, B., Witteveen, P. O., Ruijter, R., Giaccone, G., Dontabhaktuni, A., Fox, F., Katz, T., Youssoufian, H., Zhu, J., Rowinsky, E. K., & Voest, E. E., (2010). A phase I pharmacologic study of necitumumab (IMC-11F8), a fully human IgG1 monoclonal

antibody directed against EGFR in patients with advanced solid malignancies. *Clin. Cancer Res., 16,* 1915–1923.

260. Krupitskaya, Y., & Wakelee, H. A., (2009). Ramucirumab, a fully human mAb to the transmembrane signaling tyrosine kinase VEGFR-2 for the potential treatment of cancer. *Curr. Opin. Investig. Drugs, 10,* 597–605.

261. Fuchs, C. S., Tomasek, J., Yong, C. J., Dumitru, F., Passalacqua, R., Goswami, C., Safran, H., Dos Santos, L. V., Aprile, G., Ferry, D. R., Melichar, B., Tehfe, M., Topuzov, E., Zalcberg, J. R., Chau, I., Campbell, W., Sivanandan, C., Pikiel, J., Koshiji, M., Hsu, Y., Liepa, A. M., Gao, L., Schwartz, J. D., & Tabernero, J., (2014). REGARD trial investigators. ramucirumab monotherapy for previously treated advanced gastric or gastro-oesophageal junction adenocarcinoma (REGARD): an international, randomised, multicentre, placebo-controlled, phase 3 trial. *Lancet., 383,* 31–39.

262. Ueda, S., Satoh, T., Gotoh, M., Gao, L., & Doi, T., (2015). A phase ib study of safety and pharmacokinetics of ramucirumab in combination with paclitaxel in patients with advanced gastric adenocarcinomas. *Oncologist, 20*(5), 493–494.

263. Jayson, G. C., Kerbel, R., Ellis, L. M., & Harris, A. L., (2016). Antiangiogenic therapy in oncology: current status and future directions. *Lancet., pii:* S0140–6736(15)01088–01080.

264. Baselga, J., & Albanell, J., (2001). Mechanism of action of anti-HER2 monoclonal antibodies. *Ann. Oncol., 12, Suppl., 1,* 35–41.

265. Mariani, G., Fasolo, A., De Benedictis, E., & Gianni, L., (2009). Trastuzumab as adjuvant systemic therapy for HER2-positive breast cancer. *Nat. Clin. Pract. Oncol., 6,* 93–104.

266. Verma, S., Miles, D., Gianni, L., Krop, I. E., Welslau, M., Baselga, J., Pegram, M., Oh, D. Y., Diéras, V., Guardino, E., Fang, L., Lu, M. W., Olsen, S., & Blackwell, K., (2012). EMILIA Study Group. Trastuzumab emtansine for HER2-positive advanced breast cancer. *N. Engl. J. Med., 367,* 1783–1791.

267. Mazières, J., Barlesi, F., Filleron, T., Besse, B., Monnet, I., Beau-Faller, M., Peters, S., Dansin, E., Früh, M., Pless, M., Rosell, R., Wislez, M., Fournel, P., Westeel, V., Cappuzzo, F., Cortot, A., Moro-Sibilot, D., Milia, J., & Gautschi, O., (2016). Lung cancer patients with HER2 mutations treated with chemotherapy and HER2-targeted drugs: results from the European EUHER2 cohort. *Ann. Oncol., 27,* 281–286.

268. Jitawatanarat, P., & Wee, W., (2013). Update on antiangiogenic therapy in colorectal cancer: aflibercept and regorafenib. *J. Gastrointest. Oncol., 4,* 231–238.

269. Wang, T. F., & Lockhart, A. C., (2012). Aflibercept in the treatment of metastatic colorectal cancer. *Clin. Med. Insights. Oncol., 6,* 19–30.

270. Ricci, V., Ronzoni, M., & Fabozzi, T., (2015). Aflibercept a new target therapy in cancer treatment: a review. *Crit. Rev. Oncol. Hematol., 96,* 569–576.

271. Giordano, G., Febbraro, A., Venditti, M., Campidoglio, S., Olivieri, N., Raieta, K., Parcesepe, P., Imbriani, G. C., Remo, A., & Pancione, M., (2014). Targeting angiogenesis and tumor microenvironment in metastatic colorectal cancer: role of aflibercept. *Gastroenterol Res. Pract., 2014,* 526178.

272. Wilhelm, S. M., Adnane, L., Newell, P., Villanueva, A., Llovet, J. M., & Lynch, M., (2008). Preclinical overview of sorafenib, a multikinase inhibitor that targets both Raf and VEGF and PDGF receptor tyrosine kinase signaling. *Mol. Cancer Ther., 7,* 3129–3140.

273. Kane, R. C., Farrell, A. T., Saber, H., Tang, S., Williams, G., Jee, J. M., Liang, C., Booth, B., Chidambaram, N., Morse, D., Sridhara, R., Garvey, P., Justice, R., & Pazdur,

R., (2006). Sorafenib for the treatment of advanced renal cell carcinoma. *Clin. Cancer Res., 12*, 7271–7278.

274. Chowdhury, S., Larkin, J. M., & Gore, M. E., (2008). Recent advances in the treatment of renal cell carcinoma and the role of targeted therapies. *Eur. J. Cancer, 44*, 2152–2161.

275. Christensen, J. G., (2007). A preclinical review of sunitinib, a multitargeted receptor tyrosine kinase inhibitor with anti-angiogenic and antitumour activities. *Ann. Oncol., 18*, 3–10.

276. Rock, E. P., Goodman, V., Jiang, J. X., Mahjoob, K., Verbois, S. L., Morse, D., Dagher, R., Justice, R., & Pazdur, R., (2007). Food and drug administration drug approval summary: Sunitinib malate for the treatment of gastrointestinal stromal tumor and advanced renal cell carcinoma. *Oncologist, 12*, 107–113.

277. Lang, L., (2008). FDA approves sorafenib for patients with inoperable liver cancer. *Gastroenterology, 134*, 379.

278. Raymond, E., Dahan, L., Raoul, J. L., Bang, Y. J., Borbath, I., Lombard-Bohas, C., Valle, J., Metrakos, P., Smith, D., Vinik, A., Chen, J. S., Hörsch, D., Hammel, P., Wiedenmann, B., Van Cutsem, E., Patyna, S., Lu, D. R., Blanckmeister, C., Chao, R., & Ruszniewski, P., (2011). Sunitinib malate for the treatment of pancreatic neuroendocrine tumors. *N. Engl. J. Med., 364*, 501–513.

279. Grothey, A., Van Cutsem, E., Sobrero, A., Siena, S., Falcone, A., Ychou, M., Humblet, Y., Bouché, O., Mineur, L., Barone, C., Adenis, A., Tabernero, J., Yoshino, T., Lenz, H. J., Goldberg, R. M., Sargent, D. J., Cihon, F., Cupit, L., Wagner, A., & Laurent, D., (2013). CORRECT Study Group. Regorafenib monotherapy for previously treated metastatic colorectal cancer (CORRECT): an international, multicentre, randomised, placebo-controlled, phase 3 trial. *Lancet., 381*, 303–312.

280. Grothey, A., (2015). Regorafenib in metastatic colorectal cancer: optimal dosing and patient selection recommendations. *Clin. Adv. Hematol. Oncol., 13*, 514–517.

281. Pao, W., Miller, V. A., & Kris, M. G., (2004). 'Targeting' the epidermal growth factor receptor tyrosine kinase with gefitinib (Iressa) in non-small cell lung cancer (NSCLC). *Semin Cancer Biol., 14*, 33–40.

282. Cohen, M. H., Williams, G. A., Sridhara, R., Chen, G., & Pazdur, R., (2003). FDA drug approval summary: gefitinib (ZD1839) (Iressa) tablets. *Oncologist, 8*, 303–306.

283. Cohen, M. H., Johnson, J. R., Chen, Y. F., Sridhara, R., & Pazdur, R., (2005). FDA drug approval summary: erlotinib (Tarceva) tablets. *Oncologist, 10*, 461–266.

284. Gridelli, C., Bareschino, M. A., Schettino, C., Rossi, A., Maione, P., & Ciardiello, F., (2007). Erlotinib in non-small cell lung cancer treatment: current status and future development. *Oncologist, 12*, 840–849.

285. Wells, S. A. Jr., Robinson, B. G., Gagel, R. F., Dralle, H., Fagin, J. A., Santoro, M., Baudin, E., Elisei, R., Jarzab, B., Vasselli, J. R., Read, J., Langmuir, P., Ryan, A. J., & Schlumberger, M. J., (2012). Vandetanib in patients with locally advanced or metastatic medullary thyroid cancer: a randomized, double-blind phase III trial. *J. Clin. Oncol., 30*, 134–141.

286. Frampton, J. E., (2012). Vandetanib: in medullary thyroid cancer. *Drugs, 72*, 1423–1436.

287. Escudier, B., & Gore, M., (2011). Axitinib for the management of metastatic renal cell carcinoma. *Drugs R D, 11*, 113–126.

288. Rini, B. I., Garrett, M., Poland, B., Dutcher, J. P., Rixe, O., Wilding, G., Stadler, W. M., Pithavala, Y. K., Kim, S., Tarazi, J., & Motzer, R. J., (2013). Axitinib in metastatic renal

cell carcinoma: results of a pharmacokinetic and pharmacodynamic analysis. *J. Clin. Pharmacol., 53*, 491–504.

289. Habeck, M., (2002). FDA licences imatinib mesylate for CML. *Lancet. Oncol., 3*, 6.

290. Moy, B., Kirkpatrick, P., Kar, S., & Goss, P., (2007). Lapatinib. *Nat. Rev. Drug Discov., 6*, 431–432.

291. Ryan, Q., Ibrahim, A., Cohen, M. H., Johnson, J., Ko, C. W., Sridhara, R., Justice, R., & Pazdur, R., (2008). FDA drug approval summary: lapatinib in combination with capecitabine for previously treated metastatic breast cancer that overexpresses HER-2. *Oncologist, 13*, 1114–1119.

292. Nair, A., Lemery, S. J., Yang, J., Marathe, A., Zhao, L., Zhao, H., Jiang, X., He, K., Ladouceur, G., Mitra, A. K., Zhou, L., Fox, E., Aungst, S., Helms, W., Keegan, P., & Pazdur, R., (2015). FDA approval summary: Lenvatinib for progressive, radio-iodine-refractory differentiated thyroid cancer. *Clin. Cancer Res., 21*, 5205–5208.

293. Giles, F. J., & Albitar, M., (2005). Mammalian target of rapamycin as a therapeutic target in leukemia. *Curr. Mol. Med., 5*, 653–661.

294. Martelli, A. M., Tazzari, P. L., Evangelisti, C., Chiarini, F., Blalock, W. L., Billi, A. M., Manzoli, L., McCubrey, J. A., & Cocco, L., (2007). Targeting the phosphatidylinositol 3-kinase/Akt/mammalian target of rapamycin module for acute myelogenous leukemia therapy: from bench to bedside. *Curr. Med. Chem., 14*, 2009–2023.

295. Lane, H. A., Wood, J. M., McSheehy, P. M., Allegrini, P. R., Boulay, A., Brueggen, J., Littlewood-Evans, A., Maira, S. M., Martiny-Baron, G., Schnell, C. R., Sini, P., O'Reilly, T., (2009). mTOR inhibitor RAD001 (everolimus) has antiangiogenic/vascular properties distinct from a VEGFR tyrosine kinase inhibitor. *Clin. Cancer Res., 15*, 1612–1622.

296. Anargyrou, K., Dimopoulos, M. A., Sezer, O., & Terpos, E., (2008). Novel anti-myeloma agents and angiogenesis. *Leuk. Lymphoma., 49*, 677–689.

297. Armitage, J. O., Mauch P. M., Harris, N. L., Bierman, P. Non-Hodgekin's Lymphoma . In Principles and Practice of Oncology. 6th edition, Devita, V. T., Hellman, S., & Rosenberg, S. A., (2001). *Lippincott Williams and Wilkins*, Philadelphia, pp. 2256–p2316.

298. Neben, S., Hellman, S., Montgomery, M., Ferrara, J., & Mauch, P., (1993). Hematopoietic stem cell deficit of transplanted bone marrow previously exposed to cytotoxic agents. *Exp. Hematol., 21*, 156–162.

299. Mauch, P., Constine, L., Greenberger, J., Knospe, W., Sullivan, J., Liesveld, J. L., & Deeg, H. J., (1995). Hematopoietic stem cell compartment: acute and late effects of radiation therapy and chemotherapy. *Int. J. Radiat. Oncol. Biol. Phys., 31*, 1319–1339.

300. Boussios, S., Pentheroudakis, G., Katsanos, K., & Pavlidis, N., (2012). Systemic treatment-induced gastrointestinal toxicity: incidence, clinical presentation and management. *Ann. Gastroenterol., 25*, 106–118.

301. Hanahan, D., & Weinberg, R. A., (2011). Hallmarks of cancer: the next generation. *Cell, 144*, 646–674.

302. Jain, R. K., (2005). Normalization of tumor vasculature: an emerging concept in antiangiogenic therapy. *Science, 307*, 58–62.

303. Augustin, H. G., Kozian, D. H., & Johnson, R. C., (1994). Differentiation of endothelial cells: analysis of the constitutive and activated endothelial cell phenotypes. *Bioessays, 16*, 901–906.

304. Denekamp, J., (1984). Vascular endothelium as the vulnerable element in tumours. Acta. *Radiol. Oncol., 23*, 217–225.

305. Dekker, R. J., Boon, R. A., Rondaij, M. G., Kragt, A., Volger, O. L., Elderkamp, Y. W., Meijers, J. C., Voorberg, J., Pannekoek, H., & Horrevoets, A. J., (2006). KLF2 provokes a gene expression pattern that establishes functional quiescent differentiation of the endothelium. *Blood, 107,* 4354–4363.

306. Chen, H. X., & Cleck, J. N., (2009). Adverse effects of anticancer agents that target the VEGF pathway. *Nat. Rev. Clin. Oncol., 6,* 465–477.

307. Hutson, T. E., Figlin, R. A., Kuhn, J. G., & Motzer, R. J., (2008). Targeted therapies for metastatic renal cell carcinoma: an overview of toxicity and dosing strategies. *Oncologist., 13,* 1084–1096.

308. Sane, D. C., Anton, L., & Brosnihan, K. B., (2004). Angiogenic growth factors and hypertension. *Angiogenesis., 7*(3):193–201.

309. Van Heeckeren, W. J., Ortiz, J., Cooney, M. M., & Remick, S. C., (2007). Hypertension, proteinuria, & antagonism of vascular endothelial growth factor signaling: clinical toxicity, therapeutic target, or novel biomarker? *J. Clin. Oncol., 25,* 2993–2995.

310. Burger, R. A., Brady, M. F., Bookman, M. A., Fleming, G. F., Monk, B. J., Huang, H., Mannel, R. S., Homesley, H. D., Fowler, J., Greer, B. E., Boente, M., Birrer, M. J., & Liang, S. X., (2011). Gynecologic Oncology Group. Incorporation of bevacizumab in the primary treatment of ovarian cancer. *N. Engl. J. Med., 365,* 2473–2483.

311. Launay-Vacher, V., & Deray, G., (2009). Hypertension and proteinuria: a class-effect of antiangiogenic therapies. *Anticancer Drugs, 20,* 81–82.

312. Bombeli, T., Karsan, A., Tait, J. F., & Harlan, J. M., (1997). Apoptotic vascular endothelial cells become procoagulant. *Blood, 89,* 2429–2442.

313. Sugimoto, H., Hamano, Y., Charytan, D., Cosgrove, D., Kieran, M., Sudhakar, A., & Kalluri, R., (2003). Neutralization of circulating vascular endothelial growth factor (VEGF) by anti-VEGF antibodies and soluble VEGF receptor 1 (sFlt-1) induces proteinuria. *J. Biol. Chem., 278,* 12605–12608.

314. Eremina, V., Jefferson, J. A., Kowalewska, J., Hochster, H., Haas, M., Weisstuch, J., Richardson, C., Kopp, J. B., Kabir, M. G., Backx, P. H., Gerber, H. P., Ferrara, N., Barisoni, L., Alpers, C. E., & Quaggin, S. E., (2008). VEGF inhibition and renal thrombotic microangiopathy. *N. Engl. J. Med., 358,* 1129–1136.

315. Elice, F., & Rodeghiero, F., (2012). Side effects of anti-angiogenic drugs. *Thromb. Res., 129,* S50-S53.

316. Keefe, D., Bowen, J., Gibson, R., Tan, T., Okera, M., & Stringer, A., (2011). Noncardiac vascular toxicities of vascular endothelial growth factor inhibitors in advanced cancer: a review. *Oncologist., 16,* 432–444.

317. Motzer, R. J., Hutson, T. E., Tomczak, P., Michaelson, M. D., Bukowski, R. M., Rixe, O., Oudard, S., Negrier, S., Szczylik, C., Kim, S. T., Chen, I., Bycott, P. W., Baum, C. M., & Figlin, R. A., (2007). Sunitinib versus interferon alfa in metastatic renal-cell carcinoma. *N. Engl. J. Med., 356,* 115–124.

318. Spano, J. P., Chodkiewicz, C., Maurel, J., Wong, R., Wasan, H., Barone, C., Létourneau, R., Bajetta, E., Pithavala, Y., Bycott, P., Trask, P., Liau, K., Ricart, A. D., Kim, S., & Rixe, O., (2008). Efficacy of gemcitabine plus axitinib compared with gemcitabine alone in patients with advanced pancreatic cancer: an open-label randomised phase II study. *Lancet., 371,* 2101–2108.

319. Lind, J. S., & Smit, E. F., (2009). Angiogenesis inhibitors in the treatment of non-small cell lung cancer. *Ther. Adv. Med. Oncol., 1,* 95–107.

320. Gridelli, C., Maione, P., Rossi, A., De Marinis, F., (2007). The role of bevacizumab in the treatment of non-small cell lung cancer: current indications and future developments. *Oncologist, 12*, 1183–1193.
321. Kabbinavar, F., Hurwitz, H. I., Fehrenbacher, L., Meropol, N. J., Novotny, W. F., Lieberman, G., Griffing, S., & Bergsland, E., (2003). Phase II, randomized trial comparing bevacizumab plus fluorouracil (FU)/leucovorin (LV) with FU/LV alone in patients with metastatic colorectal cancer. *J. Clin. Oncol., 21*, 60–65.
322. Scappaticci, F. A., Fehrenbacher, L., Cartwright, T., Hainsworth, J. D., Heim, W., Berlin, J., Kabbinavar, F., Novotny, W., Sarkar, S., & Hurwitz, H., (2005). Surgical wound healing complications in metastatic colorectal cancer patients treated with bevacizumab. *J. Surg. Oncol., 91*, 173–180.
323. Weltermann, A., Wolzt, M., Petersmann, K., Czerni, C., Graselli, U., Lechner, K., & Kyrle, P. A., (1999). Large amounts of vascular endothelial growth factor at the site of hemostatic plug formation in vivo. *Arterioscler. Thromb. Vasc. Biol., 19*, 1757–1760.
324. Cannistra, S. A., Matulonis, U. A., Penson, R. T., Hambleton, J., Dupont, J., Mackey, H., Douglas, J., Burger, R. A., Armstrong, D., Wenham, R., & McGuire, W., (2007). Phase II study of bevacizumab in patients with platinum-resistant ovarian cancer or peritoneal serous cancer. *J. Clin. Oncol., 25*, 5180–5186.
325. Han, E. S., & Monk, B. J., (2007). Bevacizumab in the treatment of ovarian cancer. *Expert. Rev. Anticancer. Ther., 7*, 1339–1345.
326. Kamba, T., & McDonald, D. M., (2007). Mechanisms of adverse effects of anti-VEGF therapy for cancer. *Br. J. Cancer, 96*, 1788–1795.
327. Garfield, D. H., Wolter, P., Schöffski, P., Hercbergs, A., & Davis, P., (2008). Documentation of thyroid function in clinical studies with sunitinib: why does it matter? *J. Clin. Oncol., 26*, 5131–5132, author reply 5132–5133.
328. Katoh, O., Tauchi, H., Kawaishi, K., Kimura, A., & Satow, Y., (1995). Expression of the vascular endothelial growth factor (VEGF) receptor gene, KDR, in hematopoietic cells and inhibitory effect of VEGF on apoptotic cell death caused by ionizing radiation. *Cancer Res., 55*, 5687–5692.
329. Demetri, G. D., van Oosterom, A. T., Garrett, C. R., Blackstein, M. E., Shah, M. H., Verweij, J., McArthur, G., Judson, I. R., Heinrich, M. C., Morgan, J. A., Desai, J., Fletcher, C. D., George, S., Bello, C. L., Huang, X., Baum, C. M., & Casali, P. G., (2006). Efficacy and safety of sunitinib in patients with advanced gastrointestinal stromal tumour after failure of imatinib: a randomised controlled trial. *Lancet., 368*, 1329–1338.
330. Schmidinger, M., & Bellmunt, J., (2010). Plethora of agents, plethora of targets, plethora of side effects in metastatic renal cell carcinoma. *Cancer Treat. Rev., 36*, 416–424.
331. Cohen, R. B., & Oudard, S., (2012). Antiangiogenic therapy for advanced renal cell carcinoma: management of treatment-related toxicities. *Invest. New. Drugs, 30*, 2066–2079.
332. Kerbel, R. S., (2008). Tumor angiogenesis. *N. Engl. J. Med., 358*, 2039–2049.
333. Kindler, H. L., (2007). Pancreatic cancer: an update. *Curr. Oncol. Rep., 9*, 170–176.
324. Loges, S., Schmidt, T., & Carmeliet, P., (2010). Mechanisms of resistance to anti-angiogenic therapy and development of third-generation anti-angiogenic drug candidates. *Genes Cancer., 1*, 12–25.
325. Rapisarda, A., & Melillo, G., (2012). Overcoming disappointing results with antiangiogenic therapy by targeting hypoxia. *Nat. Rev. Clin. Oncol., 9*, 378–390.
326. Gacche, R. N., (2015). Compensatory angiogenesis and tumor refractoriness. *Oncogenesis., 4*, e153.

327. Giuliano, S., & Pagès, G., (2013). Mechanisms of resistance to anti-angiogenesis therapies. *Biochimie., 95*, 1110–1119.

328. Abdullah, S. E., & Perez-Soler, R., (2012). Mechanisms of resistance to vascular endothelial growth factor blockade. *Cancer, 118*, 3455–3467.

329. Crawford, Y., Kasman, I., Yu, L., Zhong, C., Wu, X., Modrusan, Z., Kaminker, J., & Ferrara, N., (2009). PDGF-C mediates the angiogenic and tumorigenic properties of fibroblasts associated with tumors refractory to anti-VEGF treatment. *Cancer Cell, 15*, 21–34.

330. Blouw, B., Song, H., Tihan, T., Bosze, J., Ferrara, N., Gerber, H. P., Johnson, R. S., & Bergers, G., (2003). The hypoxic response of tumors is dependent on their microenvironment. *Cancer Cell, 4*, 133–146.

331. Monzani, E., La Porta, C. A., (2008). Targeting cancer stem cells to modulate alternative vascularization mechanisms. *Stem Cell Rev., 4*, 51–56.

332. Donnem, T., Hu, J., Ferguson, M., Adighibe, O., Snell, C., Harris, A. L., Gatter, K. C., & Pezzella, F., (2013). Vessel co-option in primary human tumors and metastases: an obstacle to effective anti-angiogenic treatment? *Cancer Med., 2*, 427–436.

CHAPTER 5

THE TUMOUR MICROENVIRONMENT AND METASTASIS

SONIA CHADHA

Amity Institute of Biotechnology, Amity University Uttar Pradesh, Lucknow Campus, Lucknow–226028, India

CONTENTS

ABSTRACT

Metastasis consists of a number of steps that include the detachment of the cancer cells from the primary tumor, entry into the circulation, and finally seeding at secondary sites and growth. Each of these steps of metastasis is influenced by nonmalignant components of the tumor microenvironment (TME). The environment where a tumor exists includes the accompanying blood vessels, fibroblasts, various inflammatory cells, immune cells and signaling molecules, and the extracellular matrix (ECM) and is known as the tumor microenvironment. In healthy individuals, the stroma serves as a physiological barrier against tumorigenesis. But, the presence of neoplastic cells, directly or indirectly, modifies the adjacent microenvironment converting it into a pathological entity. Recent studies have shown that the TME influences tumor progression and metastasis and may direct the fate of the tumors at the site of invasion and metastasis. Survival of tumor cells at the secondary sites requires activation of the stromal cells to establish a supportive environment for the outgrowth of metastatic cells. Therefore, the understanding of the TME and its role in metastasis can result in the development of new strategies for the diagnosis, therapy, and prognosis of cancer.

5.1   INTRODUCTION

Cancer is a systemic disease involving bidirectional communication between both malignant and nonmalignant cells. The functionally supportive connective tissue framework of a biological cell is known as the stroma. It includes fibroblasts, vascular endothelial cells, and immune cells. The malignant and nonmalignant cells together with the extracellular matrix is termed as the tumor microenvironment (TME). It is a unique environment that develops due to the interaction between the stroma and tumor cells. The stroma of the normal tissues maintains the integrity of the epithelial tissues which in turn regulates normal tissue homeostasis [1]. The naïve stroma is capable of regulating immunosuppression and so is capable of possessing anticancer capabilities [2, 3]. But, on being affected by tumor-associated stimuli, the effect is reversed, and it contributes to tumor progression. The normal stroma thus possesses inherent plasticity, responds rapidly to neoplastic situations, and coevolves with the cancer cells synthesizing several cytokines, chemokines, growth factors, and proteinases, resulting in the generation of active stroma and accelerating disease progression [4]. The active stroma consists of tumor-associated fibroblasts and myofibroblasts, inflammatory cells, immune cells, endothelial cells, a remodeled matrix, and reprogrammed metabolism. Moreover, the stromal part of the TME provides a favorable environment for the cancer cells to circumvent apoptosis and to progress toward more malignant phenotypes [5].

5.2   THE TUMOR MICROENVIRONMENT

The TME contains the cancer cells together with the nonmalignant cells and noncellular components that are involved in determining the consequences of malignancy. It consists of both cellular and noncellular components. The cellular components of the TME may be hematopoietic (T cells, B cells, natural killer cells, macrophages, neutrophils and myeloid-derived suppressor cells) or mesenchymal (fibroblasts, mesenchymal stem cells, and endothelial cells) in origin. The noncellular component of the TME is known as the extracellular matrix (ECM) and consists of proteins, glycoproteins, and proteoglycans that structurally and functionally support the TME.

5.2.1   T LYMPHOCYTES

Many different T-cell populations enter the tumor microenvironment at the invasive tumor margin and in the draining lymphoid organs. Studies using immunohistochemistry have suggested that infiltration of T cells occurs in ovarian cancer, renal cell carcinoma, bladder cancer, and other solid cancers [6–8]. It has been found that infiltration of CD8+ memory T cells is associated with a good prognosis [9]. Infiltration of CD4$^+$ T helper 1 (TH1) cells (which produce cytokines interleukin-2 (IL-2) and interferon gamma (IFNγ)) in the TME also correlates with a good prognosis [9]. TH2 cells that produce IL-4, IL-5, and IL-13, or TH17 cells, are believed to promote tumor growth [9].In some cases, it has been found to be linked to a good prognosis as in the case of TH2 cells in breast cancer and TH17 cells in esophageal cancers [10, 11].

5.2.2   REGULATORY T CELLS

Regulatory T cells (Tregs) are a subpopulation of T cells that are involved in maintaining immune homeostasis and self-tolerance. They also control autoimmunity, infection, graft-versus-host disease, inflammation, fetal-maternal tolerance, and tumor immunity. The Tregs downregulate the proliferation of other T cells in the microenvironment by releasing perforins/granzymes or suppressive cytokines like interleukin-10 (IL-10) and tumor growth factor-β (TGF-β). Tregs are therefore involved in tumor progression. Higher Treg concentration with a poor prognosis is found in ovarian cancer, lung cancer glioblastoma, melanoma, and other malignancies [12–19]. Moreover, it has been found that depletion of Tregs prior to tumor resection and radiotherapy in breast cancer patient results in improved clinical outcomes [20]. Tregs play a protective role by regulating inflammation in colorectal and gastric cancers [19, 20].

Chemokines secreted by the tumor and immune cells recruit Tregs into the TME. Alternatively, the immunosuppressive Tregs may be derived from nonsuppressive CD25$^-$ conventional T cells (Tconv) under the influence of tumor-derived TGF-β. Thus, Tregs promote immune evasion and are involved in the formation of pro-tumorigenic TME.

5.2.3 B LYMPHOCYTES

B lymphocytes are the second most abundant tumor infiltrating lymphocytes and play an important role in modulating the immune response to cancer. They are commonly found in the draining lymph nodes but may also be present at the invasive margin of tumors. They inhibit tumor development by producing tumor-reactive antibodies and promoting natural killer (NK) cell-mediated tumor killing, phagocytosis by macrophages, and priming of CD8$^+$ and CD4$^+$ T cells. In contrast, B cells can also promote tumor development by production of autoantibodies and tumor growth factors. A subset of B cells–B regulatory cells (Bregs)–express cytokines such as IL-10, TGF-β, and immune regulatory ligands like programmed death ligand-1 (PD-L1). PD-L1 suppresses tumor killing by T cells and NK cells [21]. Bregs have now been identified in several human cancers including ovarian, gastric, lung, esophageal, squamous cell, colorectal, and breast carcinoma [22–27]. Infiltration of Bregs is associated with increased tumor militancy and poor prognosis. In human lymphoid malignancies, malignant B cells suppress the antitumor immune response [28, 29]. Targeting of B-regulatory functions of malignant B cells in lymphomas has shown positive results in several clinical trials [30–32].

5.2.4 NATURAL KILLER CELLS

Natural killer cells are lymphoid cells that have a natural ability to kill tumor and other infected cells [33]. Not much is known about their role in controlling solid tumor progression. Natural killer cells enter the tumor sites by extravasations through tumor vasculature [34]. The immunosuppressive effects of the TME inhibits the tumor killing function of the NK cells [33]. Dendritic cells, Tregs, myeloid derived suppressor cells, and cancer- associated fibroblasts suppress the NK cell-mediated cytotoxicity. Several studies have also revealed that tumor stroma contains NK cells having an anergic phenotype induced by malignant cell-derived TGF-β [9].

5.2.5   TUMOR-ASSOCIATED MACROPHAGES

Macrophages are a heterogenous group of terminally differentiated, tissue resident cells originating from the circulating monocytic precursors derived from the bone marrow. They exhibit plasticity and exist in two extremes of possible differentiation states - M1 and M2 [35]. M1-type macrophages play important roles in the innate response against invading pathogens, whereas M2-type macrophages are involved in tissue repair and tumor progression. M1 polarization is brought about by bacterial lipopolysaccharide, Toll-like receptor agonism, and IFNγ. M2 polarization is promoted by tumor-derived cytokines such as IL-4, IL-10, IL-13, TGF-β, and prostaglandin E2 (PGE2) [36]. The chemokine ligand CCL2 and macrophage colony-stimulating factor recruits monocytes to the tumor tissue, and then, these tumor-derived cytokines induce the monocytes to differentiate into tumor-associated macrophages (TAMs) [13]. TAMs are usually pro-tumorigenic [37]. TAMs have a very high antigen-presenting capacity but cause tumor progression. TAMs enhance proliferation, invasion, and metastasis in tumor cells. They also stimulate angiogenesis and inhibit the T cell-mediated antitumor immune response [37–40]. TME containing TAMs is associated with poor prognosis [41].

5.2.6   MYELOID-DERIVED SUPPRESSOR CELLS

More recently, it has been found that in growing tumors, there is an aberrant activation of myelopoiesis and an accumulation of immature myeloid cells known as the myeloid-derived suppressor cells (MDSC) [42]. The MDSCs suppress the T-cell responses [42, 43]. Cancer models of mouse and cancers in humans have two main MDSC subtypes: granulocytic (G-MDSC) and monocytic (M-MDSC). In humans, M-MDSC are predominantly CD14$^+$and G-MDSC are CD15$^+$, both being CD33$^+$HLA-DR$^-$[44, 45]. Several findings indicate that myeloid cells may have the plasticity to interconvert between different phenotypes, and that the TME can have a major effect on their phenotype and function [39]. G-MDSCs cause immunosuppression by producing reactive oxygen species, while the M-MDSCs do so by generating nitric oxide [46–48]. The MDSCs can also differentiate into TAMs and thereby promote tumor invasion and metastasis [49].

5.2.7 DENDRITIC CELLS

Dendritic cells (DCs) are specialized antigen-presenting cells and play an important role in the adaptive immune response. DCs are a heterogenous population of cells having high plasticity. They are derived from CD34+ bone-marrow stem cells and exist in two different developmental stages: immature and mature dendritic cells. The immature DCs reside in the peripheral tissues and function in antigen uptake and processing, while lymphoid organs harbor the mature DCs that interact with T cells and are responsible for initiating the immune response [50]. The DCs found in the TME are unable to evoke an adequate immune response against tumor antigens. The inflammatory microenvironment of the TME is responsible for impairing the functioning of the dendritic cells [51].

There are two major morphological subsets of dendritic cells, namely the myeloid or the conventional DCs and the plasmacytoid DCs. Human myeloid DCs produce IL-12 that suppresses tumor neo-angiogenesis by myeloid DCs [52]. But, the tumor microenvironment has been found to lack myeloid DCs and contain the plasmacytoid DCs, which are involved in tumor vascularization and thereby its progression [53]. The tumor-associated DCs thus favor tumor progression by initiating genomic damage, supporting neo-vascularization and stimulating tumor cell growth and spreading [54].

5.2.8 TUMOR-ASSOCIATED NEUTROPHILS

Neutrophils constitute the major inflammatory cell type in many models of cancer [55]. Neutrophils play an important role in host defense. Neutrophils that infiltrate into tumors are referred to as TANs. Interleukin-8 (IL-8), which is a chemoattractant for neutrophils, is also chiefly responsible for the recruitment of TANs into the TME [56]. The TANs may assume a pro-tumorigenic phenotype N2 or a pro-inflammatory and antitumorigenic phenotype

N1 [57].The antitumorigenic effect of TANs in the TME is decided by the dominating phenotype. Respiratory burst and granule production are inhibited in TAN. Neutrophil infiltration into the TME has been shown to be associated with metastases [58, 59]. TANs have also been shown to increase the ability of tumor cells to extravasate through endothelium, thereby increasing its metastatic potential. In contrast, some studies have also reported antitumor roles for these cells [60, 61].

5.2.9   CANCER-ASSOCIATED FIBROBLASTS

Fibroblasts are the most abundant cells in the tumor-associated stroma and are involved in the deposition of ECM and components of the basement membrane. They are involved in modulating the immune responses and homeostasis. Morphologically, the fibroblasts in cancer tissues resemble myofibroblasts, which are large spindle-shaped cells that are activated during the wound healing process. The malignant cells and the transforming factors released by them convert them into cancer-associated fibroblasts (CAFs). After the completion of the wound healing process, there is a decrease in the levels of activated myofibroblasts [62]. In contrast, the CAFs are permanently activated and do not revert to a normal phenotype nor undergo apoptosis and elimination like normal fibroblasts. The presence of CAFs correlates with poor disease prognosis in several tumors. CAFs can also be derived from resident precursors, like the endothelial cells, or mesenchymal stem cells [63, 64]. CAFs secrete various growth factors, cytokines, and chemokines, which are associated with tumor dissemination, proliferation, and metastasis. The degradation of extracellular matrix (ECM) proteins by CAFs is believed to be involved in ECM remodeling, which plays an important role during tumor dissemination. TGF-β from fibroblasts induces epithelial–mesenchymal transition (EMT) in malignant cells and contributes to the immunosuppressive microenvironment [65]. Fibroblast-produced CXCL12, a chemoattractant, causes the stromal cells to migrate into the TME [66]. In mouse models of skin, breast and pancreatic tumors, CAFs have been shown to promote tumor growth by causing neo-vascularization [66]. Fibroblasts are therefore one of the major determinants in the malignant progression of cancer and present an important target for cancer therapies.

5.2.10   VASCULAR ENDOTHELIAL CELLS

Another type of stromal cells present in the TME is the endothelial cells. Tumor growth beyond a diameter of 2–3 mm requires a proper vasculature to fulfill the energetic requirements of the tumor cell. Therefore, to continue their growth, tumor cells induce formation of new blood vessels from the existing ones by a process known as angiogenesis. Tumor angiogenesis provides the cells with nutrients and oxygen, enables the removal of metabolic wastes, and moves the cancer cells into the circulatory system. The tumor endothelial cells form the angiogenic vessels [67]. Soluble factors present in the TME, such as vascular endothelial growth factors (VEGFs), fibroblast growth factors (FGFs), platelet-derived growth factors (PDGFs), and chemokines cause activation of the endothelial cells during tumor neovascularization [68]. On sensing an angiogenic signal by a quiescent blood vessel, angiogenesis is stimulated and new blood vessels sprout from the existing vasculature [68]. The tumor vasculature is abnormal. Tumor endothelial cells are irregular in shape and size. They have uneven margins and long, fragile cytoplasmic projections that extend into the lumen. The tumor vasculature thus consists of chaotically branched vessels that are leaky and have an uneven lumen [69].

5.2.11   PERICYTES

Pericytes are multipotent perivascular cells that enwrap the endothelial cells and are involved in vasculature development. They function in angiogenesis, tissue homeostasis, vessel permeability, and blood pressure control. Malfunctioning or loss of pericytes results in increased metastasis [70, 71]. Alternatively, in several malignancies, tumor cells can circumvent intravascular invasion by adopting a pericyte-like phenotype (or pericyte mimicry) and migrate along the extravascular surface of vessels [72]. Recent studies have shown that tumor-associated pericytes have increased distance from associating blood and abnormal cytoplasmic processes and endothelial interactions [73]. This incomplete coverage and loosened endothelial–pericyte interaction results in increased vascular permeability. Lesser amount of pericytes in the tumor vasculature results in increased metastasis as shown in clinical studies of bladder and colorectal cancer [70, 74, 75]. Dissociation or loss of pericytes from their endothelial cells also results in a hypoxic tumor microenvironment, EMT, and increased tumor invasiveness [75]. Contrarily, the angiotropic tumor cells may migrate in a "pericytic-like" manner along the external surface of vascular channels without intravasation. This is known as pericyte mimicry and leads to metastasis without tumor cell entry into the blood stream. Pericyte mimicry has been seen in common malignancies of the skin, brain, pancreas, and prostate [76–78].

5.2.12 MESENCHYMAL STEM CELLS

Mesenchymal stem cells (MSCs) are nonhematopoietic pluripotent cells that give rise to a variety of connective tissue cell types. They are characterized by the expression of stromal cell markers (CD73, CD105, CD44, CD29, and CD90) [79]. MSCs can differentiate along osteogenic, adipogenic, and chondrogenic lineages when placed in the appropriate environments. Secretion of soluble factors by the tumor cells, inflammation, and a hypoxic environment recruit the MSCs to the tumor site [80]. The MSCs are capable of differentiating into cancer-associated fibroblasts (CAF), macrophages or endothelial cells and thus are responsible for tumor growth and progression [81, 82].

5.3 THE ECM OF THE TUMOR MICROENVIRONMENT

The ECM consists of a number of glycoproteins, proteins, and polysaccharides [83]. The ECM includes a compact basement membrane rich in type IV collagen, laminin and fibronectin and the interstitial matrix which consists of fibrillar collagens, proteoglycans, and glycoproteins that provide tensile strength to the tissue. The ECM provides a scaffold for cells in the TME. However, it is also involved in the evolution and spread of cancers by controlling cell adhesion to the ECM [84]. Being rich in proteins and polysaccharides, the ECM can bind to several growth factors and thereby control their signaling and binding to ligands. Additionally, the ECM may also initiate signaling [85]. Crosslinking of elastin and collagen fibers results in larger, more rigid fibrils [86]. Malignant cells, TAMs, and CAFs secrete matrix metalloproteases (MMPs) that degrade ECM proteins, and release chemokines and growth and angiogenic factors that remodel the ECM. Other proteases such as cathepsins are also unregulated, thereby aiding metastasis, angiogenesis, and inflammation [87]. Remodeling of the

ECM may lead to change in ECM dynamics, thereby affecting tumor dissemination and metastasis.

5.4   TUMOR ANGIOGENESIS

Angiogenesis is one of the hallmarks of cancer [88]. Tumor vascularization involves the co-operation of several cells of the TME such as the vascular endothelial cells, pericytes, TAMs, MSCs, and CAFs [89].

Physiological angiogenesis involves creation of the blood vessels *de novo*. This involves proliferation and assembly of angioblasts to form the primary capillary plexus, which then forms new blood vessels that sprout (new blood vessel growth from pre-existing ones) and branch. Cancer cells, however, initiate sprouting angiogenesis from the existing blood vessels of the stroma. Moreover, in tumor angiogenesis, there is an imbalance between the pro-angiogenic and anti-angiogenic factors which causes a continuous growth of new blood vessels. Moreover, the tumor vasculature is irregular, consisting of irregular, leaky and hemorrhagic blood vessels resulting in an abnormal blood flow.

Angiogenic sprouting involves release of angiogenic factors like VEGF, bFGF (basic fibroblast growth factor), angiopoietins, PDGF, and TGF β from the tumor and other cells of the TME. These diffuse to the surrounding tissues. There, they bind to the receptors present on the endothelial cells of existing blood vessels. This activates the signal transduction pathways involving RAF, p38 MAPK, and P13K. VEGF, produced by the tumor cells and the cells of the stroma, is an important regulator of angiogenesis [90]. Hypoxia increases the transcriptional activation of the VEGF gene and VEGF mRNA stability, and thus, it is involved in tumor progression and dissemination. Degradation of the basement membrane of the existing vessels is an important requirement for sprouting angiogenesis. This is initiated by bFGF and VEGF. These factors activate the endothelial cells and MMPs and induce the secretion of plasminogen activators. The ECM is degraded by the proteinases and the activated endothelial cells migrate and invade the ECM eventually differentiating into a new immature vessel. The new immature vessels are stabilized by recruitment of smooth muscle cells and pericytes, producing a vascular basal lamina. The fusion of the new blood vessel sprouts results in the built up of the final vascular system. The majority of the tumor vasculature has a basement membrane, but the pericytes are abnormal and lack their normal organization in the vessel wall.

5.5   THE METASTATIC CASCADE

Metastasis is a multistage process. It involves the spread of the cancer cells from their primary site to distant organs of the body. This process is clinically significant as approximately 90% of cancer mortality is linked to it [91].

Metastasis involves a series of steps. Angiogenesis is an important step that is required for tumor growth and for the initial progression from a pre-malignant tumor to invasive cancer. The next step is detachment from the primary tumor followed by entry into the local lymphatic and blood vessels and circulatory survival. Before extravasation and invasion, the circulating tumor cells must be capable of resisting the host immune response. The final step involves the survival of the tumor at the distant site. The TME co-evolves with the growing cancer cells. It promotes initial dissemination and subsequent invasion at the primary site and also creates a permissive niche at the distant location, thereby facilitating metastasis. Tumors select the preferential sites for metastasis and may show variable periods of dormancy in their temporary course [92]. The development of a receptive TME at the metastatic site before the arrival of disseminated tumor cells enhances metastatic efficiency [93].

5.5.1   CELL MIGRATION AND INVASION

Cell migration and invasion are the primary steps in metastasis and the propagation of cancer to distant sites. Invasion can be defined as the entry of cancer cells from the primary tumor into the surrounding stroma.

5.5.1.1   Types of Cell Migration

There are two fundamentally different patterns of cell migration, namely collective (group) cell migration and single cell migration (individual migration) [94]. The type of migration is largely determined by tissue microenvironment.

5.5.1.1.1 Collective migration

The migration of interconnected groups of cells is known as collective migration [95, 96]. In this type of migration, the cancer cells penetrate the surrounding tissues and form thin chords, clusters, or stripes [95]. Collective migration of cells has a "leading front" and the "follower" cells. The "leaders" are the mesenchymal cells having a loosened structural organization, while the "followers" form packed, rosette-like tubular structures with tight intercellular contacts. Pseudopodia formation and proteolytic degradation are carried out at the leading edge to create a space for invasion of the tumor tissue.

5.5.1.1.2 Single cell invasion or individual cell migration

This type of migration involves invasion of the surrounding tissue by individual tumor cells [97]. Single cell migration involves two different types of movements: mesenchymal and amoeboid [95, 97]. A number of researchers believe that there is a shift from one type of movement to the other (from mesenchymal to amoeboid and vice versa) in the case of single cell invasion.

Mesenchymal (fibroblast-like) cell migration: This type of movement is used by malignant cells that acquire an elongated spindle shape by losing epithelial polarity [95, 97]. The mesenchymal mechanism of invasion is a result of EMT. Mesenchymal invasion has been detected during the development of melanoma, fibrosarcoma, and other malignancies [95, 98].

Amoeboid cell migration: The amoeboid mechanism of cell migration is the most efficient mode of migration of single tumor cells. It is believed that upon destruction of the extracellular matrix and loss of adhesion molecules, the tumor cells resort to the amoeboid mechanism of invasion [95]. The malignant tumor cells undergoing amoeboid migration have a round or elliptical shape [95]. The amoeboid type of invasive growth has been observed in breast cancer, lymphoma, and melanoma [95]. In contrast to the mesenchymal movement, amoeboid mode of migration occurs when the surrounding matrix is characterized by low stiffness ("soft" matrix).

5.5.1.2 Degradation of the Extracellular Matrix

The basement membrane is first breached by the cancer cells and alteration in its organization and integrity is regarded as a hallmark of invasive carcinoma. Expression of MMPs mediates proteolytic degradation of the ECM. MMPs are a family of zinc-binding enzymes that degrade the ECM and the basement membrane. They are initially secreted as inactive zymogens and are activated by extracellular proteases.

5.5.1.3   Cell Detachment

Cell detachment is a critical step in metastasis. It involves coordinated assembly and disassembly of focal adhesions at the front and the rear of the cell. Focal adhesions are contact regions between the ECM and the cytoskeleton that are brought about by the integrin family of transmembrane proteins. The cytoplasmic region of the integrins interact with integrin-binding proteins like talin, paxillin, and focal adhesion kinase (FAK). Focal adhesion functions to support adhesion to the ECM and is also involved in signal transduction. Activation of integrins leads to the activation of signaling pathways involved in cell survival and migration. Cell detachment involves focal adhesion disassembly, detachment from integrins, and their internalization in endocytic vesicles. Detachment of cells involves loss of tight junctions or adherens junctions. Adherens junctions are constituted primarily by E-cadherens which therefore plays an important role in metastasis.

5.5.1.4   Epithelial-Mesenchymal Transition

EMT is defined as a regulated series of steps in which the epithelial cells acquire mesenchymal features. Though EMT is essential during embryonic development, wound healing and tissue regeneration, but deregulated EMT can prove to be destructive as in cancer. EMT in tumor cells is marked by a loss of E-cadherin and gain of N-cadherin. Here, the tumor cells gain mesenchymal characters and acquire a migratory phenotype and stem-like properties [99]. Cancer cells undergo EMT prior to invasion and dissemination to distant sites. On reaching those sites, the mesenchymal cells revert to an epithelial identity (mesenchymal–epithelial transition) in order to regain the ability to proliferate. The immune and stromal cells interact with the tumor at its margins [100]. TAM-derived TGF-β is responsible for increased EMT [90, 101]. Invasiveness may also be promoted through EGFR-secreted by activated TAMs [102]. IL-6 secreted from the adipocytes increases invasiveness in breast cancer. TME-associated hypoxia or inflammation also causes tumor invasion by VEGF upregulation and recruitment of MDSCs and NKs into secondary organs, thereby promoting pre-metastatic dissemination.

5.5.2   INTRAVASATION

Once the tumor cells detach from the primary tumor, they must enter the circulation in order to move to distant organs. The entry of tumor cell into the body's blood or lymphatic vessels and transportation to a new site is termed intravasation. This process is also known as transendothelial migration. Intravasation permits the cancer cells to gain access to other organs. For example, in lung cancer, transendothelial migration is facilitated by expression of integrin $\beta1$, while breast cancer intravasation is enhanced by TGF-β [103]. Conversely, intravasation has been found to be blocked in colon cancer through Notch-dependent mechanisms [104]. Cancer cells have also been found to enhance vasculature permeability by secreting factors such as angiopoietin 1, cytochrome c oxidase subunit 2, matrix metalloproteinase (MMP)-1/2/3/10, TGF-β, and VEGF in the case of lung or brain carcinoma [105]. Intravasation can occur both actively or passively.

5.5.2.1   Active Intravasation

In active intravasation, the tumor cell directly enters a blood vessel in response to chemokines, growth factors, and nutrient gradients [108]. This process is facilitated by TAMs that promote intravasation by secreting chemokines and pro-inflammatory factors. Remodeling of the ECM by TAMs facilitates tumor migration toward blood vessels. This remodeling also deregulates and detaches the pericytes, which further enables the tumor cells to bypass the blood vessel barrier [105].

5.5.2.2   Passive Intravasation

Shedding of tumor cells upon entering the bloodstream is known as passive intravasation. Increased passive intravasation occurs when the primary tumor experiences trauma. Moreover, overgrowth of the tumor cells in a restricted space results in collapse of blood and lymphatic vessels, forcing the cells into the vessels.

5.5.3   SURVIVAL IN THE CIRCULATION

After entering the blood vessels, the cancer cells can travel either through the venous or arterial circulation. The circulating tumor cells (CTCs) must survive several stresses to reach distant sites. The CTCs lack integrin-dependent adhesion to ECM and therefore undergo anoikis – an apoptosis triggered by loss of anchorage to substrate [106]. The CTCs escape anoikis by suppression of caspase-associated apoptosis by activated tropomyosin-related kinase B (TrkB) [107]. CTCs must also survive the enormous shearing forces prevailing in the blood circulation. The tumor cells that undergo EMT are found to be more resistant against these forces. The predation of tumor cells by the cells of the host's immune system is overcome by the formation of emboli by interaction with the blood platelets [108]. Coating of platelets interferes with NK cell-mediated cytotoxicity and thus impedes immune recognition.

5.5.4   EXTRAVASATION

Once the CTCs enter the microvasculature of distant organs, they form a mass that breaks the walls of containing vessels, placing the tumor cells in direct contact with the tissue parenchyma [109]. Alternatively, the tumor cells reach the tissue by penetrating through the endothelial cell and pericyte layers. It is believed that the tumor cells adopt leukocyte-like characteristics during extravasation. The process of extravasation is divided into three sequential steps.

5.5.4.1   Rolling

In the first step, the extravasating cells loosely adhere to the vascular endothelial and roll along its vascular surface. P-selectin glycoprotein ligand-1 (PSGL-1)and the E-selectin ligand-1 expression by the tumor cells helps in their rolling [110, 111]. CD24, together with sLeX, also promotes hematogenic metastasis formation, but it is less efficient than PSGL-1 [112]. Recently, the carcinoembryonic antigen (CEA), which is expressed on colon carcinoma cells, has been reported be involved in rolling [113]. Some studies have also reported the involvement of N- cadherins in the rolling of tumor cells.

5.5.4.2   Adhesion to the Vascular Endothelium

The second step of extravasation involves tight attachment of the tumor cells to the endothelium. This is mediated by selectins and cell glycoproteins. In vitro studies have shown that integrin α4β1 interacts with the vascular cell adhesion molecule *(VCAM)* [114]. These studies have shown that the metastatic capacity of melanoma cells is facilitated by the interactions of α4β1 integrin with VCAM-1. Tumor cells also express intercellular adhesion molecule-1 (ICAM-1), a ligand for β2 integrins that are found on leukocytes and not on tumor cells. This indicates that the tumor cells may use leukocytes as linkers to enable their firm adhesion to the endothelial cells. CD44 and Galectin-3, have been found to be associated with tumor- endothelial cell adhesion [115].

5.5.4.3   Diapedesis

After adhesion, the CTCs transmigrate from the endothelial barrier. This final step of the extravasation is known as diapedesis. Diapedesis is a dynamic process that involves constant formation and rupture of intercellular contacts. The CTCs develop protrusions in order to penetrate the endothelial intercellular junctions. This involves altered expressions of vascular endothelial cadherin and platelet/endothelial cell adhesion molecule (PECAM). Tumor cell diapedesis also requires the participation of cadherin. VEGF is responsible for changes in the vascular permeability of the blood vessels of the target organ [116]. Diapedisis induces irreversible damage to the endothelium because of the induction of apoptosis (loss of cell to cell contact) and due to the large size of the tumor cells as compared to the leukocytes.

5.5.5   *TUMOR ESTABLISHMENT AT THE SECONDARY SITE*

Although theoretically the CTCs have the ability to move to a wide variety of secondary locations, it has been found that individual carcinomas form metastasis in only a few target organs [117]. The layout and diameter of blood vessels may result in the arrest of CTCs at certain specific sites, for example, colorectal carcinoma cell trapped in the liver [118]. Conversely, according to the seed-and-soil hypothesis of Stephen Paget (1889), metastases is not random, but displays organ-preference [93]. The primary tumors are known to secrete factors that form a premetastatic niche that stimulates efficient metastasis. In a study in breast cancer, it was found that the expression of lysyl oxidase facilitated myeloid cell recruitment and metastasis to lung [119]. The CTCs may metastasize to specific organs via specific ligand–receptor interactions between tumor cells and the luminal walls of the microvasculature, for example, metadherin expressed in breast cancer is involved in metastasis to the lungs [120]. Recent studies have shown that the secondary microenvironment can mimic the primary TME in order to support secondary growth.

5.5.5.1   Apoptosis and Tumor Dormancy

Metastasis is considered to be an inefficient process because less than 0.01% of circulating tumor cells actually succeeds in forming secondary tumor growths. Only a few disseminated cells are competent enough to grow in the new site [11]. Many of them undergo apoptosis within a few hours of reaching the secondary site. Cancer cells at the secondary site may be destroyed by the cytotoxic mediators release by the endothelial cells at the new site or may be eliminated by immune surveillance [121]. Alternatively, the tumor cells may survive the host defense mechanisms and exist as asymptomatic micro-metastases in the body for years without detection. This is referred to as tumor dormancy. Tumor dormancy may be due to cell cycle arrest, immune surveillance, or failure to trigger angiogenesis which is necessary for tumor expansion [122].

5.5.5.2   Tumor Awakening and Metastatic Outgrowth

On escaping immune surveillance and by exiting angiogenic or cell cycle-mediated mechanisms of dormancy, the tumor cells are capable of developing lethal macrometastases. This involves immune suppression, sustained vascularization, and enhanced survival. The TAMs are believed to facilitate all these processes. Peripheral M2-polarized macrophages have been found to be associated with liver metastases in patients with pancreatic cancer

[123]. Extravasation and metastasis of cancer cells in the lung have been found to be mediated by TAMs [124]. Thus, the tumor cells that reach a new site create a favorable environment for their survival and proliferation, thus establishing secondary growth.

5.6 CONCLUSION

Metastasis is a multistage event that involves the spread of the cancer cells from their primary site to distant organs of the body. This process is clinically significant as approximately 90% of cancer mortality is linked to it. Recent studies, however, indicate that tumor invasion and metastasis are not just determined by malignant cancer cells themselves but also by the tumor microenvironment. The dynamic changes in the TME due to its various cellular and noncellular components influence the progression, dissemination, and secondary colonization of cancer. Thus, there is a need to completely understand the TME and the crosstalk between its malignant and non-malignant components. This would help in designing better therapeutic strategies for managing and treating cancer.

5.7 SUMMARY

- The cellular environment where a tumor exists is known as the tumor microenvironment.
- The tumor microenvironment includes malignant and nonmalignant cells together with non-cellular components and has an important role in modulating the metastatic capacity of most cancers.
- Metastasis is a multistage process in which the cancer cells spread from their primary site to other organs of the body. This process is clinically significant as approximately 90% of cancer mortality is linked to it.
- The various steps of metastasis involve cell migration and invasion, transendothelial migration extravasation, survival in circulation and tumor growth and proliferation at the secondary site.
- Recruitment of macrophages to the TME increases their metastatic potential.
- Tregs, bregs, TANs, and dentritic cells present in the TME have been found to be associated with a poor prognosis.

- Myeloid cell-derived suppressor cells suppress immune responses to the growing tumor and promote its metastatic potential.
- Mesenchymal stem cells are recruited to the primary site and can differentiate into cancer-associated fibroblasts (CAF), macrophages, or endothelial cells, thereby promoting tumor dissemination.
- The tumor microenvironment is thus a dynamic entity and evolves along with the tumor growth and influences tumor progression and stimulates its invasion and metastasis.

KEYWORDS

- **cancer-associated fibroblasts**
- **invasion**
- **metastasis**
- **tumor-associated macrophages**
- **tumor microenvironment**

REFERENCES

1. De Wever, O., & Mareel, M., (2003). Role of tissue stroma in cancer cell invasion. *J. Pathol., 200*, 429–447.
2. Ozdemir, B. C., Pentcheva-Hoang, T., Carstens, J. L., Zheng, X., Wu, C. C., Simpson, T. R., Laklai, H., Sugimoto, H., Kahlert, C., Novitskiy, S. V., De Jesus-Acosta, A., Sharma, P., Heidari, P., Mahmood, U., Chin, L., Moses, H. L., Weaver, V. M., Maitra, A., Allison, J. P., LeBleu, V. S., & Kalluri, R., (2014). Depletion of carcinoma-associated fibroblasts and fibrosis induces immunosuppression and accelerates pancreas cancer with reduced survival. *Cancer Cell, 25*, 719–734.
3. Rhim, A. D., Oberstein, P. E., Thomas, D. H., Mirek, E. T., Palermo, C. F., Sastra, S. A., Dekleva, E. N., Saunders, T., Becerra, C. P., Tattersall, I. W., Westphalen, C. B., Kitajewski, J., Fernandez-Barrena, M. G., Fernandez-Zapico, M. E., Iacobuzio-Donahue, C., Olive, K. P., & Stanger, B. Z., (2014). Stromal elements act to restrain, rather than support, pancreatic ductal adenocarcinoma. *Cancer Cell, 25*, 735–747.
4. Junttila, M. R., & De Sauvage, F. J., (2013). Influence of tumour micro-environment heterogeneity on therapeutic response. *Nature, 501*, 346–354.
5. Chen, F., Qi, X., Qian, M., Dai, Y., & Sun, Y., (2014). Tackling the tumor microenvironment: what challenge does it pose to anticancer therapies? *Protein Cell, 5*, 816–826.
6. Sato, E., Olson, S. H., Ahn, J., Bundy, B., Nishikawa, H., Qian, F., Jungbluth, A. A., Frosina, D., Gnjatic, S., Ambrosone, C., Kepner, J., Odunsi, T., Ritter, G., Lele, S.,

Chen, Y. T., Ohtani, H., Old, L. J., & Odunsi, K., (2005). Intraepithelial CD8+ tumor-infiltrating lymphocytes and a high CD8+/regulatory T cell ratio are associated with favorable prognosis in ovarian cancer. *Proc. Natl. Acad. Sci. USA, 102,* 18538–18543.

7. Nakano, O., Sato, M., Naito, Y., Suzuki, K., Orikasa, S., Aizawa, M., Suzuki, Y., Shin-taku, I., Nagura, H., & Ohtani, H., (2001). Proliferative activity of intratumoral CD8(+) T-lymphocytes as a prognostic factor in human renal cell carcinoma: clinicopathologic demonstration of antitumor immunity. *Cancer Res., 61,* 5132–5136.

8. Sharma, P., Shen, Y., Wen, S., Yamada, S., Jungbluth, A. A., Gnjatic, S., Bajorin, D. F., Reuter, V. E., Herr, H., Old, L. J., & Sato, E., (2007). CD8 tumor-infiltrating lympho-cytes are predictive of survival in muscle-invasive urothelial carcinoma. *Proc. Natl. Acad. Sci. USA, 104,* 3967–3972.

9. Fridman, W. H., Pages, F., Sautes-Fridman, C., & Galon, J., (2012). The immune con-texture in human tumours: impact on clinical outcome. *Nat. Rev. Cancer, 12,* 298–306.

10. Yoon, N. K., Maresh, E. L., Shen, D., Elshimali, Y., Apple, S., Horvath, S., Mah, V., Bose, S., Chia, D., Chang, H. R., & Goodglick, L., (2010). Higher levels of GATA3 predict better survival in women with breast cancer. *Hum. Pathol., 41,* 1794–1801.

11. Lv, L., Pan, K., Li, X. D., She, K. L., Zhao, J. J., Wang, W., Chen, J. G., Chen, Y. B., Yun, J. P., & Xia, J. C., (2011). The accumulation and prognosis value of tumor infil-trating IL-17 producing cells in esophageal squamous cell carcinoma. *PLoS One, 6,* e18219.

12. Curiel, T. J., Coukos, G., Zou, L., Alvarez, X., Cheng, P., Mottram, P., Evdemon-Hogan, M., Conejo-Garcia, J. R., Zhang, L., Burow, M., Zhu, Y., Wei, S., Kryczek, I., Daniel, B., Gordon, A., Myers, L., Lackner, A., Disis, M. L., Knutson, K. L., Chen, L., & Zou, W., (2004). Specific recruitment of regulatory T cells in ovarian carcinoma fosters im-mune privilege and predicts reduced survival. *Nat. Med., 10,* 942–949.

13. Leffers, N., Gooden, M. J., De Jong, R. A., Hoogeboom, B. N., Ten Hoor, K. A., Hollema, H., Boezen, H. M., Van der Zee, A. G., Daemen, T., & Nijman, H. W., (2009). Prognostic significance of tumor-infiltrating T-lymphocytes in primary and metastatic lesions of advanced stage ovarian cancer. *Cancer Immunol. Immunother, 58,* 449–459.

14. Tao, H., Mimura, Y., Aoe, K., Kobayashi, S., Yamamoto, H., Matsuda, E., Okabe, K., Matsumoto, T., Sugi, K., & Ueoka, H., (2012). Prognostic potential of FOXP3 expres-sion in non-small cell lung cancer cells combined with tumor-infiltrating regulatory T cells. *Lung. Cancer, 75,* 95–101.

15. Sayour, E. J., McLendon, P., McLendon, R., De Leon, G., Reynolds, R., Kresak, J., Sampson, J. H., & Mitchell, D. A., (2015). Increased proportion of FoxP3+ regulatory T cells in tumor infiltrating lymphocytes is associated with tumor recurrence and reduced survival in patients with glioblastoma. *Cancer Immunol. Immunother, 64,* 419–427.

16. Deleeuw, R. J., Kost, S. E., Kakal, J. A., & Nelson, B. H., (2012). The prognostic value of FoxP3+ tumor-infiltrating lymphocytes in cancer: a critical review of the literature. *Clin. Cancer Res., 18,* 3022–3029.

17. Ladoire, S., Arnould, L., Apetoh, L., Coudert, B., Martin, F., Chauffert, B., Fumoleau, P., & Ghiringhelli, F., (2008). Pathologic complete response to neoadjuvant chemo-therapy of breast carcinoma is associated with the disappearance of tumor-infiltrating foxp3+ regulatory T cells. *Clin. Cancer Res., 14,* 2413–2420.

18. Haas, M., Dimmler, A., Hohenberger, W., Grabenbauer, G. G., Niedobitek, G., & Dis-tel, L. V., (2009). Stromal regulatory T-cells are associated with a favourable prognosis in gastric cancer of the cardia. *BMC Gastroenterol, 9,* 65.

19. Salama, P., Phillips, M., Grieu, F., Morris, M., Zeps, N., Joseph, D., Platell, C., & Ia-copetta, B., (2009). Tumor-infiltrating FOXP3+ T regulatory cells show strong prognostic significance in colorectal cancer. *J. Clin. Oncol., 27*, 186–192.

20. Ladoire, S., Martin, F., & Ghiringhelli, F., (2011). Prognostic role of FOXP3+ regulatory T cells infiltrating human carcinomas: the paradox of colorectal cancer. *Cancer Immunol. Immunother, 60*, 909–918.

21. Mauri, C., & Bosma, A., (2012). Immune regulatory function of B cells. *Annu. Rev. Immunol., 30*, 221–241.

22. Zhou, X., Su, Y. X., Lao, X. M., Liang, Y. J., & Liao, G. Q., (2016). CD19(+)IL-10(+) regulatory B cells affect survival of tongue squamous cell carcinoma patients and induce resting CD4(+) T cells to CD4(+)Foxp3(+) regulatory T cells. *Oral. Oncol., 53*, 27–35.

23. Zhou, J., Min, Z., Zhang, D., Wang, W., Marincola, F., & Wang, X., (2014). Enhanced frequency and potential mechanism of B regulatory cells in patients with lung cancer. *J. Transl. Med., 12*, 304.

24. Wei, X., Jin, Y., Tian, Y., Zhang, H., Wu, J., Lu, W., & Lu, X., (2016). Regulatory B cells contribute to the impaired antitumor immunity in ovarian cancer patients. *Tumour Biol., 37*, 6581–6588.

25. Qian, L., Bian, G. R., Zhou, Y., Wang, Y., Hu, J., Liu, X., & Xu, Y., (2015). Clinical significance of regulatory B cells in the peripheral blood of patients with oesophageal cancer. *Cent. Eur. J. Immunol., 40*, 263–265.

26. Mohammed, Z. M., Going, J. J., Edwards, J., Elsberger, B., & McMillan, D. C., (2013). The relationship between lymphocyte subsets and clinico-pathological determinants of survival in patients with primary operable invasive ductal breast cancer. *Br. J. Cancer, 109*, 1676–1684.

27. Berntsson, J., Nodin, B., Eberhard, J., Micke, P., & Jirstrom, K., (2016). Prognostic impact of tumour-infiltrating B cells and plasma cells in colorectal cancer. *Int. J. Cancer, 139*, 1129–1139.

28. Wang, W. W., Yuan, X. L., Chen, H., Xie, G. H., Ma, Y. H., Zheng, Y. X., Zhou, Y. L., & Shen, L. S., (2015). CD19+CD24hiCD38hiBregs involved in downregulate helper T cells and upregulate regulatory T cells in gastric cancer. *Oncotarget, 6*, 33486–33499.

29. Shimabukuro-Vornhagen, A., Schlosser, H. A., Gryschok, L., Malcher, J., Wennhold, K., Garcia-Marquez, M., Herbold, T., Neuhaus, L. S., Becker, H. J., Fiedler, A., Scherwitz, P., Koslowsky, T., Hake, R., Stippel, D. L., Holscher, A. H., Eidt, S., Hallek, M., Theurich, S., von Bergwelt-Baildon, M. S., (2014). Characterization of tumor-associated B-cell subsets in patients with colorectal cancer. *Oncotarget, 5*, 4651–4664.

30. Westin, J. R., Chu, F., Zhang, M., Fayad, L. E., Kwak, L. W., Fowler, N., Romaguera, J., Hagemeister, F., Fanale, M., Samaniego, F., Feng, L., Baladandayuthapani, V., Wang, Z., Ma, W., Gao, Y., Wallace, M., Vence, L. M., Radvanyi, L., Muzzafar, T., Rotem-Yehudar, R., Davis, R. E., & Neelapu, S. S., (2014). Safety and activity of PD1 blockade by pidilizumab in combination with rituximab in patients with relapsed follicular lymphoma: a single group, open-label, phase 2 trial. *Lancet. Oncol., 15*, 69–77.

31. Armand, P., Nagler, A., Weller, E. A., Devine, S. M., Avigan, D. E., Chen, Y. B., Kaminski, M. S., Holland, H. K., Winter, J. N., Mason, J. R., Fay, J. W., Rizzieri, D. A., Hosing, C. M., Ball, E. D., Uberti, J. P., Lazarus, H. M., Mapara, M. Y., Gregory, S. A., Timmerman, J. M., Andorsky, D., Or, R., Waller, E. K., Rotem-Yehudar, R., & Gordon, L. I., (2013). Disabling immune tolerance by programmed death-1 blockade with pidili-

zumab after autologous hematopoietic stem-cell transplantation for diffuse large B-cell lymphoma: results of an international phase II trial. *J. Clin. Oncol.*, *31*, 4199–4206.

32. Ansell, S. M., Lesokhin, A. M., Borrello, I., Halwani, A., Scott, E. C., Gutierrez, M., Schuster, S. J., Millenson, M. M., Cattry, D., Freeman, G. J., Rodig, S. J., Chapuy, B., Ligon, A. H., Zhu, L., Grosso, J. F., Kim, S. Y., Timmerman, J. M., Shipp, M. A., & Armand, P., (2015). PD-1 blockade with nivolumab in relapsed or refractory Hodgkin's lymphoma. *N. Engl. J. Med.*, *372*, 311–319.

33. Moretta, L., Montaldo, E., Vacca, P., Del Zotto, G., Moretta, F., Merli, P., Locatelli, F., & Mingari, M. C., (2014). Human natural killer cells: origin, receptors, function, & clinical applications. *Int. Arch. Allergy. Immunol.*, *164*, 253–264.

34. Nannmark, U., Basse, P., Johansson, B. R., Kuppen, P., Kjergaard, J., & Hokland, M., (1996). Morphological studies of effector cell-microvessel interactions in adoptive immunotherapy in tumor-bearing animals. *Nat. Immun.*, *15*, 78–86.

35. Mosser, D. M., & Edwards, J. P., (2008). Exploring the full spectrum of macrophage activation. *Nat. Rev. Immunol.*, *8*, 958–969.

36. Siveen, K. S., & Kuttan, G., (2009). Role of macrophages in tumour progression. *Immunol. Lett.*, *123*, 97–102.

37. Qian, B. Z., & Pollard, J. W., (2010). Macrophage diversity enhances tumor progression and metastasis. *Cell*, *141*, 39–51.

38. Grivennikov, S. I., Greten, F. R., & Karin, M., (2010). Immunity, inflammation, & cancer. *Cell*, *140*, 883–899.

39. Biswas, S. K., & Mantovani, A., (2010). Macrophage plasticity and interaction with lymphocyte subsets: cancer as a paradigm. *Nat. Immunol.*, *11*, 889–896.

40. Mantovani, A., (2011). B cells and macrophages in cancer: yin and yang. *Nat. Med.*, *17*, 285–286.

41. Bingle, L., Brown, N. J., & Lewis, C. E., (2002). The role of tumour-associated macrophages in tumour progression: implications for new anticancer therapies. *J. Pathol.*, *196*, 254–265.

42. Gabrilovich, D. I., Ostrand-Rosenberg, S., & Bronte, V., (2012). Coordinated regulation of myeloid cells by tumours. *Nat. Rev. Immunol.*, *12*, 253–268.

43. Sica, A., & Bronte, V., (2007). Altered macrophage differentiation and immune dysfunction in tumor development. *J. Clin. Invest.*, *117*, 1155–1166.

44. Mandruzzato, S., Solito, S., Falisi, E., Francescato, S., Chiarion-Sileni, V., Mocellin, S., Zanon, A., Rossi, C. R., Nitti, D., Bronte, V., & Zanovello, P., (2009). IL4Ralpha+ myeloid-derived suppressor cell expansion in cancer patients. *J. Immunol.*, *182*, 6562–6568.

45. Poschke, I., Mougiakakos, D., Hansson, J., Masucci, G. V., & Kiessling, R., (2010). Immature immunosuppressive CD14+HLA-DR-/low cells in melanoma patients are Stat3hi and overexpress CD80, CD83, & DC-sign. *Cancer Res.*, *70*, 4335–4345.

46. Rodriguez, P. C., Ernstoff, M. S., Hernandez, C., Atkins, M., Zabaleta, J., Sierra, R., & Ochoa, A. C., (2009). Arginase I-producing myeloid-derived suppressor cells in renal cell carcinoma are a subpopulation of activated granulocytes. *Cancer Res.*, 69, 1553–1560.

47. Movahedi, K., Guilliams, M., Van den Bossche, J., Van den Bergh, R., Gysemans, C., Beschin, A., De Baetselier, P., & Van Ginderachter, J. A., (2008). Identification of discrete tumor-induced myeloid-derived suppressor cell subpopulations with distinct T cell-suppressive activity. *Blood*, *111*, 4233–4244.

48. Kusmartsev, S., Nagaraj, S., & Gabrilovich, D. I., (2005). Tumor-associated CD8+ T cell tolerance induced by bone marrow-derived immature myeloid cells. *J. Immunol.*, *175*, 4583–4592.

49. Lanzavecchia, A., & Sallusto, F., (2001). The instructive role of dendritic cells on T cell responses: lineages, plasticity and kinetics. *Curr. Opin. Immunol.*, *13*, 291–298.

50. Ma, Y., Shurin, G. V., Gutkin, D. W., & Shurin, M. R., (2012). Tumor associated regulatory dendritic cells. *Semin. Cancer Biol.*, *22*, 298–306.

51. Curiel, T. J., Cheng, P., Mottram, P., Alvarez, X., Moons, L., Evdemon-Hogan, M., Wei, S., Zou, L., Kryczek, I., Hoyle, G., Lackner, A., Carmeliet, P., & Zou, W., (2004). Dendritic cell subsets differentially regulate angiogenesis in human ovarian cancer. *Cancer Res.*, *64*, 5535–5538.

52. Conejo-Garcia, J. R., Benencia, F., Courreges, M. C., Kang, E., Mohamed-Hadley, A., Buckanovich, R. J., Holtz, D. O., Jenkins, A., Na, H., Zhang, L., Wagner, D. S., Katsaros, D., Caroll, R., & Coukos, G., (2004). Tumor-infiltrating dendritic cell precursors recruited by a beta-defensin contribute to vasculogenesis under the influence of Vegf-A. *Nat. Med.*, *10*, 950–958.

53. Ma, Y., Aymeric, L., Locher, C., Kroemer, G., & Zitvogel, L., (2011). The dendritic cell-tumor cross-talk in cancer. *Curr. Opin. Immunol.*, *23*, 146–152.

54. Mishalian, I., Bayuh, R., Levy, L., Zolotarov, L., Michaeli, J., & Fridlender, Z. G., (2013). Tumor-associated neutrophils (TAN) develop pro-tumorigenic properties during tumor progression. *Cancer Immunol. Immunother.*, *62*, 1745–1756.

55. Cortez-Retamozo, V., Etzrodt, M., Newton, A., Rauch, P. J., Chudnovskiy, A., Berger, C., Ryan, R. J., Iwamoto, Y., Marinelli, B., Gorbatov, R., Forghani, R., Novobrantseva, T. I., Koteliansky, V., Figueiredo, J. L., Chen, J. W., Anderson, D. G., Nahrendorf, M., Swirski, F. K., Weissleder, R., & Pittet, M. J., (2012). Origins of tumor-associated macrophages and neutrophils. *Proc. Natl. Acad. Sci. USA*, *109*, 2491–2496.

56. Fridlender, Z. G., Sun, J., Kim, S., Kapoor, V., Cheng, G., Ling, L., Worthen, G. S., & Albelda, S. M., (2009). Polarization of tumor-associated neutrophil phenotype by TGF-beta: "N1" versus "N2" TAN. *Cancer Cell*, *16*, 183–194.

57. Loukinova, E., Dong, G., Enamorado-Ayalya, I., Thomas, G. R., Chen, Z., Schreiber, H., & Van Waes, C., (2000). Growth regulated oncogene-alpha expression by murine squamous cell carcinoma promotes tumor growth, metastasis, leukocyte infiltration and angiogenesis by a host CXC receptor-2 dependent mechanism. *Oncogene*, *19*, 3477–3486.

58. Schaider, H., Oka, M., Bogenrieder, T., Nesbit, M., Satyamoorthy, K., Berking, C., Matsushima, K., & Herlyn, M., (2003). Differential response of primary and metastatic melanomas to neutrophils attracted by IL-8. *Int. J. Cancer*, *103*, 335–343.

59. Di Carlo, E., Forni, G., Lollini, P., Colombo, M. P., Modesti, A., & Musiani, P., (2001). The intriguing role of polymorphonuclear neutrophils in antitumor reactions. *Blood*, *97*, 339–345.

60. Suttmann, H., Riemensberger, J., Bentien, G., Schmaltz, D., Stockle, M., Jocham, D., Bohle, A., & Brandau, S., (2006). Neutrophil granulocytes are required for effective Bacillus Calmette-Guerin immunotherapy of bladder cancer and orchestrate local immune responses. *Cancer Res.*, *66*, 8250–8257.

61. De Wever, O., Demetter, P., Mareel, M., & Bracke, M., (2008). Stromal myofibroblasts are drivers of invasive cancer growth. *Int. J. Cancer*, *123*, 2229–2238.

62. Brittan, M., Hunt, T., Jeffery, R., Poulsom, R., Forbes, S. J., Hodivala-Dilke, K., Gold-man, J., Alison, M. R., & Wright, N. A., (2002). Bone marrow derivation of pericryptal myofibroblasts in the mouse and human small intestine and colon. *Gut*, *50*, 752–757.

63. Willis, B. C., Dubois, R. M., & Borok, Z., (2006). Epithelial origin of myofibroblasts during fibrosis in the lung. *Proc. Am. Thorac. Soc.*, *3*, 377–382.

64. Erez, N., Truitt, M., Olson, P., Arron, S. T., & Hanahan, D., (2010). Cancer-associated fibroblasts are activated in incipient neoplasia to orchestrate tumor-promoting inflam-mation in an NF-kappaB-dependent manner. *Cancer Cell*, *17*, 135–147.

65. Orimo, A., Gupta, P. B., Sgroi, D. C., Arenzana-Seisdedos, F., Delaunay, T., Naeem, R., Carey, V. J., Richardson, A. L., & Weinberg, R. A., (2005). Stromal fibroblasts present in invasive human breast carcinomas promote tumor growth and angiogenesis through elevated SDF-1/CXCL12 secretion. *Cell*, *121*, 335–348.

66. Chouaib, S., Kieda, C., Benlalam, H., Noman, M. Z., Mami-Chouaib, F., & Ruegg, C., (2010). Endothelial cells as key determinants of the tumor microenvironment: interac-tion with tumor cells, extracellular matrix and immune killer cells. *Crit. Rev. Immunol.*, *30*, 529–545.

67. Carmeliet, P., & Jain, R. K., (2011). Molecular mechanisms and clinical applications of angiogenesis. *Nature*, *473*, 298–307.

68. Jain, R. K., (2005). Normalization of tumor vasculature: an emerging concept in antian-giogenic therapy. *Science*, *307*, 58–62.

69. O'Keeffe, M. B., Devlin, A. H., Burns, A. J., Gardiner, T. A., Logan, I. D., Hirst, D. G., & McKeown, S. R., (2008). Investigation of pericytes, hypoxia, & vascularity in blad-der tumors: association with clinical outcomes. *Oncol. Res.*, *17*, 93–101.

70. Xian, X., Hakansson, J., Stahlberg, A., Lindblom, P., Betsholtz, C., Gerhardt, H., & Semb, H., (2006). Pericytes limit tumor cell metastasis. *J. Clin. Invest.*, *116*, 642–651.

71. Mravic, M., Asatrian, G., Soo, C., Lugassy, C., Barnhill, R. L., Dry, S. M., Peault, B., & James, A. W., (2014). From pericytes to perivascular tumours: correlation between pathology, stem cell biology, & tissue engineering. *Int. Orthop.*, *38*, 1819–1824.

72. Barlow, K. D., Sanders, A. M., Soker, S., Ergun, S., & Metheny-Barlow, L. J., (2013). Pericytes on the tumor vasculature: jekyll or hyde? *Cancer Microenviron*, *6*, 1–17.

73. Yonenaga, Y., Mori, A., Onodera, H., Yasuda, S., Oe, H., Fujimoto, A., Tachibana, T., & Imamura, M., (2005). Absence of smooth muscle actin-positive pericyte coverage of tumor vessels correlates with hematogenous metastasis and prognosis of colorectal cancer patients. *Oncology*, *69*, 159–166.

74. Cooke, V. G., LeBleu, V. S., Keskin, D., Khan, Z., O'Connell, J. T., Teng, Y., Duncan, M. B., Xie, L., Maeda, G., Vong, S., Sugimoto, H., Rocha, R. M., Damascena, A., Brentani, R. R., & Kalluri, R., (2012). Pericyte depletion results in hypoxia-associated epithelial-to-mesenchymal transition and metastasis mediated by met signaling path-way. *Cancer Cell*, *21*, 66–81.

75. Lugassy, C., Haroun, R. I., Brem, H., Tyler, B. M., Jones, R. V., Fernandez, P. M., Pati-erno, S. R., Kleinman, H. K., & Barnhill, R. L., (2002). Pericytic-like angiotropism of glioma and melanoma cells. *Am. J. Dermatopathol*, *24*, 473–478.

76. Lugassy, C., Vernon, S. E., Warner, J. W., Le, C. Q., Manyak, M., Patierno, S. R., & Barnhill, R. L., (2005). Angiotropism of human prostate cancer cells: implications for extravascular migratory metastasis. *BJU Int.*, *95*, 1099–1103.

77. Lugassy, C., Wadehra, M., Li, X., Corselli, M., Akhavan, D., Binder, S. W., Peault, B., Cochran, A. J., Mischel, P. S., Kleinman, H. K., & Barnhill, R. L., (2013). Pilot study on "pericytic mimicry" and potential embryonic/stem cell properties of angiotropic mela-

noma cells interacting with the abluminal vascular surface. *Cancer Microenviron.*, *6*, 19–29.

78. Dominici, M., Le Blanc, K., Mueller, I., Slaper-Cortenbach, I., Marini, F., Krause, D., Deans, R., Keating, A., Prockop, D., & Horwitz, E., (2006). Minimal criteria for defining multipotent mesenchymal stromal cells. The international society for cellular therapy position statement. *Cytotherapy*, *8*, 315–317.

79. Rattigan, Y., Hsu, J. M., Mishra, P. J., Glod, J., & Banerjee, D., (2010). Interleukin 6 mediated recruitment of mesenchymal stem cells to the hypoxic tumor milieu. *Exp. Cell Res.*, *316*, 3417–3424.

80. Direkze, N. C., Hodivala-Dilke, K., Jeffery, R., Hunt, T., Poulsom, R., Oukrif, D., Alison, M. R., & Wright, N. A., (2004). Bone marrow contribution to tumor-associated myofibroblasts and fibroblasts. *Cancer Res.*, *64*, 8492–8495.

81. Zhang, L., Tang, A., Zhou, Y., Tang, J., Luo, Z., Jiang, C., Li, X., Xiang, J., & Li, G., (2012). Tumor-conditioned mesenchymal stem cells display hematopoietic differentiation and diminished influx of Ca2+. *Stem Cells Dev.*, *21*, 1418–1428.

82. Ozbek, S., Balasubramanian, P. G., Chiquet-Ehrismann, R., Tucker, R. P., & Adams, J. C., (2010). The evolution of extracellular matrix. *Mol Biol. Cell*, *21*, 4300–4305.

83. Frantz, C., Stewart, K. M., & Weaver, V. M., (2010). The extracellular matrix at a glance. *J. Cell Sci.*, *123*, 4195–4200.

84. Lu, P., Takai, K., Weaver, V. M., & Werb, Z., (2011). Extracellular matrix degradation and remodeling in development and disease. *Cold Spring Harb. Perspect. Biol.*, *3*.

85. Levental, K. R., Yu, H., Kass, L., Lakins, J. N., Egeblad, M., Erler, J. T., Fong, S. F., Csiszar, K., Giaccia, A., Weninger, W., Yamauchi, M., Gasser, D. L., & Weaver, V. M., (2009). Matrix crosslinking forces tumor progression by enhancing integrin signaling. *Cell*, *139*, 891–906.

86. Lerner, I., Hermano, E., Zcharia, E., Rodkin, D., Bulvik, R., Doviner, V., Rubinstein, A. M., Ishai-Michaeli, R., Atzmon, R., Sherman, Y., Meirovitz, A., Peretz, T., Vlodavsky, I., & Elkin, M., (2011). Heparanase powers a chronic inflammatory circuit that promotes colitis-associated tumorigenesis in mice. *J. Clin. Invest.*, *121*, 1709–1721.

87. Hanahan, D., & Weinberg, R. A., (2011). Hallmarks of cancer: the next generation. *Cell*, *144*, 646–674.

88. Weis, S. M., & Cheresh, D. A., (2011). Tumor angiogenesis: molecular pathways and therapeutic targets. *Nat. Med.*, *17*, 1359–1370.

89. Du, R., Lu, K. V., Petritsch, C., Liu, P., Ganss, R., Passegue, E., Song, H., Vandenberg, S., Johnson, R. S., Werb, Z., & Bergers, G., (2008). HIF1alpha induces the recruitment of bone marrow-derived vascular modulatory cells to regulate tumor angiogenesis and invasion. *Cancer Cell*, *13*, 206–220.

90. Valastyan, S., & Weinberg, R. A., (2011). Tumor metastasis: molecular insights and evolving paradigms. *Cell*, *147*, 275–292.

91. Wan, L., Pantel, K., & Kang, Y., (2013). Tumor metastasis: moving new biological insights into the clinic. *Nat. Med.*, *19*, 1450–1464.

92. Paget, S., (1989). The distribution of secondary growths in cancer of the breast. *Cancer Metastasis. Rev.*, *8*, 98–101.

93. Friedl, P., Locker, J., Sahai, E., & Segall, J. E., (2012). Classifying collective cancer cell invasion. *Nat. Cell Biol.*, *14*, 777–783.

94. Van Zijl, F., Krupitza, G., & Mikulits, W., (2011). Initial steps of metastasis: cell invasion and endothelial transmigration. *Mutat. Res.*, *728*, 23–34.

95. Cheung, K. J., Gabrielson, E., Werb, Z., & Ewald, A. J., (2013). Collective invasion in breast cancer requires a conserved basal epithelial program. *Cell, 155*, 1639–1651.

96. Spano, D., Heck, C., De Antonellis, P., Christofori, G., & Zollo, M., (2012). Molecular networks that regulate cancer metastasis. *Semin. Cancer Biol., 22*, 234–249.

97. Yamazaki, D., Kurisu, S., & Takenawa, T., (2009). Involvement of Rac and Rho signaling in cancer cell motility in 3D substrates. *Oncogene, 28*, 1570–1583.

98. Bissell, M. J., & Hines, W. C., (2011). Why don't we get more cancer? A proposed role of the microenvironment in restraining cancer progression. *Nat. Med., 17*, 320–329.

99. Fang, H., & Declerck, Y. A., (2013). Targeting the tumor microenvironment: from understanding pathways to effective clinical trials. *Cancer Res., 73*, 4965–4977.

100. Bonde, A. K., Tischler, V., Kumar, S., Soltermann, A., & Schwendener, R. A., (2012). Intratumoral macrophages contribute to epithelial-mesenchymal transition in solid tumors. *BMC Cancer, 12*, 35.

101. Gay, L. J., & Felding-Habermann, B., (2011). Contribution of platelets to tumour metastasis. *Nat. Rev. Cancer, 11*, 123–134.

102. Reymond, N., Im, J. H., Garg, R., Vega, F. M., Borda d'Agua, B., Riou, P., Cox, S., Valderrama, F., Muschel, R. J., & Ridley, A. J., (2012). Cdc42 promotes transendothelial migration of cancer cells through beta1 integrin. *J. Cell Biol., 199*, 653–668.

103. Giampieri, S., Manning, C., Hooper, S., Jones, L., Hill, C. S., & Sahai, E., (2009). Localized and reversible TGFbeta signalling switches breast cancer cells from cohesive to single cell motility. *Nat. Cell Biol., 11*, 1287–1296.

104. Sonoshita, M., Aoki, M., Fuwa, H., Aoki, K., Hosogi, H., Sakai, Y., Hashida, H., Takabayashi, A., Sasaki, M., Robine, S., Itoh, K., Yoshioka, K., Kakizaki, F., Kitamura, T., Oshima, M., & Taketo, M. M., (2011). Suppression of colon cancer metastasis by Aes through inhibition of notch signaling. *Cancer Cell, 19*, 125–137.

105. Gerhardt, H., & Semb, H., (2008). Pericytes: gatekeepers in tumour cell metastasis? *J. Mol Med. (Berl), 86*, 135–144.

106. Guo, W., & Giancotti, F. G., (2004). Integrin signalling during tumour progression. *Nat. Rev. Mol Cell Biol., 5*, 816–826.

107. Douma, S., Van Laar, T., Zevenhoven, J., Meuwissen, R., Van Garderen, E., & Peeper, D. S., (2004). Suppression of anoikis and induction of metastasis by the neurotrophic receptor TrkB. *Nature, 430*, 1034–1039.

108. Joyce, J. A., & Pollard, J. W., (2009). Microenvironmental regulation of metastasis. *Nat. Rev. Cancer, 9*, 239–252.

109. Al-Mehdi, A. B., Tozawa, K., Fisher, A. B., Shientag, L., Lee, A., & Muschel, R. J., (2000). Intravascular origin of metastasis from the proliferation of endothelium-attached tumor cells: a new model for metastasis. *Nat. Med., 6*, 100–102.

110. Hanley, W. D., Napier, S. L., Burdick, M. M., Schnaar, R. L., Sackstein, R., & Konstantopoulos, K., (2006). Variant isoforms of CD44 are P- and L-selectin ligands on colon carcinoma cells. *FASEB J., 20*, 337–339.

111. Dimitroff, C. J., Descheny, L., Trujillo, N., Kim, R., Nguyen, V., Huang, W., Pienta, K. J., Kutok, J. L., & Rubin, M. A., (2005). Identification of leukocyte E-selectin ligands, P-selectin glycoprotein ligand-1 and E-selectin ligand-1, on human metastatic prostate tumor cells. *Cancer Res., 65*, 5750–5760.

112. Aigner, S., Ramos, C. L., Hafezi-Moghadam, A., Lawrence, M. B., Friederichs, J., Altevogt, P., & Ley, K., (1998). CD24 mediates rolling of breast carcinoma cells on P-selectin. *FASEB J., 12*, 1241–1251.

113. Thomas, S. N., Zhu, F., Schnaar, R. L., Alves, C. S., & Konstantopoulos, K., (2008). Carcinoembryonic antigen and CD44 variant isoforms cooperate to mediate colon carcinoma cell adhesion to E- and L-selectin in shear flow. *J. Biol. Chem.*, *283*, 15647–15655.

114. Okahara, H., Yagita, H., Miyake, K., & Okumura, K., (1994). Involvement of very late activation antigen 4 (VLA-4) and vascular cell adhesion molecule 1 (VCAM-1) in tumor necrosis factor alpha enhancement of experimental metastasis. *Cancer Res.*, *54*, 3233–3236.

115. Nangia-Makker, P., Sarvis, R., Visscher, D. W., Bailey-Penrod, J., Raz, A., & Sarkar, F. H., (1998). Galectin-3 and L1 retrotransposons in human breast carcinomas. *Breast Cancer Res. Treat.*, *49*, 171–183.

116. Qi, J., Chen, N., Wang, J., & Siu, C. H., (2005). Transendothelial migration of melanoma cells involves N-cadherin-mediated adhesion and activation of the beta-catenin signaling pathway. *Mol Biol. Cell.*, *16*, 4386–4397.

117. Fidler, I. J., (2003). The pathogenesis of cancer metastasis: the 'seed and soil' hypothesis revisited. *Nat. Rev. Cancer*, *3*, 453–458.

118. Gupta, G. P., & Massague, J., (2006). Cancer metastasis: building a framework. *Cell*, *127*, 679–695.

119. Erler, J. T., Bennewith, K. L., Nicolau, M., Dornhofer, N., Kong, C., Le, Q. T., Chi, J. T., Jeffrey, S. S., & Giaccia, A. J., (2006). Lysyl oxidase is essential for hypoxia-induced metastasis. *Nature*, *440*, 1222–1226.

120. Brown, D. M., & Ruoslahti, E., (2004). Metadherin, a cell surface protein in breast tumors that mediates lung metastasis. *Cancer Cell*, *5*, 365–374.

121. Granot, Z., Henke, E., Comen, E. A., King, T. A., Norton, L., & Benezra, R., (2011). Tumor entrained neutrophils inhibit seeding in the premetastatic lung. *Cancer Cell*, *20*, 300–314.

122. Hensel, J. A., Flaig, T. W., & Theodorescu, D., (2013). Clinical opportunities and challenges in targeting tumour dormancy. *Nat. Rev. Clin. Oncol.*, *10*, 41–51.

123. Yoshikawa, K., Mitsunaga, S., Kinoshita, T., Konishi, M., Takahashi, S., Gotohda, N., Kato, Y., Aizawa, M., & Ochiai, A., (2012). Impact of tumor-associated macrophages on invasive ductal carcinoma of the pancreas head. *Cancer Sci.*, *103*, 2012–2020.

124. Qian, B., Deng, Y., Im, J. H., Muschel, R. J., Zou, Y., Li, J., Lang, R. A., & Pollard, J. W., (2009). A distinct macrophage population mediates metastatic breast cancer cell extravasation, establishment and growth. *PLoS One*, *4*, e6562.

CHAPTER 6

APOPTOSIS: A REGULATORY MECHANISM IN CANCER

SUTAPA MUKHERJEE, APURBA MUKHERJEE, SOUVICK BISWAS, and MADHUMITA ROY

Department of Environmental Carcinogenesis & Toxicology, Chittaranjan National Cancer Institute, 37, S. P. Mukherjee Road, Kolkata 700 026, India, E-mail: sutapa_c_in@yahoo.com

CONTENTS

ABSTRACT

Developmental process and health of multicellular organisms are maintained by a physiological process termed as apoptosis. A balance between cell death and cell proliferation ultimately maintains the cellular homeostasis. Apoptosis is a controlled cellular death; a process that activates death-signaling pathways for deleting cells from tissues. Two major pathways execute the complex process of apoptosis. Deregulated apoptotic pathways drive normal cells toward carcinogenesis and ultimately therapy resistance. Therefore knowledge about the role of death genes, death signals, signaling pathways involved in apoptosis regulation is highly warranted. During tumorigenesis process, aberrant expression or loss of lead protein members of apoptotic pathways have been indicated. Inactivation of these proteins leads to impairment of apoptosis and contributes to cellular growth and proliferation. Such events ultimately cause a serious imbalance in growth dynamics, an essential root of cancer. Cancer cells have been reported to evolve a strategy to evade apoptosis. The present review discusses about the recent knowledge related to regulatory mechanism of apoptosis in cancer with particular emphasis on key proteins like Bcl-2 protein family, inhibitor of apoptosis protein or IAPs, p53 and caspases. Damage to DNA due to exogenous or endogenous stimuli activates and stabilizes p53 and triggers extrinsic and intrinsic apoptotic pathways. Understanding the regulatory mechanism of apoptosis in cancer from this review might expose new scopes to therapeutic approaches.

6.1   INTRODUCTION

A homeostatic balance between cell growth and death is a major responsible factor for the development and maintenance of biological systems. This balance is maintained by a physiological process termed apoptosis, which is a programmed event of cell death occurring in an orchestrated manner. This is a process found in all multicellular organisms for killing and removing specific cells not required by the system so as to maintain cellular equilibrium. It being an evolutionarily conserved process is observed from nematodes and flies to mice and humans. The process is also a pivotal constituent for the development of plant cells [1]. Apoptosis is considered as an inevitable process, essential for normal cell turnover, immune system functioning, hormone-mediated cellular atrophy, normal embryonic development, unwanted cell elimination, and homeostatic maintenance [2]. Dysregulation in cellular homeostasis due to restricted or inadequate apoptotic event may accelerate progression of cancer or development of autoimmunity. On the contrary, excessive cell death by apoptosis culminates into chronic neurodegeneration, deficiency in the immune system and impairment of fertility. Apoptotic signaling is essential for maintenance of genomic integrity; while impairment of this pathway contribute to carcinogenesis and subsequently rendering cancer cells resistant to therapy. Evasion of apoptosis, a mechanism utilized by cancerous cells, is considered as a notable indication of tumor development and metastasis [3, 4]. The present review furnishes an outline of the knowledge about apoptosis and its regulatory mechanism involved in cancer.

6.2 MORPHOLOGICAL CHANGES

Cell death may occur through either apoptosis, a physiological process or necrosis, a pathological process. Another pathological form of cell death is mitotic catastrophe. There lie distinguished differences between these death processes which are tabulated in Table 6.1.

Morphological changes as noticed during apoptosis mainly prevail at three cellular sites; they are cell membrane, nucleus, and other cytoplasmic organelles [5]. General morphological and biochemical changes occurring in these cellular organelles have been described in Table 6.2.

6.3 MECHANISM OF APOPTOSIS

Multiple factors are involved in the well organized and tightly regulated event of programmed cell death. Intrinsic mechanism of each cell governs its death or survival by apoptotic process. The cascade of event is primarily initiated by two major pathways involving either death receptor or mitochondria.

TABLE 6.1 Forms of Cell Death

Necrosis	Classic or Apoptosis	Mitotic Catastrophe
Passive	Active (ATP dependent)	Passive
Pathological	Physiological or Pathological	Pathological
Swelling, lysis	Cell shrinkage,	Swelling, lysis chromatin condensation
Dissipates	Phagocytosed	Dissipates
Inflammation	No inflammation	Inflammation
Externally induced	Internally or externally induced	Internally induced
Involvement of calpains	Involvement of caspases	Caspase dependent or independent

TABLE 6.2   Features of Apoptosis

General features	Recruitment of death receptors
	Dimerization of members of Bcl-2 family
	Cytochrome C release
	Caspase activation
	Activation of DNase
	Translocation of phosphatidylserine
	Requirement of ATP
	DNA ladder formation (internucleosomal DNA fragmentation)
Morphological features	Alteration in the cell membrane due to
	Membrane blebbing
	Clustering of organelles, formation of arrays of ribosomes, disruption of microtubule network
	Cell shrinkage, reduction in cell volume
	Condensation of entire nucleus, rather heterochromatin.
	Internucleosomal chromatin fragmentation
	Proteolysis of nuclear lamins
	Formation of apoptotic bodies
Biochemical features	Translocation of phosphatidyl serine from inner leaflet to the outer surface due to cleavage of translocase and activation of scramblase
	Cleavage of substrate proteins like PARP, actin, lamin etc Activation of Ca^{2+} and Mg^{2+} dependent endonucleases to cleave nuclear DNA
	Activation of Ca^{2+} dependent transglutaminase for membrane protein cross linking. Sustained increase in cytosolic Ca^{2+} concentration. Activation of caspases.

[Source: Ref. 6]

Both these pathways eventually activate enzymes like cysteine proteases for ultimate killing [6, 7]. Endoplasmic reticulum is also known to be involved in the process of apoptosis, although the involvement frequency is less.

6.3.1   APOPTOSIS INVOLVING DEATH RECEPTORS

This is the receptor-mediated cell death process, where ligand binds to a death receptor. Receptor–ligand binding ultimately instructs the cell to kill itself. TNF receptor (TNFR1) and Fas (CD95) are two such receptors whose ligands are TNF and Fas ligand (FasL), respectively [8]. Examples of some other receptor–ligands are DR3 (Apo3 or WSL1), DR4 (TRAIL-R1), DR5 (TRAIL-R2), and DR6 [2, 5, 8]. Death domains situated in the intracellular regions of these receptors functions in recruitment of adapter proteins like TNF receptor-associated death domain (TRADD) and Fas-associated death domain (FADD). Ligand-receptor-adaptor protein complex is known as death-inducing signaling complex (DISC), which induces procaspase 8 assembly and activation. Caspase 8 upon activation exerts its effect on its downstream effector caspases. Effector caspases subsequently involves in cleavage of specific substrate and resulting in cell death [2, 7]. Caspase 8 in some cases activates the downstream effector caspases by cleaving Bid, a proapoptotic member of the Bcl-2 family and inducing intrinsic pathway of apoptosis [7].

6.3.2   APOPTOSIS INVOLVING MITOCHONDRIA

Multiple intracellular components of the cell can recognize diverse stresses like UV or gamma radiation, heat, viral, virulence factors, deprivation of growth factors, activation of oncogenic factors, DNA damaging agents, etc. [6] and transmit the signal to the mitochondria, inculcating to perturbation in the membrane potential and mitochondrial outer membrane permeabilization [9,10]. Pro- and antiapoptotic members of the Bcl-2 family proteins are primarily responsible for membrane permeabilization and cytochrome c release. Cytochrome c after releasing from the mitochondrial inner membrane to the cytoplasm forms a complex with apoptotic protease activating factor-1 (Apaf-1) and caspase-9. This complex formed with the help of ATP is known as apoptosome, which ultimately activates caspase 3. Caspase 3 successively activates another nuclease namely caspase-activated DNase (CAD) which is implicated in fragmentation of apoptotic cell DNA at an interval of 180 bp or multiples of 180 bp. CAD remains in an inactivated state through its association with another inhibitor protein known as inhibitor of caspase-activated DNase (ICAD). Caspase 3 cleaves this ICAD protein and releases CAD [11, 12]. Caspase 3 furthermore cleaves some other proteins like protein kinases, cytoskeletal proteins (actin, lamin, vimentin) and DNA repair proteins (PARP). All these cascades of events contribute to the typical morphological features that are observed in apoptosis [7, 13]. Family members of IAPs (inhibitors of apoptosis proteins) can negatively regulate apoptosis by binding directly to caspases. A member of IAP namely XIAP (X-linked inhibitor of apoptosis protein) prevents apoptosome formation by inhibiting either caspase 9 activities or by directly binding with effector caspases-3 and -7 [14]. Two proteins residing in mitochondrial intermembrane space namely Smac (second mitochondria-derived activator of caspase) and DIABLO (direct IAP binding protein with low pI) impedes the functional activities of IAPs. Another protein also resists IAP function, namely Omi/high temperature requirement A2 (HtrA2). The NH2 terminal of these proteins serves as mitochondrial targeting signal (MLS) that helps the protein for mitochondrial transportation. Within mitochondria, this signal cleaves to form the mature protein. N-terminal ends of these mature proteins possess IAP-binding motifs, which facilitates in IAP binding and abolish the caspase-inhibitory activity of IAPs [15, 16]. Additionally, some other factors like apoptosis inducing factor (AIF) and endonuclease G are known to exert their role in inducing apoptosis. AIF, a flavoprotein localized in the mitochondria, has been reported to undergo translocation to the cytosol and nucleus to mediate caspase-independent apoptosis [17]. Endonuclease G or endoG, a mitochondria-specific nuclease, exerts nucleosomal fragmentation that is independent of caspase activation [18].

6.3.3   APOPTOSIS INVOLVING ENDOPLASMIC RETICULUM (ER)

The endoplasmic reticulum (ER) is the first halt where folding and modification of chaperone-assisted polypeptides occur to obtain the mature form of protein. The ER pathway is not well known. If the stress-induced damage to ER is very high and beyond restoration, an apoptotic response is evoked either via the response of unfolded protein or by releasing calcium into the cytoplasm [19–21]. ER is bestowed with Fas- and p53-dependent apoptosis, as a result from DNA damage and oncogene expression. Calcium release from ER can activate cytoplasmic death and sensitize mitochondria toward direct proapoptotic stimuli. Proteins associated with ER stress induced pathway are PUMA, p53, and NOXA. These proteins impart ER stress-induced apoptosis involving mitochondria and Apaf-1 [22]. Stress in the ER unleashes another pathway (independent of mitochondrial pathway) mediated via translocating Bim, another protein of the Bcl-2 family and caspase 12 activation [23]. These two ER stress response pathways evidently function independent of one another [24].

6.3.4 APOPTOSIS BY LYSOSOMAL REGULATION

Another process of regulation of apoptosis is by permeabilization of lysosomal membrane (LMP) [25]. Various signals like death receptors, reactive oxygen species (ROS) generation, inhibition of proteasome, deprivation of growth factors, and activation of p53 lead to activation of LMP [26–28]. Some reports, however, suggest that deprivation of p53 triggers LMP activation [20, 30]. Transmission of death signals to the lysosome may occur through some other factors like BID, BIM, BAX, and caspase-8. LMP consequently triggers outflow of its content like hydrolases (cathepsin) into the cytosol. Depending on the cell type, cathepsin in turn activates apoptosis (either involving caspase or independent of caspase activation). If the LMP is very profound, then it culminates into necrosis associated with permeabilization of plasma membrane. Cathepsin in some cases facilitates mitochondrial membrane potential (MOMP). LMP-induced cell death is primarily stimulated by MOMP. Cathepsin functions as an activator to cleave pro-apoptotic (Bid) or by preventing cleavage of antiapoptotic Bcl-2 proteins (Bcl-2, Bcl-XL, and Mcl-1) [26]. Caspase-independent mechanism of cathepsin mediated death on the contrary depends on AIF release from the mitochondria. AIF translocates from the mitochondria to the cytosol and ultimately to the nucleus and fosters chromatin condensation and DNA fragmentation [31]. Lysosomal pathway therefore is an important area for drug development in cancer.

6.3.5 CASPASE-INDEPENDENT APOPTOSIS

Activation of caspases is considered as the main determining factor for the induction of programmed cell death like apoptosis. However, evidence accrued from several researchers indicated the occurrence of programmed cell death in complete absence of caspases as well as independent of their activation [18, 32]. Cell death without involvement of caspase activity may occur in certain physiological and pathological situations. Caspase-independent cell death can be grouped into three main types like mitotic catastrophe, autophagy, and necrosis. The mitochondrion can play a vital role in caspase-independent apoptosis. In addition to the mitochondria, lysosomes and ERs also play their role in such type of apoptosis by releasing proteases like cathepsins and calpains [33, 34]. These type of cell deaths have diverge morphological and biochemical features depending on the cell type and kind and intensity of stimuli.

6.4 MAJOR CONTENDER IN APOPTOSIS

6.4.1 CASPASE

Caspases are a family of genes that are essential in maintenance of homeo-stasis because of their role in regulating cell death and homeostasis. The enzyme being a cysteine-rich protease cleaves the substrate after aspartic acid residue. These families of proteins are endoproteases capable of hydro-lyzing peptide bonds after aspartic acid residues in the substrate [35]. Cas-pase being central to the apoptotic mechanism can be further subclassified into initiator caspases (caspase 8 and 9) and executioner caspases (cas-pases 3, 6, and 7). Initiator caspases initiate apoptotic pathways, whereas effector caspases controls proteolysis in a coordinated fashion, resulting in breakdown of cytoplasmic and cytoskeletal proteins [35]. Proteins that are degraded by effector caspases are predominantly cytoskeletal, nuclear scaf-fold, and DNA repair proteins [35].

6.4.1.1 Regulation of Caspases in Cancer

Caspases play a pivotal role in apoptosis, and hence, deregulation of these enzymes can assist in persistence of mutated cells and foster carcinogenesis process. However, these endopeptidases have some enigmatic role in the development of tumor. Caspases can be regulated by various mechanisms like at the gene expression level, both at the transcription and posttranscrip-tion level [36]. Caspase activity may be deregulated due to alterations of spe-cific genes, methylation or alternative splicing of the caspase gene and some posttranslational modifications. Many kinases and phosphatases directly con-trol the activation of caspases. Several sites of caspase-9, including the major phosphorylation site Thr125, are phosphorylated by multiple protein kinases [36]. Direct phosphorylation of Thr125 by ERK suppresses the functional activity of caspase 9 [37]. Similarly, phosphorylation of caspase 8 by RSK2 kinase at Tyr 263 residues, manifests inhibition of apoptosis *[38]*. *S*-nitro-sylation, another regulatory modification of the catalytic site (cysteine) in caspases functions as an on/off switch to control the activity of these proteases, thereby protecting cells from apoptosis [39, 40]. Mutation and polymorphism of the CASP gene negatively influence activation of caspases, thus hinderingwith the apoptosis process and are associated with tumorigenesis [41]. Gene deletion or promoter methylation of the CASP8 gene is evident in pediatric tumors and their cell lines [42]. A correlation between loss of caspase 8 expression and amplification of Myc oncogene has been reported [42]. In a study conducted on lung cancer patients, it was observed that genetic polymorphism of caspase 9 increased the risk of the disease in the smokers but not in the nonsmokers, thus reflecting environmental influence over gene expression [43]. Somatic mutation of caspase 3 has been observed in different types of cancer [44]. Exon 3 region of the caspase-3 gene in MCF-7 breast carcinoma cells undergo somatic mutations, resulting into lack of caspase-3 protein [45]. Besides these genetic alterations, some endogenous inhibitors of caspases may control the functional activity of these enzymes. For example, Flice inhibitory protein (c-FLIP) and some of its variants have common homology with caspase 8 and 10. FLIP can compete with caspase 8 and 10 by binding with the DISC through its death domain DED and thus prevent their activities. FLIP has been reported to be overexpressed in various human tumor types [46]. Another class of protein capable of inactivating caspases are IAPs or inhibitor of apoptosis protein. Among IAPs, XIAPs in particular are very potent inhibitors of some caspases such as caspase-3 and caspase-7 [47]. Hyperactivation of some cell signaling pathways like PI3K/Akt or the Ras/MAPK drives cancer progression possibly due to caspase 9 phosphorylation [36]. Some experimental research indicated that certain exceptional mutation or silencing of caspase genes in tumor accelerates caspase-independent cell death (CID) [46, 47]. In addition to its role in apoptosis, caspases also reported to have contribution in proliferation, migration, and invasion [48–51]. Therefore, although caspases are major players in apoptosis, they are not an inevitable factor for induction of programmed cell death.

6.4.2   PROTEINS BELONGING TO BCL-2 FAMILY

So far, 19 members have been identified under this family. These proteins possess a homologous domain of BCL-2 (BH1-BH4) that functions as a major determinant in apoptosis. The family of Bcl-2 may be categorized into three functional subgroups depending on their function and existence of Bcl-2 homology. They are multidomain antiapoptotic proteins (BCL-2, BCL-XL,

BCL-W, MCL-1, BFL-1), multidomain proapoptotic proteins (BAK, BAX, BOK), and BH3-only proteins (BIM, BID, BAD, NOXA, PUMA, BMF, BIK, HRK) [52]. These proteins act as either hetero or homodimers. Mitochondrial permeability is increased by pro-apoptotic dimers (Bax). Antiapoptotic members particularly Bcl-2 and Bcl-XL by forming dimers with pro-apoptotic members inactivate their function. Bcl-2 family members primarily control apoptosis by involving mitochondria. Perturbation of the balance between pro and antiapoptotic members can results into impairment of apoptosis [53]. The apoptotic pathway regulated by BCL-2 (also known as "intrinsic," "stress," or "mitochondrial" pathway) is evolutionarily highly conserved and is regulated by interactions between the members of the Bcl-2 protein family.

6.4.2.1   Regulation of BCL-2 Proteins in Cancer

Deregulated expression of Bcl-2 and its other members of pro-survival proteins contributes in the development of tumor as well as confer therapeutic resistance [54]. Aberrant expression of some other members of the antiapoptotic Bcl-2 was recorded in human cancers and leukemias [55–57]. Bcl-2 acts at the mitochondria as well as endoplasmic reticulum (ER) via scaffolding the Bcl-2-homology or BH domain 3 (BH3) of pro-apoptotic Bcl-2- members. Disruption in this interaction leads to apoptosis. Bcl-2 by modulating Ca^{2+} signaling at ER encourages proliferation and resistance to apoptosis. Bcl-2 performs this job by directly binding and inhibiting IP3R or 1,4,5-trisphosphate receptor. Therefore, Bcl-2 regulation at both mitochondria and ER determines cancer cell survival [58]. Aberrant expression of antiapoptotic Bcl-2 members is a frequent phenomenon in human cancers of different types. Bax and Bak function as tumor suppressor proteins, and deprivation of Bax prevents apoptosis in pancreatic β-cells [59]. Several BH3-only proteins like Bad, Bim, Bid, Noxa, Puma, Bik/Blk, and Bmf impede malignancy and mediate apoptosis by functioning in an orchestrated fashion and acting as mediators of anticancer therapy [60]. Triple deletion of Bim, Puma, and Bid leads to resistance to a vast range of apoptotic stimuli [52]. Frequent gene amplification of MCL-1 is commonly observed in breast cancer, which renders the cells resistance to therapy [61]. This protein thereby aids in tumor progression and resistance [62]. Moreover, Bcl-2 family proteins are reported to be crucial in Akt-regulated cell survival in ovarian cancer resistant to cisplatin [63].

6.4.3 INHIBITOR OF APOPTOSIS PROTEIN

IAPs, a group of highly conserved proteins, primarily function in the regulation of caspases and immune signaling. Apart from inhibition of programmed cell death, these proteins are crucially involved in cellular signaling systems [64]. Apart from BIR domain; apoptosis regulatory IAPs also possess another RING finger domain at the carboxy terminal end with E3 ligase activity and thereby promote transferring of ubiquitin (Ub) to target proteins. Conjugation of Ub to the RING finger domain may occur as a single moiety or as chains of variable length [65]. Caspases are regulated by IAPs upon zymogen activation [36]. XIAP are intricately associated with regulation of caspases. BIR3 domain of XIAP by binding to the homo-dimerization surface of caspase-9 can inhibit the functional activity of the enzyme [66]. Apart from regulating the activities of caspases, IAPs also controls cellular proliferation by regulating NF-κB signal transduction and innate immune responses [67]. c-IAP functions in T cell co-stimulation and survival [68].

Migration of cell is an elementary process underlying key biological phenomena like formation and maintenance of tissue, regeneration, and ultimately cancer metastasis. IAPs are considered as major contributors in the process of endothelial cell survival and migration [69,70]. cIAP1 in cooperation with Myc propel cellular proliferation, which is achieved by ubiquitination followed by degradation of Mad1, a Myc antagonist [71]. Another study defined the role XIAP-RING domain in migration of cancer cells as it was observed that attenuation of XIAP reduces migratory ability of HCT116 colorectal carcinoma cells, which is dependent on RING domain of the XIAP protein [72]. Intermolecular cooperation between XIAP and survivin encourages tumor cell invasion by inducing metastasis. This mechanism is independent of IAP inhibition of cell death [73]. These studies indicated that this multifaceted protein functions by mechanisms like i) caspase function inhibition, ii) ubiquitination and RING E3 ligase function, and iii) cell survival signaling pathway.

6.4.3.1 Regulation of IAPs in Cancer

Several post-translational modifications of IAPs may perturb the stability of the protein by disturbing protein-protein interaction and affecting intracellular localization [74, 75]. Altered expression of IAPs are associated with resistance to therapy, cancer progression, and poor disease outcome [76]. IAP levels can be altered during crosstalk between IAP molecules [77]. Proteins having IAP-binding motif (IBM) by binding directly with BIR domains either displaces caspases or facilitates degradation of IAP [78]. Some IAPs are known to exert its function during mitosis and cytokinesis by regulating alignment and segregation of chromosome [79]. cIAP1 plays a role in controlling transcription of cyclin by regulating transcription factor E2F [80]. XIAP is considered as a regulator of death resistance and has found to be a target for personalized therapy [81]. A report of Silke et al. (2014) also suggested IAP as a potential therapeutic target in cancer [76].

6.4.4 p53

The tumor suppressor protein p53 evokes a multiple of cellular responses like protection of genomic integrity, induction of apoptosis, regulation of glycolysis, autophagy, and acceleration of cellular differentiation [82]. The protein is often termed as "guardian of the genome" or "cellular gatekeeper." Tumor suppressor gene p53 has been mapped to chromosome 17. The p53 protein binds to DNA and successively activates another gene to produce a protein called p21. p21 in turn interacts with a cell division-stimulating protein (cdk2) that prevents or stops progression of the cell to the next phase. In response to cellular stress, this tumor suppressor protein is activated and the process of activation occurs in three steps: i) p53 stabilization, ii) DNA binding at specific sequence, and iii) activation of target genes at the transcriptional level [83]. This tumor suppressor protein is composed of several domains. The central DNA-binding domain (DBD) also termed as core domain binds to response elements of target genes. Another domain denoted as TA or N-terminal transcription–activation domain is an essential site of binding for regulators of p53 gene transcription. These regulators may be positive (e.g., p300/CBP, TAFII40/60) or negative (e.g., MDM2 and MDMX) [84]. A third domain namely CTD or C-terminal oligomerization domain of p53 is contingent on alternative splicing and post-translational modification. This domain has a strong impact on DNA binding and transcriptional activity of the p53 family members [85]. p53 is a master controller of a large number of genes that imparts growth arrest at the G2-M and G1 phases. Additionally, some other compulsive roles of p53 in recognition of DNA damage, repair, apoptosis, and cellular senescence have been documented [86]. Being a key player in controlling cell growth and development, the functional regulation of p53 is highly warranted. A protein MDM2 having E3 ubiquitin ligase activity binds to TA domain of the protein and impedes transcriptional activity of p53 [87]. p53, on the other hand, also regulates MDM2 expression positively [88]. During unstressed condition, MDM2 interacts with p53 and is tightly regulated. Stressed condition leads to disruption of the p53-MDM2 complex and activates p53, thus indicating the presence of an autoregulatory loop that controls the level of active p53. p53 is associated with the intrinsic and extrinsic apoptotic pathways by transcriptional activation of PUMA, Bax, Bid, CD95, TRAIL-R2 etc. [89, 90]. Most of the target proteins of p53 are proapoptotic Bcl-2 family proteins. p53 functions not only in the nucleus but also in the cytosol [91]. The novel tumor suppressor protein has been reported to induce MOMP, thereby triggering release of proapoptotic factors. The underlying mechanism of p53-induced membrane permeabilization suggests that the protein functions like a BH3-only protein and thus activates Bax and/or Bak [91]. Transcription-independent apoptotic function of p53 has been observed in the cytoplasm and mitochondria where p53 directly activates Bax and Bak [91]. Along with apoptosis, cytoplasmic p53 is also involved in inhibition of autophagy [91].

6.4.4.1 Regulation of p53 in Cancer

Multiple post-translational modifications of p53 determine the nuclear and cytoplasmic function of this protein. Nuclear accumulation of p53 occurs due to poly (ADP) ribosylation of the protein. On the contrary, monoubiquitylation by MDM2 triggers the nuclear export of p53. p53 in the mitochondria is deubiquitylated by the mitochondrial protein HAUSP or ubiquitin-specific protease 7, thus causing the generation of non-ubiquitylated p53, which takes active part in apoptosis [92]. Human p53 possesses multiple serine (S)/threonine (T) phosphorylation sites. Multiple kinases can phosphorylate a single site at the N terminus end of p53. Similarly, multiple sites can be phosphorylated by a single kinase [93]. The most extensively studied p53 phosphorylation sites at the N terminal end are serine 15 and 20 sites. p53 phosphorylation at C-terminal serine residues either stimulates nuclear export or mitochondrial association [94]. Activation of FOXO3a, another important transcription factor, has been shown to deregulate p53 transcriptional activity. However, FOXO3a could induce apoptosis mediated by p53 but independent of p53-induced transcriptional activation. FOXO3a further-more enhances cytoplasmic accumulation of p53 and thus increases associa-tion of p53 with nuclear exporting machinery [95]. Ubiquitination, another posttranslational modification, is an important regulator of p53 stability and localization. Poly-ubiquitination of p53 protein leads to proteosomal degradation. Mono-ubiquitination, on the contrary, facilitates cytoplasmic translocation of p53 [96]. HDM2 or human double minute 2 is the crucial E3 ubiquitin ligase and a negative regulator of p53. Lysine residues residing at the C-terminal regulatory domain of p53 are ubiquitinylated by HDM2 [97]. p53 is also targeted by two other evolutionarily conserved proteins resembling like ubiquitin in their structure. These two proteins are known as SUMO or small ubiquitin-like modifier and NEDD8 or Neural precursor cell Expressed Developmentally Down-regulated protein 8. They conjugate with lysine residue of p53 [98, 99]. Sumoylation and neddylation of p53 occurs at lysine residues of C terminal ends [97]. Neddylation and sumoylation have not been manifested to affect p53 stabilization and localization.

Acetylation, another posttranslational modification of p53 is an essential event for functional activation of the protein. Acetylation is important as i) it eliminates ubiquitination on the same site and promotes protein stabiliza-tion, ii) inhibits HDM2/HDMX repressive complex to bind to target gene promoters, and iii) triggers co-factor recruitment for transcriptional activa-tion of the protein. The tumor suppressor protein p53 has nine (9) acetylation sites at its lysine residues which are acetylated by histone acetyl transfer-ase (HAT). Owing to reciprocal exclusion of acetylation and ubiquitination, sequence-specific binding of p53 to DNA occurs which results in transcrip-tional activation and protein stabilization. Balance between acetylation and deacetylation of p53 is maintained by another class of enzyme protein known as histone deacetylase (HDACs), particularly HDAC1 and Sirtuin 1 (SIRT1) [97]. A number of lysine and arginine residues in p53 are meth-ylated by either arginine methyl transferase or lysine methyl transferase. Effective outcome of p53 methylation may be either activation or repres-sion. Alterations of methylation and acetylation pattern at the lysine residues of this tumor suppressor protein increase during DNA damage. Therefore, interchange between methylation and acetylation at the same lysine residue of p53 may be the deciding factor for transcriptional activation of p53 dur-ing stress response [97]. Mutation of p53 protein or any disruption in p53 signaling pathways are commonly found in several types of human cancers. p53 mutation leads to abrogation of wild-type protein functioning [100].

Mutant p53 protein in some cases gains cancer promoting function [101–104]. Reports indicated loss of tumor suppressing function vis-a-vis gain of oncogenic function of mutant p53 cell culture system in vitro [105]. Mutant p53 binds to DNA and alters the expression of several genes. Mutant p53 binds to transcription factors and accelerates their functional activity, and interacts with protein to alter their functional activity. All these series of events culminate into gain of invasive and metastatic activity of the p53 protein [106, 107]. A very high amount of mutant p53 pool is observed in tumor cells [103]. Therefore, destabilization or inactivation of mutant p53 might be a rationale strategy. Some studies have indicated that targeting heat shock proteins through histone deacetylases might restore degradation and destabilization of mutant p53, which is mediated by MDM2 [108]. Mutant p53 has been described as enhancer of receptor tyrosine kinase proteins or RTKs in different cancer types [109]. Abnormal expression of p53 therefore renders the protein an attractive therapeutic target.

Homeostatic balance in the human body is maintained by mitosis and apoptosis. Some of the major proteins associated with apoptosis are caspases, Bcl-2 family of proteins, IAPs, and p53. Ultimate outcome of dysregulation of these key molecules is cancer, the deadliest disease. Therefore, an insight into the mechanism of these vital proteins might allow developing effective therapeutic strategies against cancer.

6.5   SUMMARY

- Homeostatic balance of a cell is regulated by cell growth and death in a complex fashion.
- Programmed cell death or apoptosis, a physiological process imparts an imperative role in maintaining cellular homeostasis, immune system functioning, hormone-dependent atrophy, development of normal embryo, and elimination of unwanted cells.
- Impairment of cellular homeostasis due to inadequate apoptotic event may undergo manifestation of cancer.
- Several pathways regulate the apoptotic process like intrinsic pathway, extrinsic pathway, and lysosomal pathway.
- Family of cysteine proteases or caspases are ultimate mediator of apoptosis. Sometimes apoptosis may progress through caspase-independent pathway.

- Apart from caspases, Bcl-2 family of proteins, IAPs, and p53 are some of the major players involved in apoptotic cascade.
- Regulation or Dysregulation of these proteins ultimately lead to either apoptosis or tumorigenesis.
- Abnormal expressions of these proteins are major contenders in cancer and are considered as potential therapeutic targets.

ACKNOWLEDGMENTS

The authors are indebted to the Director, Chittaranjan National Cancer Institute, Kolkata. There is no conflict of interest among the contributors.

KEYWORDS

- **apoptosis**
- **Bcl-2**
- **caspases**
- **IAPs**
- **p53**

REFERENCES

1. Gadjev, I., Stone, J. M., & Gechev, T. S., (2008). Programmed cell death in plants: new insights into redox regulation and the role of hydrogen peroxide. *International Review of Cell and Molecular Biology, 270,* 87–144.
2. Plati, J., Bucur, O., & Khosravi-Far, R., (2011). Apoptotic cell signaling in cancer progression and therapy. *Integr. Biol. (Camb.), 3,* 279–296.
3. Yaacoub, K., Pedeux, R., Tarte, K., & Guillaudeux, T., (2016). Role of the tumor microenvironment in regulating apoptosis and cancer progression. *Cancer Lett., 378*(2), 150–159.
4. Fernald, K., & Kurokawa, M., (2013). Evading apoptosis in cancer. *Trends Cell Biol., 12,* 620–633.
5. Sankari, S. L., Masthan, K. M., Babu, N. A., Bhattacharjee, T., & Elumalai, M., (2012). Apoptosis in cancer--an update. *Asian Pac. J. Cancer Prev., 13*(10), 4873–4878.
6. Wong, R. S. Y., (2011). Apoptosis in cancer: from pathogenesis to treatment. *J. Exp. Clin. Cancer Res., 30,* 1–14.
7. Walczak, H., (2013). Death receptor–ligand systems in cancer, cell death, & inflammation. *Cold Spring Harb. Perspect. Biol., 5*(5), a008698.

8. Rastogi, R. P., Sinha, R. P., & Sinha, R. P., (2009). Apoptosis: molecular mechanisms and pathogenicity. *EXCLI Journal, 8,* 155–181.

9. Bender, T., & Martinou, J. C., (2013). Where killers meet--permeabilization of the outer mitochondrial membrane during apoptosis. *Cold Spring Harb. Perspect. Biol., 5*(1), a011106. doi: 10. 1101/cshperspect.a011106.

10. Landes, T., & Martinou, J. C., (2011). Mitochondrial outer membrane permeabilization during apoptosis: the role of mitochondrial fission. *Biochim. Biophys. Acta., 1813*(4), 540–545.

11. Larsen, B. D., Rampalli, S., Burns, L. E., Brunette, S., et al., (2010). Caspase 3/caspase-activated DNase promote cell differentiation by inducing DNA strand breaks. *Proc. Natl. Acad. Sci. USA, 107*(9), 4230–4235.

12. Sanchez-Osuna, M., Garcia-Belinchon, M., Iglesias-Guimarais, V., Gil-Guinon, E., et al., (2014). Caspase-activated DNase is necessary and sufficient for oligonucleosomal DNA breakdown, but not for chromatin disassembly during caspase-dependent apoptosis of LN-18 glioblastoma cells. *J. Biol. Chem., 289*(27), 18752–18769.

13. Berthelet, J., & Dubrez, L., (2013). Regulation of apoptosis by inhibitors of apoptosis (IAPs). *Cells, 2*(1), 163–187.

14. Attaran-Bandarabadi, F., Abhari, B. A., Neishabouri, S. H., & Davoodi, J., (2017). Integrity of XIAP is essential for effective activity recovery of apoptosome and its downstream caspases by Smac/Diablo. *Int. J. Biol. Macromol., 17.* pii: S0141–8130(16), 33084–33087.

15. Verhagen, A. M., Kratina, T. K., Hawkins, C. J., Silke, J., et al., (2007). Identification of mammalian mitochondrial proteins that interact with IAPs via N-terminal IAP binding motifs. *Cell Death Differ., 14*(2), 348–357.

16. Zurawa-Janicka, D., Jarzab, M., Polit, A., Skorko-Glonek, J., et al., (2013). Temperature-induced changes of HtrA2(Omi) protease activity and structure. *Cell Stress Chaperones, 8*(1), 35–51.

17. Liu, G., Zou, H., Luo, T., Long, M., et al., (2016). Caspase-dependent and caspase-independent pathways are involved in cadmium-induced apoptosis in primary rat proximal tubular cell culture. *PLoS One, 11*(11), e0166823.

18. Sun, Y. S., Lv, L. X., Zhao, Z., He, X., et al., (2014). Cordycepol C induces caspase-independent apoptosis in human hepatocellular carcinoma HepG2 cells. *Biol. Pharm. Bull., 37*(4), 608–617.

19. Bhat, T. A., Chaudhary, A. K., Kumar, S., O'Malley, J., et al., (2017). Endoplasmic reticulum-mediated unfolded protein response and mitochondrial apoptosis in cancer. *Biochim. Biophys. Acta., 1867*(1), 58–66.

20. Tabas, I., & Ron, D., (2011). Integrating the mechanisms of apoptosis induced by endoplasmic reticulum stress. *Nat. Cell Biol., 13*(3), 184–190.

21. Redza-Dutordoir, M., & Averill-Bates, D. A., (2016). Activation of apoptosis signalling pathways by reactive oxygen species. *Biochim. Biophys. Acta., 1863*(12), 2977–2992.

22. Kapur, A., Felder, M., Fass, L., Kaur, J., et al., (2016). Modulation of oxidative stress and subsequent induction of apoptosis and endoplasmic reticulum stress allows citral to decrease cancer cell proliferation. *Sci. Rep., 6,* 27530.

23. Yoon, J. S., Kim, H. M., Yadunandam, A. K., Kim, N. H., et al., (2013). Neferine isolated from nelumbo nucifera enhances anti-cancer activities in Hep3B cells: molecular mechanisms of cell cycle arrest, ER stress induced apoptosis and anti-angiogenic response. *Phytomedicine, 20*(11), 1013–1022.

24. Aits, S., & Jäättelä, M. J., (2013). Lysosomal cell death at a glance. *Cell Sci.*, *126*, 1905–1912.

25. Appelqvist, H., Wäster, P., Kagedal, K., & Ollinger, K., (2013). The lysosome: from waste bag to potential therapeutic target. *J. Mol. Cell Biol.*, *5*, 214–226.

26. Denamur, S., Boland, L., Beyaert, M., Verstraeten, S. L., et al., (2016). Subcellular mechanisms involved in apoptosis induced by aminoglycoside antibiotics: Insights on p53, proteasome and endoplasmic reticulum. *Toxicol. Appl. Pharmacol.*, *309*, 24–36.

27. Messner, B., Turkcan, A., Ploner, C., Laufer, G., & Bernhard, D., (2016). Cadmium overkill: autophagy, apoptosis and necrosis signalling in endothelial cells exposed to cadmium. *Cell Mol Life Sci.*, *73*(8), 1699–1713.

28. Noutsopoulos, D., Markopoulos, G., Vartholomatos, G., Kolettas, E., et al., (2010). VL30 retrotransposition signals activation of a caspase-independent and p53-dependent death pathway associated with mitochondrial and lysosomal damage. *Cell Res.*, *20*(5), 553–562.

29. Chou, Y. W., Senadi, G. C., Chen, C. Y., Kuo, K. K., et al., (2016). Design and synthesis of pyrrolobenzodiazepine-gallic hybrid agents as p53-dependent and -independent apoptogenic signaling in melanoma cells. *Eur. J. Med. Chem.*, *109*, 59–74.

30. Rudolf, E., & Cervinka, M., (2011). Sulforaphane induces cytotoxicity and lysosome- and mitochondria-dependent cell death in colon cancer cells with deleted p53. *Toxicol. In. Vitro, 7*, 1302–1309.

31. Phang, C. W., Karsani, S. A., Sethi, G., & Abd Malek, S. N., (2016). Flavokawain C inhibits cell cycle and promotes apoptosis, associated with endoplasmic reticulum stress and regulation of MAPKs and Akt signaling pathways in HCT *116* human colon carcinoma Cells. *PLoS One*, *11*(2), e0148775.

32. Wang, L., Liu, L., Shi, Y., Cao, H., Chaturvedi, R., Calcutt, M. W., et al., (2012). Berberine induces caspase-independent cell death in colon tumor cells through activation of apoptosis-inducing factor. *PLoS One*, *7*(5), e36418. doi:10. 1371/journal.pone. 0036418.

33. Jancekova, B., Ondrouskova, E., Knopfova, L., Smarda, J., & Benes, P., (2016). Enzymatically active cathepsin D sensitizes breast carcinoma cells to TRAIL. *Tumour Biol.*, *37*(8), 10685–10696.

34. Friedman, J. R., Perry, H. E., Brown, K. C., Gao, Y., et al., (2017). Capsaicin synergizes with camptothecin to induce increased apoptosis in human small cell lung cancers via the calpain pathway. *Biochem, Pharmacol.*, *129*, 54–66.

35. Mcllwain, D. R., Berger, T., & Mak, T. W., (2013). Caspase functions in cell death and disease. *Cold Spring Harb. Perspect. Biol.*, *5*, a008656.

36. Parrish, A. B., Freel, C. D., & Kornbluth, S., (2013). Cellular mechanisms controlling caspase activation and function. *Cold Spring Harb. Perspect. Biol.*, *5*(6), pii: a008672, doi: 10. 1101/cshperspect.a008672.

37. Kitazumi, I., & Tsukahara, M., (2011). Regulation of DNA fragmentation: the role of caspases and phosphorylation. *FEBS J.*, *278*(3), 427–441.

38. Peng, C., Cho, Y. Y., Zhu, F., Zhang, J., et al., (2011). Phosphorylation of caspase-8 (Thr-263) by ribosomal S6 kinase 2 (RSK2) mediates caspase-8 ubiquitination and stability. *J. Biol. Chem.*, *286*, 6946–6954.

39. Kim, Y. M., Kim, J. H., Kwon, H. M., Lee, D. H., et al., (2013). Korean red ginseng protects endothelial cells from serum-deprived apoptosis by regulating Bcl-2 family protein dynamics and caspase S-nitrosylation. *J. Ginseng. Res.*, *37*(4), 413–424.

40. Dunne, K. A., Allam, A., McIntosh, A., Houston, S. A., Cerovic, V., et al., (2013). Increased S-nitrosylation and proteasomal degradation of caspase-3 during infection contribute to the persistence of adherent invasive Escherichia coli (AIEC) in immune cells. *PLoS One, 4, 8*(7), e68386.

41. Ghavami, S., Hashemi, M., Ande, S. R., Yeganeh, B., et al., (2009). Apoptosis and cancer: mutations within caspase genes. *J. Med. Genet., 46*(8), 497–510.

42. Olsson, M., & Zhivotovsky, B., (2011). Caspases and cancer. *Cell Death and Differentiation, 18*, 1441–1449.

43. Park, J. Y., Park, J. M., Jang, J. S., Choi, J. E., et al., (2006). Caspase 9 promoter polymorphisms and risk of primary lung cancer. *Hum. Mol Genet., 15*, 1963–1971.

44. Soung, Y. H., Lee, J. W., Kim, S. Y., Park, W. S., et al., (2004). Somatic mutations of CASP3 gene in human cancers. *Hum. Genet., 115*, 112–115.

45. Janicke, R. U., (2009). MCF-7 breast carcinoma cells do not express caspase-3. *Breast Cancer Res. Treat., 117*, 219–221.

46. Jäger, R., & Zwacka, R. M., (2010). The enigmatic roles of caspases in tumor development. *Cancers, 2*, 1952–1979.

47. Lin, Y. F., Lai, T. C., Chang, C. K., Chen, C. L., et al., (2013). Targeting the XIAP/caspase-7 complex selectively kills caspase-3-deficient malignancies. *J. Clin. Invest., 123*(9), 3861–3875.

48. Graf, R. P., Keller, N., Barbero, S., & Stupack, D., (2014). Caspase-8 as a regulator of tumor cell motility. *Curr. Mol. Med., 14*(2), 246–254.

49. Yi, C. H., & Yuan, J., (2009). The Jekyll and Hyde functions of caspases. *Dev. Cell., 16*(1), 21–34.

50. Barbero, S., Mielgo, A., Torres, V., Teitz, T., et al., (2009). Caspase-8 association with the focal adhesion complex promotes tumor cell migration and metastasis. *Cancer Res., 69*(9), 3755–3763.

51. Finlay, D., Howes, A., & Vuori, K., (2009). Critical role for caspase-8 in epidermal growth factor signaling. *Cancer Res., 69*, 5023–5029.

52. Ludwig, L. M., Nassin, M. L., Hadji, A., & LaBelle, J. L., (2016). Killing two cells with one stone: pharmacologic BCL-2 family targeting for cancer cell death and immune modulation. *Front. Pediatr., 4*, 135.

53. Jayakiran, M., (2015). Apoptosis-biochemistry: A mini review. *J. Clin. Exp. Pathol., 5*, 1.

54. Kelly, P. N., & Strasser, A., (2011). The role of Bcl-2 and its pro-survival relatives in tumourigenesis and cancer therapy. *Cell Death and Differentiation, 18*, 1414–1424.

55. Schenk, R. L., Strasser, A., & Dewson, G., (2017). BCL-2: Long and winding path from discovery to therapeutic target. *Biochem. Biophys. Res. Commun., 482*(3), 459–469.

56. Levy, M. A., & Claxton, D. F., (2017). Therapeutic inhibition of BCL-2 and related family members. *Expert. Opin. Investig. Drugs, 26*(3), 293–301.

57. Kipps, T. J., Stevenson, F. K., Wu, C. J., Croce, C. M., et al., (2017). Chronic lymphocytic leukaemia. *Nat. Rev. Dis. Primers., 3*, 16096.

58. Akl, H., Vervloessem, T., Kiviluoto, S., Bittremieux, M., et al., (2014). A dual role for the anti-apoptotic Bcl-2 protein in cancer: mitochondria versus endoplasmic reticulum. *Biochim. Biophys. Acta, 1843*(10), 2240–2252.

59. Choi, D., & Woo, M., (2010). Executioners of apoptosis in pancreatic β-cells: not just for cell death. *Am. J. Physiol. Endocrinol. Metab., 298*, E735–E741.

60. Shamas-Din, A., Brahmbhatt, H., Leber, B., & Andrews, D. W., (2011). BH3-only proteins: Orchestrators of apoptosis. *Biochimica. et Biophysica. Acta (BBA) - Molecular Cell Research, 1813*(4), 508–520.

61. Williams, M., Lee, L., Hicks, D. J., Joly, M. M., et al., (2016). Key survival factor, Mcl-1, correlates with sensitivity to combined Bcl-2/Bcl-xL Blockade. *Mol Cancer Res.*, pii: molcanres. 0280., doi: 10. 1158/1541–7786. MCR-16–0280-T.

62. Chen, L., & Fletcher, S., (2017). Mcl-1 inhibitors: a patent review. *Expert. Opin. Ther. Pat.*, *27*(2), 163–178.

63. Dai, Y., Jin, S., Li, X., & Wang, D., (2016). The involvement of Bcl-2 family proteins in Akt-regulated cell survival in cisplatin resistant epithelial ovarian cancer. *Oncotarget.*, doi: *10.* 18632/oncotarget. 13817.

64. Oberoi-Khanuja, T. K., Murali, A., & Rajalingam, K., (2013). IAPs on the move: role of inhibitors of apoptosis proteins in cell migration. *Cell Death and Disease.*, *4*(9), e784.

65. Metzger, M. B., Pruneda, J. N., Klevit, R. E., & Weissman, A. M., (2014). RING-type E3 ligases: master manipulators of E2 ubiquitin-conjugating enzymes and ubiquitination. *Biochim. Biophys. Acta.*, *1843*(1), 47–60.

66. *Silke, J., & Meier, P., (2013). Inhibitor of apoptosis (IAP) proteins – modulators of cell death and inflammation. Cold Spring Harb. Perspect. Biol.,* 5, a008730.

67. Damgaard, R. B., & Gyrd-Hansen, M., (2011). Inhibitor of apoptosis (IAP) proteins in regulation of inflammation and innate immunity. *Discov. Med.*, *11*, 221–231.

68. Giardino, T. M. L., Munitic, I., Castro, E., Herz, J., et al., (2015). *Eur. J. Immunol.*, *45*(9), 2672–2682.

69. Dubrez, L., & Rajalingam, K., (2015). IAPs and cell migration. *Semin. Cell Dev. Biol.*, *39*, 124–131.

70. Fulda, S., (2014). Regulation of cell migration, invasion and metastasis by IAP proteins and their antagonists. *Oncogene*, *33*(6), 671–676.

71. Lopez, J., John, S. W., Tenev, T., Rautureau, G. J., et al., (2011). CARD-mediated autoinhibition of cIAP1's E3 ligase activity suppresses cell proliferation and migration. *Mol Cell*, *42*, 569–583.

72. Liu, J., Zhang, D., Luo, W., Yu, J., et al., (2012). E3 ligase activity of XIAP RING domain is required for XIAP-mediated cancer cell migration, but not for its RhoGDI binding activity. *PLoS One*, *7*, e35682.

73. Mehrotra, S., Languino, L. R., Raskett, C. M., Mercurio, A. M., et al., (2010). IAP regulation of metastasis. *Cancer Cell*, *17*(1), 53.

74. Nogueira-Ferreira, R., Vitorino, R., Ferreira-Pinto, M., Ferreira, R., & Henriques-Coelho, T., (2013). Exploring the role of post-translational modifications on protein-protein interactions with survivin. *Arch. Biochem. Biophys.*, *538*(2), 64–70.

75. Marivin, A., Berthelet, J., Plenchette, S., & Dubrez, L., (2012). The inhibitor of apoptosis (IAPs) in adaptive response to cellular stress. *Cells*, *1*(4), 711–737.

76. Silke, J., & Vucic, D., (2014). IAP family of cell death and signaling regulators. *Methods Enzymol.*, *545*, 35–65.

77. Vanden, B. T., Kaiser, W. J., Bertrand, M. J., & Vandenabeele, P., (2015). Molecular crosstalk between apoptosis, necroptosis, & survival signaling. *Mol Cell Oncol.*, *2*(4), e975093. doi: 10. 4161/23723556. 2014. 975093.

78. Yeh, T. C., & Bratton, S. B., (2013). Caspase-dependent regulation of the ubiquitin-proteasome system through direct substrate targeting. *Proc. Natl. Acad. Sci. USA.*, *110*(35), 14284–14289.

79. Van der Waal, M. S., Hengeveld, R. C., Van der Horst, A., & Lens, S. M., (2012). Cell division control by the chromosomal passenger complex. *Exp. Cell. Res., 318,* 1407–1420.

80. Cartier, J., Berthelet, J., Marivin, A., Gemble, S., et al., (2011). Cellular inhibitor of apoptosis protein-1 (cIAP1) can regulate E2F1 transcription factor-mediated control of cyclin transcription. *J. Biol. Chem., 286*(30), 26406–26417.

81. Obexer, P., & Ausserlechner, M. J., (2014). X-linked inhibitor of apoptosis protein - a critical death resistance regulator and therapeutic target for personalized cancer therapy. *Front Oncol., 4,* 197.

82. Purvis, J. E., Karhohs, K. W., Mock, C., Batchelor, E., et al., (2012). p53 dynamics control cell fate. *Science, 336*(6087), 1440–1444.

83. Kruse, J. P., & Gu, W., (2009). Modes of p53 regulation. *Cell, 137*(4), 609–622.

84. Mavinahalli, J. N., Madhumalar, A., Beuerman, R. W., Lane, D. P., et al., (2010). Differences in the transactivation domains of p53 family members: a computational study. *BMC Genomics., 11*(Suppl 1):S5. 10. 1186/1471–2164–11-S1-S5.

85. Hamard, P. J., Lukin, D. J., & Manfredi, J. J., (2012). p53 basic C terminus regulates p53 functions through DNA binding modulation of subset of target genes. *J. Biol. Chem., 287*(26), 22397–22407.

86. Roos, W. P., Thomas, A. D., & Kaina, B., (2016). DNA damage and the balance between survival and death in cancer biology. *Nat. Rev. Cancer, 16*(1), 20–33.

87. Shadfan, M., Lopez-Pajares, V., & Yuan, Z. M., (2012). MDM2 and MDMX: Alone and together in regulation of P53. *Transl. Cancer Res., 1*(2), 88–89.

88. Pflaum, J., Schlosser, S., & Müller, M., (2014). p53 Family and cellular stress responses in cancer. *Front Oncol., 4,* 285.

89. Riley, T., Sontag, E., Chen, P., & Levine, A., (2008). Transcriptional control of human p53-regulated genes. *Nat. Rev. Mol Cell Biol., 9,* 402–412.

90. Beckerman, R., & Prives, C., (2010). Transcriptional regulation by p53. *Cold Spring Harb. Perspect. Biol., 2*(8), a000935.

91. Comel, A., Sorrentino, G., Capaci, V., & Sal, G. D., (2014). The cytoplasmic side of p53's oncosuppressive activities. *FEBS Letters, 588*(16), 2600–2609.

92. Park, J. H., Zhuang, J., Li, J., & Hwang, P. M., (2016). p53 as guardian of the mitochondrial genome. *FEBS Lett, 590*(7), 924–934.

93. Kruse, J. P., & Gu, W., (2009). Modes of p53 regulation. *Cell, 137*(4), 609–622.

94. Loughery, J., Cox, M., Smith, L. M., & Meek, D. W., (2014). Critical role for p53-serine 15 phosphorylation in stimulating transactivation at p53-responsive promoters. *Nucl. Acids Res., 42*(12), 7666–7680.

95. Zhang, X., Tang, N., Hadden, T. J., & Rishi, A. K., (2011). Akt, FoxO and regulation of apoptosis. *Biochimica. et Biophysica. Acta, 1813,* 1978–1986.

96. Lee, J. T., & Gu, W., (2010). The multiple levels of regulation by p53 ubiquitination. *Cell Death Differ., 17,* 86–92.

97. Dai, C., & Gu, W., (2010). p53 post-translational modification: deregulated in tumorigenesis. *Trends Mol Med., 16*(11), 528–536.

98. Ivanschitz, L., Takahashi, Y., Jollivet, F., Ayrault, O., et al., (2015). PML IV/ARF interaction enhances p53 SUMO-1 conjugation, activation, & senescence. *Proc. Natl. Acad. Sci. USA, 112*(46), 14278–14283.

99. Guihard, S., Ramolu, L., Macabre, C., Wasylyk, B., et al., (2012). The NEDD8 conjugation pathway regulates p53 transcriptional activity and head and neck cancer cell sensitivity to ionizing radiation. *Int. J. Oncol., 41*(4), 1531–1540.

100. Ren, Y. A., Mullany, L. K., Liu, Z., Herron, A. J., et al., (2016). Mutant p53 promotes epithelial ovarian cancer by regulating tumor differentiation, metastasis, & responsiveness to steroid hormones. *Cancer Res., 76*, 2206–2218.

101. Alexandrova, E. M., Mirza, S. A., Xu, S., Schulz-Heddergott, R., et al., (2017). p53 loss-of-heterozygosity is a necessary prerequisite for mutant p53 stabilization and gain-of-function in vivo. *Cell Death Dis., 8*(3), e2661.

102. Cole, A. J., Dwight, T., Gill, A. J., Dickson, K. A., et al., (2016). Assessing mutant p53 in primary high-grade serous ovarian cancer using immunohistochemistry and massively parallel sequencing. *Sci. Rep., 6*, 26191. doi: 10. 1038/srep26191.

103. Ferraiuolo, M., Di Agostino, S., Blandino, G., & Strano, S., (2016). Oncogenic intra-p53 family member interactions in human cancers. *Front Oncol., 6*, 77. doi: 10. 3389/fonc. 2016. 00077.

104. Vijayakumaran, R., Tan, K. H., Miranda, P. J., Haupt, S., & Haupt, Y., (2015). Regulation of Mutant p53 Protein Expression. *Front Oncol., 5*, 284. doi: 10. 3389/fonc. 2015. 00284.

105. Muller, P. A., & Vousden, K. H., (2013). p53 mutations in cancer. *Nat. Cell. Biol., 15*(1), 2–8.

106. Lenfert, E., Maenz, C., Heinlein, C., & Jannasch, K., (2015). Mutant p53 promotes epithelial-mesenchymal plasticity and enhances metastasis in mammary carcinomas of WAP-T mice. *Int. J. Cancer, 136*(6), 521–533.

107. Muller, P. A., Trinidad, A. G., Timpson, P., Morton, J. P., et al., (2013). Mutant p53 enhances MET trafficking and signalling to drive cell scattering and invasion. *Oncogene, 32*, 1252–1265.

108. Yan, W., Liu, S., Xu, E., Zhang, J., et al., (2013). Histone deacetylase inhibitors suppress mutant p53 transcription via histone deacetylase 8. *Oncogene, 32*(5), 599–609.

109. Wang, W., Cheng, B., Miao, L., Mei, Y., et al., (2013). Mutant p53- R273H gains new function in sustained activation of EGFR signaling via suppressing miR-27a expression. *Cell Death Dis., 4*, e574.

CHAPTER 7

CYTOPLASMIC SIGNALING CIRCUITRY: AN IMPORTANT TRAIT OF CANCER

SUBHRA DASH, K. LOHITESH, and SUDESHNA MUKHERJEE

Department of Biological Sciences, Birla Institute of Science and Technology, Pilani, Rajasthan–333031, India, E-mail: sudeshna@pilani.bits-pilani.ac.in

CONTENTS

ABSTRACT

Both inter and intracellular communication is important for proper functioning of individual cells and coordination with nearby cells, which is
dependent upon the potential of some cells to emit signals and for other
cells to respond to the received signals accordingly. Normal cells need
stimulatory signals for proliferation and differentiation, which is facilitated by transmembrane receptors present on the cell surface to which
extracellular matrix (ECM) components, cell-cell adhesion molecules,
and growth factors can bind and induce the cascade of reaction. Unlike
normal cells, cancer cells contrast strongly by showing reduced dependence on exogenous growth-promoting and growth-inhibitory factors,
evading processes like apoptosis and senescence and thereby evading
mechanisms that limit cell proliferation. In addition to this, cancer cells
can also switch the integrin receptors, and successful binding of these
receptors with ECM enables them to transduce signals into the cytoplasm,
which can influence cells by altering its motility, apoptosis, etc. These
properties of cancer cells can lead to deregulation of many signaling pathways. Many of these signaling proteins are currently under investigation
as possible targets for cancer therapy. The present chapter deals with the
various signaling pathways involved in cancer and the complexity of signal transduction that involves the cross-talk of several factors and very
few unifying principles.

7.1   INTRODUCTION

Cancer can be defined as a program that promotes uncontrolled proliferation of cells. This abnormal cellular behavior might lead us to assume that
cancer cells employ alternative and novel cellular signaling strategy to
feed their unrestrained growth and division. But the reality is that there
are subtle differences between normal and tumor cell intracellular signaling and the later actually utilizes an almost identical control circuitry. The
major difference lies in the way the tumor cells modulate the existing signaling program and bend it in their own way. Cellular signaling pathways,
in general, are not isolated from each other but are inter-connected to form
complex networks. Cells receive information from various sources via
receptors, cell-matrix, and cell-cell contacts, which is then integrated and

utilized to regulate varied cellular processes, including protein synthesis, cell growth, motility, cell architecture, polarity, differentiation, and programmed cell death. Interestingly, a single signaling molecule can act in a context-dependent manner and regulate different cellular processes with multiple signaling complexes or at different intracellular locations. The intricacy of the cellular signaling networks has major implications toward our understanding of cancer cell behavior and for our ability to use this knowledge for cancer therapy. We are gradually unraveling the intricate network of signaling and the nodes and extent of crosstalk between various molecules in the tumor cells. The present chapter described this complex signaling circuitry functional in the cellular environment of cancer cells that fuel their growth and proliferation.

7.2   RAS SIGNALING: A MASTER REGULATOR OF SIGNALING CASCADE

RAS belongs to the family of membrane-associated monomeric GTPases that conveys external signals to the cell through cell surface receptors by hydrolyzing GTP to GDP which can be exchanged (to GTP) to regulate a wide range of cellular processes [1].

The Ras subfamily consisting of K-Ras, H-Ras, N-Ras, R-Ras, R-Ras2, and M-Ras and also have other distinct members like Rap1 (A-B), Rap2 (A-B), and Ral (A-B). RAS-associated genes are frequently activated in a wide range of cancers, which is the first step in activation of mitogen-activated protein kinase (MAPK) signaling cascade involved in regulating different molecular process like differentiation, proliferation, survival, and cell death. A number of upstream signals like cytokine receptors, heterotrimeric G protein-coupled receptors, tyrosine kinase receptors, calcium channels, and integrins can stimulate the switching of GDP/GTP to facilitate RAS binding. This exchange reaction can also be facilitated by other factors like SOS (Son of sevenless), RAS guanine-releasing factor (Ras-GRF), guanine-nucleotide exchange factors (GEF), and RAS guanyl releasing protein (Ras-GRP). The GTP-bound active RAS can be inactivated by GTPase-activating proteins (GAPs) (Figure 7.1) which can interact with different target genes either to initiate or inhibit many downstream signaling pathways depending upon the signals they receive [2] (Figure 7.2).

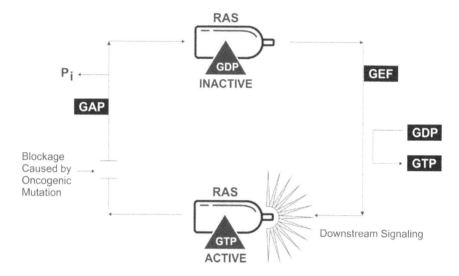

FIGURE 7.1 Activation of Ras: Tyrosine kinase receptors transduce mitogenic signals that activate guanine nucleotide exchange factor (GEF). This facilitates an inactive Ras protein to shed its GDP and bind with GTP instead. This GTP-bound Ras is an active Ras, which in turn activates its downstream targets or group of targets. Any resulting mutation can lead to the loss of GTPase activity of Ras, which results in the formation of constitutively active ras protein.

Following Ras activation, GTP linked RAS binds to RAF (the first mammalian effector of RAS to be characterized) proteins, BRAF, ARAF and c-RAF1 and activate them causing RAF translocation to the plasma membrane, which is crucial for its activation. Activated RAF then phosphorylates MAPK kinases 1 and 2 (MEK1 and MEK2) which can further phosphorylate and activate ERK1 and ERK2 (extracellular signal-regulated kinases 1 and 2). Upon activation, these are transported into the nucleus and can regulate major cellular processes like proliferation, survival, mitosis, migration, etc. [3, 4].

ERK phosphorylates c-JUN leading to the activation of AP1, which is a complex of FOS–JUN heterodimers. This stimulation enhances the expression of cyclin-D, which is a key cell cycle regulatory protein facilitating the cell to progress through the G1 phase.

Along with RAF/MAPK signaling, RAS can also interact directly with the catalytic subunit of type I phosphatidylinositol 3-kinases (PI3Ks). PI3K is known to regulate a wide range of downstream targets like PDK1

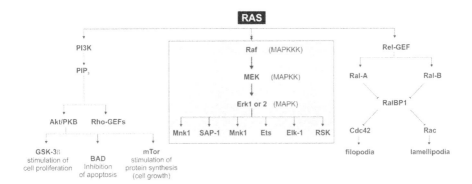

FIGURE 7.2 Ras the master controller: Ras activates three major pathways 1.The Ras Raf MAP kinase pathway that has the overall scheme of MAPKKK MAPK MAPK. Ras activates Raf kinase (MAPKK) which in turn phosphorylate and activate MEK (MAPK). MEK then activates Erk1 and 2 which are Map kinases (MAPKs). Erks can now activate other downstream targets to regulate growth and proliferation. 2. The PI3K pathway is the second effector pathway of Ras. Phosphatidylinositol-3-Kinase leads to the formation of phosphatidylinositol (3,4,5) triphosphate which in turn leads to the activation of Akt and its downstream targets. 3. The Ras-regulated pathway acts through Ral. Ras-RalGEF interaction leads to the activation of Ral proteins Ral-A and Ral-B. The GTP-bound activated Ral proteins now activates a number of downstream pathways among which Cdc42 and Rac are important for cell motility, and they mainly act by affecting the actin cytoskeleton.

(3-phosphoinositide-dependent protein kinase-1) and Akt (also known as PKB). Akt/PKB not only perform anti-apoptotic function but can also stimulate RAC, a RHO family protein that regulates the actin cytoskeleton [3]. RAS can also stimulates Ral, which along with the Akt/PKB inhibits the Forkhead transcription factors of the Foxo family and helps in the promotion of cell-cycle arrest through p27 and apoptosis through Bim and Fas ligand.

Point mutations of RAS mostly in codons 12, 13, and 61 have been found in 20% of human tumors, most frequently in KRAS (about 85%) followed by NRAS (about 15%), and then HRAS (<1%). Due to these mutations, GAPs are prevented from promoting hydrolysis of GTP, leading to the accumulation of GTP-bound Ras, i.e., the active form of RAS. Accumulating evidences Ras is found to be activated in many cancer types including breast, ovarian and stomach carcinomas due to overexpression of HER2, Neu, EGFR, etc.

7.3   AKT/PROTEIN KINASE B (PKB) SIGNALING: A CROSS POINT

Akt plays a crucial role in regulating diverse biological processes like growth, metabolism, proliferation, survival, and protein synthesis. A cascade of proteins are involved in the activation of the Akt pathway, like G-protein coupled receptors, integrins, receptor tyrosine kinases, cytokine receptors, etc. Upon activation of this pathway, phosphoinositide 3-kinase (PI3K) induces the production of phosphatidyl inositol trisphosphates (PIP3). These lipids serve as plasma membrane docking sites for proteins that harbor pleckstrin-homology (PH) domains, including Akt and its upstream activator PDK1 (Figure 7.3A). PDK1 phosphorylates Akt at Thr308 and phosphorylates it partially followed by phosphorylation at Ser473 residue by mTORC2, which activates it completely. DNA-PK, PI3K- related kinases, can also activate the Akt pathway by phosphorylating Akt at Ser473 residue. The protein phosphatase 2A (PP2A) and the PH-domain leucine-rich repeat containing

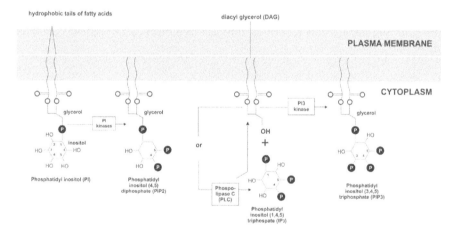

FIGURE 7.3A   Formation of PIP3: Phosphatidyl inositol is composed of three parts: two fatty acid moieties with long hydrocarbon tails integrated firmly into the plasma membrane, a glycerol moiety, and an inositol molecule attached to the glycerol through a phosphodiester bond. PI kinases add phosphates to the various hydroxyls of inositol yielding PI(4,5)-diphosphate (PIP2), which is further phosphorylated by phospholipase C yielding diacylglycerol (DAG). DAG can activate protein kinase C (PKC) and inositol (1,4,5)-triphosphate (IP3), which facilitates the release of calcium ions from intracellular stores. Otherwise, PIP2 can further be phosphorylated by PI3 kinase to yield phosphatidylinositol (3,4,5)-triphosphate (PIP3). This phosphorylated "head group" of PIP3 can attract proteins carrying PH domains, like Akt, to get hitched to the plasma membrane's inner surface.

protein phosphatases (PHLPP1/2) dephosphorylate Akt. Akt can also be inhibited by tumor suppressor phosphatase and tensin homolog (PTEN) by dephosphorylating PIP3 [5–11].

Akt isoforms share many substrates, e.g., RxRxxS/T, a consensus phosphorylation motif, and PRAS40 (proline-rich Akt substrate of 40 kDa), which are known to be phosphorylated by all three isoforms Akt1, Akt2, and Akt3, but isoform-specific Akt substrates have also been identified, e.g., actin-associated protein palladin that can only be phosphorylated by only Akt1 [8, 11].

Akt regulates cell proliferation by phosphorylating CDK inhibitors p21 and p27, and it can also regulate cell survival by either inhibiting pro-apop-

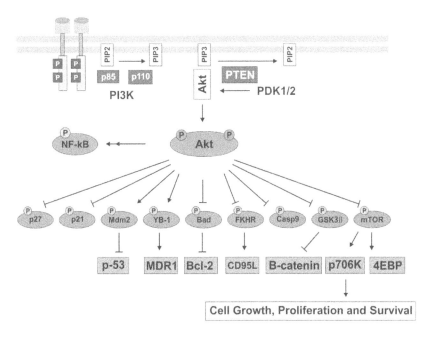

FIGURE 7.3B Akt/protein kinase B signaling: The formation of PIP3 (Figure 7.3A) by PI3K creates a docking site for cytoplasmic proteins carrying PH (pleckstrin homology) domains. Akt/PKB kinase being the most important of these. Akt/PKB is doubly phosphorylated and activated by two other kinases (PDK 1, PDK2) once docked via its PH domain inside the plasma membrane. This active Akt/PKB complex can phosphorylate a variety of substrates that regulate biological processes like cell proliferation, survival, and cell size. Some important targets of Akt includes mTOR pathway, NFκB, TGF-β etc. However, if active PTEN is present, it dephosphorylates PIP3 to PIP2 and Akt/PKB is deprived of a docking site at the plasma membrane leading to its deactivation and in turn controlled cell proliferation.

totic proteins like Bad or pro-apoptotic signals generated by protein like FoxO. Akt can regulate metabolism by activating AS160 and PFKFB2. It also contributes in cell invasion and migration by phosphorylating palladin and vimentin. Akt can phosphorylate IKKα and hence can regulate NFκB signaling. Akt has multiple targets by which it can regulate diverse cellular functions and hence can be considered as a therapeutic target for the treatment of various human diseases [8] (Figure 7.3B).

7.3.1 TYROSINE KINASE RECEPTOR MUTATION AND/OR OVEREXPRESSION

Upstream of tyrosine kinase receptor mutations or overexpression is one of the common mechanisms for Akt pathway activation in cancer. Amplified expression of critical genes like EGFR, HER2/NEU (ERBB2), FGFR, and HGFR has been found in ovarian, lung, breast, and colorectal carcinomas [12].

7.3.2 PTEN DELETION AND MUTATIONS

Dephosphorylation of phosphatidylinositol (3, 4 and 5) triphosphate (PIP3) and phosphatidylinositol (3 and 4) diphosphate by PTEN leads to inhibition of Akt. PTEN can lose its expression through various mechanisms like promoter hypermethylation, somatic mutations, deletions, etc. Cancers like prostate carcinomas, high-grade glioblastomas, and melanomas commonly exhibit loss of PTEN [12].

mTOR has a critical role in monitoring nutrient availability, cellular energy, oxygen levels, etc., and hence, in regulating cell growth and proliferation. mTOR belongs to a Ser/Thr protein kinase of the PI3K superfamily referred to as class IV PI3Ks, including ATM, ATR (ataxia telangiectasia and Rad3 related), DNA-PK, and SMG-1 (SMG1 homolog, phosphatidylinositol 3-kinase-related kinase). mTOR exists in two different complexes: mTORC1 and mTORC2. The mTORC1 complex is composed of the PRAS40 (proline-rich Akt substrate 40 kDa), the protein mLST8/GbL, and the mTOR catalytic subunit Raptor (regulatory associated protein of mTOR), while mTORC2 is composed of mTOR, mSIN1 (mammalian stress-activated protein kinase interacting protein 1), Rictor (rapamycin insensitive companion of mTOR), and mLST8/GbL. Akt phosphorylates PRAS40 and TSC2 to reduce their inhibitory effects on mTOR1 and hence activate mTOR. The association of mTORC1 with TSC1 and TSC2 provides a molecular link between mTOR and cancer. Downstream targets of mTORC1 like S6K1 (p70S6 kinase) and 4E-BP1 (4E-binding protein) are known to be involved in regulating protein synthesis; therefore, mTOR activation in tumor cells provides growth advantage. Binding of Rictor to the mTORC2 complex functions as PDK2 by phosphorylating Akt [13].

7.4   JAK-STAT SIGNALING: TRANSMISSION OF SIGNALS TO THE NUCLEUS DIRECTLY THROUGH CELL MEMBRANE

Genetic and epigenetic alterations in cancer cells lead to the activation of tyrosine kinases which can activate STAT proteins. In normal conditions, STAT proteins are known to transmit cytoplasmic signals through cytokines and growth factors for directing various cellular processes. There are seven STAT (signal transducers and activators of transcription) proteins (STAT 1A, 2A, 3A, 4A, 5A-B, and 6) and four JAK kinases in mammals [14]. JAK–STAT signaling can be broadly classified into two major pathways: canonical and non-canonical pathway [14]. Binding of a peptide ligand (e.g., cytokine) to the transmembrane receptors initiates the canonical mode of JAK–STAT signaling; this binding causes receptor dimerization that ultimately leads to cross-activation of receptor-associated JAK kinases, followed by the phosphorylation of tyrosine residues in the cytoplasmic tail. These phospho-tyrosine residues provide a docking site for the cytoplasmic STAT proteins that are phosphorylated by JAK at 700 amino acid of C-terminal tyrosine residue. Phosphorylated STAT proteins then translocate inside the nucleus where they act as transcriptional activators for many target genes. In contrast, in non-canonical pathway, STAT proteins are localized in the cytoplasm, and only a portion of the unphosphorylated pool of STAT is localized inside the nucleus in the heterochromatized form with HP1. HP1 localization and heterochromatin stability are maintained by heterochromatin-associated unphosphorylated STATs [15]. Phosphorylation of STAT causes dispersal of the heterochromatin complex, which leads to the displacement of HP1 (Figure 7.4).

STAT signaling is constitutively expressed in an increasing number of cancers due to the overactivation of one or more upstream tyrosine kinases

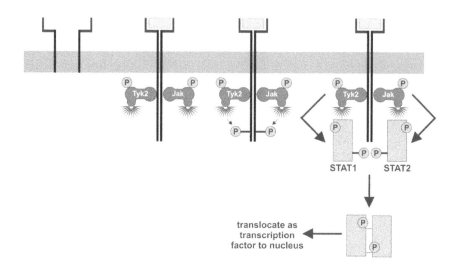

FIGURE 7.4 JAK-STAT pathway: This pathway is dependent upon the activity of JAK tyrosine kinases (e.g., JAK1, Tyk2, etc.) that are noncovalently attached to a number of cytokine receptors like interferons, thrombopoietin (TPO), erythropoietin (EPO), etc. Ligands usually activate receptors via dimerization. The JAKS (in this case JAK1 and Tyk 2) transphosphorylate each other as well as the C-terminal tails of the receptors, which then attracts different STAT proteins, like STAT1 and 2. These STAT proteins bind via their SH2 domains and are phosphorylated by the JAKS. Thereafter, the STATs dimerize and translocate to the nucleus to upregulate the expression of key genes that control proliferation.

caused by a variety of genetic and epigenetic alterations. Perhaps, the most significant indication of STAT contribution in cancer development has come from the re-engineering of Stat3 protein by introduction of a pair of cysteine residues, which causes Stat3 to dimerize spontaneously, forming stable covalent disulfide bonds. These Stat3 dimers are functional and structural mimics of the dimers that are formed normally when Stat3 is phosphorylated by JAKS. This constitutively active Stat3 protein can now function as an oncoprotein involved in transformation of NIH3T3 and some immortalized mouse cells to a tumorigenic state. Accumulating evidence from present literatures, STATs is known to be an important mediator of transformation in a variety of human cancer cell types. Src inhibition causes deactivation of Stat3 that triggers growth inhibition and apoptosis, suggesting the role of Stat3 in survival of cancer cells.

7.5   INTEGRIN SIGNALING

The proliferation of most of the cells depends on two signals: First is that the cells are correctly positioned within the tissue. This information is provided by integrins that connect the cells to the cytoskeleton. Secondly, cells require various cytokines and growth factors for proliferation. It is the precise process of these two elements that ensures the correct development and size of all the organs. When cell lose their normal cell-matrix interactions, they undergo a special type of apoptosis known as anoikis. Anoikis ensures that the misplaced cell is eliminated to prevent dysplastic growth. Anoikis also helps in physiological developmental process such as hollowing of glands and involution processes [16].

FAK can act as a signaling molecule as well as a scaffold molecule, which can recruit Src and its substrates to the site of integrin engagement. Soluble growth factors integrate with matrix-derived signals and growth factor receptor, resulting in FAK dimerization, autophosphorylation, and activation to elicit various biological responses. FAK creates high affinity binding site for the SH2 domain of Src and helps in its recruitment and activation by forming a stable FAK-Src complex, where src phosphorylates FAK at several tyrosine residues, thereby creating various phosphotyrosine binding sites that enhance its kinase activity. The FAK-Src complex facilitates the phosphorylation of FAK-associated Src substrates like p190RhoGAP,CAS, paxillin, etc., and can also recruit p85 regulatory subunit of PI3K that stimulates Grb2/Ras/MAPK and PI3K/Akt pathways, thereby enhancing cell survival and proliferation and also help in cytoskeleton remodeling and migration. PTPD1, an src-activating phosphatase, forms complex with FAK, actin, and Src, where src is recruited to cell matrix adhesion sites to regulate adhesion and migration [17] (Figure 7.5).

Tumor cells have developed various strategies to overcome anoikis. Some consists of adaptive cellular changes that help the cells to behave normally as they are in the correct environment so that the induction of anoikis process is stopped. The other way to overcome the effects of anoikis induction is by hyperactivating survival and proliferative cascade. Autophagy and entois also help the cells to overcome anoikis by rendering the cells in a dormant state until they receive a signal initiated at the extracellular matrix. In these entire situations, the final outcome is that the tumor is able to grow and metastasize [16].

In the mammary gland, a collagenous stromal layer surrounds the matrix, making it more stiffer. ECM uses rho-mediated contraction of the actin-

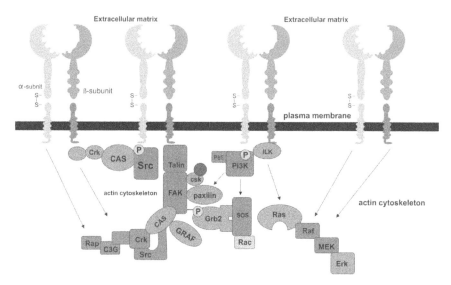

FIGURE 7.5 Integrins are generally assembled as α and β heterodimers. It links the cytoskeleton and the extracellular matrix physically. Ectodomain binding to the components of ECM triggers the association of many cytoplasmic signal transducing proteins, with focal adhesion kinase (FAK) being one of them. Resulting transphosphorylations and binding of SH2-containing signaling molecules activates many downstream signaling cascades like Ras, PI3K, and others.

myosin cytoskeleton to cope up with this stiffness. If the ECM is stiffer than the cell's ability to contract it, tensile forces that are formed facilitates clustering of integrins by assembling adhesion signaling complexes, which ultimately results in the activation of ERK, PI3K, and FAK pathways that regulate cell proliferation and survival. In the absence of focal complexes in a compliant matrix, FAK and Perk are inhibited, which helps in controlling proliferation. p53 and miR-200 members, which are known to regulate apoptosis and maintain epithelial phenotype in mammary gland, are also known to be regulated by FAK [18].

7.6   WNT SIGNALING: A KEY TO PROLIFERATION

Wnt signaling is involved in many important biological processes like development, cellular proliferation, and differentiation. These pathway components include disheveled, glycogen synthase kinase-3β (GSK 3β), β-catenin, and adenomatous polyposis coli protein (APC). These cellular proteins after interaction with each other form a complex with a protein called axin, which has an important role in regulating phosphorylation of β-catenin. Failure of such phosphorylation leads to the accumulation of β-catenin [19] (Figure 7.6A).

When the Wnt pathway is activated, glycogen synthase kinase-3β is blocked and β-catenin rescues itself from rapid destruction, thereby increasing its half-life from >20 minutes to 1–2 hours, and ultimately, a proportionate increase in its steady-state concentrations is observed. The β-catenin molecules then move to the nucleus and bind to Tcf/Lef proteins. The resulting multi-subunit transcription factor complex activates the expression of critical proteins like cyclin Dl and Myc, which are involved in cell growth and proliferation. GSK3β also phosphorylates cyclin D1 that causes its rapid destruction. Hence, the Wnt pathway modulates cyclin D1 expression at both transcriptional and posttranslational levels. This shows that Wnts can act as potent morphogens as well as mitogens, like the ligands of many tyrosine kinase receptors [20].

The alternative role of β-catenin is to maintain the cytoskeletal integrity by forming complex with E-cadherin (Figure 7.6B). The two unrelated roles of β-catenin are still unclear, i.e., whether β-catenin molecules of two pools contribute to the formation of adheren junctions and those involved in regulating transcription are in equilibrium with one another, or whether they are fully segregated in two non-equilibrating compartments in the cell. Thus, in cells that have lost their E-cadherins, the β-catenin molecules are free for nuclear translocation and transcriptional activation. However, in some cancers where E-cadherin genes are lost through mutations, the nuclear β-catenin level is not elevated above the threshold. These observations imply that the two pools of β-catenin are not interdependent. Then, there is another question: why evolution has given two unrelated functions to a single protein? These functions in worms are carried out by different proteins encoded by different genes [20].

Familial adenomatous polyposis (FAP) is an autosomal, dominantly inherited disease in which patient's shows polyps in the colon and rectum. Truncations in APC promote aberrant activation of the Wnt pathway, which leads to adenomatous lesions because of increased cell proliferation. Accumulating evidence, cancer can also be called as a stem cell disease, e.g., loss of TCF4 or DKK overexpression in the colon can result in the loss of stem cells from the colon crypts. Therefore, Wnt signaling acts as a molecular switch for stem cells to undergo proliferation or self-renewal [21].

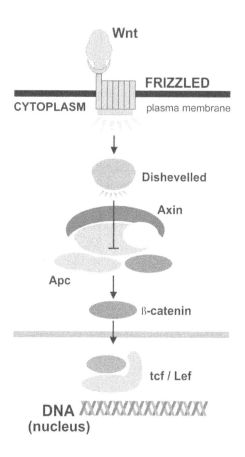

FIGURE 7.6A β-Catenin and Wnt signaling: Wnt proteins after binding to frizzled receptors, act via disheveled and inhibit glycogen synthase kinase-3β's (GSK3-β) activity, preventing GSK-3β from phosphorylation. This prevents β-catenin from degradation and accumulation in the cytoplasm and nucleus. Inside the nucleus, β-catenin associates with Tcf/Lef transcription factors to drive the expression of a number of genes that regulate major cellular processes like proliferation.

7.7   NFκB SIGNALING

NFκB is composed of a p65 and a p50 forming a heterodimeric subunit. The NFκB family in mammals is composed of five distinct members RelA (p65), RelB, Rel (cRel), NFκB1 (p50 and its precursor p105), and NFκB2 (p52 and its precursor p100). Normally, the NFκB signaling system is kept silent when sequestered in the cytoplasm by IKB (inhibitor of NFκB). However, upon receiving external stimuli, IKB kinase phosphorylates and

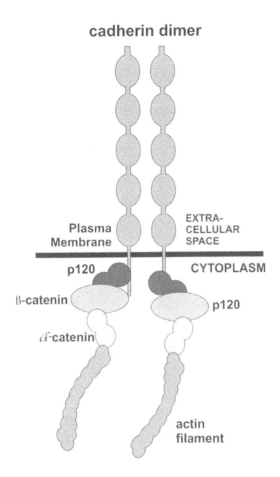

FIGURE 7.6B Different role of β-catenin: Cadherins are the transmembrane proteins like integrins, which can form attachments in the extracellular space and become linked via intermediary proteins to the actin cytoskeleton (e.g., the E-cadherin molecules projecting out from one cell can associate with E-cadherin molecules from an adjacent cell, resulting in the formation of an adherent junction between them). As evident here, β-catenin serves as one of the linkers (together with α-catenin and p120) that form the mechanical linkage between cadherins and the actin cytoskeleton.

degrades IKB. Free NFκB can now migrate inside the nucleus and activates the expression of many target genes [22], which can also influence each other [23] (Figure 7.7).

Various cellular processes like inflammation, apoptosis, cell differentiation, proliferation, and stress response are known to be regulated by the NFκB pathway. With this, it can also regulate elements of cellular regulators like growth factors, cytokines, adhesion molecules, miRNAs, etc. The regulation can be either through the canonical/classical pathway or the alternative/noncanonical pathway.

The canonical pathway applies to RelA–p50 dimers that are mostly sequestered in the cytoplasm under nonstimulated conditions in interaction with the members of the IκB family. External stimuli like genotoxic agents, TNFα, interleukin 1, and ionizing radiation leads to the phosphorylation of IκB molecules by the IKK complex at specific serine residues, which leads to ubiquitination followed by proteosomal degradation. This facilitates the

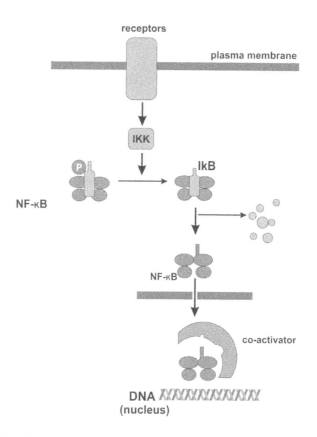

FIGURE 7.7 NFκB is a family of transcription factors that are heterodimeric in nature. This protein remains sequestered in the cytoplasm by IKB protein. IKK is activated through a variety of signaling pathways, which then phosphorylates IKB, facilitating its proteolytic degradation. The liberated NFκB can now translocate inside the nucleus, where a broad constituency of genes are activated, including anti- and pro-apoptotic genes (*not shown*).

translocation of RelA–p50 into the nucleus where it can induce the transcription of various target genes that mainly regulate inflammation and innate immunity.

The noncanonical pathway is triggered by a more stringent set of cytokines belonging to the TNF superfamily. Upstream kinase NFκB inducing kinase (nIK) activates IKKα, which leads to the phosphorylation followed by proteosomal-dependent processing of p100 (RelB inhibitor), resulting in the nuclear translocation of RelB–p52 and RelB–p50. Mostly, it regulates B cell maturation and development and functioning of secondary lymphoid organs [24].

The activation of the canonical and noncanonical NFκB pathway is decided by IKK, which phosphorylates IκB, an inhibitor of NFκB. Two catalytic complexes IKK α and β along with a regulatory subunit, IKKγ, combine together to form the IKK complex. IKKβ and γ are required for the activation of classical NFκB pathway by inflammatory signals; in contrast, RelB-p50 and RelB-p52 stimulation is absolutely dependent upon the IKKα subunit, but not on IKKβ or γ subunits [24].

In the context to cancer, once NFκB arrives in the nucleus, it can potentiate the expression of a number of key anti-apoptotic proteins like IAP(1-2), Bcl-2, etc.; at the same time, these proteins can also induce the expression of myc and cyclin Dl genes, thereby helping cells in proliferation and survival as reported in lymphoid malignancies.

7.8 NOTCH SIGNALING

Mammalian cells generally express four different types of Notch. It is a single pass transmembrane protein that acts as a cell surface receptor, binds to a ligand (NotchL), and undergoes two proteolytic cleavages, namely the ectodomain and the transmembrane domain cleavage. The transmembrane domain cleavage releases a large cytoplasmic protein fragment from its tethering to the plasma membrane. This Notch fragment then migrates to the nucleus of a targeted cell where it functions as a transcription factor with other interacting partners [20] (Figure 7.8).

The Notch pathway plays a crucial role in differentiation, survival, and proliferation of a wide range of cells and tissues. The variations in the regulation of biological processes cause the malignant transformation of cells. Humans have four notch receptors and five ligands named Jagged 1-2 and Delta-like-1,3,4 [25].

The Notch pathway is mainly linked to cancer through the recurrence of chromosomal translocation on t(7;9)(q34;q34.3), which involves the human Notch1 gene. It is mainly found in a small subset of human pre-T-cell acute lymphoblastic leukemias (T-ALL); post this discovery, notch pathway deregulation is known to be involved in many other types of human neoplasms [26].

Notch proteins also regulate the progression of epithelial to mesenchymal transition (EMT) during cardiac valve development. Overexpression of N1ICD induces EMT in immortalized porcine aortic endothelial (PAE) cells via induction of Snail and repression of VE-cadherin. In human endothelial

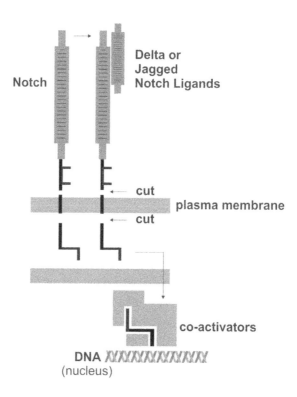

FIGURE 7.8 Notch is a transmembrane receptor that can bind ligands such as NotchL, Delta, and Jagged. Two proteolytic cleavages occurs in Notch, liberating a cytoplasmic fragment of Notch that translocates to the nucleus, where it acts as a part of the transcription factor complex that upregulate genes involved mainly in cell growth and proliferation.

cells, the activation of JAGGED1 of NOTCH receptors also promote EMT because endothelial cells either express activated NOTCH1 or NOTCH4 which represses VE-CADHERIN. NOTCH helps in tumor progression by inducing SNAI1. The human breast cell line MCF 10A showed changes in cell shape after the stable expression of N1ICD that reduces the E-CAD-HERIN protein levels [27].

Notch proteins are found to be overexpressed in cervical, squamous, and colon carcinomas. This overexpression is convoyed by the nuclear localization of cytoplasmic cleavage fragment of Notch which gives active signals to cancer cells. Ligands like Jagged and Delta are reported to be overexpressed in the cervical and prostate carcinomas [20]. In HNSCCs, numerous inactivating mutations in NOTCH1 are observed and mice with such NOTCH1 gene show skin cancer phenotype, thus confirming NOTCH1 as an important tumor suppressor gene in HNSCCs [28].

7.9   HEDGEHOG SIGNALING

Hedgehog signaling has an important role in regulating body patterning and organ development during embryogenesis. In adults, this pathway remains quiescent with the exception of roles in tissue maintenance and repair, and its inappropriate reactivation has been linked to cancer [29].

Hedgehog pathway's deregulation in cancer can be studied through three proposed models. Type I cancers harbor ligand-independent pathway activating mutations. Type II is ligand dependent and adapts autocrine mechanism where hedgehog is produced and recognized by the same or surrounding tumor cells. Type III are also dependent upon ligands but are paracrine in nature, i.e., hedgehogs are synthesized by the tumor epithelium and are received by the stromal cells. This activated stromal cells feed other signals back to the tumor for its proliferation. With this, a reverse paracrine mechanism has also been reported where hedgehog is secreted from the stromal cells to receiving cells in a tumor and activates this pathway inside the tumor [29].

Binding of the Patched to the Hedgehog causes Patched to release Smoothened protein. The activated Smoothened protein can transmit downstream signals and alter the fate of cytoplasmic Gli protein. In the absence of the Smoothened protein, Gli precursor is cleaved into two fragments, and one of these fragments move inside the nucleus and can act as a transcriptional repressor. Active smoothened inhibits cleavage of Gli protein post which intact Gli can act as a transcriptional activator for various developmental genes [30] (Figure 7.9).

Shh and Gli1 expression has been shown to affect EMT in pancreatic cancer cell lines. These observations imply that dysregulated Shh signaling is related to the severity of tumor and help in maintaining metastatic behavior. Therefore, understanding this pathway will help in the discovery of novel therapeutics for the treatment of metastatic diseases [31].

This pathway is generally found to be activated in cancers like leukemia; gastrointestinal cancer; prostate cancer; basal cell carcinomas (BCCs); medulloblastomas and ovarian, breast, and lung cancer. Specific inhibition of the hedgehog pathway may be an effective treatment of human cancer. Even more exciting is to identify a novel molecule that acts as antagonists for the hedgehog pathway [32].

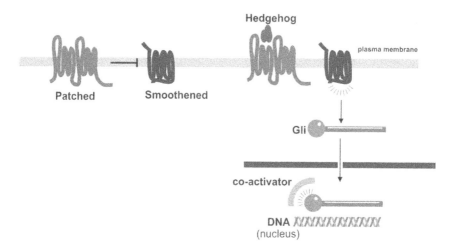

FIGURE 7.9 Patched (PTCH) is a transmembrane receptor that binds to ligands like Hedgehog. Binding of Hedgehog to PTCH causes the latter to release Smoothened. Once free, Smoothened prevents the cleavage of a Gli protein, and the latter now translocates to the nucleus, where it helps in forming functional transcription factors controlling the expression of a large number of growth regulating genes.

7.10   TGF-β SIGNALING

The transforming growth factor-β (TGF-β) superfamily is composed of three isoforms of TGF-β (TGF-β 1, 2, 3), Activins, Nodals, bone morphogenetic proteins (BMPs), growth and differentiation factor (GDF), and Mullerian inhibitory substance (MIS). TGF-β signaling starts with the dimerization of type I and II receptor serine/threonine kinases on the cell surface. Receptor II phosphorylates the kinase domain of receptor I followed by phosphorylation of smads. These smads can be broadly categorized into three domains regulatory smads (1, 2, 3, 5, and 8), co-mediator smads (smad 4), and inhibitory smads (smad 6 and 7). These heteromeric complexes are translocated into the nucleus, where in conjugation with other nuclear factors, they regulate the transcription of many target proteins. Inhibitory smads negatively regulate this signaling either by preventing the translocation of this heteromeric complex into the nucleus or by receptor degradation. Smurf E3 ubiquitin ligases and USP4/11/15 de-ubiquitinases maintains the stability of TGF-β family receptors; it is also known to regulate Smad-independent pathway like the MAPKinase (including Erk, SAPK/JNK, and p38) [33] (Figure 7.10).

TGF-β regulates different types of cellular operations like ECM production, cell growth, differentiation, angiogenesis, immunity, apoptosis, etc. The same receptor complex can induce different cellular responses depending upon the cell type and external/internal stimuli it receives. TGF-β causes growth arrest and apoptosis in epithelial type cells, but in advanced stages, it can induce EMT in cancer cells [34]. EMT is a cellular process where polarized epithelial cells loses E-cadherin, an epithelial marker, and express mesenchymal markers. TGF-β can undergo this process through both SMAD-dependent and SMAD-independent mechanisms. In pancreatic cancer, TGF-β induces phosphorylation of α-catenin and the downstream target of the Wnt pathway β-catenin in a SMAD-independent manner [35]. Mutations in genes encoding TβRI/II and decrease in phosphorylation of downstream Smad proteins are reported in many types of human cancers like pancreatic, colorectal, and gastric cancers, stating the role of TGF-β as a tumor suppressor [36].

7.11 CONCLUSION

Signal transduction in cancer cells is very complicated and involves a complex network of proteins with a variety of cross talks. The Ras-Raf-MEK pathway is most likely to be the most important mitogenic pathway in cancer pathogenesis. Most of the signaling pathways are cell specific, and in each type, the signaling cascades work in a combinatorial fashion. The pathways

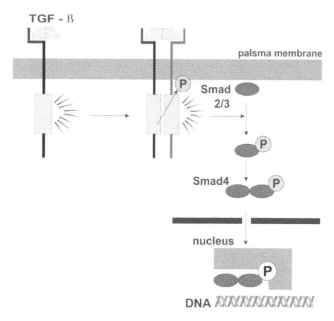

FIGURE 7.10 TGF-β comprises receptor type I and II. Binding of TGF-β ligand to type II receptor brings both the receptors together, resulting in the phosphorylation and activation of type I receptor. This in turn phosphorylates cytosolic Smad2/Smad3 and either of these phospho-Smads then form a complex with Smad4. This heterodimeric Smad complex then migrates to the nucleus, where they forms complexes with other transcription factors to regulate gene expression.

delineated in this chapter receive inputs from the growth factor receptors on the cell surface and operate in the cytoplasm. After receiving a mixture of incoming signals, these signals are emitted to molecular targets in both the cytoplasm and nucleus. There are mainly three ways in which all the major signaling pathways work. First, modulation of the intrinsic activity of the signaling molecule; second, modulation of the concentration of the molecule; and third, regulation of the intracellular localization of the signaling molecule. The kinetics of the signaling process also varies enormously in different cell types. The most predominantly deregulated are the kinase cascades like the MAP-kinase pathway. The cytoplasmic MAP kinases (MAPKs) are activated immediately within seconds after mitogen treatment. Once activated they move to the nucleus and where they phosphorylate and activate a number of transcription factor either directly or indirectly. All the signaling pathways discussed above have great significance in understanding the complexity of different types of cancers and their development.

7.12 SUMMARY

- Cancer cells are independent of external growth factors as they can communicate with each other by generating mitogenic signals endogeneuosly.
- The most important pathways involved in cancer pathogenesis are probably the Ras, Raf, MEK, and Erk pathways.
- Three main downstream signaling originating from activated Ras are the PI3K, Raf Kinase and Ral-GEF effectors.
- Raf activates MEK by phosphorylation and the activated MEK in turn activates Erk1 and 2, which again phosphorylates other substrates. So, the signaling pathway is called as the MAPK pathway.
- The phosphatidylinositol3-kinase pathway (PI3K) is mainly based on kinases phosphorylating a phospholipid. This is important for promoting cell growth and inhibiting apoptosis. The membrane-bound phosphatidylinositol is phosphorylated by PI3K and converted to PIP3.
- Akt/PKB is phosphorylated after being attracted to PIP3 by its PH domain and in turn activates a cascade of signaling that helps in proliferation. PTEN (a phosphatase) normally keeps the level of PIP3 low in normal cells. Thus, in tumors, the Akt pathway is deregulated in two ways: either by hyperactivation of PI3K or by inactivation of PTEN.
- There is a third Ras-regulated pathway where Ras communicates with Ral via Ral-GEFs'. Ral-GEFs' after binding with activated ras localizes near the inner surface of the cell membrane. This encourages a conformational change that induces Ral to activate itself by shedding its GDP and binds to GTP. The activated Ral then induces downstream targets like cdc42, Rac, etc.
- Cytokine receptors tend to lack covalently associated tyrosine kinase (TK) domains. So, they form complexes with tyrosine kinase of the Jaks which in turn phosphorylate STATs, post which it migrates to the nucleus and acts as transcription factors for cell growth and proliferation.
- In contrast to tyrosine kinase receptors that bind to growth factors (GFs), integrins mostly bind to the components of the extracellular matrix, causing the activation of focal adhesion kinase (FAK) and formation of focal adhesions. The phosphotyrosine residues on FAK act as a docking site for Src, which in turn phosphorylates more FAK ty-

rosines and finally leads to the activation of downstream targets like Ras and PI3K.

- The Wnt pathways usually acts to retain the stemness of the cell, thus maintaining the cancer cells in an undifferentiated state. Wnt acts via the frizzled receptors, maintains glycogen synthase kinase-3β (GSK-3β) in an inactivate state, which would otherwise phosphorylate key substrates like β-Catenin and CyclinD1, tagging them for destruction. The free β-catenin now moves to the nucleus and promotes the transcription of growth-inducing genes by interacting with proteins like Tcf/Lef.

- Nuclear factor-κB (NFκB) is another important signaling that depends on the homo and heterodimerization of NFκB in the cytoplasm. IKB is the inhibitor of NFκB and is involved in sequestration of NFκB in the cytoplasm. NFκB is now translocates inside the nucleus, where it activates the expression of many genes, which includes some key anti- and pro-apoptotic proteins. NFκB also functions as a growth factor by activating the expression of myc and cyclin D1 genes.

- Notch is cleaved twice after binding to one of its ligands and causes the migration of released cytoplasmic fragment to the nucleus and contributes in the formation of transcription factor complex. Thus, unlike RTKs, the Notch pathway is dependent on the breakup of the activated receptor, which means that it can fire only once, upon binding of a ligand molecule.

- Hedgehog pathway is an another pathway that helps in maintaining the stemness. Hedgehog ligand upon binding to the patched receptor helps in the release of Smoothened protein, which prevents the cleavage of cytoplasmic Gli protein. Gli now moves to the nucleus where it acts as a transcriptional activator, whereas cleaved Gli acts as a transcriptional repressor.

- TGF-β pathway involves the migration of cytoplasmic Smad transcription factors inside the nucleus where they can activate many genes. This pathway is involved in the pathogenesis of many tumors. It also plays an antagonistic role in early stages of many carcinomas by helping in growth arrest and in later stages contributes to cell invasiveness.

- The main thing to note down is that there is a huge cross-talk between the different signaling pathways. Most of the pathways work in a combined manner, ensuring that growth and proliferation are taking place at the correct time and place during development, which varies from cell to cell and is mostly tissue specific.

• Thus, in conclusion, signals are transduced through various ways: i) noncovalent modification of signaling molecules leading to change in intrinsic activity (e.g., GTP binding by Ras), covalent modification like receptor dimerization (e.g., phosphorylation of MEK by Raf); ii) alterations in the concentration of a signaling molecule (e.g., increase of PIP3 concentration by PI3K and decrease by PTEN); and iii) modulation of intracellular localization of signaling molecules (e.g., attraction of distinct SH2-containing molecules by phosphorylated RTKs, translocation of cytoplasmic molecules to the nucleus).

KEYWORDS

- **carcinogenesis**
- **cell signaling**
- **cytokines**
- **growth receptors**
- **IKB**
- **integrin**
- **JAK-STAT**
- **ligand**
- **MEK**
- **NF**κ**B**
- **notch**
- **PI3K pathway**
- **PTEN mutation**
- **RAF**
- **ras pathway**
- **receptor tyrosine kinase (RTK)**
- **sonic hedgehog**
- **TGF-β**
- **WNT**

REFERENCES

1. Sahai, E., & Marshall, C. J., (2002). RHO–GTPases and cancer. *Nature Reviews Cancer, 2,* 133–142.
2. Aoki, Y., Niihori, T., Narumi, Y., Kure, S., & Matsubara, Y., (2008). The RAS/MAPK syndromes: novel roles of the RAS pathway in human genetic disorders. *Human Mutation, 29,* 992–1006.
3. Friday, B. B., & Adjei, A. A., (2008). Advances in targeting the Ras/Raf/MEK/Erk mitogen-activated protein kinase cascade with MEK inhibitors for cancer therapy. *Clinical Cancer Research, 14,* 342–346.
4. Downward, J., (2003). Targeting RAS signalling pathways in cancer therapy. *Nature Reviews Cancer, 3*(1), 11–22.
5. Manning, B. D., & Cantley, L. C., (2007). Akt/PKB signaling: Navigating downstream. *Cell, 129,* 1261–1274.
6. Salmena, L., Carracedo, A., & Pier Paolo Pandolfi, P. P., (2008). Tenets of PTEN tumor suppression. *Cell, 133,* 403–414.
7. Bozulic, L., & Hemmings, B. A., (2009). PIKKing on PKB: regulation of PKB activity by phosphorylation. *Current Opinion in Cell Biology, 21,* 256–261.
8. Hers, I., Emma, E., Vincent, E. E., & Tavare, J. M., (2011). Akt signalling in health and disease. *Cellular Signalling, 23,* 1515–1527.
9. Bhaskar, P. T., & Hay, N., (2007). The two TORCs and Akt. *Developmental Cell, 12,* 487–502.
10. Brugge, J., Hung, M. C., & Mills, G. B., (2007). A new mutational activation in the PI3K Pathway. *Cancer Cell, 12,* 104–107.
11. Carnero, A., Aparicio, C. B., Renner, O., Link, W., & Leal, J. F. M., (2008). The PTEN/PI3K/Akt signalling pathway in cancer, therapeutic Implications. *Current Cancer Drug Targets, 8,* 187–198.
12. Cheung, M, & Testa, J. R., (2013). Diverse mechanisms of Akt pathway activation in human malignancy. *Current Cancer Drug Targets, 13,* 234–244.
13. Liu, P, Cheng, H, Roberts, T. M., & Zhao, J. J., (2009). Targeting the phosphoinositide 3-kinase (PI3K) pathway in cancer. *Nature Reviews Drug Discovery, 8,* 627–644.
14. Li, W. X., (2008). Canonical and non-canonical JAK–STAT signaling. *Trends in Cell Biology, 18,* 545–551.
15. Yu, H., & Jove, R., (2004). The STATs of cancer—new molecular targets come of age. *Nature Reviews Cancer, 4,* 97–105.
16. Guadamillas, M. C., Cerezo, A., & Del Pozo, M. A., (2011). Overcoming anoikis – pathways to anchorage independent growth in cancer. *Journal of Cell Science, 124,* 3189–3197.
17. Guarino, M., (2010). Src signaling in cancer invasion. *Journal of Cellular Physiology, 223,* 14–26.
18. Keely, P. J., (2011). Mechanisms by which the extracellular matrix and integrin signaling act to regulate the switch between tumor suppression and tumor promotion. *Journal of Mammary Gland Biology and Neoplasia, 16,* 205–219.
19. Yokota, N., Nishizawa, S., Ohta, S., Date, H., Sugimura, H., Namba, H., & Maekawa, M., (2002). Role of wnt pathway in medulloblastoma oncogenesis. *Internatioal Journal of Cancer, 101,* 198–201.
20. Robert, A., & Weinberg, S., (2007). The biology of cancer, 2nd ed., *Garland Science,* Taylor & Francis Group, LLC: United States of America.

21. Nusse, R., (2005). Wnt signaling in disease and in development. *Cell Research, 15*, 28–32.
22. Aggarwal, B. B., Shishodia, S., Sandur, S. K., Pandey, M. K., & Sethi, G., (2006). Inflammation and cancer: how hot is the link? *Biochemical Pharmacology, 72*(11), 1605–1621.
23. Hoesel, B., & Schmid, J. A., (2013). The complexity of NF-κB signaling in inflammation and cancer. *Molecular Cancer, 12*, 1.
24. Baud, V., & Karin, M., (2009). Is NF-κB a good target for cancer therapy? Hopes and pitfalls. *Nature Reviews Drug Discovery, 8*, 33–40.
25. Allenspach, E. J., Maillard, I., Aster, J. C., & Pear, W. S., (2002). Notch signaling in cancer. *Cancer Biology & Therapy, 1*, 466–476.
26. Miele, L., (2006). Notch signaling. *Clinical Cancer Research, 12*, 1074–1079.
27. Bolos, V., Bessa, J. B., & Pompa, J. L. D. L., (2014). Notch signaling in development and cancer. *Endocrine Reviews, 28*, 339–363.
28. Brakenhoff, R. H., (2011). Another notch for cancer. *Science, 333*, 1102–1103.
29. Scales, S. J., & De Sauvage, F. J., (2009). Mechanisms of hedgehog pathway activation in cancer and implications for therapy. *Trends in Pharmacological Sciences, 30*, 303–312.
30. Altaba, A. R., Sanchez, P., & Dahmane, N., (2002). Gli and Hedgehog in cancer: tumours, embryos and stem cells. *Nature Reviews Cancer, 2*, 361–372.
31. Yoo, Y. A., Kang, M. H., Lee, H. J., Kim, B. H., Park, J. K., Kim, H. K., Kim, J. S., & Oh, S. C., (2011). Sonic hedgehog pathway promotes metastasis and lymphangiogenesis via activation of Akt, EMT, & MMP-9 Pathway in gastric cancer. *Cancer Research, 71*, 7061–7070.
32. Yang, L., Xie, G., Fan, Q., & Xie, J., (2010). Activation of the hedgehog-signaling pathway in human cancer and the clinical implications. *Oncogene, 29*, 469–481.
33. Shi, Y., & Massague, J., (2003). Mechanisms of TGF-β signaling from cell membrane to the nucleus. *Cell, 113*, 685–700.
34. Korpal, M., & Kang, Y., (2010). Targeting the transforming growth factor-β signalling pathway in metastatic cancer. *European Journal of Cancer, 46*, 1232–1240.
35. Principe, D. R., Doll, J. A., Bauer, J., Jung, B., Munshi, H. G., Bartholin, L., Pasche, B., Lee, C., & Grippo, P. J., (2014). TGF-β: duality of function between tumor prevention and carcinogenesis. *Journal of the National Cancer Institute, 106*, djt369.
36. Rahimi, R. A., & Leof, E. B., (2007). TGF-0β signaling: A tale of two responses. *Journal of cellular biochemistry, 102*, 593–608.

PART II

CANCER ETIOLOGY: PHYSICAL, CHEMICAL, ENVIRONMENTAL FACTORS AND GENETIC SUSCEPTIBILITY

CHAPTER 8

CANCER: AN OVERVIEW OF RISK FACTORS

SAYALI MUKHERJEE[1] and SHABANA SIDDIQUE[2]

[1]*Amity Institute of Biotechnology, Amity University Uttar Pradesh, Lucknow Campus, Lucknow–226028, Uttar Pradesh, India*

[2]*Cancer Care Ontario, 620 University Avenue, Toronto, Ontario, Canada*

CONTENTS

ABSTRACT

Cancer is a multifactorial disease. Several etiological factors have been associated in the development of cancer. The role of some of these factors has been identified, while for others, further studies need to be done. Cancer risk increases on exposure to physical factors like ionizing radiation or ultraviolet radiation. Persistent pollutants in our environment increase the incidence of breast cancer, leukemia, etc. Air pollution and tobacco use are very important factors in increasing cancer incidence. Infectious agents like human papilloma virus or Epstein Barr virus are instrumental in the etiology of cervical cancer and Burkitt's lymphoma, respectively. Diet, obesity, and alcohol use also seems to play a very important role in the development of cancer. Several epigenetic factors like DNA methylation and histone modification may also increase the risks of developing cancer. The exact mechanism by which each of these factors is involved in the initiation and progression of cancer is still not well established. In this chapter, we will discuss some of the physical, chemical, and biological risk factors associated with the development of cancer.

8.1   INTRODUCTION

Cancer is a major disease burden worldwide. It is a problem of both developed and developing countries. According to the global cancer report, an estimation of 50% increase has been made, which would mean 15 million new cases in the year 2020 [1]. It is now well established that 5–10% of all cancers are attributed to genetic defects, but a huge role is played by environmental factors and lifestyle, which include diet (30–35%), tobacco use (25–30%), and alcohol consumption (4–6%) [2]. Among these, about two-thirds of global cancer cases and deaths are in developing countries and fall in the low- and middle-income categories. New therapeutic interventions are coming up every minute, but the concern is that the world is expected to see a significant increase in cancer morbidity and mortality in years to come. Cancer not only kills and harms cancer patients; it affects family members, coworkers, and the entire society. It is not only a health issue but also has wide social, economic, and development implications. The opportunity cost incurred by patients and those who rely on them, its mental impact, the high health expenditure it creates, and the economic loss to society that cancer creates is enormous. Research says that certain risk factors increase the chances of developing cancer; however, it fails to address the question of one person being more susceptible than the other. More than 50% of cancer cases can be prevented through reduction of cancer risk exposure and early detection. Tobacco claims about one-third of global cancer deaths (22%). The global death rate due to lung cancer, which is presumed to be caused by tobacco use, is 71%. Hepatitis B and C viruses, *Helicobacter pylori*, and human papilloma virus (HPV) infection; occupational and environmental carcinogens; and lifestyle risk factors also contribute to cancer.

In 2016, in United States, approximately, 1,685,210 new cancer cases and 595,690 cancer deaths were registered by the American Cancer Society [3]. The advancement in medical treatment and reduction in prostate cancer incidence has led to a rapid decline in cancer cases in men compared to that in women. In terms of mortality, there is less regional variability than for incidence, the rates being 15% higher in more developed than in less developed regions in men and 8% higher in women [4].

The process of carcinogenesis is complex and multistep where several genetic and molecular defects are required in order for the manifestation of the disease. The three stages of carcinogenesis are initiation, promotion, and progression, where the entire process itself is the outcome of either oncogene activation or tumor suppressor gene inactivation [5]. Identification of risk factors is very important to control the initiation and progression of the disease. Cancer is dependent on several etiological factors that may ultimately cause mutation in the genome or it may lead to cancer by some epigenetic mechanism. This chapter deals with the physical, chemical, and biological risk factors in cancer development. Lifestyle, environmental, and occupational factors will also be discussed as important factors ubiquitous in cancer risk.

8.2 PHYSICAL CAUSES OF CANCER

Physical causes of cancer primarily include radiations. Radiation (both ionizing and non-ionizing) is an ineluctable constituent of our everyday life. Ionizing radiation leads to ion pair formation by ejecting an orbital electron from a molecule or an atom. Ionizing radiation, again, can be of two types, viz., electromagnetic (X-ray and γ ray) or particulate form (α particles or neutron). Excitation is the major form of energy loss of radiation having energy 1-10eV, i.e., non-ionizing radiation like ultraviolet ray (UV), microwaves, radiofrequency, ultrasound, and electromagnetic radiation. Excitation is defined as the elevation of an electron to a higher energy state, which then returns to the ground state by emitting energy in the form of either visible light or chemical change.

8.2.1 IONIZING RADIATION

Ionizing radiation is a risk factor for various types of cancers [6]. Children are at greater susceptibility than adults for a particular dose of radiation and a longer life span with more years at cancer risks. The two most common childhood cancer/tumors that are attributed to exposure to ionizing radiation are of the central nervous system (CNS) and leukemia [7, 8]. Previous studies have reported that prenatal exposure to X-rays during diagnosis lead to 1.5 times higher incidence leukemia in children. Ionizing radiation from computed tomography (CT) scans are also associated with absorbed doses, which are much higher than those associated with conventional radiotherapy [9]. However, a study on the incidence of brain tumors have reported reduced or no risk of cancer in relation to exposure to prenatal diagnostic X-rays [10]. There are uncertainties in the risk estimates, and it is very difficult to draw a reliable conclusion regarding prenatal exposure to ionizing radiation and cancer risk.

Exposure to high levels of radiation in children increases the risk of breast cancer. Risk of thyroid cancer may increase with multiple exposures to dental X-rays [11]. Thyroid, bone marrow, and breast are most sensitive to ionizing radiation followed by the lung, colon, liver, pancreas, and lymphatic system. Organs like the kidney, bone, skin salivary gland, and brain are least sensitive to ionizing radiation. Radiotherapy for cancer may increase the incidence of secondary cancers. Genetic predisposition in association with radiation exposure may increase the risk. Some of the examples of common secondary cancers include thyroid cancer, leukemia, and sarcomas of bone and soft tissue.

Exposure to ionizing radiations also causes various types of cancer by inducing DNA alterations like change in nucleotide base or in sugar phosphate backbone [12]. Double-stranded or single-stranded DNA breaks may occur. Some of these alterations undergo base excision repair or homologous and non-homologous recombination repair mechanisms. Base excision repair is mostly error free, but the latter is error prone and large deletions and rearrangements occur in DNA which can be mutagenic or sometimes lethal. Genetic instability has been reported in cells exposed to ionizing radiation.

Ionizing radiation has also been reported to influence gene expression pattern. Radiotherapy causes molecular changes observed at the level of body fluids, which are potential biomarker candidates for the assessment of radiation exposure. Increased level of 3-hydroxybutyric acid in serum has been reported in post-treatment samples after radiotherapy [13].

8.2.2   ULTRAVIOLET RADIATION

UV radiation is the most important non-ionizing radiation around us. UV radiation may be subdivided into UVA with wavelength ranging from 313–400 nm, UVB with wavelength from 290–315 nm, and UVC with a wavelength range of 220–290 nm. UVB is most carcinogenic and more hazardous to the environment than UVC because UVC is also absorbed quickly in air. UV index indicates the extent of exposure to UV radiation, which is defined as the intensity of UV radiation that reaches our Earth's surface when sunlight is at peak and can damage skin. Most UV radiation is expected to be absorbed by the atmospheric ozone layer or it is reverted into space, but because of the depletion of the ozone layers by chlorofluorocarbons, high levels of UV radiation are penetrating the atmosphere. The main source of UV radiation is sunlight. However, several man-made sources like mercury vapor lamps, sunlamps, Black light lamps, and phototherapy for some dermatological treatment have been identified. UV radiation has been termed as "carcinogenic to humans" by The International Agency for Research on Cancer (IARC). The excitation induced by UV radiation produces chromosomal break in the sugar phosphate backbone of DNA. UV radiation can also alter gene expression similar to that by ionizing radiation.

UV radiation is known to increases skin cancer risk. Melanin, a skin pigment, normally absorbs UV radiation and protects the skin. Individuals with fair complexion have higher incidence of skin cancer because they have decreased melanin. Cancers of skin commonly include squamous cell carcinoma and basal cell cancers and affect the exposed parts of the body like head and neck. UV radiation also increases the risk of melanoma. There is a perfect correlation established for melanoma and sunlight exposure. UV radiation exposure from artificial sources like tanning, welding and metal work, and phototherapy may also lead to skin cancer. Because UV rays cannot penetrate the internal organs, cancer other than skin cancer is rare. Some studies have reported the rare incidence of cancer of the lip, carcinoma of the conjunctiva of the eye, and melanoma in eye. The health effects of UV radiation are still controversial, because it has also been reported to have a beneficial effect in cancer prevention [14].

8.3   EXPOSURE TO PERSISTENT POLLUTANTS

The industrial revolution over the last few decades has led to the production and synthesis of millions of man-made (in other words synthetic) chemicals. According to the European commission, about hundred thousand chemicals have been marketed so far, post World War II, most of which have insufficient toxicological data and control. These products are persistent toxic pollutants and are ubiquitous in the environment. Many of them are capable of acting as mutagens and/or promoters and/or carcinogens.

8.3.1   OCCUPATIONAL EXPOSURE

Cancer of the scrotum was the first documented cancer as a result of occupational exposure that was reported long back by Pott in 1775. Currently, occupational cancers represent 2–10% of all cancers, where the tendency (%) is higher in men (15–20%). To date, the different categories that these chemicals are assigned to are as follows: definite occupational carcinogens (28 chemicals), probable carcinogens (27 chemicals), and possible occupational carcinogens (113 chemicals) [15]. The classic example of a substance related to occupationally induced cancer is asbestos. Asbestos was commonly used because of its heat retaining and fireproof properties. It is reported that asbestos induces occupational cancer and accounts for 10% of lung cancer incidence [16, 17]. Wood dust-related cancers in cabinet makers are also acknowledged as occupational cancer by IARC, and benzene used linked with leukemia was recognized way back in 1997 [18], and thus, the mutagenic effects of other solvents were established, for example, the solvent trichloroethylene (TCE) has been established to be strongly associated with kidney, liver, and non-Hodgkin's lymphoma (NHL) [19]. Similarly, dye products or the by-products of aromatic amines are linked strongly with bladder cancer [20]. Cancer of the larynx, skin, and bladder has been reported from mineral oils and lubricants [21]. Post World War II, the use of phthalates has increased exponentially. Phthalates are used in various consumer and industrial products, because of their plasticizing and emulsifying properties.

Phthalates, particularly di(2-ethylhexyl)phthalate (DEHP) and butyl-benzyl-phthalate, are suspected carcinogen [22]. In vivo studies have shown that exposure to DEHP can cause liver cancer and pancreatic tumors [23]; moreover, there have been studies in workers of polyvinyl chloride (PVC) processing unit, where an elevated pancreatic cancer risk is reported [24].

8.3.2 AIR POLLUTION

Polycyclic aromatic hydrocarbons (PAHs) are produced from burning of organic substances. They are found in vehicular exhaust, waste incinerator emission, tobacco smoke, and factory smoke. They can adhere to suspended fine particulate carbon matter ($PM_{2.5}$), and therefore, can penetrate the organism more extensively and effectively. A link between exposure to air pollution and cancer has been studied in experimental animals and humans. In a survey conducted in North America, it was seen that number of deaths due to lung cancer was higher in cities with high concentration of fine particulate matter [25]. In a European study, it was seen that the percentage of lung cancer associated with vehicular pollution and Environmental Tobacco Smoke (ETS) was 5–7% in never smokers [26]. In addition to PAH and fine and ultrafine carbon particles, nitric oxide (NO_2) also plays an important role in inducing lung cancer, as is shown in animal studies by Ohyama et al. (1999) and it facilitates metastatic dissemination [27]. Nitrobenzo(a)pyrene is formed when NO_2 combines with benzo(a)pyrene, which is characterized by increased mutagenicity [28]. Also, epidemiological studies support the notion that the risk of lung cancer (in non-smokers) is increased on exposure to NO_2 [26]. Apart from lung cancer, air pollution exposure has also been linked to cancer of the larynx, nasopharynx, esophagus, oral cavity, urinary bladder, uterine cervix, breast, and leukemia and lymphoma [29–32].

A large number of carcinogens are present in emissions from vehicles, industries, and domestic use, out of which, benzene and benzo(a)pyrene are the most important, and thus, the most studied environmental carcinogen. A number of epidemiological case studies have linked chronic exposure to benzene with risk of developing leukemia. Benzene metabolites damages cellular macromolecules, which may lead to leukemia [33, 34]. A strong association has been reported to be linked with cumulative benzene exposures for acute myeloid leukemia [35]. p-Benzoquinone is the most important reactive metabolite from benzene that affects bone marrow [36]. Besides leukemia, cancer of the brain, lung, paranasal cavity, and esophagus have also been reported from benzene exposure [37]. The risk is even higher for people occupationally exposed to benzene, as is seen in traffic policemen and shoe factory workers [38, 39].

Myriads of pollutants have been reported in indoor air, which causes indoor air pollution (IAP). In addition to PAHs and fine carbon particles, indoor air accumulates ETS, biocides, formaldehyde, and other volatile organics carbons (VOCs) such as benzene and 1,3 butadiene that are known carcinogens. One of the important contributing risk factors for childhood cancers is IAP, as is shown in several population-based studies [40]. Indoor use of VOC and insecticides also increases the risk of leukemia and lymphoma [41, 42].

8.3.3   PERSISTENT ENVIRONMENTAL CONTAMINANTS

Persistent organic pollutants (POPs) consists of an array of toxic chemicals, usually synthetic chemicals, which are used for commercial purpose. POPs cause adverse effects on human health and the environment across the globe. They are capable of being easily transported by wind and water, and therefore, most POPs generated in one country can and do affect people and wildlife in a completely different place that is usually far away from the source of its production and use. They are highly persistent in the environment and have the ability to bioaccumulate and biomagnify through the food chain. Some of the most well-known POPs are PCBs, DDT, and dioxins, the exposures to which have been implicated in a number of adverse health outcomes, including cancer. Very recently, exposure to emerging persistent environmental contaminants and breast cancer risk has been reviewed [43].

8.3.3.1   Polychlorinated Biphenyls

Polychlorinated biphenyls (PCBs) are chlorinated organic pollutants that are persistent in the environment [44]. Because of their physicochemical properties, PCBs are highly stable and are used in numerous industrial products, including coolants and lubricants in transformers, dielectric in capacitors, dyes, paints, adhesives, inks, carbonless copy paper, and electromagnets. PCBs are strongly lipophilic and resistant to biological transformation; thus, they bioaccumulate in the food chain and concentrate in the fatty tissues, including breast tissue [45]. Despite PCBs being banned from use and man-ufacture since late 1970s, they are still ubiquitous in the environment. The biological effect of individual PCBs is a function of the number and positions of the chlorines in the biphenyl ring, though the mechanisms are not clearly understood; however, it can be said that perturbation in the redox environ-ment of the cell could regulate many of the biological effects [46]. Numerous studies over the decade have shown that several PCBs or their hydroxylated metabolites have estrogenic effects and are said to be endocrine disruptors that can increase the risk certain cancers and other hormone-regulated disor-ders [47]. They are also capable of producing toxic metabolites by inducing the cytochrome P450 [specially the cytochrome P450A1 (CYP1A1) gene] enzymes [47]. Carcinogenic byproducts are released from the metabolism of PCB induced by aryl hydrocarbon hydroxylase (AHH) encoded by the CYP1A1 gene [48]. The polymorphisms of the CYP1A1 gene leads to changes in enzyme activity, which in turn influences an individual's suscep-tibility to cancer.

8.3.3.2 Dioxins

Dioxins or dioxin-like compounds comprise a diverse group of polyhalo-genated aromatic hydrocarbons, which are ubiquitous in the environment [49]. According to the US EPA (2010), dioxins are produced from PVC, PCBs, and other chlorinated compounds and also from gasoline and die-sel combustion [50]. The half-life of dioxins is between 7 and 11 years in humans; therefore, they are more persistent [51]. Similar to other environ-mental contaminants, dioxins are also lipophilic, and they bioaccumulate across the food chain by localizing in the lipids of animals. Human con-suming these animals and food products are exposed to amplified concen-trations of dioxins [52]. Dioxins are known to be carcinogenic to humans. In 2000, the US EPA officially declared one of the dioxins, the 2,3,7,8-tetra chlorodibenzo para dioxin, (TCDD), to be a known carcinogen. Dioxins in general bind to the aryl hydrocarbon receptor (AHR) and elicit AHR-medi-ated biochemical and toxic responses [53]. Increased risks were reported for breast cancer in both women and men, endometrial cancer, and testicu-lar cancer in the IARC international cohort of workers [54]. Numerous in vivo studies have also shown that the endocrine system is one of the critical targets for dioxins with multiple hormone systems affected [55]. It is postulated that TCDD causes cancer by inhibiting the tumor suppressor gene and by stimulating the signaling pathway of estrogen in mammary cells [56].

8.3.3.3 Organochlorine Pesticides

Pesticides are widely used for farming or domestic purpose since several years. Many of them, in particular those belonging to the organochlorines, carbamates, and carbinols groups are designated as probable or possible carcinogen (USEPA, IARC 1991). Organochlorine pesticides (OCPs) are a class of chemicals that include chemicals such as dichlorodiphenyltrichloroethane (DDT), dieldrin, aldrin hexachlorocyclohexane (HCH), and lindane. These man-made organic chemicals were banned in the 1970s and 1980s, but even today, either the parent compound (DDT) or its metabolites [dichlorodiphenyldichloroethylene (DDE) and dichlorodiphenyldichloroethane (DDD)] are still detected in human biological samples [57]. These synthetic chemicals are persistent in the environment because they are nondegradable and have a long half-life [58]. OCPs accumulate in the food chain by binding with lipids in human adipose tissues, blood, and breast milk [59]. Human exposure increases by the consumption of dairy products, meat, and fishes [60]. Most of these chemicals act as endocrine disruptors even at very low doses and result in a number of adverse health effects in humans, including infertility and cancers [59, 61]. A number of experimental assays (both in vitro and in vivo) suggest that some POPs are endocrine disruptors [62, 63]. The well-known association between breast cancer and prolonged exposure to estrogens suggests that environmental estrogen-mimicking compounds (like DDT and its metabolites) could play a critical role in the cellular and molecular changes that occur during breast carcinogenesis [64]. In fact, the first reported assumption that there is a positive association between p,p'-DDE and breast cancer dates back to 1993 [65]. Studies in rodents have proven that these compounds bind to the estrogen receptor (ER) and not only induce tumor cell proliferation but also promote mammary tumor formation [66]. However, human epidemiological studies are inconsistent and inconclusive, where some studies do not support the association between breast cancer and OCPs [67] while others do [65, 68]. One thing to note is that the major source of exposure to DDT has shifted from the more estrogenic o,p'-DDT found in technical

DDT to the far less estrogenic p,p'-DDE, occurring via the diet [69]; this shift is one possible explanation for the lack of association. It has been recently reported that DDD, DDE, aldrin, and dieldrin induce the expression of a number of protein kinases genes that could be involved in the etiology of breast cancer [64, 70]. There have been reports on association between exposure to pesticides and risks of developing liver and prostate cancer [71, 72]. Parental exposure to carcinogenic chemicals increases the relative risk of cancer in children [73]. It has been reported that chronic paternal pesticide exposure increases the risk of leukemia and neurological tumors [74, 75].

8.4   TOBACCO USE AND CANCER

There has been an exponential increase in smokers and smokeless tobacco users worldwide despite the fact that tobacco use and its adverse impact on health have been unequivocally advertised. Lung cancer risk has been reported to be increased by cigarette smoking. Tobacco use is well documented in increasing the incidence of cancer of oral cavity [76]. Cigarette smoke contains more than 60 known carcinogens. Nitrosamines such as tobacco-specific nitrosamines (NNK and NNN) are the most common potent carcinogens in tobacco [77]. The carcinogenic chemicals present in tobacco and the type of cancer associated with tobacco smoke is presented in Table 8.1.

Most of the carcinogens in tobacco require metabolic activation in order to exert their carcinogenic effects. A balance between activation of metabolic genes and detoxifying genes is responsible for determining the cancer risk. DNA adducts formation results from metabolic activation, which may lead to cancer. Permanent mutation results from DNA adduct that escapes cellular repair mechanisms. DNA damage may lead to apoptosis of the cell or induction of mutation may lead to the conversion of a proto-oncogene into an oncogene or deactivation of a tumor suppressor gene. Numerous studies have also shown that nitrosamines present in tobacco may serve as ligands to several receptors, which lead to upregulation of cellular regulatory factors such as protein kinase B (Akt). Activation of such regulatory factors results in downregulation of apoptosis, activation of angiogenesis, and cell transformation [77, 78].

TABLE 8.1   Carcinogens Present in Tobacco Smoke and the Types of Cancer Associated with the Exposure

Class of chemical	Representative carcinogens	Types of Cancer
PAH	BaP, dibenz(a,h)anthracene	Lung, larynx, nasal, oral
Nitrosamines	NNK, NNN	cavity, esophagus, liver,
Aromatic amines	4-Aminobiphenyl, 2-napthyl-amine	pancreas, cervix, bladder, leukemia
Aldehydes	Formaldehyde, acetaldehyde	
Phenols	Catechol	
Volatile hydrocarbons	Benzene, 1,3-butadiene	
Nitro compounds	Nitromethane	
Other organics	Ethylene oxide, acrylonitrile	
Inorganic compounds	Cadmium	

[Source: Ref. 76]

8.5   INFECTIOUS AGENTS IN CANCER

Infection is a well-known factor in the etiology of cancer. It has been estimated that infectious agents are responsible for approximately 16.1% of cancers worldwide, which accounts for 2 million new cancer cases [79]. Infectious agents are the most important cause of cancer after tobacco-induced cancer. The majority of the cases of cancer due to infections occur in the developing world (22.9%) as compared to developed countries (7.4%), reflecting higher prevalence of the causative agents like human papilloma virus (HPV), hepatitis B, *Helicobacter pylori*, and human immunodeficiency virus (HIV), which cumulatively is responsible for approximately 1.9 million cancer cases, most commonly gastric cancer, liver cancer, and uterine cervix cancer.

8.5.1   *VIRUSES*

8.5.1.1   Human Papilloma Virus (HPV)

The papilloma viruses are double-stranded DNA viruses with many subtypes. Several subtypes are known to be instrumental in the development of cancer in humans. Uterine cervix cancer is the most reported cancer caused by HPV. Approximately 40 types of HPV can infect the human genital tract

[3]. Some of these are linked with benign lesions such as warts (e.g., HPV 6 and 11), while others are high risk types associated with invasive cancers and advanced precancerous lesions (e.g., HPV 16 and18) [80]. High risk types are responsible for 5% of all cancers globally [79]. Almost all cases of uterine cervix cancer are caused by HPV, and HPV type 16 and 18 are responsible for around 70 % of these cancers [81].

Genital tract infection by HPV leads to cellular alterations and neoplasia like squamous intraepithelial lesions (SIL) or cervical intraepithelial neo-plasia (CIN), which are graded according to severity based on the nuclear cytoplasmic ratio. The oncogenes coded by HPV genome are E6 and E7. E6 and E7 proteins dysregulate the normal cellular function and hence affect cell proliferation. Mutation in tumor suppressor proteins like p53 and Rb is a common fact for most of the cancers. E6 protein interferes with p53 and E7 protein interferes with Rb protein in most of the cancers related to HPV infection.

Besides cervical cancer, HPV is also known to be linked with anal cancer; oropharyngeal cancer; and cancer of the vagina, penis, and vulva. Most of these cancers are caused by HPV type 16 [82, 83].

8.5.1.2   Hepatitis B Virus (HBV)

The role of HBV is well established in the development of liver cirrhosis and liver cancer. The incidence varies with age and lifestyle and is more common in males than in females [84]. HBV causes hepatocellular carcinoma (HCC) by both direct and indirect mechanisms. The host immune system is known to be instrumental in the integration of the HBV DNA into the genome of the host. It induces both genomic instability and inserts mutation in several cancer-related genes. It has been reported that prolonged expression of the regulatory protein HBx downregulates the cellular proliferation genes and induces the oncogene expression in liver cells. HBV may also suppress the functions of p53 and modify telomerase activity. The Akt pathway and the Wnt/β-catenin pathway are often activated [85].

Transmission may occur from a person with acute infection or carrier. Individuals who are HBeAg positive are infectious and the level correlates with high titers of HBV DNA in serum. Mother to child transmission is very common.

8.5.1.3   Epstein Barr Virus (EBV)

Epstein Barr virus (EBV) was the first reported virus that was shown to be associated with cancer in humans and is involved in the pathogenesis of several cancers of lymphocytes, mesenchymal cells and epithelial cells. Infection by EBV is asymptomatic and life-long. The role of EBV is well established in the etiology of cancers like Burkitt's lymphoma, Hodgkin's lymphoma, gastric adenocarcinoma, and nasopharyngeal cancer. EBV is transmitted orally either by exchange of viral particles or infected cells in buccal fluid, and it establishes as a latent infection. Environmental factors and genetic susceptibility are important factors in the development of cancer by the virus [86]. The virus causes host genome methylation which leads to viral propagation and tumor development.

EBV has been reported in approximately 9% of gastric carcinomas [87]. In EBV-positive human gastric carcinoma, extreme hypermethylation of CpG islands in both promoter and nonpromoter CpG islands has been reported [88]. EBV colonizes resting B lymphocytes and transforms the B cells in vitro into latently infected lymphoblastoid cells (LCLs). These LCLs carry multiple copies of circular episomes and express six nuclear antigens (EBNAs 1, 2, 3A, 3B, 3C, and -LP) and three latent membrane proteins (LMPs 1, 2A, and 2B). Abundant expression of EBV-encoded small RNAs (EBER1 and EBER2) is found in all latent EBV infection, which may be targeted to detect EBV in tumor [89]. EBV normally does not infect epithelial cells but is known to be associated with undifferentiated form of nasopharyngeal carcinoma. EBV infects epithelial cells inefficiently by interacting with the viral glycoproteins present on the envelope with the integrins expressed on epithelial cells. This results in fusion of the membrane and internalization of the virus. Normal nasopharyngeal cells are resistant to latent infection by EBV, but mutations in some genes like deletion of p16 or overexpression of cyclin D1 may support latent infection in these cells [90]. The key role of EBV in the carcinogenesis process is not very clear, but new targeted therapeutic strategies can be formulated based on the behavior of the virus inside the tumor cell.

8.5.1.4   Human Herpes Virus 8 (HHV 8)

Human herpes virus, also known as Kaposi sarcoma herpes virus (KHSV), has been reported in all forms of Kaposi sarcoma and primary effusion lymphoma (PEL). Besides, KHSV is associated in the pathogenesis of several other diseases like multicentric Castleman disease (MCD) and KSHV inflammatory cytokine syndrome (KICS). The viral DNA is double stranded and present in the host cell as an episome. KHSV infects endothelial cells, monocytes, and B lymphocytes. KHSV promote carcinogenesis by evading the innate and specific immune system. The virus shows pleiotropic effects on cell signaling, e.g. it stimulates activation of the transcription factor NF-kB or promotes the Akt pathway. This leads to cell proliferation and prevention of apoptosis of the infected cell. KHSV downregulates p53 expression as its activation stimulates apoptosis of KHSV-infected host cell. KHSV genes like vFLIP, kaposin B, and a KSHV G-protein-coupled receptor [encoded by open reading frame 74 (ORF74)] increases interleukin-6 (IL-6) gene expression, which in turn activates vascular endothelial growth factor (VEGF), the main player of angiogenesis.

PEL is a rare condition associated with KHSV infection. It is a monoclonal B cell lymphoma of aggressive type. Immunoglobulin gene rearrangement takes place in these infected B cells, but the immunoglobulin is not expressed over the surface of the cell. These B lymphocytes also lack the B cell surface markers CD19, CD20, or CD79a. Immunotherapy using cytokines can be used to modulate the evasion mechanism of the host immune system by the virus.

8.5.1.5   Human T Cell Leukemia Virus (HTLV 1)

Human T cell leukemia virus (HTLV-1) is an RNA virus that affects 10 to 20 million people worldwide. The main affected areas are sub-Saharan Africa, the Caribbean, and South America and southwestern Japan. HTLV 1 has been implicated in adult T cell leukemia or lymphoma characterized by malignant transformation of regulatory T lymphocytes (Treg)/TH2 cells that express CD3/CD4/CD25/CCR4 and FoxP$_3$. The disease is characterized by lymphadenopathy and skin lesions and immunodeficiency. The prognosis of the disease is very poor. The integration of the virus to the host genome takes place at random, causing chromosomal abnormalities. HTLV-1 transactivator and oncoprotein Tax interacts with several transcription factors and regulates the transcription of different genes. Transmission can take place from breast feeding beyond 6 months, sexual transmission, or through transfusion of cellular blood products or drugs. Opportunistic infections are common in patients with T cell leukemia because of their immunocompromised state. Different therapeutic strategies have been designed to treat the disease, but no treatments have shown sufficient efficacy.

8.5.1.6   Hepatitis C Virus (HCV)

Hepatitis C virus has been reported as the causative agent of liver cancer. It is a retrovirus that cannot integrate with the host genome. HCV causes inflammation, fibrosis, and cirrhosis and ultimately leads to HCC. The carcinogenic process involves both genetic and epigenetic alterations, leading to activation of proto-oncogenes, downregulation of tumor-suppressor genes, and disruption of several signal-transduction pathways mediated by viral proteins. HCV has also been documented in the etiology of non-Hodgkin's lymphoma and papillary thyroid cancer. Genetic and environmental attributes play a key role in HCV-related extra-hepatic disorders [91].

8.5.1.7. Human Immunodeficiency Virus (HIV)

Human immunodeficiency virus (HIV) is a RNA virus known worldwide for causing Acquired Immune Deficiency Syndrome (AIDS). There is little evidence about the oncogenic effect of HIV in the development of cancer. HIV infection suppresses the immune system and makes the individual susceptible to many opportunistic infections. Previously, HIV was associated with mainly three types of cancers: non-Hodgkin lymphoma, Kaposi's sarcoma, and cervical cancer, which have infectious agents in their etiology. However, today, non-AIDS-defining malignancies (NADM) have been identified as a leading cause of mortality in HIV patients. Recent studies reported the association of HIV with lung cancer. The exact mechanism of pathogenesis is not clearly understood, but cumulative effect of immune suppression, chronic infection, and the oncogenic effects of smoking and HIV seem to play a role [92]. Anal carcinoma and anal dysplasia have also been linked to HIV infection [93]. HIV patients have a high risk of developing testicular germ cell cancer and renal cell cancer. However, a reduced risk is reported for prostrate and bladder cancer in HIV-infected subjects [94].

8.5.2   BACTERIA

8.5.2.1   Helicobacter pylori

Traditionally, bacterial infections are not associated with oncogenesis. *Helicobacter pylori* is the first bacterium identified to be linked to gastric cancer in humans by the IARC. *H. pylori* is a spiral, flagellated, gram-negative bacteria that colonizes the human gastro-intestinal tract and resides under the mucus overlying the gastric epithelium. The role of bacteria in the oncogenesis process may be attributed to induction of chronic inflammation and release of metabolites from bacteria, which may be carcinogenic. The pathogenesis is dependent on inflammation-induced cell proliferation and release of mutagenic compounds that are carcinogenic. *H. pylori* also upregulates apoptosis in gastric epithelial cells by releasing cytotoxin (VacA), monochloramine, lipopolysaccharide, and nitric oxide. The bacteria stimulate host type 1 T helper cell that lead to release of TNF-alpha and IFN-gamma, which are pro-apoptotic cytokines. Mutagenic bacterial metabolites have been implicated in some types of colon cancer. Gastric lymphoma is strongly associated with bacterial infections. Pancreatic cancer has also been reported from *H. pylori* infection [95]. Because antibiotic therapy can cure bacterial infections, the identification of cancer-causing bacteria could be useful in cancer prevention.

8.5.3   HELMINTH

Helminthes are also associated in the pathogenesis of cancer although the exact mechanism of involvement is not very clear. The helminthes mainly involved in carcinogenesis are *Schistosoma haematobium, Opisthorchis viverrini*, and *Clonorchis sinensis*. Commonly, helminth-induced cancers include liver cancer, cancer of the bile duct (cholangiocarcinoma) or urinary bladder cancer and colorectal cancer. It is postulated that the mechanism may include cell proliferation, inflammation, stimulating host immune system, modulating redox signaling, changing glucose metabolism, down-regulating tumor suppressor genes and promoting angiogenesis, invasion, and metastasis [96]. Recently, cysticerci of helminth *Taenia solium* has been reported to be associated with cerebral glioma. Decoding the mechanism of helminth-induced carcinogenesis may help in formulating preventive and therapeutic measures for cancer.

8.6   LIFESTYLE-RELATED RISKS

8.6.1   DIET

Diet and nutrition are important factors in risk of developing cancer in humans [97, 98]. The carcinogens present in our daily dietary products constitute one of the major factors other than tobacco, infections, and inflammation [99, 100]. The mutagens present in food are classified as genotoxic agents and nongenotoxic agents [99]. Genotoxic agents comprise microcomponents of nutrition, for example, PAH, heterocyclic amines (HCAs), aflatoxin, and N-nitrosamine [99, 101]. These genotoxic agents cause DNA damage by inducing mutation and chromosomal aberrations. The mode of action of non-genotoxic agents is not very well defined, but it is assumed that they indirectly affect the cell through tumor promoters. It is the combined action of nongenotoxic and genotoxic agents for a longer period of chronic and high exposure that increase the risk of carcinogenesis. Food mutagens are distributed throughout the body following oral absorption [102]. Most of the dietary carcinogens are actually procarcinogens that needs to be activated/converted by the enzymes into more potent compounds showing carcinogenicity. The body has its own mechanism to protect itself, i.e., by transforming the activated compounds into inert products that can be easily eliminated from the body [103, 104]. Many times, the chemically modified more reactive mutagens bind to DNA rather than being excreted, thereby causing coding errors during DNA replication [97, 105]. Metabolic activation predominantly occurs in the liver in the endoplasmic reticulum where there is abundance of cytochrome P_{450} enzyme. Highly reactive electrophilic products are formed, which results in forming adduct with DNA, RNA, or proteins through covalent bonding, therefore altering the structural integrity of the nucleophilic component, thereby starting a very important step in the initiation of carcinogenesis [106]. On the other hand, the nongenotoxic dietary carcinogens do not need any metabolic activation, and they act as promoters and modulate cell growth and cell death [106]. However, to note is, mutagenesis is not the sole pathway linking dietary exposure and cancer; numerous studies have shown epigenetic factors, including changes in patterns of DNA methylation, as the causative factor for the onset of carcinogenesis, and this can be modified by components in diet [97].

8.6.1.1 Polycyclic Aromatic Hydrocarbons (PAH)

PAH compounds are produced by incomplete combustion of organic matter. Smoked foods may contain PAH, which forms as a result of incomplete combustion during processing. In vivo studies have shown exposure to PAH induce foregut tumors and can also induce tumor of the lungs. Incidence of colon cancer in humans has been associated with PAH exposure. We can deduce from the in vivo and epidemiological studies that PAH is distributed to different organs in the body other than the locally exposed tissues; therefore, it is not surprising that PAH from food may increase the risk of lung cancer or breast cancer [97]. Benz (a) pyrene [BaP] is a well-studied PAH that has its source in diet. BaP is activated by CYP1A and CYP1B enzymes and hence sets in the process of carcinogenesis. BaP adduct is associated with site-specific mutations in the p53 tumor suppressor gene.

8.6.1.2 Aflatoxin B1

Aflatoxin is a type of mycotoxin produced by the mold *Aspergillus flavus* that is commonly present in legumes, rice, soybeans, milk, corns, and cheese. In vivo studies have shown AFB1 to cause liver cancer. AFB1 undergoes metabolic activation by cytochrome P450 to form the exo-8,9-epoxide. The activated AFB1 then forms DNA adducts; the adduct interacts with guanine and mutates the p53 tumor suppressor gene, thereby causing GC transition to TA at specific codon 249. This change is seen in patients diagnosed with liver cancer and with high levels of aflatoxins [97].

8.6.1.3 Heterocyclic Amines (HCA)

Heterocyclic amines are formed from amino acids, proteins, and creatinines during high temperature cooking of meat through a process called pyrolysis [107, 108]. HCA formation is influenced by type of food (beef, pork, and fish are a rich source of HCA), cooking method (frying, broiling and barbecuing), temperature of cooking (the higher the temperature, more is the formation of HCA), and the time spent for cooking. There are approximately seventeen different HCAs resulting from the cooking of red meat rich in proteins and muscles, exposure to which increase cancer risk. The most commonly and extensively studied is the 2-amino-1-methyl-6-phenylimidazole [4,5-b] pyridine (PhIP). PhIP increase the risk of developing breast, colon and prostate cancer. The mode of action of HCA carcinogens starts by bioactivation of N-hydroxylation by cytochrome P450 (CYP1A2) followed by esterification. This results in the formation of nitrenium (also called aminylium) ions (which are potent carcinogen). These nitrenium ions then binds with guanine at C8 position, thereby causing alteration in DNA sequences with subsequent base deletion, insertion, and substitution [97].

8.6.1.4   N-Nitrosamines

Nitrosamines are chemical compounds consisting of a nitroso group bonded to an amine and are formed as a result of reaction between nitrites and secondary/tertiary amine. It constitutes a large group of compounds having common carcinogenic mechanisms. The production of nitrosamines tends to increase at high temperatures (e.g., deep fried food), and high acidity (stomach acid). The source of nitrosamines can be varied, diet being one of them. The exposure to this class of compounds in humans is mainly through meats and fish products. Again, the source of N-nitrosamines can be from nicotine of tobacco smoke. Exposure to nitrosamines have been linked to cancer of the lung, liver, kidney, mammary gland, stomach, pancreas, and esophagus [109]. N-nitrosamines forms N-nitrosodimethylamine, which then undergoes enzymatic hydroxylation (by CYP2E1) to form aldehyde and monoalkylnitrosamide. These chemicals then rearrange and release a carbocation that has great affinity for DNA bases.

8.6.2   OBESITY

Excess calorie intake is associated with cancers of the breast and colon. The American Cancer Society estimated that 14% of all cancer deaths in men and 20% of all cancer deaths in women are attributed to excess body weight. Epidemiological studies have found a significant positive link between obesity and higher death rates for esophageal, colon, and stomach cancer. A meta-analysis of in vivo studies found that there was a 55% reduction in spontaneous tumors as a result of energy restriction [110]. Initially, it was hypothesized that adipokines (leptin and adiponectin) was responsible for the onset of carcinogenesis, but in vivo studies in mice devoid of adipokines ruled this factor out [111]. The other factors that play important roles in obesity-related cancers are the insulin-like growth factor I (IGF-I) and pro-inflammatory cytokines [111]. In vitro studies have shown IGF-I to increase the growth of cancer cell lines by acting directly on the cells via the IGI-I receptor, which is overexpressed in many tumors, or by acting indirectly on the p53 tumor suppressor gene. An in vivo study also suggested that diet-induced obesity leads to decreased expression of IGF binding protein-1, thereby resulting in enhanced IGF-I signaling [111].

8.6.3   ALCOHOL

A number of epidemiological studies have linked chronic alcohol use with the risk of developing cancer of the upper alimentary tract, including cancer of the oropharynx, larynx, and esophagus and of the liver. The exact mechanism of chronic alcohol use and carcinogenesis is still unknown. However, numerous in vivo studies have documented the concept that ethanol, though not a carcinogen in itself, sometimes acts as a co-carcinogen and/or tumor promoter. Ethanol is metabolized by alcohol dehydrogenase (ADH), which results in the generation of acetaldehyde and free radicals. Some previous evidence suggest that acetaldehyde in alcohol can act as a mutagen and a carcinogen. Acetaldehyde binds to DNA and proteins, destroys folate, and results in secondary hyperproliferation. Acetaldehyde directly inhibits O6 methyl-guanyltransferase, which is an important enzyme used to repair damage caused by alkylating agents which form adducts, therefore interfering with the DNA repair mechanism. Acetaldehyde is also known to cause point mutations and cause sister chromatid exchanges. Polymorphism in this gene may increase cancer risk. Alcohol use may also increases cancer risk by induction of cytochrome P4502E1 (CYP2E1), whereby there is an increase in generation of free radicals and activation of procarcinogen compounds present in alcoholic beverages, resulting in the formation of ultimate carcinogens [112]. The nutritional status in heavy drinkers is impaired because of primary and secondary malnutrition. Alcohol users are also deficient in vitamins and trace elements that have been shown to have protective effects, thereby contributing to cancer [112]. Chronic consumption of alcohol also induces liver cirrhosis, which is a major etiological risk factor for the onset of liver cancer.

8.7   EPIGENETICS AND CANCER

Extracellular vesicles include different nanoscale membranous vesicles that are released into the intercellular microenvironment by many cell types [113–115]. Very small changes in the cellular microenvironment are capable of stimulating malignant transformation of cells, and cellular microenvironment has been implicated in initiation, proliferation, and metastasis of tumor. Cancerous cells when transformed act in a paracrine or autocrine manner to disseminate bioinformation, therefore, helping in cell proliferation and metastasis. It has been demonstrated cancer cells release more extracellular vesicles than healthy normal cells, which is attributable to the activation of certain oncogenes belonging to the *ras* family [116]. Exosomes, microvesicles, and other extracellular vesicles differ in size, morphology, buoyant density, and protein composition [117]. Exosomes, microvesicles and other extracellular vesicles may contain proteins, RNA, DNA and lipids and is thus capable of delivering these factors to the intercellular environment or recipient cells [118]. Moreover, these extracellular vesicles are also transported in the biological fluids (blood, urine, ascites, and cerebrospinal fluid) and therefore can deliver their contents to neighboring as well as distant recipient cells and elicits corresponding physiological or pathological effects [119]. It is of note that epigenetic regulation constitute of processes that cause functionally relevant changes to the genome, without altering the nucleotide sequence but alteration in gene expression is seen. The genome plays a very crucial role in the tumor microenvironment, and it is this environment that influences carcinogenesis (initiation, proliferation, and metastasis) [120]. It is well documented that epigenetic processes including DNA methylation, histone modification, and microRNA (miRNA) or long non-coding (lncRNA) regulation are regulated by extracellular vesicles, and the resulting epigenetic modifications are responsible for changes in the expression of tumor promoting genes and tumor suppressing genes.

8.7.1   EXTRACELLULAR VESICLES AND DNA METHYLATION

As mentioned earlier, epigenetic modification of oncogenes, proto-onco-genes or anti-oncogenes is very important for the onset of many tumors. Variation in DNA methylation is one of the most commonly recognized factors that influence transcription of oncogenes and antioncogenes. DNA methyltranferases like DNMT1, DNMT3a, and DNMT3b add methyl groups to specific cytosines in the CpG islands of regulatory sequences, as a result of which certain genes are silenced [121]. The transcription of oncogene or antioncogenes fluctuates according to the promoter methylation status, therefore dynamically affecting tumor progression. Owing to their complex bioactive cargo, extracellular vesicles cause malignant transformation of otherwise normal cells. Hypermethylation of the promoter regions of the tumor-suppressor genes p53 and RIZ1 has been observed in cells incubated with leukemia-derived microvesicles and an increased level of DNMT3a and DNMT3b mRNA and protein is seen [122]. It was also observed that the protein and mRNA levels of activation-induced cytidine deaminase (AICDA) were increased in the recipient cells. AICDA is a deaminase actively involved in DNA initiative demethylation [122]. We can deduce from these findings that genomic instability was promoted in recipient cells which might induce leukemic transformation [122]. It has been reported that breakpoint cluster region-Abelson leukemia gene human homolog 1 (BCR-ABL1) is the dominant onco-mRNA in microvesicles released by the K562 leukemia cell line [122]. It is also reported that exosomes obtained from the serum of patients diagnosed with pancreatic cancer carry genomic double-stranded DNAs, which contained mutated KRAS and p53 genes [123]. Exo-some-associated molecular markers of gastric cancers have also been found in gastric washes and even highly acidic gastric juice [124].

8.7.2   EXTRACELLULAR VESICLES AND HISTONE MODIFICATION

Histones are the structural protein around which chromosomal DNA coils to form the basic chromatin structure. The chromatin structure is maintained or altered by histone modification. DNA methylation along with histone modification has been implicated in pathogenic expression of tumor-related genes. Posttranslational modification of specific residues in the N-terminal region of core histones, including acetylation, methylation, ubiquitination, or phosphorylation influence the chromatin shape and hence influence gene transcription [125, 126]. Gene activation is associated with methylation of H3K4, H3K48, and H3K79, whereas methylation of H3K9 and H3K27 is linked with gene inactivation [127, 128]. The enzymes histone acetyltransferase (HAT) and histone diacetylase (HDAC) regulates histone acetylation. HDAC is responsible for removing the positive charge on histones, thereby relaxing the chromatin structure and promoting gene transcription. However, the role of extracellular vesicles in histone modification is controversial. Though there are studies that show G26/24 oligodendroglioma cell line to release extracellular vesicles containing the differentiation-specific linker histone, which is not released by astrocytes under normal conditions [129].

8.7.3   EXTRACELLULAR VESICLES AND NONCODING RNA

Noncoding RNAs are the nonprotein-coding transcripts categorized as long noncoding RNAs (lncRNAs) and small noncoding RNAs including miRNAs. The miRNAs are the most abundant RNA present in exosomes. These miRNAs are small noncoding RNAs of about 22–25 nucleotides in length. It has been shown that a particular type of miRNAs is shed by metastatic cancer cells in extracellular vesicles. The microvesicles released from metastatic melanoma cells contain high levels of prominin-1, which is said to promote metastatic progression [130]. On profiling of the microRNA, 49 species of miRNA were revealed to be present in higher concentration in the metastatic melanoma-derived microvesicles than in the donor cells, and of the 49 species, 20 species were cancer-related miRNAs [131]. It is also seen that these exosome-mediated transfer of cancer-secreted miRNAs disrupt tight junctions and thus promote metastasis [132], as is seen with the exosomal transfer of miRNA-23b from the bone marrow to promote breast cancer cell dormancy in a metastatic niche, miR-210 released by metastatic cancer cells could be transported to endothelial cells and thus regulate cell metastasis [133]. It is also reported that the miRNAs in extracellular vesicles modulate tumor proliferation, and that several of these vesicles' miRNAs have been recommended for the diagnosis of cancer and/or assessment of cancer prognosis [134]. Long noncoding RNAs are nonprotein coding transcripts longer than 200 nucleotides, but they can participate in epigenetic transcriptional or posttranscriptional regulation [135]. It is also said that the extracellular content of lncRNA may reflect tumor growth, metastasis, and response to treatment, for example, lncRNA *TUC*339 is found in extracellular vesicles derived from HCC cells and has been implicated in tumor growth, adhesion, and cell cycle progression [136, 137]. *Linc-ROR* is another lncRNA enriched in extracellular vesicles from HCC that protects the cells from chemotherapy-induced apoptosis and cytotoxicity [138].

8.8 SUMMARY

- Etiological factors are very important in the development of cancer
- Exposure to ionizing radiation may increase the risk of cancer, specially brain tumors and leukemia in children.
- Ultraviolet radiation has dual health effects on humans: increases the risk of skin cancer as well as act as a source of Vitamin D
- Occupational exposure to persistent pollutants like asbestos, wood dust, benzene, mineral oils, lubricants, and phthalates increase the risk of leukemia and cancer of the skin, liver, pancreas, larynx, and kidney.
- Air pollution exposure has been linked to cancer of the lung, larynx, nasopharynx, esophagus, oral cavity, urinary bladder, uterine cervix, and breast and leukemia and lymphoma.
- Exposure to persistent organic pollutants (POPs) like PCBs, DDT, and dioxins has been implicated in a number of adverse health outcomes, including cancer
- Tobacco contains myriads of carcinogens that lead to cancer, and it can provide a classic example of a model for understanding mechanism of cancer induction by exogenous chemical carcinogens.
- Infectious agents like viruses, bacteria, and helminths have been implicated in cancer risk.
- Diet and nutrition play an important role in cancer development
- Excess calorie intake has been shown to contribute to increase risk of several cancers like breast, colon, and prostate cancer.
- Chronic alcohol use with the risk of developing cancer of the upper alimentary tract, including cancer of the oropharynx, larynx, and esophagus and of the liver.
- Epigenetic modification of oncogenes, proto-oncogenes, or anti-oncogenes is very important for the onset of many tumors.

KEYWORDS

- cancer
- epigenetics
- etiology
- infectious agents
- pollutants
- tobacco use

REFERENCES

1. WHO, World Health Organisation, 2003.
2. Anand, P., Kunnumakkara, A. B., Sundaram, C., Harikumar, K. B., Tharakan, S. T., Lai, O. S., et al. Cancer is a preventable disease that requires major lifestyle changes. *Pharmaceutical Research*, *25*(9), 2097–2116.
3. Society, A. C., (2014). *Cancer Facts & Figures*.
4. (IARC) IAfRiC, (2012). Globocan 2012: Estimated cancer incidence, Mortality and prevalence worldwide in 2012.
5. Hursting, S. D. W. Q., Sturgis, E. M., & Clinton, S. K., (1999). *The Cancer related Genes: Oncogenes, Tumor Suppressor Genes, & the DNA Damage-Responsive Genes*. California: Academic Press, 11–27.
6. Radiation, UUNSCotEoA. Annex B: Effects of radiation exposure of children. In: UNSCEAR Report (2013). Sources, effects and risks of ionizing radiation, Vol. II. New York:United nations scientific committee on the effects of atomic radiation (UNSCEAR), United Nations.
7. Belson, M., Kingsley, B., & Holmes, A., (2007). Risk factors for acute leukemia in children: a review. *Environmental Health Perspectives*, *115*(1), 138–145.
8. Wiemels, J., (2012). Perspectives on the causes of childhood leukemia. Chemico-biological interactions *196*(3), 59–67.
9. Baysson, H., Journy, N., Roue, T., Ducou-Lepointe, H., Etard, C., & Bernier, M. O., (2016). [Exposure to CT scans in childhood and long-term cancer risk: A review of epidemiological studies]. *Bulletin Du Cancer*, *103*(2), 190–198.
10. Stalberg, K., Haglund, B., Axelsson, O., Cnattingius, S., Pfeifer, S., & Kieler, H., (2008). Prenatal ultrasound and the risk of childhood brain tumour and its subtypes. *British Journal of Cancer*, *98*(7), 1285–1287.
11. Memon, A., Godward, S., Williams, D., Siddique, I., & Al-Saleh, K., (2010). Dental x-rays and the risk of thyroid cancer: a case-control study. *Acta. Oncologica.*, *49*(4), 447–453.
12. JL S., (1995). *Radiation Carcinogenesis and the Development of Radiation Injury Boston*: Springer International, 473–508.
13. Ros-Mazurczyk, M., Wojakowska, A., Marczak, L., Polanski, K., Pietrowska, M., Jelonek, K., et al., (2017). Ionizing radiation affects profile of serum metabolites: in-

creased level of 3-hydroxybutyric acid in serum of cancer patients treated with radiotherapy. *Acta Biochimica Polonica, 64*(1), 189–193.

14. Krause, R., Matulla-Nolte, B., Essers, M., Brown, A., & Hopfenmuller, W., (2006). UV radiation and cancer prevention: what is the evidence? *Anticancer Research, 26*(4A), 2723–2727.

15. Clapp, R., Howe, G., & LeFevre, M., (2005). *Environmental and Occupational Causes of Cancer*:Review of recent scientific literature.

16. Belpomme, D., Irigaray, P., Hardell, L., Clapp, R., Montagnier, L., Epstein, S., et al., (2007). The multitude and diversity of environmental carcinogens. *Environmental Research, 105*(3), 414–429.

17. Belpomme, D., Irigaray, P., Sasco, A. J., Newby, J. A., Howard, V., Clapp, R., et al., (2007). The growing incidence of cancer: role of lifestyle and screening detection (Review). *International Journal of Oncology, 30*(5), 1037–1049.

18. Surralles, J., Autio, K., Nylund, L., Jarventaus, H., Norppa, H., Veidebaum, T., et al., (1997). Molecular cytogenetic analysis of buccal cells and lymphocytes from benzene-exposed workers. *Carcinogenesis, 18*(4), 817–823.

19. Raaschou-Nielsen, O., Hansen, J., McLaughlin, J. K., Kolstad, H., Christensen, J. M., Tarone, R. E., et al., (2003). Cancer risk among workers at Danish companies using trichloroethylene: a cohort study. *American Journal of Epidemiology, 158*(12), 1182–1192.

20. Cantor, K. P. WMH., Moore, L., & Lubin, J., (2006). *Water Contaminants*. Dordrecht, Kluwer Academic Publisher, 149–169.

21. Mackerer, C. R., Griffis, L. C., Grabowski, Jr .J. S., & Reitman, F. A. Petroleum mineral oil refining and evaluation of cancer hazard. *Applied Occupational and Environmental Hygiene, 18*(11), 890–901.

22. Shea, K. M., (2003). American academy of pediatrics committee on environmental H. Pediatric exposure and potential toxicity of phthalate plasticizers. *Pediatrics, 111*(6 Pt 1), 1467–1474.

23. Rao, M.S., Yeldandi, A. V., & Subbarao, V., (1990). Quantitative analysis of hepatocellular lesions induced by di(2-ethylhexyl)phthalate in F-344 rats. *Journal of Toxicology and Environmental Health, 30*(2), 85–89.

24. Selenskas, S., Teta, M. J., & Vitale, J. N., (1995). Pancreatic cancer among workers processing synthetic resins. *American Journal of Industrial Medicine, 28*(3), 385–398.

25. Pope, C. A., Burnett, R. T., Thun, M. J., Calle, E. E., Krewski, D., Ito, K., et al., (2002). Lung cancer, cardiopulmonary mortality, & long-term exposure to fine particulate air pollution. *Jama., 287*(9), 1132–1141.

26. Vineis, P., Hoek, G., Krzyzanowski, M., Vigna-Taglianti, F., Veglia, F., Airoldi, L., et al., (2007). Lung cancers attributable to environmental tobacco smoke and air pollution in non-smokers in different European countries: a prospective study. *Environmental Health : A Global Access Science Source, 6*, 7.

27. Ohyama, K., Ito, T., & Kanisawa, M., (1999). The roles of diesel exhaust particle extracts and the promotive effects of NO2 and/or SO2 exposure on rat lung tumorigenesis. *Cancer Letters, 139*(2), 189–197.

28. Tokiwa, H., Sera, N., Nakashima, A., Nakashima, K., Nakanishi,Y., & Shigematu, N., (1994). Mutagenic and carcinogenic significance and the possible induction of lung cancer by nitro aromatic hydrocarbons in particulate pollutants. *Environmental Health Perspectives, 102, Suppl. 4*, 107–110.

29. Kuper, C. F., Arts, J. H., & Feron, V. J., (2003). Toxicity to nasal-associated lymphoid tissue. *Toxicology Letters, 140–141*, 281–285.

30. Sasco, A. J., Secretan, M. B., & Straif, K., (2004). Tobacco smoking and cancer: a brief review of recent epidemiological evidence. *Lung Cancer, 45 Suppl. 2*, 3–9.

31. Guo, J., Kauppinen, T., Kyyronen, P., Heikkila, P., Lindbohm, M. L., & Pukkala, E., (2004). Risk of esophageal, ovarian, testicular, kidney and bladder cancers and leukemia among finnish workers exposed to diesel or gasoline engine exhaust. *International Journal of Cancer, 111*(2), 286–292.

32. Johnson, K. C., (2005). Accumulating evidence on passive and active smoking and breast cancer risk. *International Journal of Cancer, 117*(4), 619–628.

33. Whysner, J., Reddy, M. V., Ross, P. M., Mohan, M., & Lax, E. A., (2004). Genotoxicity of benzene and its metabolites. *Mutation Research, 566*(2), 99–130.

34. Faiola, B., Fuller, E. S., Wong, V. A., Pluta, L., Abernethy, D. J., Rose, J., et al., (2004). Exposure of hematopoietic stem cells to benzene or 1, 4-benzoquinone induces gender-specific gene expression. *Stem Cells, 22*(5), 750–758.

35. Descatha, A., Jenabian, A., Conso, F., & Ameille, J., (2005). Occupational exposures and haematological malignancies: overview on human recent data. *Cancer Causes & Control: CCC, 16*(8), 939–953.

36. Xie, Z., Zhang, Y., Guliaev, A. B., Shen, H., Hang, B., Singer, B., et al., (2005). The p-benzoquinone DNA adducts derived from benzene are highly mutagenic. *DNA Repair, 4*(12), 1399–1409.

37. Beach, J., & Burstyn, I., (2006). Cancer risk in benzene exposed workers. *Occupational and Environmental Medicine, 63*(1), 71–72.

38. Seniori, C. A., Quinn, M., Consonni, D., & Zappa, M., (2003). Exposure to benzene and risk of leukemia among shoe factory workers. *Scandinavian Journal of Work, Environment & Health, 29*(1), 51–59.

39. Wiwanitkit, V., Suwansaksri, J., & Soogarun, S., (2005). Cancer risk for Thai traffic police exposed to traffic benzene vapor. *Asian Pacific Journal of Cancer Prevention: APJCP, 6*(2), 219–220.

40. Zhang, J., & Smith, K. R., (2003). Indoor air pollution: a global health concern. *British Medical Bulletin, 68*, 209–225.

41. Viegi, G., & Simoni, M., (2004). Scognamiglio A, Baldacci S, Pistelli F, Carrozzi L, et al. Indoor air pollution and airway disease. The international journal of tuberculosis and lung disease: *The Official Journal of the International Union Against Tuberculosis and Lung Disease, 8*(12), 1401–1415.

42. Menegaux, F., Baruchel, A., Bertrand, Y., Lescoeur, B., Leverger, G., Nelken, B., et al., (2006). Household exposure to pesticides and risk of childhood acute leukaemia. *Occupational and Environmental Medicine, 63*(2), 131–134.

43. Siddique. S., Kubwabo, C., & Harris, S. A., (2016). A review of the role of emerging environmental contaminants in the development of breast cancer in women. *Emerging Contaminants, 2*(4), 204–219.

44. DeCastro, B. R., Korrick, S. A., Spengler, J. D., & Soto, A. M., (2006). Estrogenic activity of polychlorinated biphenyls present in human tissue and the environment. *Environmental Science & Technology 40*(8), 2819–2825.

45. Quinsey, P. M., Donohue, D. C., & Ahokas, J. T., (1995). Persistence of organochlorines in breast milk of women in Victoria, Australia. Food and chemical toxicology : *An International Journal Published for the British Industrial Biological Research Association, 33*(1), 49–56.

46. Venkatesha, V. A., Venkataraman, S., Sarsour, E. H., Kalen, A. L., Buettner, G. R., Robertson, L. W., et al., (2008). Catalase ameliorates polychlorinated biphenyl-induced cytotoxicity in nonmalignant human breast epithelial cells. *Free Radical Biology & Medicine, 45*(8), 1094–1102.
47. Negri, E., Bosetti, C., Fattore, E., La Vecchia, C., (2003). Environmental exposure to polychlorinated biphenyls (PCBs) and breast cancer: a systematic review of the epidemiological evidence. *European Journal of Cancer Prevention : The Official Journal of the European Cancer Prevention Organisation, 12*(6), 509–516.
48. Craig, Z. R., Wang, W., & Flaws, J. A., (2011). Endocrine-disrupting chemicals in ovarian function: effects on steroidogenesis, metabolism and nuclear receptor signaling. *Reproduction, 142*(5), 633–646.
49. Linden, J., Lensu, S., Tuomisto, J., & Pohjanvirta, R., (2010). Dioxins, the aryl hydrocarbon receptor and the central regulation of energy balance. *Frontiers in Neuroendocrinology, 31*(4), 452–478.
50. U. S. EPA. (2013). Update to An inventory of sources and environmental releases of dioxin-like compounds in the united states for the years (1987), (1995) & (2000), External Review Draft). U. S. Environmental Protection Agency, Washington, DC, EPA/600/R-11/005A. http://cfpub.epa.gov/ncea/CFM/nceaQFind.cfm?keyword=Dioxin.
51. Schecter, A., Birnbaum, L., Ryan, J. J., & Constable, J. D., (2006). Dioxins: an overview. *Environmental Research, 101*(3), 419–428.
52. Kulkarni, P. S., Crespo, J. G., & Afonso, C. A., (2008). Dioxins sources and current remediation technologies--a review. *Environment International, 34*(1), 139–153.
53. Beischlag, T. V., Luis Morales, J., Hollingshead, B. D., & Perdew, G. H., (2008). The aryl hydrocarbon receptor complex and the control of gene expression. *Critical Reviews in Eukaryotic Gene Expression, 18*(3), 207–250.
54. Kogevinas, M., Becher, H., Benn, T., Bertazzi, P. A., Boffetta, P., Bueno-de-Mesquita, H. B., et al., (1997). Cancer mortality in workers exposed to phenoxy herbicides, chlorophenols, & dioxins. An expanded and updated international cohort study. *American Journal of Epidemiology, 145*(12), 1061–1075.
55. Birnbaum, L. S., & Tuomisto, J., (2000). Non-carcinogenic effects of TCDD in animals. *Food Additives and Contaminants, 17*(4), 275–288.
56. Seifert, A., Taubert, H., Hombach-Klonisch, S., Fischer, B., Navarrete Santos, A., (2009). TCDD mediates inhibition of p53 and activation of ERalpha signaling in MCF-7 cells at moderate hypoxic conditions. *International Journal of Oncology, 35*(2), 417–424.
57. Pestana, D., Teixeira, D., Faria, A., Domingues, V., Monteiro, R., & Calhau, C., (2013). Effects of environmental organochlorine pesticides on human breast cancer: Putative involvement on invasive cell ability. *Environmental Toxicology.*
58. Xu, X., Dailey, A. B., Talbott, E. O., Ilacqua, V. A., Kearney, G., & Asal, N. R., (2010). Associations of serum concentrations of organochlorine pesticides with breast cancer and prostate cancer in US adults. *Environmental Health Perspectives*, 60–66.
59. Shakeel, M. K., George, P. S., Jose, J., Jose, J., & Mathew, A., (2010). Pesticides and breast cancer risk: a comparison between developed and developing countries. *Asian Pacific Journal of Cancer Prevention: APJCP, 11*(1), 173–180.
60. Lee, S. A., Dai, Q., Zheng, W., Gao, Y. T., Blair, A., Tessari, J. D., et al., (2007). Association of serum concentration of organochlorine pesticides with dietary intake and other lifestyle factors among urban Chinese women. *Environment International, 33*(2), 157–163.

61. Ociepa-Zawal, M., Rubis, B., Wawrzynczak, D., Wachowiak, R., & Trzeciak, W. H., (2010). Accumulation of environmental estrogens in adipose tissue of breast cancer patients. *Journal of Environmental Science and Health Part A, Toxic/Hazardous Substances & Environmental Engineering, 45*(3), 305–312.

62. Casals-Casas, C., & Desvergne, B., (2011). Endocrine disruptors: from endocrine to metabolic disruption. *Annual Review of Physiology, 73*, 135–162.

63. Steinmetz, R., Young, P. C., Caperell-Grant, A., Gize, E. A., Madhukar, B. V., Ben-Jonathan, N., et al., (1996). Novel estrogenic action of the pesticide residue β-hexachlorocyclohexane in human breast cancer cells. *Cancer Research, 56*(23), 5403–5409.

64. Valerón, P. F., Pestano, J. J., Luzardo, O. P., Zumbado, M. L., Almeida, M., & Boada, L. D., (2009). Differential effects exerted on human mammary epithelial cells by environmentally relevant organochlorine pesticides either individually or in combination. *Chemico-Biological Interactions, 180*(3), 485–491.

65. Wolff, M. S., Toniolo, P. G., Lee, E. W., Rivera, M., & Dubin, N., (1993). Blood levels of organochlorine residues and risk of breast cancer. *Journal of the National Cancer Institute 85*(8), 648–652.

66. George, J., & Shukla, Y., (2011). Pesticides and cancer: Insights into toxicoproteomic-based findings. *Journal of Proteomics, 74*(12), 2713–2722.

67. Ward, E. M., Schulte, P., Grajewski, B., Andersen, A., Patterson, D. G., Jr. Turner, W., et al., (2000). Serum organochlorine levels and breast cancer: a nested case-control study of Norwegian women. *Cancer Epidemiology, Biomarkers & Prevention* : A publication of the American Association for Cancer Research, cosponsored by the American Society of Preventive Oncology, *9*(12), 1357–1367.

68. Cohn, B. A., Wolff, M. S., Cirillo, P. M., & Sholtz, R. I., (2007). DDT and breast cancer in young women: new data on the significance of age at exposure. *Environmental Health Perspectives, 115*(10), 1406–1414.

69. Soto, A. M., Sonnenschein, C., Chung, K. L., Fernandez, M. F., Olea, N., & Serrano, F. O., (1995). The E-SCREEN assay as a tool to identify estrogens: an update on estrogenic environmental pollutants. *Environmental Health Perspectives, 103, Suppl., 7*, 113–122.

70. Boada, L. D., Zumbado, M., Henríquez-Hernández, L. A., Almeida-González, M., Álvarez-León, E. E., Serra-Majem, L., et al., (2012). Complex organochlorine pesticide mixtures as determinant factor for breast cancer risk: a population-based case-control study in the Canary Islands (Spain). *Environmental Health, 11*(1), 28.

71. Vo Pham, T., Bertrand, K. A., Hart, J. E., Laden, F., Brooks, M. M., Yuan, J. M., et al., (2017). Pesticide exposure and liver cancer: a review. *Cancer Causes & Control: CCC, 28*(3), 177–190.

72. Lewis-Mikhael, A. M., Olmedo-Requena, R., Martínez-Ruiz, V., Bueno-Cavanillas, A., & Jiménez-Moleón, J. J., (2015). Organochlorine pesticides and prostate cancer, Is there an association? A meta-analysis of epidemiological evidence. *Cancer Causes & Control, 26*(10), 1375–1392.

73. Zahm, S. H., & Ward, M. H., (1998). Pesticides and childhood cancer. *Environmental Health Perspectives, 106, Suppl., 3*, 893–908.

74. Ma, X., Buffler, P. A., Gunier, R. B., Dahl,G., Smith, M. T., Reinier, K., et al., (2002). Critical windows of exposure to household pesticides and risk of childhood leukemia. *Environmental Health Perspectives, 110*(9), 955–960.

75. Cordier, S., Mandereau, L., Preston-Martin, S., Little, J., Lubin, F., Mueller, B., et al., (2001). Parental occupations and childhood brain tumors: results of an international case-control study. *Cancer Causes & Control: CCC, 12*(9), 865–874.
76. Wogan, G. N., Hecht, S. S., Felton, J. S., Conney, A. H., & Loeb, L. A., (2004). Environmental and chemical carcinogenesis. *Seminars in Cancer Biology, 14*(6), 473–486.
77. Hecht, S. S., (2002). Human urinary carcinogen metabolites: biomarkers for investigating tobacco and cancer. *Carcinogenesis, 23*(6), 907–922.
78. Hecht, S. S., (2003). Tobacco carcinogens, their biomarkers and tobacco-induced cancer. *Nature Reviews Cancer, 3*(10), 733–744.
79. De Martel, C., Ferlay, J., Franceschi, S., Vignat, J., Bray, F., Forman, D., et al., (2012). Global burden of cancers attributable to infections in 2008: a review and synthetic analysis. *The Lancet Oncology, 13*(6), 607–615.
80. Lowy, D. R., & Schiller, J. T., (2012). Reducing HPV-associated cancer globally. *Cancer Prevention Research, 5*(1), 18–23.
81. Winer, R. L., Hughes, J. P., Feng, Q., O'Reilly, S., Kiviat, N. B., Holmes, K. K., et al., (2006). Condom use and the risk of genital human papillomavirus infection in young women. *The New England Journal of Medicine, 354*(25), 2645–2654.
82. Gillison, M. L., Chaturvedi, A. K., & Lowy, D. R., (2008). HPV prophylactic vaccines and the potential prevention of noncervical cancers in both men and women. *Cancer, 113(10 Suppl)*, 3036–3046.
83. Chaturvedi, A. K., Engels, E. A., Pfeiffer, R. M., Hernandez, B. Y., Xiao, W., Kim, E., et al., (2011). Human papillomavirus and rising oropharyngeal cancer incidence in the United States. *Journal of Clinical Oncology : Official Journal of the American Society of Clinical Oncology, 29*(32), 4294–4301.
84. Leung, N., (2005). HBV and liver cancer. *The Medical journal of Malaysia, 60, Suppl. B.*, 63–66.
85. Guerrieri, F., Belloni, L., Pediconi, N., & Levrero, M., (2013). Molecular mechanisms of HBV-associated hepatocarcinogenesis. *Seminars in Liver Disease, 33*(2), 147–156.
86. Kushekhar, K., Van den Berg, A., Nolte, I., Hepkema, B., Visser, L., & Diepstra, A., (2014). Genetic associations in classical hodgkin lymphoma: a systematic review and insights into susceptibility mechanisms. *Cancer Epidemiology, Biomarkers & Prevention* : a publication of the American Association for Cancer Research, cosponsored by the American Society of Preventive Oncology, *23*(12), 2737–2747.
87. Murphy, G., Pfeiffer, R., Camargo, M. C., & Rabkin, C. S., (2009). Meta-analysis shows that prevalence of Epstein-Barr virus-positive gastric cancer differs based on sex and anatomic location. *Gastroenterology, 137*(3), 824–833.
88. Qu, Y., Dang, S., & Hou, P., (2013). Gene methylation in gastric cancer. *Clinica Chimica acta, International Journal of Clinical Chemistry, 424*, 53–65.
89. Tao, Q., Young, L. S., Woodman, C. B., & Murray, P. G., (2006). Epstein-Barr virus (EBV) and its associated human cancers--genetics, epigenetics, pathobiology and novel therapeutics. *Frontiers in bioscience : A Journal and Virtual Library, 11*, 2672–2713.
90. Tsang, C. M., Deng, W., Yip, Y. L., Zeng, M. S., Lo, K. W., & Tsao, S. W., (2014). Epstein-Barr virus infection and persistence in nasopharyngeal epithelial cells. *Chinese Journal of Cancer, 33*(11), 549–555.
91. Ferri, C., Sebastiani, M., Giuggioli, D., Colaci, M., Fallahi, P., Piluso, A., et al., (2015). Hepatitis C virus syndrome: A constellation of organ- and non-organ specific autoimmune disorders, B-cell non-Hodgkin's lymphoma, & cancer. *World Journal of Hepatology 7*(3), 327–343.

92. Kiderlen, T. R., Siehl, J., & Hentrich, M., (2017). HIV-Associated Lung Cancer. *Oncology Research and Treatment, 40*(3), 88–92.

93. Oette, M., Mosthaf, F. A., Sautter-Bihl, M. L., & Esser, S., (2017). HIV-Associated anal dysplasia and anal carcinoma. *Oncology Research and Treatment, 40*(3), 100–105.

94. Hentrich, M., & Pfister, D., (2017). HIV-Associated urogenital malignancies. *Oncology Research and Treatment, 40*(3), 106–112.

95. Guo, Y., Liu, W., & Wu, J., (2016). Helicobacter pylori infection and pancreatic cancer risk: A meta-analysis. *Journal of Cancer Research and Therapeutics, 12 (Supplement)*, 229–232.

96. Van Tong, H., Brindley, P. J., Meyer, C. G., & Velavan, T. P., (2017). Parasite infection, carcinogenesis and human malignancy. *E. Bio. Medicine, 15*, 12–23.

97. Goldman, R., & Shields, P. G., (2003). Food mutagens. *The Journal of Nutrition, 133, Suppl., 3*, 965–973.

98. Sutandyo, N., (2010). Nutritional carcinogenesis. *Acta Medica Indonesiana, 42*(1), 36–42.

99. Sugimura, T., (2000). Nutrition and dietary carcinogens. *Carcinogenesis, 21*(3), 387–395.

100. Schottenfeld, D. F. J., (1996). *Cancer Epidemiology and Prevention*. New York, Oxford University Press, 438–461.

101. Oliveira, P. A., Colaco, A., Chaves, R., Guedes-Pinto, H., De-La-Cruz, P. L., & Lopes, C., (2007). Chemical carcinogenesis. *Anais da Academia Brasileira de Ciencias, 79*(4), 593–616.

102. Van Leeuwen, I. M., & Zonneveld, C., (2001). From exposure to effect: a comparison of modeling approaches to chemical carcinogenesis. *Mutation Research, 489*(1), 17–45.

103. Luch, A., (2005). Nature and nurture - lessons from chemical carcinogenesis. Nature reviews, *Cancer, 5*(2), 113–125.

104. Klaunig, J. E., Kamendulis, L. M., & Xu, Y., (2000). Epigenetic mechanisms of chemical carcinogenesis. *Human & Experimental Toxicology, 19*(10), 543–555.

105. Poirier, M. C., Santella, R. M., & Weston, A., (2000). Carcinogen macromolecular adducts and their measurement. *Carcinogenesis, 21*(3), 353–359.

106. Williams, G. M., (2001). Mechanisms of chemical carcinogenesis and application to human cancer risk assessment. *Toxicology, 166*(1–2), 3–10.

107. Park, B. K., Kitteringham, N. R., Maggs, J. L., Pirmohamed, M., & Williams, D. P., (2005). The role of metabolic activation in drug-induced hepatotoxicity. *Annual Review of Pharmacology and Toxicology, 45*, 177–202.

108. Knize, M. G., Salmon, C. P., Pais, P., & Felton, J. S., (1999). Food heating and the formation of heterocyclic aromatic amine and polycyclic aromatic hydrocarbon mutagens/carcinogens. *Advances in Experimental Medicine and Biology, 459*, 179–193.

109. W, L., (1999). *In Vivo Testing for Carcinogenicity*. Berlin: Springer-Verlag, 179–209.

110. Calle, E. E., Rodriguez, C., Walker-Thurmond, K., & Thun, M. J., (2003). Overweight, obesity, & mortality from cancer in a prospectively studied cohort of U. S. adults. *The New England Journal of Medicine, 348*(17), 1625–1638.

111. Hursting, S. D., Nunez, N. P., Varticovski, L., & Vinson, C., (2007). The obesity-cancer link: lessons learned from a fatless mouse. *Cancer Research, 67*(6), 2391–2393.

112. Poschl, G., & Seitz, H. K., (2004). Alcohol and cancer. *Alcohol and Alcoholism, 39*(3), 155–165.

113. Van der, V. E. J., Nolte-'t Hoen, E. N., Stoorvogel, W., Arkesteijn, G. J., & Wauben, M. H., (2012). Fluorescent labeling of nano-sized vesicles released by cells and subsequent

quantitative and qualitative analysis by high-resolution flow cytometry. *Nature Protocols, 7*(7), 1311–1326.

114. Raposo, G., & Stoorvogel, W., (2013). Extracellular vesicles: exosomes, microvesicles, & friends. *The Journal of Cell Biology, 200*(4), 373–383.

115. Gouveia de Andrade, A. V., Bertolino, G., Riewaldt, J., Bieback, K., Karbanova, J., Odendahl, M., et al., (2015). Extracellular vesicles secreted by bone marrow- and adipose tissue-derived mesenchymal stromal cells fail to suppress lymphocyte proliferation. *Stem Cells and Development, 24*(11), 1374–1376.

116. Rechavi, O., Goldstein, I., & Kloog, Y., (2009). Intercellular exchange of proteins: the immune cell habit of sharing. FEBS letters, *583*(11), 1792–1799.

117. Bobrie, A., Colombo, M., Raposo, G., & Thery, C., (2011). Exosome secretion: molecular mechanisms and roles in immune responses. *Traffic, 12*(12), 1659–1668.

118. Mathivanan, S., Ji, H., & Simpson, R. J., (2010). Exosomes: extracellular organelles important in intercellular communication. *Journal of Proteomics, 73*(10),1907–1920.

119. Smalley, D. M., Sheman, N. E., Nelson, K., & Theodorescu, D., (2008). Isolation and identification of potential urinary microparticle biomarkers of bladder cancer. *Journal of Proteome Research, 7*(5), 2088–2096.

120. Jaenisch, R., & Bird, A., (2003). Epigenetic regulation of gene expression: how the genome integrates intrinsic and environmental signals. *Nature Genetics, 33,* 245–254.

121. Robertson, K. D., Uzvolgyi, E., Liang, G., Talmadge, C., Sumegi, J., Gonzales, F. A., et al., (1999). The human DNA methyltransferases (DNMTs) 1, 3a and 3b: coordinate mRNA expression in normal tissues and overexpression in tumors. *Nucleic Acids Research, 27*(11), 2291–2298.

122. Zhu, X., You, Y., Li, Q., Zeng, C., Fu, F., Guo, A., et al., (2014). BCR-ABL1-positive microvesicles transform normal hematopoietic transplants through genomic instability: implications for donor cell leukemia. *Leukemia, 28*(8), 1666–1675.

123. Kahlert, C., Melo, S. A., Protopopov, A., Tang, J., Seth, S., Koch, M., et al., (2014). Identification of double-stranded genomic DNA spanning all chromosomes with mutated KRAS and p53 DNA in the serum exosomes of patients with pancreatic cancer. *The Journal of Biological Chemistry, 289*(7), 3869–3875.

124. Yoshida, Y., Yamamoto, H., Morita, R., Oikawa, R., Matsuo, Y., Maehata, T., et al., (2014). Detection of DNA methylation of gastric juice-derived exosomes in gastric cancer. *Integrative Molecular Medicine, 1,* 17–21.

125. Munshi, A., Shafi, G., Aliya, N., & Jyothy, A., (2009). Histone modifications dictate specific biological readouts. *Journal of Genetics and Genomics = Yi Chuan Xue Bao, 36*(2), 75–88.

126. Lee, K. K., & Workman, J. L., (2007). Histone acetyltransferase complexes: one size doesn't fit all. *Nature Reviews Molecular Cell Biology, 8*(4), 284–295.

127. Hou, H., & Yu, H., (2010). Structural insights into histone lysine demethylation. *Current Opinion in Structural Biology, 20*(6), 739–748.

128. Gallinari, P., Di Marco, S., Jones, P., Pallaoro, M., & Steinkuhler, C., (2007). HDACs, histone deacetylation and gene transcription: from molecular biology to cancer therapeutics. *Cell Research, 17*(3), 195–211.

129. Schiera, G., Di Liegro, C. M., Saladino, P., Pitti, R., Savettieri, G., Proia, P., et al., (2013). Oligodendroglioma cells synthesize the differentiation-specific linker histone H1 and release it into the extracellular environment through shed vesicles. *International Journal of Oncology, 43*(6), 1771–1776.

130. Lorico, A., Mercapide, J., & Rappa, G., (2013). Prominin-1 (CD133) and Metastatic melanoma: current knowledge and therapeutic perspectives. *Advances in Experimental Medicine and Biology, 777*, 197–211.

131. Rappa, G., Mercapide, J., Anzanello, F., Le, T. T., Johlfs, M. G., Fiscus, R. R., et al., (2013). Wnt interaction and extracellular release of prominin-1/CD133 in human malignant melanoma cells. *Experimental Cell Research, 319*(6), 810–819.

132. Zhou, W., Fong, M. Y., Min, Y., Somlo, G., Liu, L., Palomares, M. R., et al., (2014). Cancer-secreted miR-105 destroys vascular endothelial barriers to promote metastasis. *Cancer Cell, 25*(4), 501–515.

133. Kosaka, N., Iguchi, H., Hagiwara, K., Yoshioka, Y., Takeshita, F., & Ochiya, T., (2013). Neutral sphingomyelinase 2 (nSMase2)-dependent exosomal transfer of angiogenic microRNAs regulate cancer cell metastasis. *The Journal of Biological Chemistry, 288*(15), 10849–10859.

134. Kogure, T., Lin, W. L., Yan, I. K., Braconi, C., & Patel, T., (2011). Intercellular nanovesicle-mediated microRNA transfer: a mechanism of environmental modulation of hepatocellular cancer cell growth. *Hepatology, 54*(4), 1237–1248.

135. Perkel, J. M., (2013). Visiting "noncodarnia". *BioTechniques, 54*(6), 301, 303–304.

136. Kogure, T., Yan, I. K., Lin, W. L., & Patel, T., (2013). Extracellular Vesicle-Mediated Transfer of a Novel Long Noncoding RNA TUC339: A Mechanism of Intercellular Signaling in Human Hepatocellular Cancer. *Genes & Cancer, 4*(7–8), 261–272.

137. Braconi, C., Valeri, N., Kogure, T., Gasparini, P., Huang, N., Nuovo, G. J., et al., (2011). Expression and functional role of a transcribed noncoding RNA with an ultraconserved element in hepatocellular carcinoma. *Proceedings of the National Academy of Sciences of the United States of America, 108*(2), 786–791.

138. Takahashi, K., Yan, I. K., Kogure, T., Haga, H., & Patel, T., (2014). Extracellular vesicle-mediated transfer of long non-coding RNA ROR modulates chemosensitivity in human hepatocellular cancer. *FEBS Open Bio, 4*, 458–467.

CHAPTER 9

SINGLE NUCLEOTIDE POLYMORPHISMS AS SUSCEPTIBILITY MARKERS FOR CANCER

SURESH KUMAR YADAV and SOMALI SANYAL

Amity Institute of Biotechnology, Amity University Uttar Pradesh, Lucknow Campus, Lucknow, Uttar Pradesh, 226028, India, E-mail: ssanyal@lko.amity.edu

CONTENTS

ABSTRACT

Cancer develops due to exposure to several chemical and physical carcinogens that cause DNA damage. However, every individual who is exposed to such risk factors does not develop cancer. Similarly, many individuals develop the disease without being exposed to any of the known risk factors. This indicates a differential susceptibility to develop cancer. Such discrepancies in disease development arise from genetically predetermined inter-individual variation in susceptibility. The susceptibility may be low or high, and genetic characteristics, which determine an individual's susceptibility to cancer, are modulated by genetic polymorphisms, for example, by single nucleotide polymorphism (SNP). Genes involved in carcinogen metabolism, DNA repair, cell cycle regulation, and apoptosis coordinate to facilitate the initial defense against cancer development. Metabolic enzymes detoxify carcinogens to provide the first line of defense. The DNA repair protein repairs the damaged DNA and prevents the consequences of mutagenic exposure of cell. During the process of DNA repair, cell cycle regulatory proteins keep the cell arrested at a specific phase of cell cycle. If the damage remains unrepaired, the cell undergoes apoptosis. Polymorphisms that cause subtle alteration in carcinogen metabolism, DNA repair, and cell cycle regulatory and apoptotic protein can influence these processes and consequently the individual's susceptibility to carcinogens; therefore, they are postulated to serve as "susceptibility marker" of cancer.

9.1   INTRODUCTION

The genomes of any two human individuals are almost 99.9% identical and have only 0.1% variation. This 0.1% variation is mainly attributed to the presence of single nucleotide polymorphism (SNP) in the human genome. SNP is a change in single nucleotide in the DNA sequence that results in alternative forms of DNA sequences or polymorphic DNA. This change in sequence may be either by transition: purine-purine (A<->T)/ pyrimidine-pyrimidine (G<->C) or by transversion: purine-pyrimidine/pyrimidine-purine. The possibility of change by transversion is twice than the change by transition. The majority of SNPs are not of biological use, and only a small fraction of the substitutions have biological significance and form the basis for the diversity found in humans [1]. A variation is termed as SNP only when it is genetically stable and is propagated within the population. Apart from the genetic stability, the variation should be present within at least 1% of total population.

SNPs are present throughout the genome and vary from coding to noncoding regions. SNPs in noncoding regions form synonymous (similar) proteins, i.e., the amino acid sequence of the protein remained unchanged, and thus, the same protein is formed. SNPs present in coding regions may form nonsynonymous (different) proteins, i.e., the amino acid sequence of the protein is changed and a different protein is formed. Apart from changing the amino acid sequence of the protein, SNPs in the coding region may also alter the amount of mRNA formed within the cell. Effect of SNPs can also occur at the transcription level or at the posttranslational level. For example, if there is an SNP in the promoter region, then the binding of the transcription factor will be affected. As a result, less mRNA will be formed and finally less protein will be formed (Figure 9.1). The decreased levels of mRNA may also lead to less levels of enzyme formation and eventually reduced metabolic activities within the cell and vice-versa. Nonsynonymous SNPs can also affect posttranslational modifications such as protein phosphorylation, which is a crucial step in signal transduction. On the other hand, if the SNP is present in the non-coding regions of RNA, this may lead to alternative splicing and thus form an alternate protein.

9.2 MAPPING OF SNP

Huge numbers of SNPs were generated by two main methods: Shotgun sequencing and sequence comparison. In the Shotgun method, mixture of 24 ethnically different individuals' genome was sequenced with reduced representation sequencing approach [2]. This was done by The SNP Consortium (TSC) which comprised biotechnology and pharmaceutical firms. In the sequence comparison method, the overlapping regions between large inserts in Bacterial Artificial Chromosome (BAC) were sequenced. This was done in the Human Genome Project (HGP). The mapping of SNPs was done by comparing sequences with the assembled human genome sequence. Till February 2001, a total of 1.42 million SNPs were mapped, with an average density of 1 in every 1.91 kb [3].

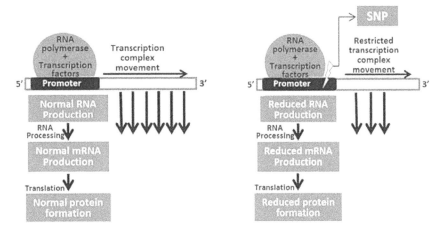

FIGURE 9.1 Impact of SNP on gene expression.

Several researchers worldwide might find the same SNP, and when these SNPs are submitted in the database, they may result in huge repetition in the database because of the same SNP sequence. To avoid this repetition, a unique RS number is given to each SNP. The RS number for SNP stands for Reference SNP cluster ID. It is a unique accession number used by scientists, researchers, and databases to refer to specific SNPs. The RS IDs are used to reduce redundancy in the sequences identified by different researchers and scientists. Whenever researchers identify a SNP, they send the sequence surrounding the SNP to the SNP database. If overlapping sequences are sent, they are merged to the same SNP Id, which in turn makes it nonredundant, and thus, a unique Reference SNP cluster ID is created. There are several databases of SNPs, like dbSNP, ExPASy, EBI, GeneSNPs, Clinvar, Geneatlas, Gene Cards Database, Genome Variation server, HOWDY, HGMD, jSNP, The Human Genome Database, OMIM, SNP-Database, Seattle SNPs, etc.

9.3   GENOTYPING OF SNPS

SNP genotyping involves two key steps: i) formation of allele-specific products and ii) separation and identification of the allele-specific products. Following are different techniques that are used for SNP genotyping.

9.3.1   POLYMERASE CHAIN REACTION AND RESTRICTION FRAGMENT LENGTH POLYMORPHISM TECHNIQUE

The DNA fragment of interest with the SNP is amplified with the PCR technique. This is followed by a restriction enzyme digestion of the amplified fragments with appropriate restriction endonucleases, which specifically recognize and cut either the variant or the common sequences. Finally, the digested products are resolved by gel electrophoresis and visualized using ethidium bromide under UV light.

9.3.2   SINGLE STRAND DNA CONFORMATION AND HETERODUPLEXES

Single strand conformation polymorphism (SSCP) can also be used for SNP detection. It is based on folding conformation specificity of ssDNA, when kept in non-denaturing conditions. Even a single base change in DNA fragment of 300 base pair will significantly change the conformation in such a way that it can be detected by polyacrylamide gel electrophoresis (PAGE). Currently, denaturing high performance liquid chromatography (DHPLC) technique is being utilized for the separation of the heteroduplex and homoduplex strands [4].

9.3.3 PRIMER EXTENSION

In this technique, oligonucleotides (also known as primers) are used to facilitate in vitro DNA synthesis either by PCR or by other sequencing methods. Two main variations exist in this technique. In the first technique, two allele-specific and complementary oligonucleotides are used to facilitate the DNA polymerase activity. In the second technique, a single base extension (SBE) primer is used, such that its 3' end is located just before the SNP to be tested. The DNA polymerase then incorporates differently fluorescent dye-labeled ddNTPs. The results may be obtained on a florescent plate reader by utilizing any method that differentiates incorporated labeled oligonucleotides from nonincorporated ones.

In these methods, simultaneously genotyped different loci are separated by gel electrophoresis [5] or by hybridization [6]. Recently, matrix-assisted laser desorption/ionization time-of-flight mass spectrometry (MALDI-TOF) is being used to differentiate genotypes.

9.3.4 OLIGONUCLEOTIDE LIGATION ASSAY (OLA)

In this technique, two, each allele specific and differentially labeled on one side of SNP, oligonucleotides are designed in such a way that they attach themselves at the position of polymorphism to be tested. These alleles can be detected either by using colorimetric methods or by gel electrophoresis.

9.3.5 PYROSEQUENCING

Pyrosequencing is a new and fast technology. It is based on the measurement of pyrophosphate (PPi) released when template complementary nucleotides are incorporated by a DNA polymerase. The four nucleotides are added sequentially in the reaction mixture and the sequence of successful incor-porations of nucleotide is recorded on a pyrogram, which finally gives the sequence. By comparing the pyrograms's sequence with the reference, we can detect the SNPs [7]. Pyrosequencing is an excellent method to detect new polymorphisms.

9.3.6   EXONUCLEASE DETECTION (TAQMAN)

In this technique, Taq DNA Polymerase's 5'->3' exonuclease activity is utilized to degrade an internal FRET (florescence resonance energy trans-fer) probe. Due to this degradation, the fluorescence is not quenched by the quencher, and thus, the fluorescence is emitted and measured. Two different internal FRET probes specific for two different alleles are used for the deter-mination of genotype [8].

9.3.7   INVADER ASSAY

This assay utilizes the invasive cleavage of oligonucleotide probes. It uses FENs (Flap Endonucleases) that removes redundant portions from 5' end downstream DNA fragment overlapping an upstream DNA fragment. This upstream fragment is also known as invader. An invader is designed in such a way that its 3' has the polymorphism under investigation. Two invaders are designed such that they overlap the polymorphic site and each correspond to one allele. This cleaved fragment is monitored as this invader probe cleaves the FRET probe. There is no requirement of PCR amplification, and the results are obtained on a fluorescence plate reader.

9.4   SNP AS SUSCEPTIBILITY MARKER

9.4.1   POLYMORPHISMS OF THE METABOLIC GENES AND SUSCEPTIBILITY TO CANCER

At an early stage, most cancers are initiated by carcinogens or xenobiotics. Tobacco smoke, food, and environmental pollutants are source of exogenous carcinogens. Most of these exogenous carcinogens require metabolic activa-tion prior to their reaction with biomolecules like DNA. Enzymes involved in carcinogen metabolism are classified as phase I and phase II enzymes. The phase I detoxification system, composed of cytochrome P450 super-familiy of enzymes, is generally the first enzymatic defense against foreign compound. The phase I enzyme besides increasing the solubility of the carcinogen also make them more reactive by reduction, oxidation, or hydrolysis reaction. Phase II enzymes detoxify the metabolites generated by phase I reaction. This group of enzymes conjugate ionized groups (e.g., glutathione, methyl, or acetyl) to the activated metabolites and convert those into less reactive, more water soluble, and excretal. Polymorphisms in phase I and phase II metabolic gene influence the induction and functioning of metabolic enzymes and hence alter individual carcinogen and drug metabolic capacity. Examples of association of genetic polymorphism in the metabolic gene with the risk of cancer have been discussed in the following sections.

9.4.1.1 Cytochrome P450

Cytochrome P450 (CYP450) enzymes are the most important phase I metabolic enzymes. They are mostly involved in deactivation of endogenous compounds and xenobiotics. They also convert procarcinogens to ultimate carcinogens by oxidation. There are several modes by which CYP450s activate procarcinogens such as: 1) CYP1A1 and CYP1B1 mediate the formation of epoxide and diol-epoxides intermediates, 2) CYP2A6, CYP2A13, and CYP2E1 mediates the activation of most nitrosamines to unstable metabolites, which can rearrange to give diazonium ions, and 3) CYP2E1 is involved in activation of tetrachloromethane to produce free radicals. For CYP2B6 and CYP2D6, only a minor role has been found in procarcinogen activation. Polymorphisms of CYP1A1 (-3801T/C and -4889A/G), CYP1A2 (- 163C/A and -2467T/delT), CYP1B1 (-48G/C, -119G/T and -432G/C), and CYP2E1 (-1293G/C and -1053 C/T) were found to be associated with an increased risk of lung cancer. Polymorphisms in CYP1A1 (-3801T/C and -4889A/G) and CYP2E1 (PstI/Rsa and 9-bp insertion) have an association with higher risk of colon cancers, whereas CYP1A2 (-163C/A and -3860G/A) polymorphisms are found to be protective. The risk of breast cancer has been found to be increased with the CYP1A1 (-3801T/C and -4889A/G), CYP1B1 -432G/C, and CYP2B6 (-516G/T and -785A/G) polymorphisms. In conclusion, CYP1A1, CYP1A2, CYP1B1, CYP2A6, and CYP2E1 are responsible for most of the procarcinogens activation, and their gene polymorphisms are associated with the risk of cancers [9].

9.4.1.2   Glutathione S Transferase P1

The glutathione S-transferase (GSTs) are a family of protein that conjugate electrophilic molecules with glutathione to convert them into less toxic substances and belong to phase II metabolic enzymes. Carcinogen detoxified by GSTs include polycyclic aromatic hydrocarbons present in diet and tobacco smoke. Besides, a variety of anticancer drugs are also metabolized by the member of this group. Thus, genetic polymorphisms in these enzymes have high relevance for cancer susceptibility. In humans, GSTs have been grouped into seven main classes and glutathione transferase P1 (GSTP1) is one of them. The GSTP1 gene belongs to pi class, is present on chromosome 11q13, and shows nonsynonymous SNPs. Among the different nonsynonymous SNPs on the GSTP1 gene, the I105V polymorphism (rs1695), which affects the kinetic property of the enzyme, is well explored in context with the risk of cancer. This GSTP1 polymorphism showed a significant association with prostate cancer [10]. Similarly, the V allele was also found to increase risk for oral cancer susceptibility in case of East Asians and Euro Caucasians [11] and lung cancer in Asians [12]. This variant allele for this polymorphism also showed increased susceptibility for bladder cancer [13] and gastric cancer in East Asians [14]. It has also been reported to increase risk for malignant melanoma [15].

9.4.1.3   Methylenetetrahydrofolate Reductase (Mthfr)

Beside phase I and phase II metabolism, folate metabolism also plays a vital role in cancer development. Folate metabolism is required for nucleic acid synthesis, regeneration of methionine, and shuttling and redox reactions of one carbon units required for normal metabolism and regulation. The transfer of one carbon units required in various biochemical reactions is mediated by folates. It plays an important role in the synthesis of S-adenosylmethionine (SAM), which serves as the methyl group donor in several methylation reactions like DNA, RNA, and protein methylation. DNA methylation in turn is a critical epigenetic determinant in DNA stability, DNA integrity, and mutagenesis as well as in gene expression. Thus, altered distribution of methyl groups due to abnormal folate metabolism affects both methylation and DNA synthesis-processes that play an essential role in the development of cancers [16].

Methylenetetrahydrofolate reductase (Mthfr) is a protein encoding gene located on chromosome number 1p36.3. The enzyme coded by this gene is important for folate metabolism, which is an essential process for cell metabolism. It also catalyzes the conversion of 5,10-methylenetetrahydrofolate to 5-methyltetrahydrofolate, which is a co-substrate for homocysteine remethylation to methionine. MTHFR 2572C>A (rs4846049), 4869C>G (rs1537514), and 5488C>T(rs3737967) polymorphisms were associated with increased susceptibility of colorectal cancer [17]. MTHFR C677T (rs1801133) polymorphism showed its association with an increased risk of esophageal cancer and stomach cancer in Asians [18]. It also showed increased risk to develop acute myeloid leukemia [19] as well as oral cancer [20]. Similarly, it also showed an increased risk for cervical cancer [21].

9.4.2 POLYMORPHISMS OF THE DNA REPAIR GENES AND SUSCEPTIBILITY TO CANCER

DNA is continuously exposed to a range of damaging agents, which include reactive cellular metabolites, environmental chemicals, and ionizing and UV radiation. DNA damage resulting from these exposures obstruct normal transcription and replication, which results in cellular malfunctioning and cell death and in the long run contributes in cellular aging. If the damage remains unrepaired due to inaccurate repair mechanisms, it becomes fixed into mutation and thus can cause cancer. A set of genome surveillance, namely nucleotide excision repair, base excision repair, homologous recombination repair, nonhomologous end joining, and mismatch repair mechanisms, collectively counteract the genomic insults. SNPs can alter the functionality of proteins that are involved in the DNA repair and thus affect the DNA repair capacity of the cell. Deficit DNA repair may result in cancer, and polymorphisms in DNA repair genes are reported to alter the risk of many different cancers, which is discussed in the following sections.

9.4.2.1 Xeroderma Pigmentosum Group C (XPC)

The xeroderma pigmentosum group C (XPC) gene spans 33 kb on chromosome 3 and contains 16 exons. The XPC protein binds to HR23B and play a key role in global genomic nucleotide excision repair (NER). Studies have shown an association of XPC polymorphisms with several cancers. The Val allele for XPC Ala499Val (rs2228000) polymorphism is associated with an increased risk of breast cancer, especially in the case of postmenopausal females [22]. This substitution also increases the risk of urinary bladder cancer [23]. Similarly, the Gln allele for XPC Lys939Gln (rs2228001 A>C) polymorphism showed a significant association with an increased risk of colorectal cancer in subjects with age of 57 years or younger [24]. It also increases the risk of local disease relapse by 6 folds in the case of head and neck cancer [25]. In contrary, the same allele from XPC Lys939Gln polymorphism showed an association with reduced risk for prostate cancer thus acts as a protective factor [26]. XPC rs1870134 GG genotype increases the risk of hepatocellular cancer [27].

9.4.2.2   Xeroderma Pigmentosum Group D

Xeroderma pigmentosum group D (XPD) or XRCC2 is a protein encoding gene located on chromosome number 19q13.3. It codes for protein XPD, which is a part of human transcriptional initiation factor TFIIH. It also has a ATP-dependent helicase activity. It is involved in the NER pathway. It opens the DNA around the damaged area. Several studies have suggested the association of XPD polymorphisms with the susceptibility to several cancers. XPD (rs50872) polymorphism was associated with an increased risk of breast cancer. Studies revealed that XPD rs11615, rs1800975, and rs50872 polymorphisms are related to different grades of breast cancer [22]. Lys751Gln (rs13181) is the most studied polymorphism of XPD that is associated with many different cancers. Zafeer et al. showed increased risk of head and neck cancer with Gln allele for XPD Lys751Gln polymorphisms [28]. Similarly, the Gln allele also increases the risk of renal cell carcinoma [29] and thyroid cancer [30]. This polymorphism also contributes to the susceptibility of esophageal cancer and nasopharyngeal carcinoma [31, 32]. It also contributes to the increased risk of hepatocellular carcinoma, especially in East Asian populations [33]. On the contrary, this allele shows protective association against oral squamous cell carcinoma (OSCC) [34]. The variant Asn allele for another XPD Asp312Asn (rs1799793) polymorphism showed increased risk for bladder[35] and gastric cancer [36]. Another nonsynonymous XPD polymorphism Arg156Arg (rs238406 C>A) was found to modulate the risk of arsenic-induced skin cancer [37].

9.4.2.3 Xeroderma Pigmentosum Complementation Group G

Xeroderma pigmentosum complementation group G (XPG) is a protein encoding gene present on chromosome number 13q33. It codes for a single strand-specific DNA endonuclease that is involved in repair of UV-induced DNA damage. It acts as a cofactor for DNA glycosylase that removes oxidized pyrimidines from DNA. Studies have revealed an association of XPG polymorphisms with several cancers. The variant alleles T and C respectively from XPG polymorphisms C>T (rs2094258) and G>A (rs873601) were found to increase the risk of colorectal cancer [38]. XPG (rs17655) polymorphism was found to be associated with an elevated risk of gastric cancer [39]. The variant allele His for XPG Asp1104His polymorphism showed an association with increased risk of lung cancer, especially in Asian population [40]. Similarly, it is also a risk factor for head and neck cancer, especially for laryngeal cancer in Asian population [41]. It is also associated with an increased risk of gastrointestinal cancers [42].

9.4.2.4 X-ray Repair Cross-Complementing 1

X-ray repair cross-complementing 1 (XRCC1) is a protein encoding gene located on chromosome number 19q13.2. The XRCC1 protein lacks enzymatic activity, but it acts as a scaffolding protein that interacts with DNA ligase III, polymerase beta, and poly (ADP-ribose) polymerase to participate in the base excision repair pathway. It is involved in single-strand DNA break re-joining. Several SNPs have been identified in the XRCC1 gene, and many of them showed an association with susceptibility to several cancers. The variant Arg allele for XRCC1 Gln399Arg (rs25487) polymorphism showed an association with susceptibility to lung cancer [43]. The variant allele of XRCC1 Arg280His polymorphism showed increased risk of laryngeal cancer [44]. Similarly, the variant allele of XRCC1 Arg194Trp polymorphism is associated with increased susceptibility to gastric cancer in the Chinese population [45]. It also constitutes a risk factor for thyroid carcinoma [45].

9.4.2.5 8-Oxoguanine DNA Glycosylases

The 8-oxoguanine DNA glycosylases (OGG1) gene is located on chromosome 3p26.2. It encodes for a DNA repair enzyme that is involved in the excision repair of 8-hydroxy-2'-deoxyguanine (8-OH-dG) from oxidatively damaged DNA. Several SNPs have been found on the OGG1 gene and were evaluated as susceptibility markers for several cancers. OGG1 Ser326Cys polymorphism was found to be associated with the increased susceptibility of orolaryngeal cancer [46] and colorectal cancer [47]. Similarly, it also showed increased susceptibility to develop upper aero-digestive and gastrointestinal tract cancer, breast cancer, and esophageal cancer[48]. It has also been reported to be associated with increased risk of lung, digestive system, and head and neck cancers [49].

9.4.3   POLYMORPHISMS OF THE CELL CYCLE REGULATORY GENES AND SUSCEPTIBILITY OF CANCER

Mammalian cell usually remain in the resting (G0) state and proliferate only under the influence of extracellular growth signals, such as growth factors and hormones. Growth signals received at the cell membrane reaches the nucleus by several transducer molecules that are either membrane bound or cytoplasmic. These growth signals cause cell division via a tightly regulated and timely coordinated process, referred to as cell cycle. In eukaryotes, cell cycle is divided into four phases, namely the synthesis (S) phase, the mitotic (M) phase, and two gap phases (G1 and G2). G1 precede the S phase, while G2 precede the M phase. Progression of cell cycle stops at two checkpoints, namely G1/S and G2/M, unless certain criteria are fulfilled. Unlike normal cells, a cancer cell divides in the absence of growth signals and often lose the two checkpoints of the cell cycle. Losses in cell cycle checkpoints promote carcinogenesis by allowing expansion of cell carrying mutation in critical genes. A number of regulatory proteins regulate the movement of the cell beyond these check points. Some promote movement of the cell from one phase to other, such as cyclins and cyclin-dependent kinases (CDKs), while some other inhibit the movement of the cell from one phase to other, such as members of the CDKN2A and Cip/Kip family. Polymorphisms that alter the function of cell cycle regulatory proteins can modulate cellular proliferation and thus alter the risk of cancer. In the following sections, SNP in several cell cycle regulatory genes are discussed in the context of risk of different cancers.

9.4.3.1 Cyclin D1

The gene for cyclin D1 or CCND1 is located on chromosome number 11q13.3 and codes for cyclin D1 protein. Cyclin D1 acts as a regulatory subunit of CDK4/CDK6, which is required for G1/S transition in cell cycle. It also interacts with the tumor suppressor protein retinoblastoma (Rb). Mutations and overexpression of this gene alters cell cycle progression, which is frequently observed in several tumors and thus contributes to tumorigenesis. Several studies have also established the association of SNPs of the CCND1 gene with different cancers. The A allele of CCND1 G870A (rs9344) polymorphism was found to significantly increase the risk of multiple myeloma. Similar association was also found with lung carcinoma, breast cancer, and acute lymphoblastic leukemia [50]. Increased susceptibility was also observed for oral cancer and colorectal cancer with the variant allele for CCND1 G870A (rs9344) polymorphism [51]. It also showed a significant association with increased susceptibility for nasopharyngeal carcinoma [52].

9.4.3.2 Tumor Protein 53

The tumor protein 53 (TP53) gene is located on chromosome number 17p13.1. It codes for tumor suppressor protein (p53). This protein has DNA binding, transcriptional activators, and oligomerization domains. It is involved in apoptosis, negative regulation of cell cycle, senescence, DNA repair, and cellular metabolism. Apoptosis is mediated either by repression of Bcl-2 expression or by BAX/FAS antigen expression. Cell cycle regulation is done by producing CDK inhibitors. For DNA repair, it prevents CDK7 activity after associating itself with the CAK complex. It is a protein that responds to various cellular stresses by either regulating its cellular levels or by posttranslational modification. P53 show anticancer activity, and it does this by one of the several mechanisms: it can activate DNA repair mechanism in case of severe DNA damage; can arrest cell cycle at G1/S transition in case of DNA damage; can initiate apoptosis in case of irreparable DNA damage; and can generate senescence response in case of short telomeres. Several SNPs in the p53 gene have been documented, and some of these have been evaluated as susceptibility markers for cancer. The most studied one is p53 Arg72Pro (rs1042522) polymorphism. This variant Pro allele for this P53 gene polymorphism was associated with an increased risk of *Helicobacter pylori*-associated gastric cancer in Korean population and with an increased risk of esophageal cancer [53, 54]. It was also significantly associated with an increased risk of developing breast cancer [55]. It also showed an association with increased risk to develop thyroid cancer especially under the recessive model [56]. It also influences the development of stomach cancer in northeast (Mizoram) Indian population [57] and contributes to increased risk of bladder cancer development, especially in Asian population [58].

9.4.3.3 Protein P21

The gene for protein p21 is located on chromosome number 11q14.1. It encodes for PAK proteins. These proteins are members of the serine/threonine p21-activating kinase family. There are six PAK isoforms, namely PAK1, PAK2, and PAK3 (group A) and PAK4, PAK5, and PAK6 (group B). These PAK proteins are involved in signaling pathways and play a crucial role in cytoskeleton dynamics, cell adhesion, apoptosis, cell proliferation, cell migration, mitosis, and vesicle-mediated cellular transport processes. The p21 protein binds to and thus inhibits the activity of CDK2, CDK1, and CDK4/6, thereby regulating the cell cycle progression at the G1/S phase. p21 can also bind with proliferating cell nuclear antigen (PCNA) and plays a key role in S phase DNA replication and DNA damage repair. It can phosphorylate BAD and thus can protect the cell from apoptosis. It is activated by interaction of CDC42 and RAC1. p21 also phosphorylates and thereby activates MAP2K1, and hence, it mediates the activation of downstream MAP kinases. Its activity is inhibited in the cells undergoing apoptosis, due to the binding of CDC2L1 and CDC2L2. The gene that synthesize p21 harbor many different SNPs, and some of those have shown association with the risk of different cancers. p21 3' UTR (rs1059234) polymorphism showed an association with increased risk of squamous cell carcinoma of the head and neck (SCCHN) [59]. The variant allele for p21 C98A (rs1801270) polymorphism was associated with an increased risk for uterine leiomyoma [60]. Another p21 polymorphism that replaces serine for arginine at codon 31 (Ser31Arg) was associated with susceptibility for the development of cervical lesions, gastrointestinal tract tumor, and breast cancer [61, 62]. In contrast, significantly decreased risks were found for oesophageal cancer and gastric cancer among Asians [63] with the variant allele for Ser31Arg polymorphism.

9.4.4 POLYMORPHISMS OF THE APOPTOTIC GENES AND SUSCEPTIBILITY TO CANCER

Programmed cell death, i.e., apoptosis, has been accounted in various aspects of cancer development. Apoptotic capacity varies between two individuals, which is largely attributed to hereditary traits. SNPs located within an apoptotic gene may influence susceptibility to cancer in various ways. Low apoptotic activity may favor cancer development because of the failure to eliminate cellular clones carrying damaged DNA, but at the same time may also protect against malignancy by preserving the antitumor immune cells [64]. Molecular and epidemiological evidence demonstrate that altered gene expression and SNPs in the genes of apoptotic pathway are associated with many cancers and is discussed in the following sections.

9.4.4.1 B-Cell Lymphoma 2

B-Cell lymphoma 2 (Bcl-2) is a protein encoding gene located on chromosome number 18q21.33. This gene encodes for an integral outer mitochondrial membrane protein that plays a crucial role in promoting cellular survival. Bcl-2 proteins regulate apoptosis or programmed cell death either by inducing pro-apoptotic proteins or by inhibiting antiapoptotic proteins. Bcl-2 is specifically considered as an important antiapoptotic protein. It regulates apoptosis by controlling the mitochondrial membrane permeability. It appears to function in a feedback loop system with caspases, and it inhibits caspase activity either by binding to the apoptosis-activating factor (APAF-1) or by preventing the release of cytochrome c from the mitochondria. Several polymorphisms have been documented in the Bcl-2 gene, which are possible susceptibility markers for different cancers. Bcl2 (-938C>A) (rs2279115) polymorphism was shown to be associated with an increased risk for breast cancer development [65]. The gene also showed a significant association with the increased risk of glioma [66] and potential association with increased susceptibility to gastric cancer [67]. It has also been reported to increase the susceptibility for developing esophageal cancer and acute myeloid leukemia [68, 69]. Another Bcl-2 (rs17757541) C>G polymorphism was associated with an increased risk of gastric cardiac adenocarcinoma [70].

9.4.4.2 Caspases

Cysteinyl aspartate proteases (Caspase) are protein encoding genes. Caspase 7 and caspase 9 are located on chromosome numbers 10q25.3 and 1p36.21, respectively. Caspases encode for cysteine-aspartic acid proteases. They are involved in the signaling pathways of apoptosis, inflammation, and necrosis. They play a crucial role in the execution of cell apoptosis by following a cascade mechanism. These enzymes are divided into initiators and effectors. Caspases exist in the form of inactive pro-enzymes, and these are proteolytically cleaved at conserved aspartic residues and produce one large and one small subunit. These subunits dimerize to form the active enzymes. Caspase 7 cleaves and activates the sterol regulatory element binding proteins (SREBPs). It also proteolytically cleaves poly(ADP-ribose) polymerase (PARP) at the 216-Asp-Gly-217 bond. Caspase 9 is involved in the activation cascade of caspases. Caspase 9 binds to Apaf-1, which in turn leads to the activation of the protease that cleaves and activates caspase-3. Caspase 9 also promotes DNA damage-induced apoptosis in an ABL1/c-Abl-dependent manner. It also proteolytically cleaves poly (ADP-ribose) polymerase (PARP). It is also thought to be a tumor suppressor.

Caspase7 (rs2227310) polymorphism was shown to be associated with an increased risk of lung cancer [71]. Another caspase7 polymorphism (rs7907519) was shown to have a significant interaction with gastro-esophageal reflux disease, and it plays an important role in esophageal adenocarcinoma [72]. Caspase 7 (rs12416109 and rs3814231) polymorphisms were associated with an increased risk of childhood leukemia [73]. Several other SNPs of Caspase7 including rs11593766, rs3124740, rs11196445, rs11196418, rs4353229, and rs10787498 have been reported to be associated with an increased risk for endometrial and cervical cancer[74, 75]. On the contrary, caspase 7 (rs4353229) polymorphism showed a protective association with gastric cancer [76]. Caspase 7 (rs2227310) and caspase 9 (rs4645981) are associated with an increased susceptibility to lung cancer [77]. The variant allele for caspase 9 -1263 polymorphism was shown to increase susceptibility to pancreatic cancer [78], while a protective association of the same allele was observed with colorectal, prostate, bladder, and gastric cancer [79–82].

9.4.4.3 FAS Cell Surface Death Receptor

Fas cell surface death receptor (FAS/FasR) is a protein encoding gene located on chromosome number 10q23.31. It is also known as apoptosis antigen 1 (APT or APO-1). It is a receptor for TNFSF6/FASLG. The adapter molecule FADD facilitates the binding of caspase 8 to the activated receptor. This results in the formation of death-inducing signaling complex (DISC), which comprises Fas-associated death domain protein (FADD), caspase 8, and caspase 10. DISC activates caspase 8, which eventually activates the rest of the cascade for apoptosis. This receptor activates NF-κB, MAPK3/ERK1, and MAPK8/JNK, and is involved in transducing the proliferating signals in normal diploid fibroblast as well as in T cells. Several polymorphisms in the FAS gene have been reported to alter the risk of many different cancers. Fas-670 (rs1800682) polymorphisms were shown to have a significant associations with prostate, hepatocellular, and esophageal cancers [83, 84]. Fas-1377 (rs2234767) polymorphism was shown to significantly increase the risk for breast, lung, and gastric cancers, especially in Asians [85–87]. It also showed an increased susceptibility to bladder cancers in Turkish population [88]. Fas-16 (rs10898853) polymorphism was found to be significantly associated with papillary thyroid cancer [89].

9.4.4.4 Akt Serine/Threonine Kinase 2

Akt Serine/Threonine Kinase 2 (Akt2) is a protein encoding gene located on chromosome number 19q13.2. It codes for a serine/threonine kinase that regulates cell metabolism, proliferation, cell survival, angiogenesis, and tumor formation. It also regulates apoptosis via the phosphorylation of MAP3K5 (apoptosis signal-related kinase). Phosphorylation decreases MAP3K5 kinase activity stimulated by the oxidative stress, and thus, it prevents the apoptosis process. Akt2 (rs7254617) polymorphism was shown to be associated with an increased risk of prostate cancer [90]. Akt2 polymorphisms were also shown to have an increased risk for developing gastric cancer and lung cancer [91].

9.5 SUMMARY

- Cancer arises due to exposure to physical and chemical carcinogens that causes DNA damage

- Carcinogens are metabolized to less toxic substances with phase I and phase II metabolic enzymes, and if not metabolized properly, they damage different biomolecules including DNA.
- SNPs in genes that synthesize metabolic enzymes can alter their efficiency and thus their metabolic capacity. Several studies have depicted polymorphisms in metabolic enzymes as susceptibility markers for several cancers.
- Damaged DNA is repaired by different DNA repair pathways in which a plethora of DNA repair proteins are involved.
- SNPs in DNA repair genes might influence their DNA repair capacity and have been reported to alter the risk of many different cancers.
- During the process of DNA repair, a cell needs to take a halt at the cell cycle, and proteins that are involved in the cell cycle checkpoint regulate this process.
- SNPs in cell cycle regulatory genes modulate the functions of cell cycle regulatory proteins and have been documented as susceptibility markers for several cancers.
- If the damaged induced in DNA is not repaired due to faulty DNA repair system, the cell moves to apoptosis.
- However, due to SNPs in apoptotic genes, the antiapoptotic proteins become inefficient while the proapoptotic proteins become more efficient.
- Studies have shown association of several SNPs in the apoptotic genes to modulate the risk of cancer.

KEYWORDS

- **cancer**
- **SNP**
- **susceptibility**

REFERENCES

1. Collins, F. S., Guyer, M. S., & Charkravarti, A., (1997). Variations on a theme: cataloging human DNA sequence variation. *Science, 278*, 1580–1581.

2. Collins, F. S., Brooks, L. D., & Chakravarti, A., (1998). A DNA polymorphism discovery resource for research on human genetic variation. *Genome Res, 8*, 1229–1231.

3. Sachidanandam, R., Weissman, D., Schmidt, S. C., Kakol, J. M., Stein, L. D., Marth, G., Sherry, S., Mullikin, J. C., Mortimore, B. J., Willey, D. L., Hunt, S. E., Cole, C. G., Coggill, P. C., Rice, C. M., Ning, Z., Rogers, J., Bentley, D. R., Kwok, P. Y., Mardis, E. R., Yeh, R. T., Schultz, B., Cook, L., Davenport, R., Dante, M., Fulton, L., Hillier, L., Waterston, R. H., McPherson, J. D., Gilman, B., Schaffner, S., Van Etten, W. J., Reich, D., Higgins, J., Daly, M. J., Blumenstiel, B., Baldwin, J., Stange-Thomann, N., Zody, M. C., Linton, L., Lander, E. S., & Altshuler, D., (2001). A map of human genome sequence variation containing 1. 42 million single nucleotide polymorphisms. *Nature, 409*, 928–933.

4. Liu, W., Smith, D. I., Rechtzigel, K. J., Thibodeau, S. N., & James, C. D., (1998). Denaturing high performance liquid chromatography (DHPLC) used in the detection of germline and somatic mutations. *Nucleic Acids Res, 26*, 1396–1400.

5. Lindblad-Toh, K., Winchester, E., Daly, M. J., Wang, D. G., Hirschhorn, J. N., Laviolette, J. P., Ardlie, K., Reich, D. E., Robinson, E., Sklar, P., Shah, N., Thomas, D., Fan, J. B., Gingeras, T., Warrington, J., Patil, N., Hudson, T. J., & Lander, E. S., (2000). Large-scale discovery and genotyping of single-nucleotide polymorphisms in the mouse. *Nat. Genet., 24*, 381–386.

6. Hirschhorn, J. N., Sklar, P., Lindblad-Toh, K., Lim, Y. M., Ruiz-Gutierrez, M., Bolk, S., Langhorst, B., Schaffner, S., Winchester, E., & Lander, E. S., (2000). SBE-TAGS: an array-based method for efficient single-nucleotide polymorphism genotyping. *Proc. Natl. Acad. Sci. USA, 97*, 12164–12169.

7. Ronaghi, M., (2001). Pyrosequencing sheds light on DNA sequencing. *Genome Res, 11*, 3–11.

8. Lee, L. G., Connell, C. R., & Bloch, W., (1993). Allelic discrimination by nick-translation PCR with fluorogenic probes. *Nucleic Acids Res., 21*, 3761–3766.

9. He, X., & Feng, S., (2015). Role of metabolic enzymes P450 (CYP) on activating procarcinogen and their polymorphisms on the risk of cancers. *Curr. Drug Metab., 16*, 850–863.

10. Yu, Z., Li, Z., Cai, B., Wang, Z., Gan, W., Chen, H., Li, H., & Zhang, P., (2013). Association between the GSTP1 Ile105Val polymorphism and prostate cancer risk: a systematic review and meta-analysis. *Tumour Biol., 34*, 1855–1863.

11. Yan, J., Xie, L. M., Shen, G. F., Yu, D. D., & Wang, Y. L., (2014). [GSTP1 Ile105Val polymorphism confer susceptibility to oral cancer:a meta-analysis]. *Shanghai Kou Qiang Yi Xue, 23*, 498–504.

12. Xu, C. H., Wang, Q., Zhan, P., Qian, Q., & Yu, L. K., (2014). GSTP1 Ile105Val polymorphism is associated with lung cancer risk among Asian population and smokers: an updated meta-analysis. *Mol Biol. Rep., 41*, 4199–4212.

13. Safarinejad, M. R., Safarinejad, S., & Shafiei, N., (2013). Association of genetic polymorphism of glutathione S-transferase (GSTM1, GSTT1, GSTP1) with bladder cancer susceptibility. *Urol. Oncol., 31*, 1193–1203.

14. Ma, Y., Wei, X., Han, G., Xue, M., Li, G., & Li, Y., (2013). Glutathione S-transferase P1 Ile105Val polymorphism contributes to increased risk of gastric cancer in East Asians. *Tumour Biol., 34*, 1737–1742.

15. Ibarrola-Villava, M., Martin-Gonzalez, M., Lazaro, P., Pizarro, A., Lluch, A., & Ribas, G., (2012). Role of glutathione S-transferases in melanoma susceptibility: association with GSTP1 rs1695 polymorphism. *Br. J. Dermatol., 166*, 1176–1183.

16. Nazki, F. H., Sameer, A. S., & Ganaie, B. A., (2014). Folate: metabolism, genes, polymorphisms and the associated diseases. *Gene, 533*, 11–20.

17. Jeon, Y. J., Kim, J. W., Park, H. M., Kim, J. O., Jang, H. G., Oh, J., Hwang, S. G., Kwon, S. W., Oh, D., & Kim, N. K., (2015). Genetic variants in 3'-UTRs of methylenetetrahydrofolate reductase (MTHFR) predict colorectal cancer susceptibility in Koreans. *Sci. Rep., 5*, 11006.

18. Tang, M., Wang, S. Q., Liu, B. J., Cao, Q., Li, B. J., Li, P. C., Li, Y. F., Qin, C., & Zhang, W., (2014). The methylenetetrahydrofolate reductase (MTHFR) C677T polymorphism and tumor risk: evidence from *134* case-control studies. *Mol Biol. Rep., 41*, 4659–4673.

19. Huang, L., Deng, D., Peng, Z., Ye, F., Xiao, Q., Zhang, B., Ye, B., Mo, Z., Yang, X., Liu, Z. Polymorphisms in the methylenetetrahydrofolate reductase gene (MTHFR) are associated with susceptibility to adult acute myeloid leukemia in a Chinese population. *Cancer Epidemiol., 39*, 328–333.

20. Tsai, C. W., Hsu, C. F., Tsai, M. H., Tsou, Y. A., Hua, C. H., Chang, W. S., Lin, C. C., & Bau, D. T., (2011). Methylenetetrahydrofolate reductase (MTHFR) genotype, smoking habit, metastasis and oral cancer in Taiwan. *Anticancer Res., 31*, 2395–2399.

21. Botezatu, A., Socolov, D., Iancu, I. V., Huica, I., Plesa, A., Ungureanu, C., & Anton, G., (2013). Methylenetetrahydrofolate reductase (MTHFR) polymorphisms and promoter methylation in cervical oncogenic lesions and cancer. *J. Cell Mol Med., 17*, 543–549.

22. He, B. S., Xu, T., Pan, Y. Q., Wang, H. J., Cho, W. C., Lin, K., Sun, H. L., Gao, T. Y., & Wang, S. K., (2016). Nucleotide excision repair pathway gene polymorphisms are linked to breast cancer risk in a Chinese population. *Oncotarget, 7*, 84872–84882.

23. Sankhwar, M., Sankhwar, S. N., Bansal, S. K., Gupta, G., & Rajender, S., (2016). Polymorphisms in the XPC gene affect urinary bladder cancer risk: a case-control study, meta-analyses and trial sequential analyses. *Sci. Rep., 6*, 27018.

24. Hua, R. X., Zhu, J., Jiang, D. H., Zhang, S. D., Zhang, J. B., Xue, W. Q., Li, X. Z., Zhang, P. F., He, J., & Jia, W. H., (2016). Association of XPC gene polymorphisms with colorectal cancer risk in a southern chinese population: A case-control study and meta-analysis. *Genes (Basel)., 7*.

25. Stur, E., Agostini, L. P., Garcia, F. M., Peterle, G. T., Maia, L. L., Mendes, S. O., Anders, Q. S., Reis, R. S., Santos, J. A., Ventorim, D. P., Carvalho, M. B., Tajara, E. H., Santos, M., Paula, F., Silva-Conforti, A. M., & Louro, I. D., (2015). Prognostic significance of head and neck squamous cell carcinoma repair gene polymorphism. *Genet Mol Res., 14*, 12446–12454.

26. Kahnamouei, S. A., Narouie, B., Sotoudeh, M., Mollakouchekian, M. J., Simforoosh, N., Ziaee, S. A., Samzadeh, M., Afshari, M., Jamaldini, S. H., Imeni, M., & Hasanzad, M., (2016). Association of XPC gene polymorphisms with prostate cancer risk. *Clin. Lab., 62*, 1009–1015.

27. Wang, B., Xu, Q., Yang, H. W., Sun, L. P., Yuan, Y. (2016) The association of six polymorphisms of five genes involved in three steps of nucleotide excision repair pathways with hepatocellular cancer risk. *Oncotarget, 7*, 20357–20367.

28. Zafeer, M., Mahjabeen, I., & Kayani, M. A., (2016). Increased expression of ERCC2 gene in head and neck cancer is associated with aggressive tumors: a systematic review and case-control study. *Int. J. Biol. Markers., 31*, 17–25.

29. Loghin, A., Banescu, C., Nechifor-Boila, A., Chibelean, C., Orsolya, M., Tripon, F., Voidazan, S., & Borda, A., (2016). XRCC3 Thr241Met and XPD Lys751Gln gene polymorphisms and risk of clear cell renal cell carcinoma. *Cancer Biomark, 16*, 211–217.

30. Shkarupa, V. M., Henyk-Berezovska, S. O., Palamarchuk, V. O., Talko, V. V., & Klymenko, S. V., (2015). Research of DNA repair genes polymorphism XRCC1 and XPD and the risks of thyroid cancer development in persons exposed to ionizing radiation after the Chornobyl disaster. *Probl. Radiac. Med. Radiobiol., 20,* 552–571.

31. Guo, X. F., Wang, J., Lei, X. F., Zeng, Y. P., & Dong, W. G., (2015). XPD Lys751Gln polymorphisms and the risk of esophageal cancer: an updated meta-analysis. *Intern. Med., 54,* 251–259.

32. Lye, M. S., Visuvanathan, S., Chong, P. P., Yap, Y. Y., Lim, C. C., & Ban, E. Z., (2015). Homozygous wildtype of XPD K751Q polymorphism is associated with increased risk of nasopharyngeal carcinoma in malaysian population. *PLoS One, 10,* e0130530.

33. Peng, Q., Li, S., Lao, X., Chen, Z., Li, R., & Qin, X., (2014). Association between XPD Lys751Gln and Asp312Asn polymorphisms and hepatocellular carcinoma risk: a systematic review and meta-analysis. *Medicine (Baltimore), 93,* e330.

34. Dos Santos Pereira, J., Fontes, F. L., De Medeiros, S. R., De Almeida Freitas, R., De Souza, L. B., & Da Costa Miguel, M. C., (2016). Association of the XPD and XRCC3 gene polymorphisms with oral squamous cell carcinoma in a northeastern Brazilian population: A pilot study. *Arch. Oral. Biol., 64,* 19–23.

35. Savina, N. V., Nikitchenko, N. V., Kuzhir, T. D., Rolevich, A. I., Krasny, S. A., & Goncharova, R. I., (2016). The cellular response to oxidatively induced DNA damage and polymorphism of some DNA repair genes associated with clinicopathological features of bladder cancer. *Oxid. Med. Cell Longev., 5710403.*

36. Ji, H. X., Chang, W. S., Tsai, C. W., Wang, J. Y., Huang, N. K., Lee, A. S., Shen, M. Y., Chen, W. Y., Chiang, Y. C., Shih, T. C., Hsu, C. M., & Bau, D. T., (2015). Contribution of DNA repair xeroderma pigmentosum group D genotype to gastric cancer risk in Taiwan. *Anticancer Res., 35,* 4975–4981.

37. Hsu, L. I., Wu, M. M., Wang, Y. H., Lee, C. Y., Yang, T. Y., Hsiao, B. Y., & Chen, C. J., (2015). Association of environmental arsenic exposure, genetic polymorphisms of susceptible genes, & skin cancers in Taiwan. *Biomed Res. Int., 892579.*

38. Hua, R. X., Zhuo, Z. J., Zhu, J., Zhang, S. D., Xue, W. Q., Zhang, J. B., Xu, H. M., Li, X. Z., Zhang, P. F., He, J., & Jia, W. H., (2016). XPG gene polymorphisms contribute to colorectal cancer susceptibility: A two-stage case-control study. *J. Cancer, 7,* 1731–1739.

39. Feng, Y. B., Fan, D. Q., Yu, J., & Bie, Y. K., (2016). Association between XPG gene polymorphisms and development of gastric cancer risk in a Chinese population. *Genet. Mol Res., 15.*

40. Zhou, B., Hu, X. M., & Wu, G. Y., (2016). Association between the XPG gene Asp1104His polymorphism and lung cancer risk. *Genet Mol Res., 15.*

41. Jiang, H. Y., Zeng, Y., Xu, W. D., Liu, C., Wang, Y. J., & Wang, Y. D., (2015). Genetic association between the XPG Asp1104His polymorphism and head and neck cancer susceptibility: evidence based on a meta-analysis. *Asian Pac. J. Cancer Prev., 16,* 3645–3651.

42. Luo, J. F., Yan, R. C., & Zou, L., (2014). XPG Asp1104His polymorphism and gastrointestinal cancers risk: a meta-analysis. *Int. J. Clin. Exp. Med., 7,* 4174–4182.

43. Liu, H. X., Li, J., & Ye, B. G., (2016). Correlation between gene polymorphisms of CYP1A1, GSTP1, ERCC2, XRCC1, & XRCC3 and susceptibility to lung cancer. *Genet. Mol Res., 15.*

44. Wu, W. Q., Zhang, L. S., Liao, S. P., Lin, X. L., Zeng, J., & Du, D., (2016). Association between XRCC1 polymorphisms and laryngeal cancer susceptibility in a Chinese sample population. *Genet. Mol Res., 15.*

45. Chen, S., Zhu, X. C., Liu, Y. L., Wang, C., & Zhang, K. G., (2016). Investigating the association between XRCC1 gene polymorphisms and susceptibility to gastric cancer. *Genet. Mol Res., 15*.

46. Elahi, A., Zheng, Z., Park, J., Eyring, K., McCaffrey, T., & Lazarus, P., (2002). The human OGG1 DNA repair enzyme and its association with orolaryngeal cancer risk. *Carcinogenesis, 23*, 1229–1234.

47. Lai, C. Y., Hsieh, L. L., Tang, R., Santella, R. M., Chang-Chieh, C. R., & Yeh, C. C., (2016). Association between polymorphisms of APE1 and OGG1 and risk of colorectal cancer in Taiwan. *World J. Gastroenterol., 22*, 3372–3380.

48. Das, S., Nath, S., Bhowmik, A., Ghosh, S. K., & Choudhury, Y., (2016). Association between OGG1 Ser326Cys polymorphism and risk of upper aero-digestive tract and gastrointestinal cancers: a meta-analysis. *Springerplus, 5*, 227.

49. Zhou, P. T., Li, B., Ji, J., Wang, M. M., & Gao, C. F., (2015). A systematic review and meta-analysis of the association between OGG1 Ser326Cys polymorphism and cancers. *Med. Oncol., 32*, 472.

50. Bedewy, A. M., Mostafa, M. H., Saad, A. A., El-Maghraby, S. M., Bedewy, M. M., Hilal, A. M., & Kandil, L. S., (2013). Association of cyclin D1 A870G polymorphism with two malignancies: acute lymphoblastic leukemia and breast cancer. *J. BUON, 18*, 227–238.

51. Sameer, A. S., Parray, F. Q., Dar, M. A., Nissar, S., Banday, M. Z., Rasool, S., Gulzar, G. M., Chowdri, N. A., & Siddiqi, M. A., (2013). Cyclin D1 G870A polymorphism and risk of colorectal cancer: a case control study. *Mol Med. Rep., 7*, 811–815.

52. Liao, D., Wu, Y., Pu, X., Chen, H., Luo, S., Li, B., Ding, C., Huang, G. L., & He, Z., (2014). Cyclin D1 G870A polymorphism and risk of nasopharyngeal carcinoma: a case-control study and meta-analysis. *PLoS One, 9*, e113299.

53. Kim, N., Cho, S. I., Lee, H. S., Park, J. H., Kim, J. H., Kim, J. S., Jung, H. C., & Song, I. S., (2010). The discrepancy between genetic polymorphism of p53 codon 72 and the expression of p53 protein in Helicobacter pylori-associated gastric cancer in Korea. *Dig. Dis. Sci., 55*, 101–110.

54. Zhao, Y., Wang, F., Shan, S., Qiu, X., Li, X., Jiao, F., Wang, J., & Du, Y., (2010). Genetic polymorphism of p53, but not GSTP1, is association with susceptibility to esophageal cancer risk - a meta-analysis. *Int. J. Med. Sci., 7*, 300–308.

55. Liu, J., Tang, X., Li, M., Lu, C., Shi, J., Zhou, L., Yuan, Q., & Yang, M., (2013). Functional MDM4 rs4245739 genetic variant, alone and in combination with P53 Arg72Pro polymorphism, contributes to breast cancer susceptibility. *Breast Cancer Res. Treat., 140*, 151–157.

56. Wu, B., Guo, D., & Guo, Y., (2014). Association between p53 Arg72Pro polymorphism and thyroid cancer risk: a meta-analysis. *Tumour Biol., 35*, 561–565.

57. Malakar, M., Devi, K. R., Phukan, R. K., Kaur, T., Deka, M., Puia, L., Sailo, L., Lalhmangaihi, T., Barua, D., Rajguru, S. K., Mahanta, J., & Narain, K., (2014). p53 codon 72 polymorphism interactions with dietary and tobacco related habits and risk of stomach cancer in Mizoram, India. *Asian Pac. J. Cancer Prev., 15*, 717–723.

58. Gallais, A., (1990). Quantitative genetics of doubled haploid populations and application to the theory of line development. *Genetics, 124*, 199–206.

59. Li, J., Li, Z., Kan, Q., Sun, S., Li, Y., & Wang, S., (2015). Association of p21 3' UTR gene polymorphism with cancer risk: Evidence from a meta-analysis. *Sci. Rep., 5*, 13189.

60. Salimi, S., Hajizadeh, A., Yaghmaei, M., Rezaie, S., Shahrakypour, M., Teimoori, B., Parache, M., Naghavi, A., & Mokhtari, M., (2016). The effects of p21 gene C98A polymorphism on development of uterine leiomyoma in southeast Iranian women. *Tumour Biol., 37*, 12497–12502.

61. Lima, G., Santos, E., Angelo, H., Oliveira, M., Heraclio, S., Leite, F., De Melo, C., Crovella, S., Maia, M., & Souza, P., (2016). Association between p21 Ser31Arg polymorphism and the development of cervical lesion in women infected with high risk HPV. *Tumour Biol., 37*, 10935–10941.

62. Dong, Y., Wang, X., Ye, X., Wang, G., Li, Y., Wang, N., Yang, Y., Chen, Z., & Yang, W., (2015). Association between p21 Ser31Arg polymorphism and gastrointestinal tract tumor risk: A meta-analysis. *Technol. Cancer Res. Treat., 14*, 627–633.

63. Liu, F., Li, B., Wei, Y., Chen, X., Ma, Y., Yan, L., & Wen, T., (2011). P21 codon 31 polymorphism associated with cancer among white people: evidence from a meta-analysis involving 78, 074 subjects. *Mutagenesis, 26*, 513–521.

64. Imyanitov, E. N., (2009). Gene polymorphisms, apoptotic capacity and cancer risk. *Hum. Genet., 125*, 239–246.

65. Bhushann, M. P., Jarjapu, S., Vishwakarma, S. K., Nanchari, S. R., Cingeetham, A., Annamaneni, S., Mukta, S., Triveni, B., & Satti, V., (2016). Influence of BCL2–938 C>A promoter polymorphism and BCL2 gene expression on the progression of breast cancer. *Tumour Biol., 37*, 6905–6912.

66. Li, W., Qian, C., Wang, L., Teng, H., & Zhang, L., (2014). Association of BCL2–938C>A genetic polymorphism with glioma risk in Chinese Han population. *Tumour Biol., 35*, 2259–2264.

67. Mou, X., Li, T., Wang, J., Ali, Z., Zhang, Y., Chen, Z., Deng, Y., Li, S., Su, E., Jia, Q., He, N., Ni, J., & Cui, D., (2015). Genetic variation of BCL2 (rs2279115), NEIL2 (rs804270), LTA (rs909253), PSCA (rs2294008) and PLCE1 (rs3765524, rs10509670) genes and their correlation to gastric cancer risk based on universal tagged arrays and Fe3O4 magnetic nanoparticles. *J. Biomed. Nanotechnol., 11*, 2057–2066.

68. Liu, Z., Sun, R., Lu, W., Dang, C., Song, Y., Wang, C., Zhang, X., Han, L., Cheng, H., Gao, W., Liu, J., & Lei, G., (2012). The -938A/A genotype of BCL2 gene is associated with esophageal cancer. *Med. Oncol., 29*, 2677–2683.

69. Cingeetham, A., Vuree, S., Dunna, N. R., Gorre, M., Nanchari, S. R., Edathara, P. M., Meka, P., Annamaneni, S., Digumarthi, R., Sinha, S., & Satti, V., (2015). Influence of BCL2–938C>A and BAX-248G>A promoter polymorphisms in the development of AML: case-control study from South India. *Tumour Biol., 36*, 7967–7976.

70. Li, Q., Yin, J., Wang, X., Wang, L. M., Shi, Y. J., Zheng, L., Tang, W. F., Ding, G. W., Liu, C., Liu, R. P., Gu, H. Y., Sun, J. M., & Chen, S. C., (2013). B-cell Lymphoma 2 rs17757541 C>G polymorphism was associated with an increased risk of gastric cardiac adenocarcinoma in a Chinese population. *Asian Pac. J. Cancer Prev., 14*, 4301–4306.

71. Lee, W. K., Kim, J. S., Kang, H. G., Cha, S. I., Kim, D. S., Hyun, D. S., Kam, S., Kim, C. H., Jung, T. H., & Park, J. Y., (2009). Polymorphisms in the caspase7 gene and the risk of lung cancer. *Lung Cancer, 65*, 19–24.

72. Wu, I. C., Zhao, Y., Zhai, R., Liu, C. Y., Chen, F., Ter-Minassian, M., Asomaning, K., Su, L., Heist, R. S., Kulke, M. H., Liu, G., & Christiani, D. C., (2011). Interactions between genetic polymorphisms in the apoptotic pathway and environmental factors on esophageal adenocarcinoma risk. *Carcinogenesis, 32*, 502–506.

73. Park, C., Han, S., Lee, K. M., Choi, J. Y., Song, N., Jeon, S., Park, S. K., Ahn, H. S., Shin, H. Y., Kang, H. J., Koo, H. H., Seo, J. J., Choi, J. E., & Kang, D., (2012). Association between CASP7 and CASP14 genetic polymorphisms and the risk of childhood leukemia. *Hum. Immunol., 73*, 736–739.

74. Xu, H. L., Xu, W. H., Cai, Q., Feng, M., Long, J., Zheng, W., Xiang, Y. B., & Shu, X. O., (2009). Polymorphisms and haplotypes in the caspase-3, caspase-7, & caspase-8 genes and risk for endometrial cancer: a population-based, case-control study in a Chinese population. *Cancer Epidemiol. Biomarkers. Prev., 18*, 2114–2122.

75. Shi, T. Y., He, J., Wang, M. Y., Zhu, M. L., Yu, K. D., Shao, Z. M., Sun, M. H., Wu, X., Cheng, X., & Wei, Q., (2015). CASP7 variants modify susceptibility to cervical cancer in Chinese women. *Sci. Rep., 5*, 9225.

76. Wang, M. Y., Zhu, M. L., He, J., Shi, T. Y., Li, Q. X., Wang, Y. N., Li, J., Zhou, X. Y., Sun, M. H., Wang, X. F., Yang, Y. J., Wang, J. C., Jin, L., & Wei, Q. Y., (2013). Potentially functional polymorphisms in the CASP7 gene contribute to gastric adenocarcinoma susceptibility in an eastern Chinese population. *PLoS One, 8*, e74041.

77. Lee, S. Y., Choi, Y. Y., Choi, J. E., Kim, M. J., Kim, J. S., Jung, D. K., Kang, H. G., Jeon, H. S., Lee, W. K., Jin, G., Cha, S. I., Kim, C. H., Jung, T. H., & Park, J. Y., (2010). Polymorphisms in the caspase genes and the risk of lung cancer. *J. Thorac. Oncol., 5*, 1152–1158.

78. Theodoropoulos, G. E., Michalopoulos, N. V., Panoussopoulos, S. G., Taka, S., & Gazouli, M., (2010). Effects of caspase-9 and survivin gene polymorphisms in pancreatic cancer risk and tumor characteristics. *Pancreas, 39*, 976–980.

79. Theodoropoulos, G. E., Gazouli, M., Vaiopoulou, A., Leandrou, M., Nikouli, S., Vassou, E., Kouraklis, G., & Nikiteas, N., (2011). Polymorphisms of caspase 8 and caspase 9 gene and colorectal cancer susceptibility and prognosis. *Int. J. Colorectal Dis., 26*, 1113–1118.

80. Kesarwani, P., Mandal, R. K., Maheshwari, R., & Mittal, R. D., (2011). Influence of caspases 8 and 9 gene promoter polymorphism on prostate cancer susceptibility and early development of hormone refractory prostate cancer. *BJU Int., 107*, 471–476.

81. Gangwar, R., Mandhani, A., & Mittal, R. D., (2009). Caspase 9 and caspase 8 gene polymorphisms and susceptibility to bladder cancer in north Indian population. *Ann. Surg. Oncol., 16*, 2028–2034.

82. Liamarkopoulos, E., Gazouli, M., Aravantinos, G., Tzanakis, N., Theodoropoulos, G., Rizos, S., & Nikiteas, N., (2011). Caspase 8 and caspase 9 gene polymorphisms and susceptibility to gastric cancer. *Gastric Cancer, 14*, 317–321.

83. Liu, T., Zuo, L., Li, L., Yin, L., Liang, K., Yu, H., Ren, H., Zhou, W., Jing, H., Liu, Y., & Kong, C., (2014). Significant association among the Fas -670 A/G (rs1800682) polymorphism and esophageal cancer, hepatocellular carcinoma, & prostate cancer susceptibility: a meta-analysis. *Tumour Biol., 35*, 10911–10918.

84. Lima, L., Morais, A., Lobo, F., Calais-da-Silva, F. M., Calais-da-Silva, F. E., & Medeiros, R., (2008). Association between FAS polymorphism and prostate cancer development. *Prostate. Cancer Prostatic. Dis., 11*, 94–98.

85. Geng, P., Li, J., Ou, J., Xie, G., Wang, N., Xiang, L., Sa, R., Liu, C., Li, H., & Liang, H., (2014). Association of Fas -1377 G/A polymorphism with susceptibility to cancer. *PLoS One, 9*, e88748.

86. Wu, Z., Wang, H., Chu, X., Chen, J., & Fang, S., (2013). Association between FAS-1377 G/A polymorphism and susceptibility to gastric cancer: evidence from a meta-analysis. *Tumour Biol., 34*, 2147–2152.

87. Li, K., Li, W., Zou, H., & Zhao, L., (2014). Association between FAS 1377G>A polymorphism and breast cancer susceptibility: a meta-analysis. *Tumour Biol., 35*, 351–356.

88. Verim, L., Timirci-Kahraman, O., Akbulut, H., Akbas, A., Ozturk, T., Turan, S., Yaylim, I., Ergen, A., Ozturk, O., & Isbir, T., (2014). Functional genetic variants in apoptosis-associated FAS and FASL genes and risk of bladder cancer in a Turkish population. *In. Vivo, 28*, 397–402.

89. Eun, Y. G., Chung, D. H., Kim, S. W., Lee, Y. C., Kim, S. K., & Kwon, K. H., (2014). A Fas-associated via death domain promoter polymorphism (rs10898853, -16C/T) as a risk factor for papillary thyroid cancer. *Eur. Surg. Res., 52*, 1–7.

90. Chen, J., Shao, P., Cao, Q., Li, P., Li, J., Cai, H., Zhu, J., Wang, M., Zhang, Z., Qin, C., & Yin, C., (2012). Genetic variations in a PTEN/Akt/mTOR axis and prostate cancer risk in a Chinese population. *PLoS One, 7*, e40817.

91. Soung, Y. H., Lee, J. W., Nam, S. W., Lee, J. Y., Yoo, N. J., & Lee, S. H., (2006). Mutational analysis of Akt1, Akt2 and Akt3 genes in common human carcinomas. *Oncology, 70*, 285–289.

PART III

CANCER PREVENTION AND CONVENTIONAL THERAPIES

DIETARY PHYTOCHEMICALS IN THE PREVENTION AND THERAPY OF CANCER: MODULATION OF MOLECULAR TARGETS

SHAMEE BHATTACHARJEE

Dept. of Zoology, West Bengal State University, Berunanpukuria, P.O. Malikapur, Kolkata–700126, India, E-mail: shamee1405@gmail.com

CONTENTS

ABSTRACT

Cancer incidence and mortality continue to increase globally. The existing anticancer therapies are inadequate and have limited clinical success due to their severe toxic side effects and huge cost. The protective effect of consuming plant foods in the form of fruits, vegetables, spices, and beverages, as evident from epidemiological studies, has led to the identification of their specific phytochemical constituents that have beneficial effects as anticancer agents. These dietary phytochemicals have been proven to exert their effect on various "hallmark" features of cancer cells, such as evasion of apoptosis, uncontrolled proliferation, sustained angiogenesis, invasion, and metastasis, through modulating several key signaling pathways such as intrinsic and extrinsic apoptotic cascade, the Ras-Raf-MEK-ERK pathway, the PI-3/Akt/mTOR pathway, the NF-κB pathway, the VEGF signaling pathway, etc. However, unfortunately, the promising activities of dietary phytochemicals in rodent models and in vitro studies have not been translated into clinical success till date. This may be due to several reasons like poor bioavailability of some potent anticancer dietary phytochemicals, unexpected toxicity, difficulty in determining the appropriate dose for clinical investigation, complexity in choosing efficacy biomarkers in clinical studies due to the pleiotropic action of phytochemicals, and so on. All these factors have led scientists to hypothesize that a purified phytochemical might not have the same health benefits as the whole food, and it is the complex mixture of phytochemicals present in fruits and vegetables that act in an additive and/or synergistic manner to exert their protective effect on human health.

The aim of this chapter is to provide a comprehensive review on the existing knowledge of some common anticancer dietary phytochemicals with an emphasis on their molecular targets and mechanism of actions. The challenges in translating phytochemicals into tangible clinical benefit are also discussed.

10.1   INTRODUCTION

"Let food be thy medicine and medicine be thy food." Hippocrates, the father of modern medicine, had quoted this famous statement way back in 431 BC. This underscores the fact that the beneficial effects of food on human health

have been known since antiquity. However, the question of the continuum between food and medicine has also been of great interest throughout history as is evident from a report where Socrates distinguishes between two categories: that of drug/medicament (pharmakon) and that of food (sition) and indicates that one can easily be dissimulated as the other [1].

Although knowledge about the importance of diet has been handed down from generation to generation for millennia, scientific studies about the link between diet and health are only a few decades old. A large number of epidemiological studies have attempted to elucidate the impact of diet on health and disease [2], and overwhelming evidence indicates that plant-based diet can reduce the risk of several chronic diseases including cancer [3]. A review of such studies suggests that plant foods have chemopreventive potential and that dietary differences between populations account for a significant proportion of the variation in cancer occurrence in different parts of the world [4, 5].

Asians have a much lower risk of colon, prostate, and breast cancers than populations in the Western countries. This is largely attributed to the consumption of more vegetables, fruits, and tea by the Asians, thus emphasizing the role of these plant foods as natural chemopreventive and chemotherapeutic agents [6]. It is reported that a significant proportion of cancer incidences are preventable by consuming a healthy diet consisting of vegetables and fruits [7]. The rising evidence in favor of the ability of plant foods to inhibit, delay, or reverse the process of carcinogenesis [8], coupled with the inadequacies of existing anticancer therapies has led to an increased interest in dietary phytochemicals [9].

According to the latest GLOBOCAN report produced by the International Agency for Research on Cancer (IARC), about 14.1 million new cancer cases and 8.2 million deaths occurred in 2012 worldwide [10]. Current clinical therapies including radiotherapy and chemotherapy elicit severe toxic reactions [11] because the majority of the antineoplastic agents target rapidly proliferating cells non-specifically, including both cancer and normal cells [12]. Drug resistance of solid tumors also adds to the limitations of chemotherapy [13]. Therefore, there is an increased focus on alternate remedies and their possible combination with conventional anticancer drugs to treat or prevent this dreadful disease and improve quality of life in cancer patients.

Natural product repertoire is a potential source for novel drugs. A total of 11% of the drugs considered as basic and essential by the World Health

Organization (WHO) are exclusively of plant origin, and a significant number are synthetic drugs obtained from natural precursors [14]. Potent sources of such natural compounds are foods such as vegetables, fruits, spices, and plant roots [15].

According to various *in vivo, in vitro*, and clinical trial data, the health promoting effects of plant-based diet is contributed mainly by the biologically active compounds or "phytochemicals" [16]. "Bioactive compounds" or phytochemicals are secondary plant metabolites that are extra-nutritional constituents and typically occur in small quantities in plant foods [17]. These secondary metabolites can be unique to specific species or genera and do not play any role in the plants' primary metabolic requirements, but rather, they increase their overall ability to survive and overcome local challenges by allowing them to interact with their environment [18]. The primary metabolites, in contrast, such as phytosterols, acyl lipids, nucleotides, amino acids, and organic acids, are found in all plants and perform metabolic roles that are essential and usually evident. Due to their large biological activities, plant secondary metabolites have been used for centuries in traditional medicine. Thus, they represent an important source of active pharmaceuticals [19].

10.2 DIETARY PHYTOCHEMICALS

Phytochemicals are usually classified according to their biosynthetic pathways [20] into the following types:

10.2.1 POLYPHENOLS

Polyphenols are ubiquitous plant secondary metabolites characterized by the presence of more than one phenol unit per molecule. These phytochemicals can be divided into several classes according to the number of phenol rings that they contain and the structural elements that bind these rings to one another [21]. The main groups of polyphenols are flavonoids, phenolic acids, phenolic alcohols, stilbenes, lignans, coumarins, and tannins [22] (Table 10.1)

Among these, the largest and best studied polyphenols are flavonoids, which comprise several thousands of compounds, including flavonols, flavones, catechins, flavanones, anthocyanidins, and isoflavones [23]. Epidemi-

TABLE 10.1 Example of Some Dietary Polyphenols

Polyphenol	Subclass	Structure	Major Dietary Sources
Catechins (catechin.epigallicatechin, epi-gallocatechingallate)	Flavonoids	(−)-Epicatechin (EC) (−)-Epigallocatechin (EGC) (−)-Epicatechin-3-gallate (ECG) (−)-Epigallocatechin-3-gallate (EGCG)	Green tea, Black Tea
Quercetin	Flavonoids		Apples. citrus fruits. onions. parsley, red wine and tea

TABLE 10.1 (Continued)

Polyphenol	Subclass	Structure	Major Dietary Sources
Gensitein & daidzein	Flavonoids	**Genistein** **Daidzein**	Soyabean, soymilk, soy flour
Kaempferol	Flavonoids	**Kaempferol**	Endive, broccoli, kale, green beans, leeks

Myricetin

Flavonoids

Walnut, berries, red wine

Naringenin

Flavonoids

Citrus fruits

TABLE 10.1 (Continued)

Polyphenol	Subclass	Structure	Major Dietary Sources
Gallic Acid	Phenolic acid	Gallic Acid	Wine, mangoes, gree tea and black tea
Curcumin	Chalcones	CURCUMIN	Turmeric
Resveratrol	Stilbenes	Resveratrol	peanuts, grapes, red wine, and cranberries, blueberries

[Sources: Refs. 22 and 59]

ological studies have revealed an inverse association between consumption of polyphenol-rich diet and occurrence of cancer [24–28].

10.2.2 TERPENOIDS AND CAROTENOIDS

Terpenoids, also referred to as terpenes or isoprenoids, are synthesized from two five-carbon building blocks. Based on the number of building blocks, i.e., the number of isoprene units, terpenoids are classified as monoterpenes, sequiterpenes, diterpenes, sesterterpenes, triterpenes, tetraterpenes, and polyterpenes [29] (Table 10.2).

Monoterpenes are found in the essential oils of citrus fruits, peppermints, and many other plants. Experimental and epidemiological evidence suggests that many of these dietary monoterpenes, including d-limonene which is a precursor to a large number of oxygenated monocyclic monoterpenes such as carveol, carvone, menthol, perillyl alcohol and perillaldehyde, has chemopreventive activity against several cancers [30, 31].

Carotenoids, nature's most widespread pigments, belong to the category of tetraterpenoids, and are classified into hydrocarbons (carotenes) and their oxygenated derivatives (xanthophylls), with a 40-carbon skeleton of isoprene units. By virtue of their role as provitamins and their antioxidant effects, carotenoids have received considerable attention [32]. The carotenoids that are most frequently found in fruits, vegetables, and human blood plasma are α- and β-carotene, lycopene, β-cryptoxanthin, zeaxanthin, and lutein [33]. Epidemiologically, a high-carotenoid intake via a fruit- and vegetable-rich diet is associated with a decreased risk of various forms of cancer [34].

10.2.3 ALKALOIDS

Alkaloids constitute an important class of structurally diversified compounds that have nitrogen atom in the heterocyclic ring and are derived from amino acids. In plants, alkaloids may exist in the free state, as salts or as amine or alkaloid N-oxides. Depending upon their biosynthetic precursor and heterocyclic ring system, alkaloids have been classified into different categories including indole, tropane, piperidine, purine, imidazole, pyrrolizidine, pyrrolidine, quinolizidine, and isoquinoline alkaloids [35]. Vinblastine and vincristine are the first significant anticancer alkaloid, isolated from *Vinca rosea* and *Catharanthus roseus* (Apocynacea), respectively, which intro-

TABLE 10.2 Examples of Some Dietary Terpenoids

Dietary Terpenoid	Subclass	Structure	Dietary Source
D-limonene	Monoterpene		peel of citrus fruits,
Perillyl alcohol	Monoterpene		Cherries, spearmint, sage, and celery seeds.
Carvacrol	Monoterpenes		Oregano, thyme
Geraniol	Monoterpene		Nutmeg, lavender, Blueberries
Linalool	Monoterpene		Coriander seeds

Dietary Terpenoid	Subclass	Structure	Dietary Source
Anethole	Monoterpene		Anise seed, Fennel
Cucurbetanes	Triterpenoid		Bitter melon
Oleananes	Triterpenoids		Olive

TABLE 10.2 (Continued)

Dietary Terpenoid	Subclass	Structure	Dietary Source
Lycopene	Carotenoid		Tomato
α-carotene and β-carotene	Carotenoid	α-carotene β-carotene	Pumpkin, carrots,

[Sources: Refs. 33 and 29]

duced new era in anticancer drug discovery [36]. Some prominent dietary alkaloids that have drawn extensive attention in therapeutics are piperine, berberine, caffeine, etc. (Table 10.3).

10.2.4 ORGANOSULFUR COMPOUNDS

Organosulfur compounds are found most commonly in plants belonging to Brassicaceae (e.g., cruciferous vegetables such as broccoli, cabbage, cauliflower, mustard, etc.) and those belonging to Liliaceae (e.g., *Allium* vegetables such as onion, leeks, and garlic) and confer the characteristic flavor of these vegetables. Organosulfur compounds contain sulfur atoms that are bound to a cyanate group or a carbon atom in a cyclic or non-cyclic configuration. Because of the nonpolar characteristic and low molecular weight of some sulfur-containing metabolites, these molecules are often volatile [37].

The organosulfides in *Alliums* are classified into two major groups: (1) oil-soluble polysulfides and (2) water-soluble thiosulfinates, the intermediate formed upon the reaction of the vacuolar enzyme alliinase with the non-volatile S-alk(en)yl-l-cysteine-sulfoxides present in the cell cytoplasm when *Alliums* are crushed. The volatile sulfur compounds that include diallyl trisulfide (DATS), diallyl disulfide (DADS), and diallyl sulfide (DAS) in *Allium* vegetables such as garlic are generated through enzymatic reactions of alliinase on non-volatile precursors (allylcysteine sulfoxide (alliin) and γ-glutamylcysteine) [38]. Water-soluble organosulfur compounds such as S-allylcysteine are derived enzymatically from γ-glutamylcysteines as in aged garlic extract [39] (Table 10.4).

Cruciferous vegetables are rich sources of glucosinolates, the hydrolysis of which by a class of plant enzymes called myrosinase results in the formation of biologically active compounds such as indoles and isothiocyanates [40]. Intense in vitro and in vivo research has not only identified the contribution of the abovementioned dietary phytochemicals in mediating the anticancer effects of fruits and vegetables, but the possible mechanisms by which these bioactive food components prevent cancer have also been elucidated.

Tumorigenesis is considered to be a multistep process, i.e., cells evolve progressively from normalcy through a series of pre-malignant states into invasive cancers [41]. It is suggested that six essential alterations in cell physiology collectively dictate malignant growth: self-sufficiency in growth

TABLE 10.3   Examples of Some Dietary Alkaloids

Dietary Alkaloid	Subclass	Structure	Dietary Source
Caffeine	Purine Alkaloid	Caffeine	Coffee beans
Papaverine	Isoquino-line Alka-loid		Opium
Berberine	Isoquino-line alka-loid		Oregon grape
Piperine	Piperidine alkaloid		Black pepper
Capsaicin	Amide type alkaloid		Chili peppers belonging to genus *Capsicum*

[Sources: Refs. 35 and 106]

signals, insensitivity to growth-inhibitory (antigrowth) signals, evasion of programmed cell death (apoptosis), limitless replicative potential, sustained angiogenesis, and tissue invasion and metastasis. Phytochemicals have been reported to target different stages of multistep carcinogenesis, thereby contributing to cancer prevention [42, 43]. The present chapter reviews current knowledge on the cancer preventive and therapeutic potential of some

TABLE 10.4 Examples of Some Dietary Organosulfur Compounds.

Dietary organosulfur	Structure	Dietary Source
DAS, DADS, DATS	DAS DADS DATS	Garlic Onion
S-allyl cysteine		Garlic
Phenyl isothiocyanate	NCS	Broccoli Cabbage
Allyl isothiocyanate	NCS	Mustard
Sulforaphane		Broccoli sprouts

[Source: Ref. 38]

common dietary phytochemicals, with a particular focus on their molecular targets related to some hallmark features of cancer.

However, it may be noted that a voluminous amount of literature is available on anticancer dietary phytochemicals and their plausible mechanism of action. But due to space constraints, the chapter had to be restricted to some of the more common dietary phytochemicals only. My sincere apologies to those scientists whose work could not be cited here.

10.3   INDUCTION OF APOPTOSIS BY DIETARY PHYTOCHEMICALS

Apoptosis is triggered through two well-characterized pathways in mammalian cells. The first one is the extrinsic pathway that depends on triggering of death receptors (e.g., TNF) and transmembrane proteins expressed on the cell surface, and the second one is the intrinsic pathway that is mediated by molecules released from the mitochondria (e.g., Bcl-2 protein family) [44]. A hallmark of cancer is resistance to apoptosis, with both the loss of proapoptotic signals and the gain of antiapoptotic mechanisms contributing to tumorigenesis. Therefore, induction of apoptosis in cancer cells is one of the key approaches to fight against cancer. Activation of caspases, induction of proapoptotic proteins, and downregulation of antiapoptotic proteins are the most common ways by which phytochemicals inhibit cancer cell growth.

10.3.1   POLYPHENOLS

Dietary polyphenols exert their anticancer effect by multiple molecular mechanisms of action on apoptosis signaling pathways in cancer cells [45].

An expanding body of evidence suggest that epigallocatechin-3-gallate (EGCG) (major polyphenol of green tea) [46–48], curcumin (active ingredient of turmeric) [49–51], resveratrol (a phytoalexin found in grapes, red wine, and mulberries) [52, 53], genistein (found in soya) [54, 55], and quercetin and luteolin [56] induced apoptosis in a diverse range of cancer cells such as renal cell carcinoma cell line 786-0, mouse lymphoma cells (L5178Y), human prostate carcinoma cells (DU145), human epidermoid carcinoma cells (A431), human nonsmall cell lung carcinoma cell line (A549), human prostate carcinoma cells (LNCaP), human myelogenous leukemia (HL-60) cell line, HepG2, and MCF7 cell line.

EGCG is reported to induce apoptosis through multiple mechanisms. The tea polyphenol inhibited the expression of antiapoptotic Bcl-2 and Bcl-XL and induced the expression of proapoptotic Bax, Bak, Bcl-XS, and PUMA followed by caspase 3 activation [57] in various cancer cells [58]. EGCG-induced apoptosis in tumor cells may be mediated through NF-κB inactivation [59] and stabilization of p53 [60], which decreases the expression of Bcl-2 [61]. Many recent studies demonstrated that EGCG induced apoptosis through generation of ROS and caspase 3 and caspase 9 activation [62].

Curcumin has been reported to induce apoptosis by activation of extrinsic and intrinsic pathways of apoptosis. The p53-independent induction of apoptosis by curcumin in human melanoma cells through the Fas receptor/caspase 8 pathway was demonstrated for the first time by Bush et al. [63]. There are also several reports of curcumin-induced modulation of proteins involved in the intrinsic pathway of apoptosis such as upregulation of Bax, Bim, Bak, Puma, and Noxa; downregulation of the antiapoptotic proteins Bcl-2 and Bcl-xL; increase in caspase 3 level; and release of cytochrome c, leading to apoptosis in cancer cells [64]. Generation of oxidative stress and increased endoplasmic reticulum stress in transformed cells have also been implicated in the induction of apoptosis by curcumin [65, 66]. Moreover, curcumin is reported to be a strong inhibitor of NF-κB and potentiates TNF-induced apoptosis [67].

Like curcumin, resveratrol has been reported to induce apoptosis in vitro and in vivo by activating both extrinsic and intrinsic pathways of cell death machinery [52] and inhibiting the activity of NF-κB [68]. Resveratrol was shown to sensitize various cancer cells to TNF-related apoptosis-inducing ligand (TRAIL)-dependent cell death via stimulation of both death receptors (TRAIL/DR4 and TRAIL-R2/DR5) and mitochondrial apoptotic signaling pathways [69]. One study demonstrated that resveratrol induces apoptosis in prostate cancer cells through inhibition of the PI3K/Akt and mTOR pathway and activation of FOXO transcription factors that play important roles in regulation of cell cycle and apoptosis [70].

Genistein regulates multiple regulatory factors to modulate apoptosis. It is reported to activate the ATM/p53-p21$^{wafl\ cipl}$cross-talk regulatory network, which is implicated in apoptosis [71]. Increased Bax:Bcl-2 ratio; mitochondrial release of cytochrome c; and activation of caspase 9, caspase 12, and caspase 3 has been implicated in the induction of apoptosis by genistein [72]. Genistein is also reported to upregulate TNF-α, FasL, TRADD, and FADD and activate caspase 8, thereby triggering the extrinsic apoptotic pathway

[73]. The soy isoflavone has also been reported to be a potent inhibitor of pro-survival signaling pathways such as the NF-κB and Akt pathways [74].

Laboratory investigations have shown that quercetin generates intracellular ROS and induces apoptosis through controlling the AMPK/ASK1 pathway and inhibition of the mTOR pathway in p53 mutant cells [75, 76]. Aalinkeel et al. [77] reported that quercetin-induced apoptosis in prostate cancer cells is characterized by downregulation of the expression of Hsp90 while exerting no quantifiable effect on normal prostate epithelial cells.

10.3.2   TERPENOIDS AND CAROTENOIDS

Monoterpenes like carvacrol, a major component of oregano and thyme essential oils, induced colon cancer cell apoptosis in a dose-dependent manner. At the molecular level, carvacrol downregulated the expression of Bcl-2 and upregulated the expression of Bax and c-Jun N-terminal kinase78. Linalool, the active component of coriander, and anethole (active component of anise and fennel) have also been reported to induce apoptosis in vitro and in vivo in sarcom-180 cancer cells [79, 80]. Geraniol potently induced apoptosis and autophagy. At the molecular level, geraniol inhibited Akt signaling and activated AMPK signaling, resulting in mTOR inhibition [81]. Perillyl alcohol was shown to induce apoptosis in a wide variety of cancer cell lines including human glioblastoma cell lines (U87 and A172) and a primary cell culture derived from a human glioblastoma tumor specimen (GBM-1) [82].

Two main natural carotenoids of the spice saffron, crocin and crocetin, have potent antitumor effects both in vitro and in vivo [83]. Crocin has been reported to induce apoptosis in several cancer cell lines such as human pancreatic cancer cell line (BxPC-3) [84], human gastric adenocarcinoma AGS cells [83], and so on. Lutein, as well as all-trans-retinoic acid, induced apoptosis in SV-40-transformed mammary cells and MCF-7 human mammary carcinoma cells [86].

Carotenoids are reported to induce apoptosis by both intrinsic and extrinsic pathways of apoptosis. Apoptosis induced by β-carotene was characterized by chromatin condensation and nuclear fragmentation, DNA degradation, PARP cleavage, and caspase 3 activation [34]. β-Carotene has been postulated to act as a pro-oxidant and increase intracellular ROS, which may be responsible for mitochondrial dysfunction and cytochrome c release [87]. One study suggested that ROS-mediated loss of Ku pro-

teins might be the underlying mechanism for β-carotene-induced apoptosis in gastric cancer AGS cells [88]. β-carotene can regulate apoptosis by
other mechanisms also. For e.g., one study suggested that nuclear loss of
ATM may be the underlying mechanism of beta-carotene-induced apoptosis of gastric cancer cells [89]. Another important carotenoid, lycopene,
has been investigated for its capability to induce apoptosis in lung [90],
colon [91], prostate [92], and mammary cancer cells [93]. Most mechanistic studies on lycopene-induced apoptosis have been done with prostate
cancer cells, which suggests that lycopene reduces mitochondrial transmembrane potential and induced the release of mitochondrial cytochrome
c. Lycopene has also been reported to induce apoptosis in LNCaP prostate
cancer and MDA-MB-468- triple negative breast cancer cells by decreasing phosphorylation of Akt and increasing the apoptotic Bax and antiapoptotic Bcl-2 ratio. Lycopene can also block growth factor-mediated
antiapoptotic signals by directly inhibiting growth factor receptor binding
or by inhibiting downstream components of the PI3K–Akt–mTOR pathway [94].

10.3.3   ALKALOIDS

Black pepper (*Piper nigrum*), a very widely used spice that is known for its
pungent piperidine alkaloid constituent, piperine, is known to inhibit growth
of cancer cells and has been shown to induce apoptosis in a vast array of
cancer cells such as triple-negative breast cancer cells [95], HRT-18 rectal
cancer cells [96], A549 lung cancer cells [97], melanoma SK MEL 28 cells,
B16 F0 cells [98], etc. Capsaicin, a pungent phytochemical in a variety of
red peppers of the genus *Capsicum*, trigger apoptosis in several types of
human cancer cells, including breast cancer and gastric cancer [99, 100].
Similarly, long-term exposure to capsaicin for 36–72 hours also produces
robust apoptosis in nonsmall cell lung cancer (NSCLC), T-cell leukemia,
esophageal carcinoma, astroglioma, and prostate and colon cancer cells in
cell culture models [101].

A well-known dietary alkaloid, caffeine (purine alkaloid), found abundantly in cocoa beans, coffee beans, cola nuts, and tea leaves, has been reported
to exert anticancer effect through induction of apoptosis in a large number of
cancer cells such as U251 cells (human glioma cell line) [102], HTB182 and
CRL5985 lung cancer cells [103], human H358 cell line [104], etc.

Another dietary alkaloid, berberine (isoquinoline alkaloid), has been reported to cause significant apoptosis in human glioblastoma T98G cells [105], androgen-sensitive LNCaP and androgen-insensitive DU145 prostate cancer cells, human epidermoid carcinoma A431 cells [106], human breast cancer MCF7 cell line [107], etc.

Treatment with all the alkaloids discussed above has been shown to promote apoptosis through a mitochondria-dependent pathway by increasing the levels of cytoplasmic cytochrome c, caspase 3 and caspase 9 activity and cleavage of PARP along with elevated ratio of Bax/Bcl-2 [95, 108–111]. Additionally, mechanisms that induce the intrinsic apoptotic pathway are also being elucidated for the alkaloids. For e.g., caffeine-induced apoptosis has also been found to be mediated by an increase in the expression of FoxO1 and its proapoptotic target Bim [102]. Piperine was found to inhibit survival-promoting Akt activation in cancer cells [95]. Generation of ROS has also been implicated to play a vital role in piperine-mediated apoptosis [96]. A recent study has shown a direct link between ROS generation and Chk-1 activation through DNA damage, leading to G1 cell cycle arrest and apoptosis [98]. The apoptotic activity of capsaicin has been found to be mediated via the transient receptor potential vanilloid (TRPV) receptors (specifically TRPV1 and 6) in cancer cells. Binding to the TRPV receptors induced the stimulation of both extrinsic and intrinsic pathways of apoptosis [101].

10.3.4 ORGANOSULFUR COMPOUNDS

Organosulfurs such as diallyl sulfide (DAS), diallyl disulfide (DADS), diallyl trisulfide (DATS), SAMC, and S-allyl cysteine (SAC), which are mostly found in *Allium* vegetables, induce apoptosis in a variety of cancer cell lines such as SW480 human colon cancer cells, PC-3 and DU145 human prostate cancer cells, T24 human bladder cancer cells, human acute myeloid leukemia cells (HL-60), lung carcinoma cells (A549), human breast cancer cells (MCF-7), HepG2 hepatoma cells, and so on. Many studies have also reported the proapoptotic activity of allicin in human ovarian cells (SKOV3) and in human glioblastoma multiforme cells (U87MG) and that of ajoene in HL-60 cells [112].

The majority of organosulfur compounds activate the so-called intrinsic or mitochondria-mediated pathway in the execution of apoptosis, which involves loss of mitochondrial membrane potential and release of apopto-genic molecules from the mitochondria to the cytosol. SAMC and DADS bind to tubulin directly, suppress microtubule dynamics and disrupt microtu-bule assembly, interfere with mitotic spindle formation, arrest cells in mito-sis, and trigger signaling pathways that lead to apoptosis [113]. Experimental evidence support a critical role of ROS as an intermediary of organosulfur compound-induced apoptosis [112].

10.4 INHIBITION OF CELLULAR PROLIFERATION BY DIETARY PHYTOCHEMICALS

Uncontrolled cell proliferation is a hallmark of cancer. Unregulated prolifer-ation of cells is the fundamental abnormality that results in the development of cancer. This is associated with altered expression and/or activity of cell cycle-related proteins. In normal cells, there is a delicate balance between growth promoting signals and growth inhibitory signals. Cancer cells, how-ever, are self-sufficient to generate their own growth signals (e.g., mitogen-activated protein kinase (MAPK), Ras/Raf/MEK/ERK and PI3K/PTEN/Akt signaling cascades) and become insensitive to antigrowth signals (e.g., p53, phosphatase and tensin homolog (PTEN), retinoblastoma protein (Rb), lead-ing to their uncontrolled proliferation [114]. Overwhelming evidence from experiments suggest the antiproliferative effects of phytochemicals, indicat-ing their ability to inhibit the growth of several types of cancers.

10.4.1 POLYPHENOLS

Several studies have elucidated the antiproliferative activity of polyphe-nols in vitro and in vivo. Some prominent polyphenols such as the poly-hydroxylated flavonoid quercetin [5], the major green tea catechin EGCG [115–119], the polyphenolic phytoalexin resveratrol [120], curcumin [121], and soy isoflavones genistein and biochanin A [122, 123] exerted potent growth inhibitory effects on several malignant tumor cells such as HeLa cells, gastric cancer cells (HGC-27, NUGC-2, MKN-7, and MKN-28), colon cancer cells (COLO 320 DM, HCT-116, and SW-480), human breast cancer MDA-MB-231 cells, prostate cancer cells PC-3, human epidermoidal can-cer (A431), human liver cancer cells (HepG2), melanoma cell lines (C32, G-361, and WM 266-4), and human pancreatic cancer cells. Haddad et al.

have screened a representative subgroup of 26 flavonoids for antiproliferative effect on the human PCa (LNCaP and PC3), breast cancer (MCF-7), and normal prostate stromal cell lines (PrSC), and the majority of these flavonoids showed potent antiproliferative activity [124]. The effect of eight polyphenols (quercetin, chrysin, apigenin, emodin, aloe-emodin, rhein, cis-stilbene, and trans-stilbene) was studied on cell proliferation, cell cycle, and apoptosis in four lymphoid and four myeloid leukemic cells lines, together with normal hematopoietic control cells [125].

Attenuation of the activity of various tyrosine kinase pathways such as the PI3K/Akt/mTOR pathway, EGFR tyrosine kinase, focal adhesion kinase (FAK), STAT3, and the MAPK pathway has been suggested to be a distinct mechanism underlying the action of majority of the polyphenols (quercetin, genistein, resveratrol, curcumin, EGCG, myricetin, kaempferol, anthocyanidins, etc.) on tumor cell proliferation [5, 125–131].

Antiproliferative effects of many dietary polyphenols (curcumin, EGCG, resveratrol, and genistein) is also mediated by regulating the two important and interlinked signaling pathways, viz., Wnt/β-catenin and NF-κB signaling [129, 131–134].

In addition, there are also other mechanisms employed by various phytochemicals to inhibit cell proliferation. For e.g., EGCG impairs cell signaling via effects on membrane lipids [135], induces $G_0 G_1$ cell cycle arrest via increasing the expression of p21, p18, and p53; and reduces the expression of cyclins D1 and E as well as cyclin-dependent kinase CDK-2, 4, and 6 [127, 136]. EGCG showed antiproliferative activity against HeLa cells through depolymerization of cellular microtubule. EGCG also prevented the reformation of the cellular microtubule network distorted by cold treatment and inhibited polymerization of tubulin in a cell-free system [137]. EGCG has also been shown to bind to both estrogen receptor alpha (ERα) and estrogen receptor beta (ERβ) and to inhibit proliferation of the estrogen-sensitive MCF-7 breast cancer cell line [138, 139].

Resveratrol upregulates the expression of PTEN and decreases the phosphorylation of Akt1/2 [128, 132]. Resveratrol was also found to inhibit translation of fatty acid synthase (FASN) in HER2-positive breast cancer [140].

The antiproliferative effects of curcumin is accompanied by the inhibition of signaling proteins, including transcription factors (activator protein-1 and early growth response-1), cytokines such as tumor necrosis factor, cell cycle proteins such as cyclin D, cell surface adhesion molecules, as well as cyclooxygenase 2, nitric oxide synthase, matrix metalloproteinase-9, urinary plasminogen activator, and so on [129].

Genistein has been found to inhibit cell proliferation by promoting tumor suppressor FOXO3 activity, thereby promoting FOXO3 interaction with mutated p53, leading to increased expression of the p27kip1 cell cycle inhibitor [130]. Biochanin-A has been reported to mediate its antiproliferative activity by preventing phosphorylation and degradation of IκBα, thereby blocking NF-κB activation, which in turn leads to decreased expression of iNOS, thus inhibiting proliferation [123].

10.4.2 TERPENOIDS AND CAROTENOIDS

Dietary isoprenic derivatives such as carotenoids, retinoids, perillyl alcohol, limonene, geraniol, farnesol, etc. have been demonstrated to interfere with cell proliferation by modulating molecular targets including Rho, nuclear receptors, c-myc, connexin43, NF-κB, and Nrf2 [141]. The monoterpene perillyl alcohol inhibits cell proliferation by impairing the Ras-Raf-MEK-ERK pathway in U87 and U343 glioblastoma cells [142]. Inhibition of isoprenylation of prenylated proteins such as Ras by monoterpenes might account for the antitumor activity of some monoterpenes [143].

Several triterpenoids have been shown to exert antiproliferative effect against a number of cancer cells. The inhibition of STAT3 leading to the suppression of gene products involved in proliferation (cyclin D1) and survival (Bcl-2, Bcl-xL, and Mcl-1) has been proposed to be the antiproliferative mechanism of action of the triterpenoids [144, 145].

An investigation conducted by Kotake-Nara et al. [146] to examine the cytotoxicity of 15 different carotenoids in prostate cancer cell lines found that cell viability was significantly reduced by acyclic carotenoids and the most potent antiproliferative carotenoid was lycopene. Another study demonstrated that beta-carotene significantly suppressed cell viability and cell proliferation and thus significantly reduced the growth of three different prostate cancer cell lines, namely PC-3, Du 145, and LNCaP [147]. Beta-carotene and lycopene inhibited the growth of both estrogen-receptor (ER)-positive MCF-7 and ER-negative Hs578T/MDA-MB-231 human breast cancer cells [148]. Studies have shown that lycopene is a more potent inhibitor of cancer cell proliferation than other carotenoids like alpha-carotene or beta-carotene [149]. Studies have demonstrated that lycopene inhibits the growth of different types of human cancers including prostate, breast, and lung cancer [150].

According to Hirsh et al. [151], carotenoids, including lycopene, suppress malignant cell proliferation by inhibition of estrogen activity of 17-β-estradiol in hormone-dependent cancerous cells. The ability of lycopene to inhibit DNA synthesis, reduce the expression of cell cycle regulatory proteins such as cyclins (cyclin D1 and E) and cyclin-dependent kinases 2 and 4, and suppress insulin-like growth factor (IGF-1) accounts for its inhibitory effect on cell proliferation [152].

Yang et al. [153] showed that lycopene induced activation of the PPARγ-LXRα-ABCA1 pathway was associated with its anti-proliferative effects in LNCaP cells.

Inhibition of telomerase has also been recently suggested to be a novel mechanism of anticancer activity of some carotenoids like lycopene and crocin [154, 155].

10.4.3 ALKALOIDS

Prominent dietary alkaloids like the piperidine alkaloid piperine and the isoquinoline alkaloids berberine and papaverine have been reported to exhibit antitumor activities in vitro and in vivo. Piperine inhibited the proliferation of osteosarcoma HOS and U2OS cells [156]; SW480 and HT-29 cells [157]; human prostate cancer DU145, PC-3 and LNCaP cells [158]; triple-negative breast cancer (TNBC) cells; and TNBC xenografts in immunodeficient mice [159]. The antiproliferative effect of berberine has been tested in A431 cells [160], PANC-1 and MiaPaca-2 pancreatic cancer cells, PDAC tumor xenografts [161], LnCaP and PC-3 human prostate cancer cells [162], mouse (IMCE) and human (HT-29) colon tumor cells and HT-29 cell xenograft model [163], primary effusion lymphoma [164], and so on. Papaverine has been reported to inhibit cell proliferation in HepG2 hepatocarcinoma cells [165] and MCF-7 and MDA-MB-231 cell lines [166].

Inhibition of DNA synthesis, mTORC1 activity, ERK activation, and the EGFR signaling pathway have been proposed to be responsible for the suppression of mitogenic signaling in PDAC cells by berberine treatment [161, 162]. Furthermore, another study showed that EGFR inactivation by berberine was mediated by the activation of ubiquitin ligase Cbl and Cbl's interaction with EGFR, followed by EGFR ubiquitinylation and downregulation in the presence or absence of EGF treatment [163].

Induction of cell cycle arrest [164], suppression of Wnt/β-catenin signaling [167], and that of NF-κB activity [164] are also some other possible mechanisms of antiproliferative activity of berberine. Inhibition of telomerase activity by berberine and papaverine is also reported [165].

Various mechanisms like causing cell cycle arrest at G2/M and G_0/G1 (accompanied by decreased expression of corresponding cyclins such as cyclin B1, cyclin D, and cyclin A and increased phosphorylation of CDK-1 and checkpoint kinase 2 (Chk2) have been documented upon piperine treatment [158]. Moreover, the level of p21 (Cip1) and p27 (Kip1) was increased dose-dependently by piperine treatment [156, 168]. In addition, piperine treatment also inhibited phosphorylation of Akt and interfered with the c-Jun N-terminal kinase (c-JNK) and p38 mitogen-activated protein kinase (MAPK) signaling pathways [157, 169].

10.4.4   ORGANOSULFUR COMPOUNDS

In vitro and in vivo studies have reported that organosulfur compounds are able to suppress the proliferation of various tumor cells [170]. Studies have shown that the various organosulfur compounds can suppress cancer cell proliferation by inducing cell cycle arrest, mainly in the G2/M phase. DADS-mediated time- and dose-dependent G2/M phase arrest was demonstrated for the first time by Milner and colleagues and was found to be accompanied by decreased kinase activity of CDK1/cyclin B complex, reduction in complex formation between CDK1 and cyclin B, and a decrease in the Cdc25C protein level [171]. It has also been postulated that these dietary phytochemicals might inhibit the cell division cycle (Cdc) 25 phosphatases, which are crucial enzymes of the cell cycle progression [172]. More recent studies have revealed that DATS-mediated cell cycle arrest is linked to c-JNK- dependent generation of ROS [173]. The antiproliferative effect of organosulfur compounds has been proposed to be dependent on the allyl and sulfur groups, i.e., as the number of sulfur atoms in the lipid compounds increased, so did their ability to suppress cell proliferation [174].

10.5   INHIBITING ANGIOGENESIS BY DIETARY PHYTOCHEMICALS

Angiogenesis, the development of new blood vessels from pre-existing ones, is essential for tumor growth and metastasis. Therefore, suppression of angiogenesis constitutes an important target for the control of tumor progression [175]. The angiogenic process is tightly controlled by a delicate balance between pro- and antiangiogenic factors. Examples of some pro-angiogenic factors are i) growth factors such as vascular endothelial growth factor (VEGF), basic fibroblast growth factor (FGF), platelet-derived growth factor (PDGF), epidermal growth factor (EGF), and their receptors and ii) transcription factors such as NF-κB and hypoxia-inducible factor-1α (HIF-1α) [176], etc. Some endogenous antiangiogenic factors are angiostatin, endostatin, thrombospondin, etc. A great deal of evidence suggests that chemopreventive phytochemicals can target and modulate different mechanistic aspects of the angiogenesis process [177].

10.5.1 POLYPHENOLS

Flavonoids including green tea catechins (EGCG, epigallocatechin (EGC), and epicatechin-gallate (ECG)), quercetin, genistein, apigenin, anthocyanidins, kaempferol, luteolin, etc. have been found to inhibit angiogenesis in vitro and in vivo [178]. Other polyphenols, namely resveratrol and curcumin, have also been found to suppress tumor angiogenesis [179–181].

Polyphenols, namely resveratrol, delphinidin, genistein, diadzein, apigenin, and curcumin, exert their antiangiogenic effect mainly by downregulation of the angiogenic factors (VEGF) and upregulation of tissue inhibitor metalloproteinases (TIMP)-1, which lead to reduction of tumor cell invasion and blood vessel growth [182–184]. In addition, EGCG inhibits receptor tyrosine kinase signaling including VEGF and ERK1/2 signaling and suppresses VEGF promoter activity and protein expression in colon carcinoma HT29 cells. Catechin-3-gallate and epicatechin-3-gallate also possess similar activities [184]. The flavonoid luteolin inhibits VEGF-induced phosphorylation of PI3K, leading to the inhibition of HUVEC survival and proliferation [185]. Curcumin and genistein suppress TGF-β induced expression of VEGF in human HT-1080 fibrosarcoma [186]. Resveratrol, genistein, and apigenin are found to decrease the expression of HIF-1 [187]. Apigenin inhibited the expression of HIF-1 and VEGF via the PI3K/Akt/p70S6K1 and HDM2/p53 pathways [188, 189]. A recent study has shown that resveratrol at lower concentrations stimulates proliferation and protects human umbilical vein endothelial cells (HUVECs) against spontaneous apoptosis by suppressing endogenous PKG kinase activity and decreasing the expression of cell-survival proteins [190].

10.5.2   TERPENOIDS AND CAROTENOIDS

The monoterpene perillyl alcohol, which has been experimentally proven to have cancer chemopreventive activity, has been reported to interfere with the angiogenic process also. It prevented new blood vessel growth in the in vivo chicken embryo chorioallantoic membrane assay and also effectively inhibited differentiation of endothelial cells into capillary-like networks. Perillyl alcohol was observed to downregulate VEGF expression in cancer cell lines and upregulate the release of Ang2 from endothelial cells [191]. Lupeol, an important dietary triterpenoid, has also been shown to target angiogenesis by transcriptional modulation of angiogenic genes like MMP-2 and MMP-9, HIF-1α, VEGFA, and Flt-1 [192].

Antiangiogenic activity has been proposed to be one of the putative anticancer actions of lycopene in several in vitro and in vivo studies. The carotenoid has been found to inhibit in vitro angiogenesis in HUVECs as well as in rat aortic rings at physiological concentrations [193, 194]. Chorioallantoic membrane assay and matrigel plug assay in mice demonstrated the antiangiogenic effect of lycopene in vivo [195]. These studies have shown that lycopene inhibited invasion, migration, and tubule formation in HUVECs. Moreover, it has also been reported that reduction of tumor growth by high-dose lycopene treatment is accompanied by decreased circulating levels of VEGF [196]. Zu et al. [197] has hypothesized that the consumption of a diet rich in lycopene-containing foods reduces the aggressive potential of prostate cancer by inhibiting the neoangiogenesis that occurs in tumor development.

The antiangiogenic property of lycopene is evident from its inhibitory effect on the activities of MMP-2, urokinase-type plasminogen activator, and expression of Rac1. Lycopene also enhances the expression of inhibitors of angiogenesis such as TIMP-2 and plasminogen activator inhibitor-1. Moreover, lycopene has also been found to attenuate VEGF receptor-2 (VEGFR2)-mediated phosphorylation of extracellular signal-regulated kinase (ERK), p38, and Akt as well as protein expression of PI3K [198]. In addition to VEGF and MMPs, a recent study has also reported the significant reduction of (HIF)-1α and CD-31 by lycopene-enriched tomato extract in N-nitrosodiethylamine (NDEA)-induced hepatocellular carcinoma [199].

Contrary to the role of lycopene in angiogenesis, previous studies indicate that β-carotene has proangiogenic activity [200, 201], which can be related to the potent activation of chemotaxis and changes in the expression of genes mediating cell adhesion and matrix assembly in HUVECs. The downregulation of cellular adhesion molecules such as VCAM-1, ICAM, and selectin E by β-carotenoids in human aortic endothelium stimulated with IL-β1 was suggested to be responsible for the modulatory effect on inflammatory response [202] and may reflect the anti-inflammatory, protective effect of β-carotenoids on endothelium [200].

10.5.3   ALKALOIDS

Piperine and capsaicin are reported to inhibit angiogenesis by modulating different aspects of the angiogenic process, including proliferation, migration, and tubule formation in HUVECs. Both the alkaloids also inhibited in vivo angiogenesis [203, 204]. The mechanism of action of piperine has been shown to be the inhibition of phosphorylation of Ser 473 and Thr 308 residues of Akt (protein kinase B), which is a key regulator of endothelial cell function and angiogenesis [203] and that of capsaicin involves blocking the downstream events of VEGF-induced KDR/Flk-1 signaling, such as activation of p38 mitogen-activated protein kinase and p125 FAK tyrosine phosphorylation, which are requisite for the mitogenic activity of VEGF in endothelial cells. However, its molecular target is distinct from the VEGF receptor KDR/Flk-1 per se [204].

Berberine is known to reduce tumor-induced angiogenesis *in vitro* and *in vivo* [205–207]. The alkaloid was found to inhibit the capability of HCC to stimulate HUVEC's proliferation, migration, and endothelial tubule formation [208]. Berberine is also found to induce the degradation of HIF-1 [187]. It has been hypothesized that the antiangiogenic activity of berberine is mainly mediated through the inhibition of various proinflammatory and proangiogenic factors and the major ones are HIF, VEGF, COX-2, NO, NF-κB, and proinflammatory cytokines [205, 206].

10.5.4   ORGANOSULFUR COMPOUNDS

Isothiocyanates, found abundantly in cruciferous vegetables, have been reported to exert antiangiogenic effect in vivo and in vitro. Both allyl isothiocyanate (AITC) and phenyl isothiocyanate (PITC) significantly inhibited endothelial cell proliferation, survival, migration, invasion, and tubule formation in vitro [209, 210]. Studies have shown that reduction in tumor growth in mice is mediated by the antiangiogenic activity of isothiocyanates [211, 212]. Both the thiocyanates were found to significantly suppress VEGF secretion and cause downregulation of VEGF receptors [210, 212]. Apart from modulating serum VEGF, AITC and PITC are suggested to act as angiogenesis inhibitors through downregulation of proinflammatory cytokines such as IL-1β, IL-6, GM-CSF, and TNF-α and upregulation of IL-2 and TIMP [209]. Additionally, downregulation of serum NO and TNF-α level (which is a mediator of NO synthesis) by AITC and PITC in angiogenesis-induced animals has been proposed to contribute to their antiangiogenic activity [213]. Sulforaphane and aliphatic isothiocyanate present in cruciferous vegetables decrease newly formed microcapillaries in vitro in HMEC1 (an immortalized human microvascular endothelial cell line) and also inhibits hypoxia-induced transcription of VEGF, HIF-1α, and c-myc along with the suppression of VEGF receptor KDR/flk1 and MMP-2 [214, 215].

Organosulfur compounds found in *Allium* vegetables, such as allin and allyl sulfides, have also been reported to inhibit migration and capillary-like tube formation in HUVECs as well as cause inhibition of *ex vivo* neovascularization in chick chorioallantoic membrane assay [216]. The antiangiogenic effects of alliin were mediated partly by increase in cellular nitric oxide and p53 expression [217] and that of DATS correlated with the suppression of VEGF secretion, downregulation of VEGF receptor-2, and inactivation of Akt [218].

10.6   INHIBITING CELL MIGRATION AND INVASION BY DIETARY PHYTOCHEMICALS

Invasive capacity of a cancer cell is the single most important trait that distinguishes benign from malignant lesions [219]. The abilities of tumor cells to invade the host and to induce endothelial cell invasion and neovascularization are central to malignant progression. During the metastatic cascade, changes in cell-cell and cell-matrix adhesion are of paramount importance. The metastatic cascade is therefore dependent on the loss of adhesion between cells, which results in the dissociation of the cell from the primary tumor, and subsequently the ability of the cell to attain a motile phenotype via changes in cell to matrix interaction. Matrix metalloproteinases (MMPs) are an important component of cell invasion that are capable of degrading a range of extracellular matrix proteins, thereby allowing cancer cells to migrate and invade. It is now increasingly recognized that these processes–

cell motility and invasion–might provide a rich source of novel targets for cancer therapy and that appropriate inhibitors may restrain both metastasis and neoangiogenesis [220]. The potential inhibitory effect of phytochemicals on cancer cell invasion and metastasis is being increasingly explored by the scientific community [221].

10.6.1 POLYPHENOLS

Dietary treatment of grape polyphenols (resveratrol, quercetin, and catechin) in nude mice, injected with MDA-MB-435 bone metastatic variant, inhibited metastatic mammary tumor progression to bone and liver [222]. The mechanism by which resveratrol inhibits invasion and metastasis has been shown to be mediated by regulating a long non-coding RNA-MALAT1, which in turn alters the nuclear localization of β-catenin, resulting in lowered Wnt/β-catenin signaling and eventual decrease in expression of several target genes known to play a pivotal role in invasion and metastasis, such as c-myc and MMP-7 [223]. Inhibition of NF-κB activation and subsequent downregulation of the expression of MMP-2 and MMP-9 have also been reported to be responsible for resveratrol-induced reduced migratory and invasive abilities of A549 lung cancer cells [224].

The inhibitory effect of curcumin on metastasis and invasion of different types of cancers such as melanoma, breast, prostate, lung, etc. has been reported in a number of studies [225, 226]. Mechanistically, curcumin has been shown to interrupt an important positive feedback loop between the inflammatory cytokines CXCL1 and -2 and NF-κB that is responsible for the activation of several mediators of metastasis [227]. Additionally, a novel mechanism involving the induction of DnaJ-like heat shock protein 40, HLJ1, by curcumin, through activation of the c-Jun NH_2-kinase (JNK)/JunD pathway, thereby modulating E-cadherin expression, has been suggested to inhibit lung cancer cell invasion and metastasis [228].

Several other dietary polyphenols such as quercetin [229], luteolin [230], genistein [231], apigenin, catechin gallate [232], etc., were also found to inhibit cancer migration and invasion by influencing the level of MMPs in different ways [6]. Interestingly, the inhibitory effect on MMP-2 and MMP-9 was positively correlated with the number of hydroxyl groups in the flavonoids [233].

10.6.2   TERPENOIDS AND CAROTENOIDS

Perillyl alcohol treatment has been reported to significantly inhibit cell invasion and migration in hepatoma cells (HepG2, SMMC-7721, and MHCC97H), murine glial C6 cells [234]. The mechanism of action includes decreasing the activity of the Notch signaling pathway and increasing E-cadherin expression regulated by Snail [235].

Several studies have demonstrated that carotenoids, including lycopene, β-carotene, and α-carotene, exhibits antimetastatic effects [236–238]. Additionally, at the same concentration, lycopene was found to be more effective than β-carotene in reducing cell invasion [239]. The antimigration and anti-invasion activities of lycopene against SK-Hep-1cells are associated with its induction of the antimetastatic gene *nm23-H1* [239]. In addition, Kozuki et al. [237] suggested that the antioxidative property of lycopene may partly explain its anti-invasive action.

10.6.3   ALKALOIDS

Piperine has been reported to inhibit lung metastasis of B16F-10 melanoma cells in mice [240]. The anti-invasive effects of piperine on fibrosarcoma, osteosarcoma, and 4T1 breast cancer have also been demonstrated in vitro and in vivo [241–243].

The antimetastatic effect of piperine is reported to be mediated by increased expression of TIMP-1/-2 and downregulation of MMP-2/-9/-13 [242, 243]. Furthermore, piperine-mediated suppression of MMP-9 in tumor cells was found to occur through the inhibition of PKCα and ERK phosphorylation and reduction of NF-κB and AP-1 activation [241].

The antimigration and anti-invasion activity of capsaicin has been demonstrated in highly metastatic B16-F10 melanoma cells [244], HuCCT1 cholangiocarcinoma cells [245], prostate tumors [246], and so on. Capsaicin has been proposed to suppress migration and invasion of cancer cells by inhibiting NF-κB p65 via the AMPK-SIRT1 and AMPK-IκBα signaling pathways, leading to subsequent suppression of MMP-9 expression [245]. Moreover, its antimetastatic role has also been correlated with the inhibition of activity of phosphatidylinositol 3-kinase (PI3-K) and its downstream targets Akt and Rac1 [245].

Inhibition of invasion, motility, and filopodia formation in the nasopharyngeal carcinoma cell line 5-8F was observed after treatment with berberine [247]. Berberine has also been reported to suppress in vitro migration and invasion of human SCC-4 tongue squamous cancer cells through inhibition of FAK, IKK, NF-κB, u-PA, and MMP-2 and MMP-9 [248].

10.6.4   ORGANOSULFUR COMPOUNDS

ICAM-1 expression in human umbilical endothelial cells, induced by TNF-α, was found to be inhibited by allicin [249]. Two organosulfur compounds, S-allylcysteine and S-allylmercaptocysteine, isolated from garlic, were found to suppress the invasive potential of androgen-independent prostate cancer cells [250] through restoration of E-cadherin expression. Inhibition of MMP-2 and MMP-9 mRNA and protein expression has been reported to be mediated by AITC in human hepatoma SK-Hep1 cells *in vitro* [251]. The anti-invasiveness and antimetastatic potential of allylsulfides (DADS and DATS) have also been evaluated in many studies [252, 253]. Inhibitory effects of DADS on cell motility and invasiveness were found to be associated with increased tightness of the tight junctions and inhibition of MMP-2 and MMP-9.

10.7   DIETARY PHYTOCHEMICALS AS EPIGENETIC MODULATORS: AN EMERGING AREA OF RESEARCH

Epigenetics refers to heritable but reversible changes in gene expression that do not involve alterations in the DNA sequences [254]. Epigenetic alterations are considered to be promising targets for cancer prevention strategies as they occur early during carcinogenesis and represent potentially initiating events for cancer development [255]. In recent years, "nutri-epigenetics," which focuses on the influence of dietary agents on epigenetic mechanism(s), has emerged as an exciting novel area in epigenetics research [256]. The major epigenetic mechanisms for the regulation of gene expression are DNA methylation, histone modifications, and post-transcriptional gene regulation by non-coding microRNAs.

Evidence suggests that polyphenols such as green tea polyphenols (especially EGCG), curcumin, genistein, resevratrol, quercetin, etc., exert their anticancer effects by correcting epigenetic alterations in cancer cells. All the polyphenols mentioned above have been found to inhibit DNA

methyltransferase (DNMT) to various extents. Inhibition of DNMTs ultimately results in DNA hypomethylation and restoration of tumor suppressor gene expression in cancer cells [256]. Reactivation of the tumor suppressor genes *p21CIP1/WAF1, RARβ, MGMT*, and *p16INK4a* through promoter hypomethylation and active chromatin modifications have been reported after treatment with various polyphenols [256, 257]. Treatment with EGCG has also been shown to mediate demethylation of the *hTERT* promoter, which results in the recruitment of gene repressor complexes, thereby down-regulating hTERT.

Similarly, other phytochemicals like sulforaphane and phenethyl isothiocyanate (PEITC) (components of cruciferous vegetables) has been reported to modulate DNA methylation. Sulforaphane has been shown to downregulate DNMT in cancer cells and cause site-specific CpG demethylation within the first exon of the hTERT gene, leading to telomerase inhibition. PEITC demethylated the hypermethylated promoter of the GSTP1 gene, reactivating GSTP1 in androgen-dependent and androgen-independent prostate cancer cells. Demethylation of GSTP1 promoter has also been observed with lycopene treatment in breast cancer cells [258].

Phytochemicals have been shown to cause histone modification due to their ability to modulate the activity of HATs and HDACs enzymes. Many studies have demonstrated modulation of HDAC activity by EGCG treatment, which led to the re-expression of tumor suppressor genes [257]. Curcumin was also shown to inhibit HDAC activity, which led to decreased activity of NF-κB and Notch1 and inhibition of cell proliferation, cell cycle arrest, and apoptosis [259, 260]. Soy isoflavones like genistein, daidzein, and equol (a daidzein metabolite) also possesses histone modifying activity, leading to reactivation of tumor suppressor genes such as PTEN, p53, p21/waf1/cip1, and p16INK4a [256]. In both in vitro and in vivo studies resveratrol could decrease the acetylation of histone H3K9 by inducing SIRT1 expression and inhibit survivin expression to elicit a profound inhibitory effect on BRCA1 mutant cancer cells. Apart from polyphenols, treatment with organosulfur compounds like DADS was found to result in hyperacetylation of histones, upregulation of p21, arrest of cell cycle, and induction of differentiation and apoptosis in a variety of cancer cell lines. DADS, allyl mercaptan, S-allylmercaptocysteine, or allyl isothiocyanate treatment was also found to decrease HDACs in cancer cells.

Alterations in expression profiles of miRNAs are also mediated by phytochemicals as evident by a number of investigations. Green tea polyphenols were found to modify the expression of miRNAs in various human cancers. The expression of a number of miRNAs was found to be altered with EGCG treatment in various cancer cells such as HepG2, MCF-7, LNCaP, etc. [256]. Similarly, other polyphenols like curcumin, quercetin, genistein, and resveratrol were shown to modulate miRNAs in several cancer cells. These phytochemicals have been demonstrated to downregulate several oncogenic miRNAs (e.g. miR-17, miR-21, miR-25, miR-92a-2. etc.) which are known to be target genes for NF-κB, COX-2, mesenchymal markers such as ZEB1, slug, vimentin, and the key effectors of the TGFβ signaling pathway. Expression of several tumor suppressor miRNAs including the let-7 family members, miR-26a, miR-146a, miR-101, miR-200b/c, etc., have been reported to be induced by the phytochemicals. Although PEITC have been found to prevent the downregulation of miRNAs induced by cigarette smoke, no study on the effect of PEITC on miRNA expression in cancer has been reported so far. However, indole-3-carbinol (I3C), which is also obtained from cruciferous vegetables, was found to increase the expression of epithelial markers and decrease the expression of mesenchymal and proliferative markers by regulating miRNA expression in cancer cells [256, 257].

Other plant phytochemicals that can modify epigenetic events and may have potential to be developed as effective chemopreventive and/or therapeutic agents are under investigation.

10.8   DIETARY PHYTOCHEMICALS IN CLINICAL TRIALS

Among the innumerable phytochemicals that have been studied for their probable anticancer activity, only a few of them are under clinical trials. Based on literature search, curcumin, green tea polyphenols, lycopene, and certain organosulfur compounds have shown promise in clinical settings. In a phase II clinical trial of curcumin, significant tumor regression was observed in curcumin-treated pancreatic cancer patients [261]. Cheng et al. [262] showed that this compound improved histologic parameters in 1 out of 2 patients with resected bladder cancer, 1 out of 6 patients with intestinal metaplasia of the stomach, and 1 out of 4 patients with uterine cervical intraepithelial neoplasm. Consumption of more than five cups of green tea per day by breast cancer patients resulted in lower recurrence rate and a longer disease-free period than patients who consumed fewer than four cups per day [263]. Consumption of green tea catechin capsules inhibited the progression of high-grade prostate intraepithelial neoplasia to cancer [264]. In a phase II trial, 113 men diagnosed with prostate cancer were randomized to consume six cups daily of brewed green tea, black tea (BT), or water (control) prior to radical prostatectomy (RP). Evidence of a systemic antioxidant effect was observed (reduced urinary 8OHdG) with only green tea consumption. Green tea, but not BT or water, also led to a small but statistically significant decrease in serum prostate-specific antigen (PSA) levels [265]. Administration of resveratrol to patients with colorectal adenocarcinoma reduces tumor cell proliferation [266]. In patients with colorectal cancer and hepatic metastases, resveratrol increases caspase 3 in malignant hepatic tissue compared with the tissue from the placebo-treated patients [267]. The results suggest that consumption of resveratrol induces anticarcinogenic effects in the human gastrointestinal tract.

Lycopene supplements reduced tumor size and PSA level in localized prostate cancers, accompanied by downregulation of nuclear translocation of the androgen receptor [268].

10.9   CHALLENGES AND FUTURE DIRECTION

According to the World Cancer Report issued by the International Agency for Research on Cancer (IARC), cancer incidence would increase dramatically by 50% to almost 15 million in the year 2020. Cytotoxic chemotherapies, molecularly targeted drugs, immunotherapies, and hormonal therapies are the major therapeutic options to treat cancer. In spite of the great promise of the molecularly targeted therapies, single-target therapies are not adequate to achieve significant clinical success. Moreover, all these treatment modalities are either extremely toxic or expensive or sometimes both. Thus, cancer continues to mystify clinical treatment efforts, and the search for effective therapies continues. As discussed in the chapter above, a voluminous number of experimental and epidemiological evidence suggests that an increased consumption of fruit and vegetables is a relatively easy and practical strategy to reduce significantly the incidence of chronic diseases such as cancer. Based on these studies of compounds isolated from plants, which were tested for their anticancer activity in vitro and in vivo, it is suggested that phytochemicals present in fruits and vegetables can modulate key cellular signaling pathways that regulate cell proliferation, apoptosis, angiogenesis, cell migration, and invasion, leading to potent anticancer effects. The high potency, low toxicity and cost-effectiveness of phytochemicals as compared to synthetic anticancer agents have made them a compelling alternative treatment strategy against cancer. However, the nontoxic therapeutic effects have not yet been substantiated by clinical trials or in long-term randomized controlled trials. The enthusiasm surrounding the cancer preventive effect of the consumption of fruits and vegetables began to dampen in the late 1990s when the results of large prospective cohort studies of diet and cancer did not confirm the strong inverse associations found in most case–control studies [269]. Nevertheless, a few studies do provide strong evidence in favor of the benefit of fruits and vegetable consumption for some types of cancers [270]. Liu reviewed some investigations showing an inverse relation between cancer risk and consumption of whole foods such as fruits and vegetables. However, the same cancer preventive effect has not been observed for the purifed bioactive phytochemicals [271]. The isolated pure compound either loses its bioactivity or there are issues of poor oral bioavailability of dietary phytochemicals, which have hindered progress in cancer prevention and therapy. For instance, although curcumin is thought to have potent anticancer properties, it is poorly absorbed from the gut, which is coupled with the high degree of its metabolism in the liver and its rapid elimination in the bile, accounting for its poor bioavailability [272]. Therefore, a key question that baffles scientists today is whether a purified phytochemical has the same health benefit as the whole food or a mixture of foods.

Under such a scenario, a new approach to cancer prevention and therapeutics known as the "broad-spectrum" approach, involving combinations of phytochemicals with proven anticancer properties, has been proposed by scientists [273]. However, given the pleiotropic biological effects of phytochemicals, there are several challenges for the translation of phytochemicals to the clinic. For e.g., the selection of an appropriate dose, which must be based on the trade-off between efficacy and toxicity, is an important issue. The choice of the stage of carcinogenesis most effectively targeted by phytochemicals is also a concern. Moreover, the identification of reliable, clinically valid biomarkers to predict response has been a major challenge. All these factors, in addition to the poor bioavailability and unanticipated side effects of some phytochemicals, are responsible for the limited clinical success in developing phytochemicals as effective anticancer drugs.

However, despite all the challenges and skepticism facing drug discovery from plant origin, phytochemicals from dietary sources remain potential candidates for novel anticancer drugs. There is a wealth of dietary phytochemicals that have shown convincing anticancer property in laboratory animals with potential for clinical translation. Perhaps, a rational design of studies aimed at defining the "right" doses, long-term preclinical studies with realistic concentrations that are achievable in human tissues, a thorough understanding of the compounds and their pharmacological effects, and use of validated surrogate biomarkers to predict treatment outcome would be essential for natural phytochemicals' druggability and their transition from bench top to patients' bedside [274].

10.10 SUMMARY

- Epidemiological studies prove that diet rich in fruits and vegetables have cancer-preventive properties
- Fruits and vegetables are rich sources of different phytochemicals such as polyphenols, terpenoids, alkaloids, organosulfur compounds, etc.
- These phytochemicals can modulate key signaling pathways that regulate cellular processes such as proliferation, apoptosis, angiogenesis, and metastasis.
- Multitargeted therapy is considered to be a more efficient approach in cancer treatment, and therefore, a combination of different phytochemicals can be a novel strategy.
- However, there are several challenges in applying these phytochemicals to human clinical trials, such as their low bioavailability and unpredicted toxicity.

KEYWORDS

- **angiogenesis**
- **anticancer**
- **apoptosis**
- **cell proliferation**
- **dietary phytochemical**
- **metastasis**
- **molecular targets**
- **signaling pathways**

REFERENCES

1. Totelin, L., (2015). When foods become remedies in ancient Greece: The curious case of garlic and other substances. *J. Ethnopharmacol., 167*, 30–37.
2. Michels, K. B., (2003). Nutritional epidemiology--past, present, future. *Int. J. Epidemiol., 32*, 486–488.
3. Donaldron, M. S., (2004). Nutrition and cancer A review of the evidence for an anticancer diet. *Nutrition Journal, 3*, 1–21.
4. World Cancer Research Fund, (2007), American Institute for Cancer Research Food, nutrition, physical activity, & the prevention of cancer: a global perspective Second Expert Report. Washington, DC: AICR.
5. Benetou, V., Orfanos, P., Lagiou, P., Trichopoulos, D., Boffetta, P., & Trichopoulou, A., (2008). Vegetables and fruits in relation to cancer risk: evidence fromthe Greek EPIC cohort study *Cancer Epidemiol. Biomarkers. Prev., 17*, 387–392.
6. Kanadaswami, C., Lee, L., Lee, P. H., Hwang, J., Ke, F. C., Huang, Y. T., & Lee, M. T., (2005). The antitumor activities of flavonoids. *In. Vivo, 19*, 895–910.
7. Key, T. J., Schatzkin, A., Willett, W. C., Allen, N. E., Spencer, E. A., & Travis, R. C., (2004). Diet, nutrition and the prevention of cancer *Public Health Nutr., 7*, 187–200.
8. Pratheeshkumar, P., Sreekala, C., Zhang, Z., Budhraja, A., Ding, S., Son, Y. O., Wang, X., Hitron, A., Hyun-Jung, K., Wang, L., Lee, J. C., & Shi, X., (2012). Cancer prevention with promising natural products: mechanisms of action and molecular targets. *Anticancer Agents Med. Chem., 12*, 1159–1184.
9. Neergheen, V. S., Bahorun, T., Taylor, E. W., Jen, L. S., & Aruoma, O. I., (2010). Targeting specific cell signaling transduction pathways by dietary and medicinal phytochemicals in cancer chemoprevention. *Toxicology., 278*, 229–241.
10. Torre, L. A. Bray, F., Siegel, R. L., Ferlay, J., Lortet-Tieulent, J., & Jemal, A., (2012). Global cancer statistics. *CA. Cancer J. Clin., 65*, 87–108.
11. Metri, K., Bhargav, H., Chowdhury, P., & Koka, P. S., (2013). Ayurveda for chemoradiotherapy induced side effects in cancer patients. *J. Stem. Cells., 8*, 115–129.
12. De Almeida, V. L., Leitao, A., Reina, L. C. B. Montanari, C. A., Donnici, C. L., & Lopes, M. T. P., (2005). Cancer e agentes antineoplásicos especificos e ciclo-celular nao especificos que interagem com o DNA: uma introducao. *Quimica. Nova., 28*, 118–129.
13. De Oliveira, R. B., & Alves, R. J., (2002). Agentes antineoplasicos biorredutiveis: uma nova alternativa para o tratamento de tumores solidos. *Quimica. Nova., 25*, 976–984.
14. Rates, S. M., (2001). Plants as source of drugs. *Toxicon., 39*, 603–613.
15. Gullett, N. P., Ruhul Amin, A. R., Bayraktar, S., Pezzuto, J. M., Shin, D. M., Khuri, F. R., Aggarwal, B. B., Surh, Y. J., & Kucuk, O., (2010). Cancer prevention with natural compounds. *Semin. Oncol., 37*, 258–281.
16. Upadhyay, S., & Dixit, M., (2015). Role of polyphenols and other phytochemicals on molecular signaling. *Oxid. Med. Cell Longev., 504253*.
17. Kris-Etherton, P. M., Hecker, K. D., Bonanome, A., Coval, S. M., Binkoski, A. E., Hilpert, K. F., Griel, A. E., & Etherton, T. D., (2002). Bioactive compounds in foods: their role in the prevention of cardiovascular disease and cancer *Am. J. Med., 113, Suppl.* 9B, 71–88.
18. Demain, A. L., & Fang, A., (2000). The natural functions of secondary metabolites. *Adv. Biochem. Eng. Biotechnol., 69*, 1–39.
19. Rao, S. R., & Ravishankar, G. A., (2002). Plant cell cultures: Chemical factories of secondary metabolites. *Biotechnol. Adv., 20*, 101–153.

20. Wink, M., (2010). Introduction: Biochemistry, physiology and ecological functions of secondary metabolites, in annual plant reviews volume *40*: *Biochemistry of Plant Secondary Metabolism,* second edition (ed. Wink, M.), Wiley-Blackwell, Oxford, UK.

21. Stevenson, D. E., & Hurst, R. D., (2007). Polyphenolic phytochemicals--just antioxidants or much more? *Cell Mol. Life Sci., 64,* 2900–2916.

22. D'Archivio, M., Filesi, C., Di Benedetto, R., Gargiulo, R., Giovannini, C., & Masella, R., (2007). Polyphenols, dietary sources and bioavailability. *Ann. Ist. Super. Sanita., 43,* 348–361.

23. Lotito, S. B., & Frei, B., (2006). Consumption of flavonoid-rich foods and increased plasma antioxidant capacity in humans: cause, consequence, or epiphenomenon? *Free Radic. Biol. Med., 41,* 1727–1746.

24. Zhou, Y., Zheng, J., Li, Y., Xu, D. P., Li, S., Chen, Y. M., & Li, H. B., (2016). Natural polyphenols for prevention and treatment of cancer *Nutrients, 8,* pii: E515.

25. Knekt, P., Kumpulainen, J., Jarvinen, R., Rissanen, H., Heliovaara, M., Reunanen, A., Hakulinen, T., & Aromaa, A., (2002). Flavonoid intake and risk of chronic diseases. *Am. J. Clin. Nutr., 76,* 560–568.

26. Zhong, L., Goldberg, M. S., Gao, Y. T., Hanley, J. A., Parent, M. E., & Jin, F., (2001). A population-based case-control study of lung cancer and green tea consumption among women living in Shanghai, China. *Epidemiology, 12,* 695–700.

27. Hui, C., Qi, X., Qianyong, Z., Xiaoli, P., Jundong, Z., & Mantian, M., (2013). Flavonoids, flavonoid subclasses and breast cancer risk: A meta-analysis of epidemiologic studies. *PLoS One, 8,* e54318. doi:10. 1371/journal.pone. 0054318.

28. Rossi, M., Garavello, W., Talamini, R., La Vecchia, C., Franceschi, S., Lagiou, P., Zambon, P., Dal Maso, L., Bosetti, C., & Negri, E., (2007). Flavonoids and risk of squamous cell esophageal cancer *Int. J. Cancer, 120,* 1560–1564.

29. Bishayee, A., Ahmed, S., Brankov, N., & Perloff, M., (2011). Triterpenoids as potential agents for the chemoprevention and therapy of breast cancer *Front. Biosci. (Landmark Ed), 16,* 980–996.

30. Shojaei, S., Kiumarsi, A., Moghadam, A. R., Alizadeh, J., Marzban, H., & Ghavami, S., (2014). Perillyl alcohol (Monoterpene Alcohol), Limonene. *Enzymes, 36,* 7–32.

31. Chen, T. C., Fonseca, C. O., & Schönthal, A. H., (2015). Preclinical development and clinical use of perillyl alcohol for chemoprevention and cancer therapy. *Am. J. Cancer Res., 5,* 1580–1593.

32. Liu, R. H., (2004). Potential synergy of phytochemicals in cancer prevention: mechanism of action. *J. Nutr., 134,* 3479S–85S.

33. Elisabet, F. G., Irene, C. L., Manuel, J. G., Juan, G. F., Antonio, P. G., & Dámaso, H. M., (2012). Carotenoids bioavailability from foods: From plant pigments to efficient biological activities. *Food Research International, 46,* 438–450.

34. Müller, K., Carpenter, K. L., Challis, I. R., Skepper, J. N., & Arends, M. J., (2002). Carotenoids induce apoptosis in the T-lymphoblast cell line Jurkat E6. 1. *Free. Radic. Res., 36,* 791–802.

35. Kaur, R., & Arora, S., (2015). Alkaloids-important therapeutic secondary metabolites of plant origin. *J. Crit. Rev., 2,* 1–8.

36. Cragg, G. M., & Newman, D. J., (2005). Plants as source of anticancer agents. *J. Ethnopharmacol., 100,* 72–99.

37. Iranshahi, M., (2012). A review of volatile sulfur-containing compounds from terrestrial plants: biosynthesis, distribution and analytical methods. *Journal of Essential Oil Research, 24,* 393–434.

38. Tocmo, R., Liang, D., Lin, Y., & Huang, D., (2015). Chemical and biochemical mechanisms underlying the cardioprotective roles of dietary organopolysulfides. *Frontiers in Nutrition, 2*, 1.

39. Colín-González, A. L., Santana, R. A., Silva-Islas, C. A., Chánez-Cárdenas, M. E. Santamaría, A., & Maldonado, P. D., (2012). The antioxidant mechanisms underlying the aged garlic extract- and S-Allylcysteine-induced protection. *Oxidative Medicine and Cellular Longevity, 2012*, 907162.

40. Holst, B., & Williamson, G., (2004). A critical review of the bioavailability of glucosinolates and related compounds. *Nat. Prod. Rep., 21*, 425–447.

41. Chaffer, C. L., & Weinberg, R. A., (2015). How does multistep tumorigenesis really proceed? *Cancer Discovery, 5*, 22–24.

42. Hanahan, D., & Weinberg, R. A., (2011). Hallmarks of cancer: the next generation. *Cell, 144*, 646–674.

43. Kroemer, G., & Pouyssegur, J., (2008). Tumor cell metabolism: cancer's Achilles' heel. *Cancer Cell, 13*, 472–482.

44. Green, D. R., (2000). Apoptotic pathways: paper wraps stone blunts scissors. *Cell, 102*, 1–4.

45. Szliszka, E., & Krol, W., (2011). The role of dietary polyphenols in tumor necrosis factor-related apoptosis inducing ligand (TRAIL)-induced apoptosis for cancer chemoprevention. *Eur. J. Cancer Prev., 20*, 63–69.

46. Gu, B., Ding, Q., Xia, G., & Fang, Z., (2009). EGCG inhibits growth and induces apoptosis in renal cell carcinoma through TFPI-2 overexpression. *Oncol. Rep., 21*, 635–640.

47. Rahmani, A. H., Al, Shabrmi, F. M., Allemailem, K. S., Aly, S. M., & Khan, M. A., (2015). Implications of green tea and its constituents in the prevention of cancer via the modulation of cell signalling pathway. *Biomed. Res. Int.*, 925640.

48. Singh, B. N., Shankar, S., & Srivastava, R. K., (2011). Green tea catechin, epigallocatechin-3-gallate (EGCG): mechanisms, perspectives and clinical applications. *Biochem. Pharmacol., 82*, 1807–1821.

49. Bush, J. A., Cheung, K. J., & Jr. Li, G., (2001). Curcumin induces apoptosis in human melanoma cells through a Fas receptor/caspase-8 pathway independent of p53. *Exp. Cell Res., 271*, 305–314.

50. Mukhopadhyay, A., Bueso-Ramos, C., Chatterjee, D., Pantazis, P., & Aggarwal, B. B., (2001). Curcumin downregulates cell survival mechanisms in human prostate cancer cell lines. *Oncogene, 20*, 7597–7609.

51. Anto, R. J., Mukhopadhyay, A., Denning, K., & Aggarwal, B. B., (2002). Curcumin (diferuloylmethane) induces apoptosis through activation of caspase-8, BID cleavage and cytochrome c release: its suppression by ectopic expression of Bcl-2 and Bcl-xl. *Carcinogenesis, 23*, 143–150.

52. Fulda, S., & Debatin, K. M., (2006). Resveratrol modulation of signal transduction in apoptosis and cell survival: a mini-review. *Cancer Detect. Prev., 30*, 217–223.

53. Kundu, J. K., & Surh, Y. J., (2008). Cancer chemopreventive and therapeutic potential of resveratrol: mechanistic perspectives. *Cancer Lett., 269*, 243–261.

54. Zhang, J., Su, H., Li, Q., Li, J., & Zhao, Q., (2017). Genistein decreases A549 cell viability via inhibition of the PI3K/Akt/HIF1α/VEGF and NF**κB/COX**2 signaling pathways. *Mol. Med. Rep.,* doi: 10. 3892/mmr. 2017, 6260. [Epub ahead of print].

55. Su, S. J., Chow, N. H., Kung, M. L., Hung, T. C., & Chang, K. L., (2003). Effects of soy isoflavones on apoptosis induction and G2-M arrest in human hepatoma cells in-

volvement of caspase-3 activation, Bcl-2 and Bcl-XL downregulation, & Cdc2 kinase activity. *Nutr. Cancer*, *45*, 113–123.

56. Yamashita, N., & Kawanishi, S., (2000). Distinct mechanisms of DNA damage in apoptosis induced by quercetin and luteolin. *Free Radic. Res., 33*, 623–633.

57. Smith, D. M., Wang, Z., Kazi, A., Li, L. H., Chan, T. H., & Dou, Q. P., (2002). Synthetic analogs of green tea polyphenols as proteasome inhibitors. *Mol. Med., 8*, 382–392.

58. Aggarwal, B. B., & Shishodia, S., (2006). Molecular targets of dietary agents for prevention and therapy of cancer *Biochem. Pharmacol., 71*, 1397–1421.

59. Singh, B. N., Shankar, S., & Srivastava, R. K., (2011). Green tea catechin, epigallocatechin-3-gallate (EGCG): mechanisms, perspectives and clinical applications. *Biochem. Pharmacol., 82*, 1807–1821.

60. Hastak, K., Gupta, S., Ahmad, N., Agarwal, M. K., Agarwal, M. L., & Mukhtar, H., (2003). Role of p53 and NF-kappaB in epigallocatechin-3-gallate-induced apoptosis of LNCaP cells. *Oncogene, 22*, 4851–4859.

61. Fujiki, H., Suganuma, M., Okabe, S., Sueoka, E., Sueoka, N., Fujimoto, N., Goto, Y., Matsuyama, S., Imai, K., & Nakachi, K., (2001). Cancer prevention with green tea and monitoring by a new biomarker, hnRNP B1. *Mutat. Res., 480–481*, 299–304.

62. Shankar, S., Suthakar, G., & Srivastava, R. K., (2007). Epigallocatechin-3-gallate inhibits cell cycle and induces apoptosis in pancreatic cancer *Front. Biosci., 12*, 5039–5051.

63. Bush, J. A., Cheung, Jr. K. J., & Li, G., (2001). Curcumin induces apoptosis in human melanoma cells through a Fas receptor/caspase-8 pathway independent of p53. *Exp. Cell Res., 271*, 305–314.

64. Reuter, S., Eifes, S., Dicato, M., Aggarwal, B. B., & Diederich, M., (2008). Modulation of anti-apoptotic and survival pathways by curcumin as a strategy to induce apoptosis in cancer cells. *Biochem. Pharmacol., 76*, 1340–1351.

65. Atsumi, T., Tonosaki, K., & Fujisawa, S., (2006). Induction of early apoptosis and ROS-generation activity in human gingival fibroblasts (HGF) and human submandibular gland carcinoma (HSG) cells treated with curcumin. *Arch. Oral. Biol., 51*, 913–921.

66. Pae, H. O., Jeong, S. O., Jeong, G. S., Kim, K. M., Kim, H. S., Kim, S. A., Kim, Y. C., Kang, S. D., Kim, B. N., & Chung, H. T., (2007). Curcumin induces pro-apoptotic endoplasmic reticulum stress in human leukemia HL-60 cells. *Biochem. Biophys. Res. Commun., 353*, 1040–1045.

67. Bharti, A. C., Donato, N., Singh, S., & Aggarwal, B. B., (2003). Curcumin (diferuloylmethane) down-regulates the constitutive activation of nuclear factor-kappa B and IkappaBalpha kinase in human multiple myeloma cells, leading to suppression of proliferation and induction of apoptosis. *Blood, 101*, 1053–1062.

68. Estrov, Z., Shishodia, S., Faderl, S., Harris, D., Van, Q., Kantarjian, H. M., Talpaz, M., & Aggarwal, B. B., (2003). Resveratrol blocks interleukin-1beta-induced activation of the nuclear transcription factor NF-kappaB, inhibits proliferation, causes S-phase arrest, & induces apoptosis of acute myeloid leukemia cells. *Blood, 102*, 987–995.

69. Fulda, S., & Debatin, K. M., (2005). Resveratrol-mediated sensitisation to TRAIL-induced apoptosis depends on death receptor and mitochondrial signalling, *Eur. J. Cancer, 41*, 786– 798.

70. Zanella, F., Link, W., & Carnero, A., (2010). Understanding FOXO, new views on old transcription factors. *Curr. Cancer Drug. Targets, 10*, 135–146.

71. Zhang, Z., Wang, C. Z., Du, G. J., Qi, L. W., Calway, T., He, T. C., Du, W., & Yuan, C. S., (2013). Genistein induces G2/M cell cycle arrest and apoptosis via ATM/p53-dependent pathway in human colon cancer cells. *Int. J. Oncol., 43*, 289–296.

72. Das, A., Banik, N. L., & Ray, S. K., (2006). Mechanism of apoptosis with the involvement of calpain and caspase cascades in human malignant neuroblastoma SH-SY5Y cells exposed to flavonoids. *Int. J. Cancer, 119*, 2575–2585.

73. George, J., Banik, N. L., & Ray, S. K., (2010). Genistein induces receptor and mitochondrial pathways and increases apoptosis during BCL-2 knockdown in human malignant neuroblastoma SK-N-DZ cells. *J. Neurosci. Res., 88*, 877–886.

74. Li, Y., & Sarkar, F. H., (2002). Inhibition of nuclear factor kappaB activation in PC3 cells by genistein is mediated via Akt signaling pathway. *Clin. Cancer Res., 8*, 2369–2377.

75. Lee, Y. K., Hwang, J. T., Kwon, D. Y., Surh, Y. J., & Park, O. J., (2010). Induction of apoptosis by quercetin is mediated through AMPKalpha1/ASK1/p38 pathway. *Cancer Lett., 292*, 228–236.

76. Lee, Y. K., Park, S. Y., Kim, Y. M., Lee, W. S., & Park, O. J., (2009). AMP kinase/cyclooxygenase-2 pathway regulates proliferation and apoptosis of cancer cells treated with quercetin. *Exp. Mol. Med., 41*, 201–207.

77. Aalinkeel, R., Bindukumar, B., Reynolds, J. L., Sykes, D. E., Mahajan, S. D., Chadha, K. C., & Schwartz, S. A., (2008). The dietary bioflavonoid, quercetin, selectively induces apoptosis of prostate cancer cells by down-regulating the expression of heat shock protein 90. *Prostate, 68*, 1773–1789.

78. Fan, K., Li, X., Cao, Y., Qi, H., Li, L., Zhang, Q., & Sun, H., (2015). Carvacrol inhibits proliferation and induces apoptosis in human colon cancer cells. *Anticancer Drugs, 26*, 813–823.

79. Jana, S., Patra, K., Sarkar, S., Jana, J., Mukherjee, G., Bhattacharjee, S., & Mandal, D. P., (2014). Antitumorigenic potential of linalool is accompanied by modulation of oxidative stress: an in vivo study in sarcoma-180 solid tumor model. *Nutr. Cancer, 66*, 835–848.

80. Jana, S., Patra, K., Mukherjee, G., Bhattacharjee, S., & Mandal, D. P., (2015). Antitumor potential of anethole singly and in combination with cyclophosphamide in murine Sarcoma-180 transplantable tumor model. *RSC Adv., 5*, 56549–56559.

81. Kim, S. H., Park, E. J., Lee, C. R., Chun, J. N., Cho, N. H., Kim, I. G., Lee, S., Kim, T. W., Park, H. H., So, I., & Jeon, J. H., (2012). Geraniol induces cooperative interaction of apoptosis and autophagy to elicit cell death in PC-3 prostate cancer cells. *Int. J. Oncol., 40*, 1683–1690.

82. Fernandes, J., Da, Fonseca, C. O., Teixeira, A., & Gattass, C. R., (2005). Perillyl alcohol induces apoptosis in human glioblastoma multiforme cells. *Oncol. Rep., 13*, 943–947.

83. Bolhassani, A., Khavari, A., Bathaie, S. Z. (2014) Saffron and natural carotenoids: Biochemical activities and anti-tumor effects. *Biochim . Biophys. Acta, 1845*, 20–30.

84. Bakshi, H., Sam, S., Rozati, R., Sultan, P., Islam, T., Rathore, B., Lone, Z., Sharma, M., Triphati, J., & Saxena, R. C., (2010). DNA fragmentation and cell cycle arrest: a hallmark of apoptosis induced by crocin from kashmiri saffron in a human pancreatic cancer cell line. *Asian Pac. J. Cancer Prev., 11*, 675–679.

85. Hoshyar, R., Bathaie, S. Z., & Sadeghizadeh, M., (2013). Crocin triggers the apoptosis through increasing the Bax/Bcl-2 ratio and caspase activation in human gastric adenocarcinoma, AGS, cells. *DNA Cell Biol., 32*, 50–57.

86. Sumantran, V. N., Zhang, R., Lee, D. S., & Wicha, M. S., (2000). Differential regulation of apoptosis in normal versus transformed mammary epithelium by lutein and retinoic acid. *Cancer Epidemiol. Biomarkers Prev., 9*, 257–263.

87. Cui, Y., Lu, Z., Bai, L., Shi, Z., Zhao, W. E., & Zhao, B., (2007). Beta-Carotene induces apoptosis and up-regulates peroxisome proliferator-activated receptor gamma expres-

sion and reactive oxygen species production in MCF-7 cancer cells. *Eur. J. Cancer, 43,* 2590–2601.

88. Park, Y., Choi, J., Lim, J. W., & Kim, H., (2015). β-Carotene induced apoptosis is mediated with loss of Ku proteins in gastric cancer AGS cells. *Genes Nutr., 10,* 467.

89. Jang, S. H., Lim, J. W., & Kim, H., (2009). Mechanism of beta-carotene-induced apoptosis of gastric cancer cells: involvement of ataxia-telangiectasia-mutated. *Ann. New York Acad. Sci., 1171,* 156–162.

90. Liu, C., Lian, F., Smith, D. E., Russell, R. M., & Wang, X. D., (2003). Lycopene supplementation inhibits lung squamous metaplasia and induces apoptosis via up-regulating insulin-like growth factor-binding protein 3 in cigarette smoke-exposed ferrets. *Cancer Res., 63,* 3138–3144.

91. Teodoro, A. J., Oliveira, F. L., Martins, N. B., Maia Gde, A., Martucci, R. B., & Borojevic, R., (2012). Effect of lycopene on cell viability and cell cycle progression in human cancer cell lines. *Cancer Cell Int., 12,* 36.

92. Ivanov, N. I., Cowell, S. P., Brown, P., Rennie, P. S., Guns, E. S., & Cox, M. E., (2007). Lycopene differentially induces quiescence and apoptosis in androgen-responsive and -independent prostate cancer cell lines. *Clin. Nutr., 26,* 252–263.

93. Takeshima, M., Ono, M., Higuchi, T., Chen, C., Hara, T., & Nakano, S., (2014). Antiproliferative and apoptosis-inducing activity of lycopene against three subtypes of human breast cancer cell lines. *Cancer Sci., 105,* 252–257.

94. Ono, M., Takeshima, M., & Nakano, S., (2015). Mechanism of the anticancer effect of lycopene (Tetraterpenoids). *Enzymes, 37,* 139–166.

95. Greenshields, A. L., Doucette, C. D., Sutton, K. M., Madera, L., Annan, H., Yaffe, P. B., Knickle, A. F., Dong, Z., & Hoskin, D. W., (2015). Piperine inhibits the growth and motility of triple-negative breast cancer cells. *Cancer Lett., 357,* 129–140.

96. Yaffe, P. B., Doucette, C. D., Walsh, M., & Hoskin, D. W., (2013). Piperine impairs cell cycle progression and causes reactive oxygen species-dependent apoptosis in rectal cancer cells. *Exp. Mol. Pathol., 94,* 109–114.

97. Lin, Y., Xu, J., Liao, H., Li, L., & Pan, L., (2014). Piperine induces apoptosis of lung cancer A549 cells via p53-dependent mitochondrial signaling pathway. *Tumour Biol., 35,* 3305–3310.

98. Fofaria, N. M., Kim, S. H., & Srivastava, S. K., (2014). Piperine causes G1 phase cell cycle arrest and apoptosis in melanoma cells through checkpoint kinase-1 activation. *PLoS One, 9,* e94298.

99. Chow, J., Norng, M., Zhang, J., & Chai, J., (2007). TRPV6 mediates capsaicin-induced apoptosis in gastric cancer cells--Mechanisms behind a possible new "hot" cancer treatment. *Biochim. Biophys. Acta, 1773,* 565–576.

100. Sarkar, A., Bhattacharjee, S., & Mandal, D. P., (2015). Induction of apoptosis by eugenol and capsaicin in human gastric cancer AGS cells--Elucidating the role of p53. *Asian. Pac. J. Cancer Prev., 16,* 6753–6759.

101. Lau, J. K., Brown, K. C., Dom, A. M., Witte, T. R., Thornhill, B. A., Crabtree, C. M., Perry, H. E., Brown, J. M., Ball, J. G., Creel, R. G., Damron, C. L., Rollyson, W. D., Stevenson, C. D., Hardman, W. E., Valentovic, M. A., Carpenter, A. B., & Dasgupta, P., (2014). Capsaicin induces apoptosis in human small cell lung cancer via the TRPV6 receptor and the calpain pathway. *Apoptosis, 19,* 1190–1201.

102. Sun, F., Han, D. F., Cao, B. Q., Wang, B., Dong, N., & Jiang, D. H., (2016). Caffeine-induced nuclear translocation of FoxO1 triggers Bim-mediated apoptosis in human glioblastoma cells. *Tumour Biol., 37,* 3417–3423.

103. Wang, G., Bhoopalan, V., Wang, D., Wang, L., & Xu, X., (2015). The effect of caffeine on cisplatin-induced apoptosis of lung cancer cells. *Exp. Hematol. Oncol., 4*, 5.

104. Dubrez, L., Coll, J. L., Hurbin, A., Solary, E., & Favrot, M. C., (2001). Caffeine sensitizes human H358 cell line to p53-mediated apoptosis by inducing mitochondrial translocation and conformational change of BAX protein. *J. Biol. Chem., 276*, 38980–38987.

105. Eom, K. S., Kim, H. J., So, H. S., Park, R., & Kim, T. Y., (2010). Berberine-induced apoptosis in human glioblastoma T98G cells is mediated by endoplasmic reticulum stress accompanying reactive oxygen species and mitochondrial dysfunction. *Biol. Pharm. Bull., 33*, 1644—1649.

106. Mantena, S. K., Sharma, S. D., & Katiyar, S. K., (2006). Berberine inhibits growth, induces G1 arrest and apoptosis in human epidermoid carcinoma A431 cells by regulating Cdki-Cdk-cyclin cascade, disruption of mitochondrial membrane potential and cleavage of caspase 3 and PARP. *Carcinogenesis, 27*, 2018–2027.

107. Barzegar, E., Fouladdel, S., Movahhed, T. K., Atashpour, S., Ghahremani, M. H., Ostad, S. N., & Azizi, E., (2015). Effects of berberine on proliferation, cell cycle distribution and apoptosis of human breast cancer T47D and MCF7 cell lines. *Iran. J. Basic. Med. Sci., 18*, 334–342.

108. Liu, J. D., Song, L. J., Yan, D. J., Feng, Y. Y., Zang, Y. G., & Yang, Y., (2015). Caffeine inhibits the growth of glioblastomas through activating the caspase-3 signaling pathway in vitro. *Eur Rev. Med. Pharmacol. Sci., 19*, 3080–3088.

109. Mantena, S. K., Sharma, S. D., & Katiyar, S. K., (2006). Berberine, a natural product, induces G1-phase cell cycle arrest and caspase-3-dependent apoptosis in human prostate carcinoma cells. *Mol. Cancer Ther., 5*, 296–308.

110. Patil, J. B., Kim, J., & Jayaprakasha, G. K., (2010). Berberine induces apoptosis in breast cancer cells (MCF-7) through mitochondrial-dependent pathway. *Eur. J. Pharmacol., 645*, 70–78.

111. Lin, C. H., Lu, W. C., Wang, C. W., Chan, Y. C., & Chen, M. K., (2013). Capsaicin induces cell cycle arrest and apoptosis in human KB cancer cells. *BMC. Complement. Altern. Med., 13*, 46.

112. Herman-Antosiewicz, A., Powolny, A. A., & Singh, S. V., (2007). Molecular targets of cancer chemoprevention by garlic-derived organosulfides. *Acta Pharmacol. Sin., 28*, 1355–1364.

113. Xiao, D., Pinto, J. T., Gundersen, G. G., & Weinstein, I. B., (2005). Effects of a series of organosulfur compounds on mitotic arrest and induction of apoptosis in colon cancer cells. *Mol. Cancer Ther., 4*, 1388–1398.

114. Hanahan, D., & Weinberg, R. A., (2000). The hallmarks of cancer. *Cell, 100*, 57–70.

115. Chakrabarty, S., Ganguli, A., Das, A., Nag, D., & Chakrabarti, G., (2015). Epigallocatechin-3-gallate shows anti-proliferative activity in HeLa cells targeting tubulin-microtubule equilibrium. *Chem. Biol. Interact., 242*, 380–389.

116. Baker, K. M., & Bauer, A. C., (2015). Green tea catechin, EGCG, suppresses PCB 102-induced proliferation in estrogen-sensitive breast cancer cells. *Int. J. Breast. Cancer, 163591*.

117. Thangapazham, R. L., Singh, A. K., Sharma, A., Warren, J., Gaddipati, J. P., & Maheshwari, R. K., (2007). Green tea polyphenols and its constituent epigallocatechin gallate inhibits proliferation of human breast cancer cells in vitro and in vivo. *Cancer Lett., 245*, 232–241.

118. Yu, H. N., Shen, S. R., & Yin, J. J., (2007). Effects of interactions of EGCG and Cd (2+) on the growth of PC-3 cells and their mechanisms. *Food Chem. Toxicol., 45*, 244–249.

119. Du, G. J., Zhang, Z., Wen, X. D., Yu, C., Calway, T., Yuan, C. S., & Wang, C. Z., (2012). Epigallocatechin Gallate (EGCG) is the most effective cancer chemopreventive polyphenol in green tea. *Nutrients, 4*, 1679–1691.

120. Kundu, J. K., & Surh, Y. J., (2008). Cancer chemopreventive and therapeutic potential of resveratrol: mechanistic perspectives. *Cancer Lett., 269*, 243–261.

121. Aggarwal, B. B., Kumar, A., & Bharti, A. C., (2003). Anticancer potential of curcumin: preclinical and clinical studies. *Anticancer Res., 23*, 363–398.

122. Qi, W., Weber, C. R., Wasland, K., & Savkovic, S. D., (2011). Genistein inhibits proliferation of colon cancer cells by attenuating a negative effect of epidermal growth factor on tumor suppressor FOXO3 activity. *BMC Cancer, 11*, 219.

123. Kole, L., Giri, B., Manna, S. K., Pal, B., & Ghosh, S., (2011). Biochanin-A, an isoflavone, showed anti-proliferative and anti-inflammatory activities through the inhibition of iNOS expression, p38-MAPK and ATF-2 phosphorylation and blocking NFκB nuclear translocation. *Eur. J. Pharmacol., 653*, 8–15.

124. Haddad, A. Q., Venkateswaran, V., Viswanathan, L., Teahan, S. J., Fleshner, N. E., & Klotz, L. H., (2006). Novel antiproliferative flavonoids induce cell cycle arrest in human prostate cancer cell lines. *Prostate Cancer Prostatic Dis., 9*, 68–76.

125. Mahbub, A. A., Le Maitre, C. L., Haywood-Small, S. L., McDougall, G. J., Cross, N. A., & Jordan-Mahy, N., (2013). Differential effects of polyphenols on proliferation and apoptosis in human myeloid and lymphoid leukemia cell lines. *Anticancer Agents. Med. Chem., 13*, 1601–1613.

126. Hou, Z., Lambert, J. D., Chin, K. V., & Yang, C. S., (2004). Effects of tea polyphenols on signal transduction pathways related to cancer chemoprevention. *Mutat. Res., 555*, 3–19.

127. Manson, M. M., (2005). Inhibition of survival signalling by dietary polyphenols and indole-3-carbinol. *Eur. J. Cancer, 41*, 1842–1853.

128. Liu, Y. Z., Wu, K., Huang, J., Liu, Y., Wang, X., Meng, Z. J., Yuan, S. X., Wang, D. X., Luo, J. Y., Zuo, G. W., Yin, L. J., Chen, L., Deng, Z. L., Yang, J. Q., Sun, W. J., & He, B. C., (2014). The PTEN/PI3K/Akt and Wnt/β-catenin signaling pathways are involved in the inhibitory effect of resveratrol on human colon cancer cell proliferation. *Int. J. Oncol., 45*, 104–112.

129. Siwak, D. R., Shishodia, S., Aggarwal, B. B., & Kurzrock, R., (2005). Curcumin-induced antiproliferative and proapoptotic effects in melanoma cells are associated with suppression of IkappaB kinase and nuclear factor kappaB activity and are independent of the B-Raf/mitogen-activated/extracellular signal-regulated protein kinase pathway and the Akt pathway. *Cancer, 104*, 879–890.

130. Qi, W., Weber, C. R., Wasland, K., & Savkovic, S. D., (2011). Genistein inhibits proliferation of colon cancer cells by attenuating a negative effect of epidermal growth factor on tumor suppressor FOXO3 activity. *BMC Cancer, 11*, 219.

131. Kang, N. J., Shin, S. H., Lee, H. J., & Lee, K. W., (2011). Polyphenols as small molecular inhibitors of signaling cascades in carcinogenesis. *Pharmacol. Ther., 130*, 310–324.

132. Vanamala, J., Reddivari, L., Radhakrishnan, S., & Tarver, C., (2010). Resveratrol suppresses IGF-1 induced human colon cancer cell proliferation and elevates apoptosis via suppression of IGF-1R/Wnt and activation of p53 signaling pathways. *BMC Cancer, 10*, 238.

133. Takahashi, M., & Wakabayashi, K., (2004). Gene mutations and altered gene expression in azoxymethane-induced colon carcinogenesis in rodents. *Cancer Sci., 95*, 475–480.

134. Bhatia, D., Thoppil, R. J., Mandal, A., Samtani, K. A., Darvesh, A. S., & Bishayee, A., (2013). Pomegranate bioactive constituents suppress cell proliferation and induce apoptosis in an experimental model of hepatocellular carcinoma: Role of Wnt/ β -catenin signaling pathway. *Evid. Based Complement Alternat. Med., 371813*.

135. Adachi, S., Nagao, T., Ingolfsson, H. I., Maxfield, F. R., Andersen, O. S., Kopelovich, L., & Weinstein, I. B., (2007). The inhibitory effect of (-)-epigallocatechin gallate on activation of the epidermal growth factor receptor is associated with altered lipid order in HT29 colon cancer cells. *Cancer Res., 67*, 6493–6501.

136. Hou, Z., Lambert, J. D., Chin, K. V., & Yang, C. S., (2004). Effects of tea polyphenols on signal transduction pathways related to cancer chemoprevention. *Mutat. Res., 555*, 3–19.

137. Chakrabarty, S., Ganguli, A., Das, A., Nag, D., & Chakrabarti, G., (2015). Epigallocatechin-3-gallate shows anti-proliferative activity in HeLa cells targeting tubulin-microtubule equilibrium. *Chem. Biol. Interact., 242*, 380–389.

138. Farabegoli, F., Barbi, C., Lambertini, E, & Piva, R., (2007). (-)-Epigallocatechin-3-gallate downregulates estrogen receptor alpha function in MCF-7 breast carcinoma cells. *Cancer Detect. Prev., 31*, 499–504.

139. Goodin, M. G., Fertuck, K. C., Zacharewski, T. R., & Rosengren, R. J., (2002). Estrogen receptor-mediated actions of polyphenolic catechins in vivo and in vitro. *Toxicol. Sci., 69*, 354–361.

140. Khan, A., Aljarbou, A. N., Aldebasi, Y. H., Faisal, S. M., & Khan, M. A., (2014). Resveratrol suppresses the proliferation of breast cancer cells by inhibiting fatty acid synthase signaling pathway. *Cancer Epidemiol., 38*, 765–772.

141. Ong, T. P., Cardozo, M. T., De Conti, A., & Moreno, F. S., (2012). Chemoprevention of hepatocarcinogenesis with dietary isoprenic derivatives: cellular and molecular aspects. *Curr. Cancer Drug Targets, 12*, 1173–1190.

142. Afshordel, S., Kern, B., Clasohm, J., Konig, H., Priester, M., Weissenberger, J., Kogel D., & Eckert, G. P., (2015). Lovastatin and perillyl alcohol inhibit glioma cell invasion, migration, & proliferation--impact of Ras-/Rho-prenylation. *Pharmacol. Res., 91*, 69–77.

143. Yadav, V. R., Prasad, S., Sung, B., Kannappan, R., & Aggarwal, B. B., (2010). Targeting inflammatory pathways by triterpenoids for prevention and treatment of cancer. *Toxins, 2*, 2428–2466.

144. Petronelli, A, Pannitteri, G., & Testa, U., (2009). Triterpenoids as new promising anticancer drugs. *Anticancer Drugs, 20*, 880–892.

145. Kotake-Nara, E., Kushiro, M., Zhang, H., Sugawara, T., Miyashita, K., & Nagao, A., (2001). Carotenoids affect proliferation of human prostate cancer cells. *J. Nutr., 131*, 3303–3306.

146. Williams, A. W., Boileau, T. W., Zhou, J. R., Clinton, S. K., Erdman, J. W Jr., (2000). Beta-carotene modulates human prostate cancer cell growth and may undergo intracellular metabolism to retinol. *J. Nutr., 130*, 728–732.

147. Prakash, P., Russell, R. M., & Krinsky, N. I., (2001). In vitro inhibition of proliferation of estrogen-dependent and estrogen-independent human breast cancer cells treated with carotenoids or retinoids. *J. Nutr., 13*, 1574–1580.

148. Barber, N. J., & Barber, J., (2002). Lycopene and prostate cancer. *Prostate Cancer Prostatic. Dis., 5,* 6–12.

149. Ono, M., Takeshima, M., & Nakano, S., (2015). Mechanism of the anticancer effect of lycopene (Tetraterpenoids). *Enzymes, 37,* 139–166.

150. Hirsch, K., Atzmon, A., Danilenko, M., Levy, J., & Sharoni, Y., (2007). Lycopene and other carotenoids inhibit estrogen activity of 17beta-estradiol and genistein in cancer cells. *Breast Cancer Res. Treat., 104,* 221–230.·.

151. Teodoro, A. J., Oliveira, F. L., Martins, N. B., Maia Gde, A., Martucci, R. B., & Borojevic, R., (2012). Effect of lycopene on cell viability and cell cycle progression in human cancer cell lines. *Cancer Cell Int., 12,* 36.

152. Yang, C. M., Lu, I. H., Chen, H. Y., & Hu, M. L., (2012). Lycopene inhibits the proliferation of androgen-dependent human prostate tumor cells through activation of PPARγ-LXRα-ABCA1 pathway. *J. Nutr. Biochem., 23,* 8–17.

153. Gharib, A., & Faezizadeh, Z., (2014). In vitro anti-telomerase activity of novel lycopene-loaded nanospheres in the human leukemia cell line K562. *Pharmacogn. Mag., 10,* 157–163.

154. Noureini, S. K., & Wink, M., (2012). Antiproliferative effects of crocin in HepG2 cells by telomerase inhibition and hTERT down-regulation. *Asian Pac. J. Cancer Prev.,* 2305–2309.

155. Zhang, J., Zhu, X., Li, H., Li, B., Sun, L., Xie, T., Zhu, T., Zhou, H., & Ye, Z., (2015). Piperine inhibits proliferation of human osteosarcoma cells via G2/M phase arrest and metastasis by suppressing MMP-2/-9 expression. *Int. Immunopharmacol., 24,* 50–58.

156. Hou, X. F., Pan, H., Xu, L. H., Zha, Q. B., He, X. H., & Ouyang, D. Y., (2015). Piperine suppresses the expression of CXCL8 in lipopolysaccharide-activated SW480 and HT-29 cells via downregulating the mitogen-activated protein kinase pathways. *Inflammation, 38,* 1093–1102.

157. Ouyang, D. Y., Zeng, L. H., Pan, H., Xu, L. H., Wang, Y., Liu, K. P., & He, X. H., (2013). Piperine inhibits the proliferation of human prostate cancer cells via induction of cell cycle arrest and autophagy. *Food Chem. Toxicol., 60,* 424–430.

158. Greenshields, A. L., Doucette, C. D., Sutton, K. M., Madera, L., Annan, H., Yaffe, P. B., Knickle, A. F., Dong, Z., & Hoskin, D. W., (2015). Piperine inhibits the growth and motility of triple-negative breast cancer cells. *Cancer Lett., 357,* 129–140.

159. Li, D. X., Zhang, J., Zhang, Y., Zhao, P. W. Yang, L. M., (2015). Inhibitory effect of berberine on human skin squamous cell carcinoma A431 cells. *Genet. Mol. Res., 14,* 10553–10568.

160. Ming, M., Sinnett-Smith, J., Wang, J., Soares, H. P., Young, S. H., Eibl, G., & Rozengurt, E., (2014). Dose-dependent AMPK-dependent and independent mechanisms of berberine and metformin inhibition of mTORC1, ERK, DNA synthesis and proliferation in pancreatic cancer cells. *PLoS One, 9,* e114573.

161. Huang, Z. H., Zheng, H. F., Wang, W. L., Wang, Y., Zhong, L. F., Wu, J. L., & Li, Q. X., (2015). Berberine targets epidermal growth factor receptor signaling to suppress prostate cancer proliferation in vitro. *Mol. Med. Rep., 11,* 2125–2128.

162. Wang, L., Cao, H., Lu, N., Liu, L., Wang, B., Hu, T., Israel, D. A., Peek, R. M. Jr, Polk, D. B., & Yan, F., (2013). Berberine inhibits proliferation and down-regulates epidermal growth factor receptor through activation of Cbl in colon tumor cells. *PLoS One, 8,* e56666.

163. Goto, H., Kariya, R., Shimamoto, M., Kudo, E., Taura, M., Katano, H., & Okada, S., (2012). Antitumor effect of berberine against primary effusion lymphoma via inhibition of NF-κB pathway. *Cancer Sci.*, *103*, 775–781.

164. Noureini, S. K., & Wink, M., (2014). Antiproliferative effect of the isoquinoline alkaloid papaverine in hepatocarcinoma HepG-2 cells--inhibition of telomerase and induction of senescence. *Molecules, 19*, 11846–11859.

165. Sajadian, S., Vatankhah, M., Majdzadeh, M., Kouhsari, S. M., Ghahremani, M. H., & Ostad, S. N., (2015). Cell cycle arrest and apoptogenic properties of opium alkaloids noscapine and papaverine on breast cancer stem cells. *Toxicol. Mech. Methods., 25*, 388–395.

166. Wu, K., Yang, Q., Mu, Y., Zhou, L., Liu, Y., Zhou, Q., & He, B., (2012). Berberine inhibits the proliferation of colon cancer cells by inactivating Wnt/β-catenin signaling. *Int. J. Oncol., 41*, 292–298.

167. Ouyang, D. Y., Zeng, L. H., Pan, H., Xu, L. H., Wang, Y., Liu, K. P., & He, X. H., (2013). Piperine inhibits the proliferation of human prostate cancer cells via induction of cell cycle arrest and autophagy. *Food Chem. Toxicol., 60*, 424–430.

168. Do, M. T., Kim, H. G., Choi, J. H., Khanal, T., Park, B. H., Tran, T. P., Jeong, T. C., & Jeong, H. G., (2013). Antitumor efficacy of piperine in the treatment of human HER2-overexpressing breast cancer cells. *Food Chem., 141*, 2591–2599.

169. Knowles, L. M., & Milner, J. A., (2001). Possible mechanism by which allyl sulfides suppress neoplastic cell proliferation. *J. Nutr., 131*, 1061S-1066S.

170. Herman-Antosiewicz, A., Powolny, A. A., & Singh, S. V., (2007). Molecular targets of cancer chemoprevention by garlic-derived organosulfides. *Acta Pharmacol. Sin., 28*, 1355–1364.

171. Viry, E., Anwar, A., Kirsch, G., Jacob, C., Diederich, M., & Bagrel, D., (2011). Antiproliferative effect of natural tetrasulfides in human breast cancer cells is mediated through the inhibition of the cell division cycle 25 phosphatases. *Int. J. Oncol., 38*, 1103–1111.

172. Antosiewicz, J., Herman-Antosiewicz, A., Marynowski, S. W., & Singh, S. V., (2006). c-Jun NH(2)-terminal kinase signaling axis regulates diallyl trisulfide-induced generation of reactive oxygen species and cell cycle arrest in human prostate cancer cells. *Cancer Res., 66*, 5379–5386.

173. Omar, S. H., & Al-Wabel, N. A., (2010). Organosulfur compounds and possible mechanism of garlic in cancer. *Saudi Pharm. J., 18*, 51–58.

174. Ferrara, N., & Kerbel, R. S., (2005). Angiogenesis as a therapeutic target. *Nature, 15*, 438, 967–974.

175. Strieter, R. M., (2005). Masters of angiogenesis. *Nat. Med., 11*, 925–927.

176. Bhat, T. A., & Singh, R. P., (2008). Tumor angiogenesis--a potential target in cancer chemoprevention. *Food Chem. Toxicol., 46*, 1334–1345.

177. Mojzis, J., Varinska, L., Mojzisova, G., Kostova, I., & Mirossay, L., (2008). Antiangiogenic effects of flavonoids and chalcones. *Pharmacol. Res., 57*, 259–265.

178. Kraft, T. E., Parisotto, D., Schempp, C., & Efferth, T., (2009). Fighting cancer with red wine? Molecular mechanisms of resveratrol. *Crit. Rev. Food. Sci. Nutr., 49*, 782–799.

179. Brakenhielm, E., Cao, R., & Cao, Y., (2001). Suppression of angiogenesis, tumor growth, & wound healing by resveratrol, a natural compound in red wine and grapes. *FASEB J., 15*, 1798–1800.

180. Gupta, S. C., Kim, J. H., Prasad, S., & Aggarwal, B. B., (2010). Regulation of survival, proliferation, invasion, angiogenesis, & metastasis of tumor cells through modulation of inflammatory pathways by nutraceuticals. *Cancer Metastasis. Rev., 29*, 405–434.

181. Kim, M. H., Jeong, Y. J., Cho, H. J., Hoe, H. S., Park, K. K., Park, Y. Y., Choi, Y. H., Kim, C. H., Chang, H. W., Park, Y. J., Chung, I. K., & Chang, Y. C., (2017). Delphinidin inhibits angiogenesis through the suppression of HIF-1α and VEGF expression in A549 lung cancer cells. *Oncol Rep., 37*, 777–784.

182. Tosetti, F., Ferrari, N., De Flora, S., & Albini, A., (2002). Angioprevention: angiogenesis is a common and key target for cancer chemopreventive agents. *FASEB. J., 16*, 2–14.

183. Jung, Y. D., Kim, M. S., Shin, B. A., Chay, K. O., Ahn, B. W., Liu, W., Bucana, C. D., Gallick, G. E., & Ellis, L. M., (2001). EGCG, a major component of green tea, inhibits tumour growth by inhibiting VEGF induction in human colon carcinoma cells. *Br. J. Cancer, 84*, 844–850.

184. Bagli, E., Stefaniotou, M., Morbidelli, L., Ziche, M., Psillas, K., Murphy, C., & Fotsis, T., (2004). Luteolin inhibits vascular endothelial growth factor-induced angiogenesis, inhibition of endothelial cell survival and proliferation by targeting phosphatidylinositol 3'-kinase activity. *Cancer Res., 64*, 7936–7946.

185. Shih, S. C., & Claffey, K. P., (2001). Role of AP-1 and HIF-1 transcription factors in TGF-beta activation of VEGF expression. *Growth Factors, 19*, 19–34.

186. López-Lázaro, M., (2006). Hypoxia-inducible factor 1 as possible target for cancer chemoprevention. *Cancer Epidemiol. Biomarkers Prev., 15*, 2332–2335.

187. Liu, L. Z., Fang, J., Zhou, Q., Hu, X., Shi, X., & Jiang, B. H., (2005). Apigenin inhibits expression of vascular endothelial growth factor and angiogenesis in human lung cancer cells: implication of chemoprevention of lung cancer *Mol. Pharmacol., 68*, 635–634.

188. Fang, J., Xia, C., Cao, Z., Zheng, J. Z., Reed, E., & Jiang, B. H., (2005). Apigenin inhibits VEGF and HIF-1 expression via PI3K/Akt/p70S6K1 and HDM2/p53 pathways. *FASEB. J., 19*, 342–353.

189. Wong, J. C., & Fiscus, R. R., (2015). Resveratrol at anti-angiogenesis/anticancer concentrations suppresses protein kinase G signaling and decreases IAPs expression in HUVECs. *Anticancer Res., 35*, 273–281.

190. Loutrari, H., Hatziapostolou, M., Skouridou, V., Papadimitriou, E., Roussos C., Kolisis, F. N., & Papapetropoulos, A., (2004). Perillyl alcohol is an angiogenesis inhibitor. *J. Pharmacol. Exp. Ther., 311*, 568–575.

191. Vijay, A. B. R., Prabhu, T., Ramesh, C. K., Vigneshwaran, V., Riaz, M., Jayashree, K., & Prabhakar, B. T., (2014). New role of lupeol in reticence of angiogenesis, the cellular parameter of neoplastic progression in tumorigenesis models through altered gene expression. *Biochem. Biophys. Res. Commun., 448*, 139–144.

192. Sahin, M., Sahin, E., & Gumuslu, S., (2012). Effects of lycopene and apigenin on human umbilical vein endothelial cells in vitro under angiogenic stimulation. *Acta Histochem., 114*, 94–100.

193. Elgass, S., Cooper, A., & Chopra, M., (2012). Lycopene inhibits angiogenesis in human umbilical vein endothelial cells and rat aortic rings. *Br. J. Nutr., 108*, 431–439.

194. Chen, M. L., Lin, Y. H., Yang, C. M., & Hu, M. L., (2012). Lycopene inhibits angiogenesis both in vitro and in vivo by inhibiting MMP-2/uPA system through VEGFR2-mediated PI3K-Akt and ERK/p38 signaling pathways. *Mol. Nutr. Food. Res., 56*, 889–899.

195. Trejo-Solís, C., Pedraza-Chaverrí, J., Torres-Ramos, M., Jiménez-Farfán, D., Cruz, Salgado, A., Serrano-García, N., Osorio-Rico, L., & Sotelo, J., (2013). Multiple molecular and cellular mechanisms of action of lycopene in cancer inhibition. *Evid. Based Complement Alternat. Med., 705121*.

196. Zu, K., Mucci, L., Rosner, B. A., Clinton, S. K., Loda, M., Stampfer, M. J., & Giovan-nucci, E., (2014). Dietary lycopene, angiogenesis, & prostate cancer: a prospective study in the prostate-specific antigen era. *J. Natl. Cancer Inst., 106*(2).

197. Chen, M. L., Lin, Y. H., Yang, C. M., & Hu, M. L., (2012). Lycopene inhibits angio-genesis both in vitro and in vivo by inhibiting MMP-2/uPA system through VEG-FR2-mediated PI3K-Akt and ERK/p38 signaling pathways. *Mol. Nutr. Food Res., 56*, 889–899.

198. Bhatia, N., Gupta, P., Singh, B., & Koul, A., (2015). Lycopene enriched tomato extract inhibits hypoxia, angiogenesis, & metastatic markers in early stage N-nitrosodiethyl-amine induced hepatocellular carcinoma. *Nutr. Cancer, 67*, 1268–1275.

199. Dembinska-Kiec, A., Polus, A., Kiec-Wilk, B., Grzybowska, J., Mikolajczyk, M., Hart-wich, J., Razny, U., Szumilas, K., Banas, A., Bodzioch, M., Stachura, J., Dyduch, G., Laidler, P., Zagajewski, J., Langman, T., & Schmitz, G., (2005). Proangiogenic activity of beta-carotene is coupled with the activation of endothelial cell chemotaxis. *Biochi-mica. Et. Biophysica. Acta, 1740*. 222–239.

200. Razny, U., Polus, A., Kiec-Wilk, B., Wator, L., Hartwich, J., Stachura, J., Tomaszewska, R., Dyduch, G., Laidler, P., Schmitz, G., Goralczyk, R., Wertz, K., Riss, G., Franssen-van Hal, N. L., Keijer, J., & Dembinska-Kiec, A., (2010). Angiogenesis in Balb/c mice under beta-carotene supplementation in diet. *Genes Nutr., 5*, 9–16.

201. Martin, K. R., Wu, D., & Meydani, M., (2000). The effects of carotenoids on the ex-pression of cell surface adhesion molecules and binding of monocytes to human aortic endothelial cells, *Atherosclerosis*, 265–274.

202. Doucette, C. D., Hilchie, A. L., Liwski, R., & Hoskin, D. W., (2013). Piperine, a dietary phytochemical, inhibits angiogenesis. *J. Nutr. Biochem., 24*, 231–239.

203. Gupta, S. C., Kim, J. H., Prasad, S., & Aggarwal, B. B., (2010). Regulation of survival, proliferation, invasion, angiogenesis, & metastasis of tumor cells through modulation of inflammatory pathways by nutraceuticals. *Cancer Metastasis. Rev., 29*, 405–434.

204. Pierpaoli, E., Damiani, E., Orlando, F., Lucarini, G., Bartozzi, B., Lombardi, P., Salva-tore, C., Geroni, C., Donati, A., & Provinciali, M., (2015). Antiangiogenic and antitu-mor activities of berberine derivative NAX014 compound in a transgenic murine model of HER2/neu-positive mammary carcinoma. *Carcinogenesis, 36*, 1169–1179.

205. Chu, S. C., Yu, C. C., Hsu, L. S., Chen, K. S., Su, M. Y., & Chen, P. N., (2014). Ber-berine reverses epithelial-to-mesenchymal transition and inhibits metastasis and tumor-induced angiogenesis in human cervical cancer cells. *Mol. Pharmacol., 8*, 609–623.

206. Hamsa, T. P., & Kuttan, G., (2012). Antiangiogenic activity of berberine is mediated through the downregulation of hypoxia-inducible factor-1, VEGF, & proinflammatory mediators. *Drug Chem. Toxicol., 35*, 57–70.

207. Jie, S., Li, H., Tian, Y., Guo, D., Zhu, J., Gao, S., & Jiang, L., (2011). Berberine inhibits angiogenic potential of Hep G2 cell line through VEGF down-regulation in vitro. *J. Gastroenterol. Hepatol., 26*, 179–185.

208. Thejass, P., & Kuttan, G., (2007). Inhibition of endothelial cell differentiation and pro-inflammatory cytokine production during angiogenesis by allyl isothiocyanate and phe-nyl isothiocyanate. *Integr. Cancer Ther., 6*, 389–399.

209. Xiao, D., & Singh, S. V., (2007). Phenethyl isothiocyanate inhibits angiogenesis in vitro and ex vivo. *Cancer Res., 67*, 2239–2246.

210. Kumar, A., D'Souza, S. S., Tickoo, S., Salimath, B. P., & Singh, H. B., (2009). Antian-giogenic and proapoptotic activities of allyl isothiocyanate inhibit ascites tumor growth in vivo. *Integr. Cancer Ther., 8*, 75–87.

211. Davaatseren, M., Hwang, J. T., Park, J. H., Kim, M. S., Wang, S., & Sung, M. J., (2014). Allyl isothiocyanate ameliorates angiogenesis and inflammation in dextran sulfate sodium-induced acute colitis. *PloS One, 9,* e102975.

212. Thejass, P., & Kuttan, G., (2007). Allyl isothiocyanate (AITC) and phenyl isothiocyanate (PITC) inhibit tumour-specific angiogenesis by downregulating nitric oxide (NO) and tumour necrosis factor-alpha (TNF-alpha) production. *Nitric Oxide, 16,* 247–257.

213. Xu, C., Shen, G., Chen, C., Gélinas, C., & Kong, A. N., (2005). Suppression of NF-kappaB and NF-kappaB-regulated gene expression by sulforaphane and PEITC through IkappaBalpha, IKK pathway in human prostate cancer PC-3 cells. *Oncogene, 24,* 4486–4495.

214. Bertl, E., Bartsch, H., & Gerhäuser, C., (2006). Inhibition of angiogenesis and endothelial cell functions are novel sulforaphane-mediated mechanisms inchemoprevention. *Mol. Cancer Ther., 5,* 575–585.

215. Powolny, A. A., & Singh, S. V., (2008). Multitargeted prevention and therapy of cancer by diallyl trisulfide and related Allium vegetable-derived organosulfur compounds. *Cancer Lett., 269,* 305–314.

216. Mousa, A. S., & Mousa, S. A., (2005). Anti-angiogenesis efficacy of the garlic ingredient alliin and antioxidants: role of nitric oxide and p53. *Nutr. Cancer, 53,* 104–110.

217. Xiao, D., Li, M., Herman-Antosiewicz, A., Antosiewicz, J., Xiao, H., Lew, K. L., Zeng, Y., Marynowski, S. W., & Singh, S. V., (2006). Diallyl trisulfide inhibits angiogenic features of human umbilical vein endothelial cells by causing Akt inactivation and downregulation of VEGF and VEGF-R2. *Nutr. Cancer, 55,* 94–107.

218. Eccles, S. A., Box, C., & Court, W., (2005). Cell migration/invasion assays and their application in cancer drug discovery. *Biotechnol. Annu. Rev., 11,* 391–421.

219. Livant, D. L., (2005). Targeting invasion induction as a therapeutic strategy for the treatment of cancer. *Curr. Cancer Drug Targets, 5,* 489–503.

220. Weng, C. J., & Yen, G. C., (2012). Chemopreventive effects of dietary phytochemicals against cancer invasion and metastasis: phenolic acids, monophenol, polyphenol, & their derivatives. *Cancer Treat. Rev., 38,* 76–87.

221. Castillo-Pichardo, L., Martínez-Montemayor, M. M., Martínez, J. E., Wall, K. M., Cubano, L. A., & Dharmawardhane, S., (2009). Inhibition of mammary tumor growth and metastases to bone and liver by dietary grape polyphenols. *Clinical. & Experimental. Metastasis., 26,* 505–516.

222. Ji, Q., Liu, X., Fu, X., Zhang, L., Sui, H., Zhou, L., Sun, J., Cai, J., Qin, J., Ren, J., & Li, Q., (2013). Resveratrol inhibits invasion and metastasis of colorectal cancer cells via MALAT1 mediated Wnt/β-catenin signal pathway. *PloS ONE, 8,* e78700. doi:10. 1371/journal.pone. 0078700.

223. Liu, P. L., Tsai, J. R., Charles, A. L., Hwang, J. J., Chou, S. H., Ping. Y. H., Lin, F. Y., Chen, Y. L. Hung. C. Y., Chen, W. C., Chen, Y. H., & Chong, I. W., (2010). Resveratrol inhibits human lung adenocarcinoma cell metastasis by suppressing heme oxygenase 1-mediated nuclear factor-kappaB pathway and subsequently downregulating expression of matrix metalloproteinases. *Mol. Nutr. Food Res., 54,* 196–204.

224. Maheshwari, R. K., Singh, A. K., Gaddipati, J., & Srimal, R. C., (2006). Multiple biological activities of curcumin: a short review. *Life Sci., 78,* 2081–2087.

225. Curcumin inhibits proliferation, invasion, angiogenesis and metastasis of different cancers through interaction with multiple cell signaling proteins, (2008). *Cancer Lett,. 269,* 199–225.

226. Killian, P. H., Kronski, E., Michalik, K. M., Barbieri, O., Astigiano, S., Sommerhoff, C. P., Pfeffer, U., Nerlich, A. G., & Bachmeier, B. E., (2012). Curcumin inhibits prostate cancer metastasis in vivo by targeting the inflammatory cytokines CXCL1 and -2. *Carcinogenesis*, *33*, 2507–2519.

227. Chen, H. W., Lee, J. Y., Huang, J. Y., Wang, C. C., Chen, W. J., Su, S. F., Huang, C. W., Ho, C. C., Chen, J. J., Tsai, M. F., Yu, S. L., & Yang, P. C., (2008). Curcumin inhibits lung cancer cell invasion and metastasis through the tumor suppressor HLJ1. *Cancer Res.*, *68*, 7428–7438.

228. Zhang, X. M., Huang, S. P., & Xu, Q., (2004). Quercetin inhibits the invasion of murine melanoma B16-BL6 cells by decreasing pro-MMP-9 *via* the PKC pathway. *Cancer Chemother. Pharmacol.*, *53*, 82–88.

229. Lin, Y. C., Tsai, P. H., Lin, C. Y., Cheng, C. H., Lin, T. H., Lee, K. P., Huang, K. Y., Chen, S. H., Hwang, J. J., Kandaswami, C. C., & Lee, M. T., (2013). Impact of flavonoids on matrix metalloproteinase secretion and invadopodia formation in highly invasive A431-III cancer cells. *PLoS One.*, *8*, e71903.

230. Pavese, J. M., Krishna, S. N., & Bergan, R. C., (2014). Genistein inhibits human prostate cancer cell detachment, invasion, & metastasis. *Am. J. Clin. Nutr.*, *100*, Suppl 1:431S-6S.

231. Lee, S. J., Lee, K. W., Hur, H. J., Chun, J. Y., Kim, S. Y., & Lee, H. J., (2007). Phenolic phytochemicals derived from red pine (*Pinus densiflora*) inhibit the invasion and migration of SK-Hep-1 human hepatocellular carcinoma cells. *Ann. New York. Acad. Sci.*, *1095*. 536–544.

232. Ende, C., & Gebhardt, R., (2004). Inhibition of matrix metalloproteinase- 2 and -9 activities by selected flavonoids. *Planta. Med.*, *70*, 1006–1008.

233. Teruszkin, B. I., Alves de Paulo, S., Henriques, S. N., Curié, C. M., Gibaldi, D., Bozza, M., Orlando da Fonseca, C., Da, Glória da, & Costa Carvalho, M., (2002). Effects of perillyl alcohol in glial C6 cell line in vitro and anti-metastatic activity in chorioallantoic membrane model. *Int. J. Mol. Med.*, *10*, 785–788.

234. Ma, Y., Bian, J., & Zhang, F., (2016). Inhibition of perillyl alcohol on cell invasion and migration depends on the Notch signaling pathway in hepatoma cells. *Mol. Cell Biochem.*, *411*, 307–315.

235. Huei-Yan, C., Chih-Min, Y., Jen-Yin, C., Te-Cheng, Y., & Miao-Lin, Hu., (2015). Multicarotenoids at physiological levels inhibit metastasis in human hepatocarcinoma SK-Hep-1 Cells. *Nutr. Cancer*, *67*, 676–686.

236. Kozuki, Y., Miura, Y., & Yagasaki, K., (2001). Inhibitory effects of carotenoids on the invasion of rat ascites hepatoma cells in culture. *Cancer Lett.*, *151*, 111–115.

237. Pradeep, C. R., & Kuttan, G., (2003). Effect of beta-carotene on the inhibition of lung metastasis in mice. *Phytomedicine.*, *10*, 159–164.

238. Huang, C. S., Shih, M. K., Chuang, C. H., & Hu, M. L., (2005). Lycopene inhibits cell migration and invasion and upregulates Nm23-H1 in a highly invasive hepatocarcinoma, SK-Hep-1 cells. *J. Nutr.*, *135*, 2119–2123.

239. Pradeep, C. R., & Kuttan, G., (2002). Effect of piperine on the inhibition of lung metastasis induced B16F-10 melanoma cells in mice. *Clin. Exp. Metastasis.*, *19*, 703–708.

240. Hwang, Y. P., Yun, H. J., Kim, H. G., Han, E. H., Choi, J. H., Chung, Y. C., & Jeong, H. G., (2011). Suppression of phorbol-12-myristate-13-acetate-induced tumor cell invasion by piperine via the inhibition of PKCalpha/ERK1/2-dependent matrix metalloproteinase-9 expression. *Toxicol. Lett.*, *203*, 9–19.

241. Zhang, J., Zhu, X., Li, H., Li, B., Sun, L., Xie, T., Zhu, T., Zhou, H., & Ye, Z., (2015). Piperine inhibits proliferation of human osteosarcoma cells via G2/M phase arrest and metastasis by suppressing MMP-2/-9 expression. *Int. Immunopharmacol., 24*, 50–58.

242. Lai, L., Fu, Q., Liu, Y., Jiang, K., Guo, Q., Chen, Q., & Shen, J., (2012). Piperine suppresses tumor growth and metastasis *in vitro* and *in vivo* in a 4T1 murine breast cancer model. *Acta Pharmacologica. Sinica., 33*, 523–530.

243. Shin, D. H., Kim, O. H., Jun, H. S., & Kang, M. K., (2008). Inhibitory effect of capsaicin on B16-F10 melanoma cell migration via the phosphatidylinositol 3-kinase/Akt/Rac1 signal pathway. *Exp. Mol. Med., 40*, 486–494.

244. Lee, G. R., Jang, S. H., Kim, C. J., Kim, A. R., Yoon, D. J., Park, N. H., & Han, I. S., (2014). Capsaicin suppresses the migration of cholangiocarcinoma cells by down-regulating matrix metalloproteinase-9 expression via the AMPK-NF-κB signaling pathway. *Clin. Exp. Metastasis., 31*, 897–907.

245. Venier, N. A., Yamamoto, T., Sugar, L. M., Adomat, H., Fleshner, N. E., Klotz, L. H., & Venkateswaran, V., (2015). Capsaicin reduces the metastatic burden in the transgenic adenocarcinoma of the mouse prostate model. *Prostate, 75*, 1300–1311.

246. Tang, F., Wang, D., Duan, C., Huang, D., Wu, Y., Chen, Y., Wang, W., Xie, C., Meng, J., Wang, L., Wu, B., Liu, S., Tian, D., Zhu, F., He, Z., Deng, F., & Cao, Y., (2009). Berberine inhibits metastasis of nasopharyngeal carcinoma 5–8F cells by targeting Rho kinase-mediated Ezrin phosphorylation at threonine 567. *J. Biol. Chem., 284*, 27456–27466.

247. Ho, Y. T., Lu, C. C., Yang, J. S., Chiang, J. H., Li, T. C., Ip, S. W., Hsia TC, Liao, C. L., Lin, J. G., Wood, W. G., & Chung, J. G., (2009). Berberine induced apoptosis via promoting the expression of caspase-8, -9 and -3, apoptosis-inducing factor and endonuclease G in SCC-4 human tongue squamous carcinoma cancer cells. *Anticancer Res., 29*, 4063–4070.

248. Mo, S. J., Son, E. W., Rhee, D. K., & Pyo, S., (2003). Modulation of TNF-alpha-induced ICAM-1 expression, NO and H_2O_2 production by alginate, allicin and ascorbic acid in human endothelial cells. *Arch. Pharm. Res., 26*, 244–251.

249. Chu, Q., Ling, M. T., Feng, H., Cheung, H. W., Tsao, S. W., Wang, X., & Wong, Y. C., (2006). A novel anticancer effect of garlic derivatives: Inhibition of cancer cell invasion through restoration of E-cadherin expression. *Carcinogenesis, 27*, 2180–2189.

250. Hwang, E. S., & Lee, H. J., (2006). Allyl isothiocyanate and its *N*-acetylcysteine conjugate suppress metastasis via inhibition of invasion, migration, & matrix metalloproteinase-2/-9 activities in SK-Hep 1 human hepatoma cells. *Exp. Biol. Med (Maywood), 231*, 421–430.

251. Shin, D. Y., Kim, G. Y., Kim, J. I., Yoon, M. K., Kwon, T. K., Lee, S. J., Choi, Y. W., Kang, H. S., Yoo, Y. H., & Choi, Y. H., (2010). Anti-invasive activity of diallyl disulfide through tightening of tight junctions and inhibition of matrix metalloproteinase activities in LNCaP prostate cancer cells. *Toxicol. In. Vitro., 24*, 1569–1576.

252. Singh, S. V., Powolny, A. A., Stan, S. D., Xiao, D., Arlotti, J. A., Warin, R., Hahm, E. R., Marynowski, S. W., Bommareddy, A., Potter, D. M., & Dhir, R., (2008). Garlic constituent diallyl trisulfide prevents development of poorly differentiated prostate cancer and pulmonarymetastasis multiplicity in TRAMP mice. *Cancer Res., 15, 68*, 9503–9511.

253. Perri, F., Longo, F., Giuliano, M., Sabbatino, F., Favia, G., Ionna, F., Addeo, R., Della V. S. G., Di Lorenzo, G., & Pisconti, S., (2017). Epigenetic control of gene expression: Potential implications for cancer treatment. *Crit. Rev. Oncol. Hematol., 111*, 166–172.

254. Gerhauser, C., (2013). Cancer chemoprevention and nutriepigenetics: state of the art and future challenges. *Top. Curr. Chem.*, *329*, 73–132.

255. Thakur, V. S., Deb, G., Babcook, M. A., & Gupta, S., (2014). Plant phytochemicals as epigenetic modulators: role in cancer chemoprevention. *AAPS. J.*, *16*, 151–163.

256. Shukla, S., Meeran, S. M., & Katiyar, S. K., (2014). Epigenetic regulation by selected dietary phytochemicals in cancer chemoprevention. *Cancer Lett.*, *355*, 9–17.

257. King-Batoon, A., Leszczynska, J. M., & Klein, C. B., (2008). Modulation of gene methylation by genistein or lycopene in breast cancer cells. *Environ. Mol. Mutagen.*, *49*, 36–45.

258. Chen, Y., Shu, W., Chen, W., Wu, Q., Liu, H., & Cui, G., (2007). Curcumin, both histone deacetylase and p300/CBP-specific inhibitor, represses the activity of nuclear factor kappa B and Notch-1 in Raji cells. *Basic Clin. Pharmacol. Toxicol.*, *101*, 427–433.

259. Lee, S. J., Krauthauser, C., Maduskuie, V., Fawcett, P. T., Olson, J. M., & Rajasekaran, S. A., (2011). Curcumin-induced HDAC inhibition and attenuation of medulloblastoma growth in vitro and in vivo. *BMC. Cancer*, *11*, 144.

260. Dhillon, N., Aggarwal, B. B., Newman, R. A., Wolff, R. A., Kunnumakkara, A. B., Abbruzzese, J. L., Ng, C. S., Badmaev, V., & Kurzrock, R., (2008). Phase II trial of curcumin in patients with advanced pancreatic cancer *Clin. Cancer Res.*, *14*, 4491–4499.

261. Cheng, A. L., Hsu, C. H., Lin, J. K., Hsu, M. M., Ho, Y. F., Shen, T. S., Ko, J. Y., Lin, J. T., Lin, B. R., Ming-Shiang, W., Yu, H. S., Jee, S. H., Chen, G. S., Chen, T. M., Chen, C. A., Lai, M. K., Pu, Y. S., Pan, M. H., Wang, Y. J., Tsai, C. C., & Hsieh, C. Y., (2001). Phase I clinical trial of curcumin, a chemopreventive agent, in patients with high-risk or pre-malignant lesions. *Anticancer Res.*, *21*, 2895–2900.

262. Nakachi, K., Matsuyama, S., Miyake, S., Suganuma, M., & Imai, K., (2000). Preventive effects of drinking green tea on cancer and cardiovascular disease: epidemiological evidence for multiple targeting prevention. *Biofactors.*, *13*, 49–54.

263. Bettuzzi, S., Brausi, M., Rizzi, F., Castagnetti, G., Peracchia, G., & Corti, A., (2006). Chemoprevention of human prostate cancer by oral administration of green tea catechins in volunteers with high-grade prostate intraepithelial neoplasia: a preliminary report from a one year proof-of-principle study. *Cancer Res.*, *66*, 1234–1240.

264. Henning, S. M., Wang, P., Said, J. W., Huang, M., Grogan, T., Elashoff, D., Carpenter, C. L., Heber, D., & Aronson, W. J., (2015). Randomized clinical trial of brewed green and black tea in men with prostate cancer prior to prostatectomy. *Prostate*, *75*, 550–559.

265. Patel, K. R., Brown, A., Jones, D. J. L., Britton, R. G., Hemingway, D., Miller, A. S., West, K. P., Booth, T. D., Perloff, M., Crowell, J. A., Brenner, D. E., Steward, W. P., Gescher, A. J., & Brown, K., (2010). Clinical pharmacology of Resveratrol and its metabolites in colorectal cancer patients. *Cancer Res.*, *70*, 7392–7399.

266. Howells, L. M., Berry, D. P., Elliott, P. J., Jacobson, E. W., Hoffmann, E., Hegarty, B., Brown, K., Steward, W. P., & Gescher, A. J., (2011). Phase I randomized, double-blind pilot study of micronized resveratrol (SRT501) in patients with hepatic metastases-safety, pharmacokinetics, & pharmacodynamics. *Cancer Prev. Res.*, *4*, 1419–1425.

267. Kucuk, O., Sarkar, F. H., Djuric, Z., Sakr, W., Pollak, M. N., Khachik, F., Banerjee, M., Bertram, J. S., & Wood D. P. Jr., (2002). Effects of lycopene supplementation in patients with localized prostate cancer. *Exp. Biol. Med.*, *227*, 881–885.

268. Willett, W. C., (2010). Fruits, vegetables, & cancer prevention: turmoil in the produce section. *J. Natl. Cancer Inst.*, *102*, 510–511.

269. Lee, J. E., Mannisto, S., Spiegelman, D., et al., (2009). Intakes of fruit, vegetables, & carotenoids and renal cell cancer risk: a pooled analysis of 13 prospective studies *Cancer Epidemiol. Biomarkers Prev., 186*, 1730–1739.

270. Liu, R. H., (2003). Health benefits of fruit and vegetables are from additive and synergistic combinations of phytochemicals. *Am. J. Clin. Nutr., 78*, 517S-520S.

271. Anand, P., Kunnumakkara, A. B., Newman, R. A., & Aggarwal, B. B., (2007). Bioavailability of curcumin: problems and promises. *Mol. Pharm., 4*, 807–818.

272. Yim, C. Y., Mao, P., & Spinella, M. J., (2014). Headway and hurdles in the clinical development of dietary phytochemicals for cancer therapy and prevention: lessons learned from vitamin A derivatives. *AAPS. J., 16*, 281–288.

273. Wang, H., Khor, T. O., Shu, L., Su, Z., Fuentes, F., Lee, J. H., & Kong, A. N. T., (2012). Plants against cancer: A review on natural phytochemicals in preventing and treating Cancers and their druggability. *Anticancer Agents Med. Chem., 12*, 1281–1305.

CHAPTER 11

HEALTH BENEFITS AND PREVENTIVE EFFECTS OF COMMON BEVERAGES IN CANCER

VIVEK KUMAR GAUR,[1,2] SANJAY GUPTA,[3] and
JANMEJAI KUMAR SRIVASTAVA[1]

[1.]Amity Institute of Biotechnology, Amity University Uttar Pradesh, Lucknow Campus, Lucknow–226028, Uttar Pradesh, India

[2.]CSIR-Indian Institute of Toxicology Research, M.G. Road, Lucknow, India

[3.]Department of Urology, Case Western Reserve University, 10900 Euclid Avenue, Cleveland, Ohio, USA

CONTENTS

ABSTRACT

A number of products can be obtained from a common source by varying the composition and concentration of one or more of the constituents, depending on which they can be disease causing or healthful. Beverages are liquid drinks other than water, although the major constituents in most of the beverages is water. Beverages are widespread in the market and are highly consumed because of their taste and because they provide nutrition, replenish ions, and offer protection against many diseases. Different beverages have different effects on the human body, and one must be cautious while selecting a drink. The relative amount of a constituent is also the determinant of the effect of a beverage on the human body, as a low concentration of caffeine is effective as stress relevant but its high concentration may even cause death. In this chapter, we have summarized the major beverages obtained from different sources, including animal, plant, and synthetically derived. The plant-derived beverages are found to contain bioactive components from them, many of which have been shown to have anti-inflamatory, antioxidant, immunomodulatory, and anticancerous properties. Concentration of these bioactive components in the beverages can also vary depending on the processing and preparation methodology, which then determines its properties.

11.1   INTRODUCTION

The word beverage has been defined as a liquid drink that is not water and is intended for consumptions by humans. Though all beverages include water, water itself is not considered as a beverage, and the role of water in beverages is only to prevent dehydration by maintaining the body balance. Beverages are not only limited to human needs, but they have also become a part of human society in a cultural aspect. Depending on the presence and absence of alcohol content, beverages can be divided into two broad classes, namely alcoholic beverages and nonalcoholic beverages. Flavor and the stimulant effect are the two major factors on which alcohol drinks are being judged. Alcoholic beverages are the oldest beverages in human history to be associated with human culture, and they can be marked by the presence of more than 5% alcohol. On the other hand, nonalcoholic beverages are the ones in which alcohol is absent or may be present in very low concentration. Beverages can be classified based on their alcoholic content, followed by their source of origin (Figure 11.1). In addition to being a good refreshing agent, they may also provide the user with increased energy, immunity, and various nutrients, such as energy drinks, milk, and cocoa, respectively. Owing to these properties, they are receiving increasing interest and are currently most widely consumed other than water. Artificial coloring and flavoring agents are also added to certain drinks in order to enhance their taste and properties. Beverages apart from being an integral part of the human society also impart harmful or beneficial effects depending on the source of the beverage and its constituents, and the benefits from the consumption of a beverage can be accessed by limiting their utilization according to the regulatory guidelines. An optimal consumption of some beverages may contribute to anti-inflammatory, antioxidants, immune boosting, antidiabetic, antidiuretic, and anticancer property in humans.

11.2   BIOLOGICAL BEVERAGE

11.2.1   MAMMALIAN MILK

Mammalian milk is the first food/source of energy for mammals in the postnatal period and is the only food to be given in this period; thus, it contains all the essential nutrients and energy required for proper growth and development. The consumption of mammalian milk generally stops after the weaning period. There are several factors that influence the production of milk, such as animal's nutritional status, species, lactation stage, environmental condition, and genetics [1, 2]. The most frequently consumed mammalian milk is from cow, goat, and sheep (in decreasing order). The major constituents of milk are water, lactose, fat, protein, minerals, and vitamins [3, 4].

11.2.1.1   Protein

The important protein source of human diet is milk, which contains soluble proteins (20% of total proteins) and insoluble proteins (80%) [3, 5]. To meet amino acid requirement in human a good quality protein (in terms of bioavailability and digestiblity) is required; milk proteins can be considered as good quality proteins [6, 7], exhibiting beneficial role. Serum albumin, β-lactoglobulin, lactoperoxidase, α-85 lactoalbumin, lysozyme immunoglobulins, lactoferrin, transferrin, and proteose-peptone constitutes the solu-

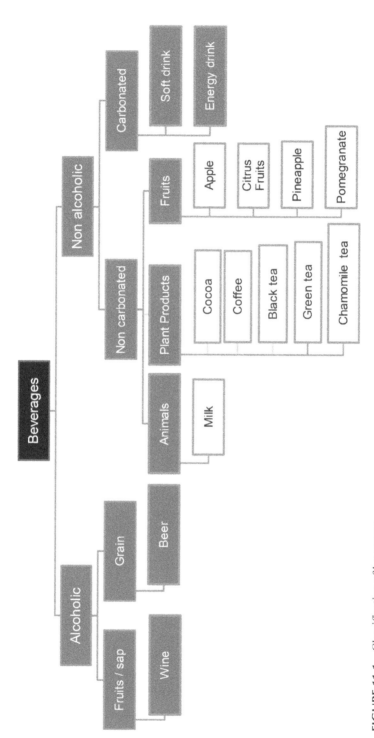

FIGURE 11.1   Classification of beverages.

ble fraction of milk proteins [5]. Colostrum was found to contain 100 times more immunoglobulins than milk, thus imparting immunity to infants after birth [8, 9]. Casein is the major protein of the insoluble fraction, and it functions as a mineral binding agent by forming coagulum for phosphorus and calcium, thereby increasing their stomach digestibility [10]. Function and relative differences in cow and human milk protein composition are shown in Table 11.1 [11, 12].

11.2.1.2   Fatty Acids

Triglycerides, cholesterol, phospholipid, diacylglycerol, and free fatty acids are the milk fatty acid constituents, of which triglycerides constitute the major fraction. Milk contains the fat fraction in a globular form; these globules can only be digested by pancreatic lipolysis if they are first exposed to gastric digestion [13]. Milk fatty acids are the results of animal feed or the activity of microorganisms in the lumen, and their amount depends on mastatis, lactation stage, ruminal fermentation, and feed-related factors [12].

TABLE 11.1   Relative Concentration and Function of Important Milk Proteins in Cow and Human Milk

Protein	Function	Concentration (g/l) in Cow	Concentration (g/l) in Human
Total caseins	Mineral transport	26.0	2.7
Total whey proteins	(Ca, PO4, Fe, Zn, Cu	6.3	67.3
β -Lactoglobulin	Retinol and fatty acids binding	3.2	Absent
α-Lactoalbumin	Lactose production, calcium transport, immunomodulator; anticarcinogen	1.2	1.9
Imunoglobulin (A, M, E, G)	Immune protection	0.7	1.3
Lactoferrin	Antioxidant Immunomodulator, iron absorption, anticarcinogen	0.1	1.5
Lactoperoxidase	Antimicrobial	0.03	0.0007
Lysozyme		0.0004	0.1

[Sources: Refs. 11 and 12]

11.2.1.3 Vitamins and Minerals

Milk has a specific micronutrient composition of minerals and vitamins. Among the minerals, calcium is most abundant, and hence, milk is considered as a privileged source for calcium; the other minerals present are magnesium, phosphorus, selenium, and zinc [14]. Vitamins present in milk are both water soluble (like thiamine and riboflavin) and liposoluble (vitamins A, D, and E). Milk product fortification can be done for betterment of nutritional status and increasing vitamin A concentration [15].

11.2.1.4 Health Beneficial Properties

Myristic, palmitic, and lauric acids were found to increase total cholesterol, low density lipoproteins, and high density lipoprotein, respectively, whereas stearic acid decreases cholesterol/high density lipoprotein ratio, there by exhibiting protective effects [16]. Regardless of high fat content, milk consumption has not been linked to cardiovascular disease risks [17, 18]. Milk offer several protective effects, including antihypertensive and antithrombotic actions [19], immunomodulatory and cytomodulatory effects[20], and as antioxidant [21] imparting actions in the nervous, immune, cardiovascular, and digestive systems.

There are contradictory results for the role of milk in cancer. Few studies suggest that the consumption of moderate milk has no or inverse effect on breast [22, 23], colorectal [24, 25], bladder [26], and prostate cancer [27], while some other epidemiological evidence suggests the cancer preventive properties against colorectal cancer [25].

11.3 FRUIT BEVERAGES

Fruits represent an important part of world agriculture production. According to FAO, fruit juice is a pure filtered form of squeezed pulp when nothing is added to it. Sodium benzoate can be used as a preservative in fruit juices to extend the shelf life, but it is not mandatory. In 2015–2016, India was the largest producer of papayas (44.03%), mangoes (including mangosteens and guavas) (37.57%), and bananas (22.94%), creating a fortune of Rs. 3,524.50 crores (APEDA report). Mangoes, walnuts, grapes, bananas and pomegranates share a larger portion of exported fruits of the country.

Fruits are also considered as super foods as they contain health-promoting vitamins, minerals, and natural components that enhance or fortify the nutritional value of conventional foods. They can enhance health and reduce the risk of many acute and chronic diseases. Most fruits can be used to make juice. This section describes the fruits, their constituents, and their health beneficial properties

11.3.1 APPLES

Apples are the pomaceous fruit of apple tree *Malus domestica*, and have long been associated with the biblical story of Adam and Eve. The fruit originated in the Middle East just about 4000 years ago, and is one of the most favorite and popular fruits ever known. As with the well-known adage "An apple a day keeps the doctor away," the fruit has been doing much good for people who are health conscious. It furnishes many health benefits on human health as it contains high levels of polyphenols and other phytochemicals [28, 29]. Main structural classes of apple constituents include hydroxycinnamic acids, dihydrochalcones, flavonols (quercetin, glycosides), catechins and oligomeric procyanidins, as well as triterpenoids in apple peel and anthocyanins in red apples [30].

The nutritional composition of apple juice is quite similar to that of apples [31]. Photochemical compounds found in apples protect the brain from Parkinson's and Alzheimer's diseases [32]: flavonols (quercetin glycosides) acts as an anti-inflammatory and antiallergic agent, while epicatechins and catechins reduce plaque buildup in the arteries [33]. Procynidin present in apples is beneficial in the prevention of coronary diseases and diabetes [33]. Apple is a low glycemic food with a high fiber content of both soluble and insoluble nature, which aids in digestion, weight management, and controls rapid rise in blood sugar. Apple's fiber helps in cleansing of the liver and therefore prevents obesity, heart diseases, intestinal diseases such as ulcerative colitis, hemorrhoids, and inflammatory bowel disease [34]. Several studies have specifically linked apple consumption with a reduced risk for cancer, especially lung cancer in women [35]; it is also associated with a decreased risk of asthma and a decrease in bronchial hypersensitivity [33].

11.3.2 CITRUS FRUITS

Citrus fruit belongs to the family Rutaceae, which comprises about 140 genera and 1,300 species; it is commonly found throughout the globe. The fruits of this class are highly nutritious, and each and every part of these fruits is useful in some form. It can be used for the production of juices, concentrates, marmalade, jams, etc. Citrus is well known for its high vitamin C content, vitamin A, thiamin, folate, potassium, fiber, proteins, magnesium, copper, hesperidin, flavonoids, a variety of other trace vitamins and minerals, making it one of the most valuable fruit.

11.3.3 SWEET ORANGE (Citrus sinensis)

Since ancient time oranges and lemons are gaining popularity for their refreshing taste, thirst quenching properties, and several health benefits. *The origin of sweet orange is from southeast Asia; they are mainly cultivated in China and referred to as* "Chinese Apple." *In Sanskrit,* oranges and lemon *are named as* "Nagrunga" and "Nimbu," respectively, and their extracts are used for medicin*al and drin*k*ing purposes.* Today, it is grown almost all across the globe and used as a food product for humans because of its high *n*utritive *v*alues in terms of vitamins, minerals, etc. *[36].* Nutritive profile of the fruit is very impressive, as it consist of glycemic and non-glycemic constituents like carbohydrate (sugars and fiber), potassium, folate, vitamin B6, phosphorus, magnesium, calcium, thiamin, niacin, copper, riboflavin, pantothenic acid, and other phytochemicals including carotenoids, isohesperidin, terpineol, naringin, limonin, flavonoids, hesperidin, and limonene, which are responsible for the bitter taste of some grape fruits, lemons, and oranges [37]. The average energy value of fresh fruit is also low, as cholesterol is not found in this fruit because of the absense of fat and sodium; hence, it can be used a super food for people with excess body weight [37]. Limonoids stimulate the secretion of a detoxifying enzyme, glutathione S-transferase (GST), which inhibits tumor formation in the body [38]. Anticancer properties were observed from flavonoids and limonene, while quercetin imparts a variety of health beneficial properties such antitumor and anti-inflammatory properties [39], thus preventing prostatitis, allergies/inflammations, heart diseases, respiratory diseases such as bronchitis and asthma, cataract, and cancer [40]. Hesperidin is a flavonoid glycoside present abundantly in citrus fruits that reduces cholesterol and also possesses anti-inflammatory effect [41]. Orange oil is used to treat chronic bronchitis. Dried orange flower tea stimulates the nervous system [41]. Feeding of orange oils, rich in limonene, seemed to inhibit tumors of stomach, lung, and mammary tumors [39].

11.3.4   TANGERINE TREE (Citrus reticulata)

Tangerine or mandarin oranges, member of the citrus family, are a tasty and refreshing citrus fruit loaded with goodness of many nutritious compounds, including flavonoids, vitamin C, vitamin A, potassium, and folate [42]. They consist of tengeritin, a polymethoxylated flavone, which is an anti-cancer agent and strengthens the cell wall and protects it from invasion [43]. Flavonoids prevent the growth of cancerous cells and arrests proliferation of tumor cells. It neutralizes free radicals, have potential to protect against the development of heart disease by promoting better blood flow in arteries, prevents clot formation in arteries, and prevents "Bad Cholesterol" formation [40]. Vitamin C is a potent antioxidant that helps to fight against free radical damage and is crucial for the synthesis of collagen in the body [39]. Vitamin A boosts immune function, vision, reproductive health, and signal transduction between nerves [44]. Folate maintains health of new cells by building DNA and RNA. Folate is a crucial vitamin during periods of rapid growth, such as pregnancy and infancy [45] and is essential for the production of red blood cells [46]. Phytochemicals such as limonoids (triterpenes), monoterpenes, flavanoids, hydroxycinnamic acid and carotenoids have been found in ample amount in citrus fruits [47]. Hydroxyethylrutosides (HER) have properties of curing capillary permeability, ease bruising, and relieves hemorrhoids; varicose veins can also be treated using HER [48, 49].

11.3.5   APPLE CIDER

Cider also called as "Soft Cider" or "Apple Cider" is a non-alcoholic apple-derived beverage, which is inexpensive and easy to prepare. Apple cider offers a major advantage of being free from the insecticide pyridaben, which may be usually present in apple juice if not properly processed. This removal or decrease is achieved during apple cider processing as washing can not reduce pyridaben level because of its lipophilic nature. During cider processing, the choring and peeling process contribute significantly in0 the reduction of the insecticide [50]. The organoleptic qualities of apple cider, such as flavor, color, astringency, and bitterness, are atributed to polyphenols present in apple cider, which determine the "mouth feel" of apple cider [51–54]. Polyphenols also contribute to health protective properties of apple ciders, such as antioxidant, anti-inflammatory, neutralizing capacity, free-radical scavenging, and anticancer activity and coronary heart disease prevention [55–58]. Besides, polyphenols also provide aroma to the cider by fermentation and hence prevents its spoilage [53, 59, 60]. Phenols are also found to interact with proteins, thereby improving the coloidal stability [51, 61, 62].

11.3.6 PINEAPPLE

Pineapple (*Ananas comosus*) is sometimes called the "King of Fruit" [63]. It is also known as the queen of fruits due to its excellent flavor and taste [64]. Pineapple typically contains water, protein, fat, carbohydrate, fiber, ash, calcium, phosphorus, iron, sodium, potassium, sugar, bromelain (a protein digesting enzyme), citric acid, malic acid, and vitamins A and B [65, 66]. Pineapple fruits are an excellent source of vitamins and minerals and have minimal fat and sodium content [67]. *A. comosus* leaves have anti-hyperglycemic and analgesic properties [68]. Bromelain has a significant amount of fibrinolytic, antiedematous, antithrombotic, and anti-inflammatory activities. Bromelain accounts for many therapeutic benefits like treatment of sinusitis, angina pectoris, surgical trauma, bronchitis, debridement of wounds, thrombophlebitis, and enhanced absorption of drugs, particularly antibiotics. It also relieves diarrhea, osteoarthritis, and various cardiovascular disorders. Bromelain was also found to promote apoptotic cell death and anticancer activities [69]. It has been used to treat rheumatoid arthritis [70], diabetic ulcers and speeds up the recovery mechanism of tissues during general surgery.

Bromelain prevents or minimizes the severity of transient ischemic attack (TIA) and angina pectoris. It is also found useful in the prevention and treatment of thrombophlebitis. It may also breakdown cholesterol plaques and exerts a potent fibrinolytic activity [71]. Pineapple reduces blood clotting, and it helps in the removal of plaque from arterial walls [72]. It cures bronchitis and throat infections. Pineapple acts as cerebral toner and combats loss of memory [64].

11.3.7 POMEGRANATE

Pomegranate (*Punica granatum L.*) belongs to the Punicaceae family and is among the oldest recognized edible fruit. Pomegranate is the valuable source of bioactive compounds like phenol [73, 74], flavonols, tannins, and anthocyanins [75]. The mesocarp and fruit peel of pomegranate is the major source of these bioactive compounds [76]. Maturity status, climatic conditions, and juice extraction methods influence the composition and concentration of bioactive compounds in pomegranate juice [77–83]. When the juice is derived from the whole fruit and not only from arils, a higher amount of hydrolyzable tannins and polyphenol was found [76]. The health promoting properties include protection against the risk of diabetes, atherosclerosis, neurodegenerative disorders, and cancer [75, 84]. Punicalagin and ellagic acid (polyphenol) in pomegranate has antioxidant activity [85, 86], imparting antimutagenic property against direct and indirect procarcinogens and mutagens [87]. Antiproliferative effects of a specific pomegranate juice on PC-3 and HeLa cancer cells lines were recently reported [88]. Further biochemical studies are required to fully elucidate the chemopreventive mechanisms of action for antimutagenicity of pomegranate juice.

11.4 PLANT-BASED BEVERAGES

Plant-based beverages are the beverages manufactured from the plant constituents. Because the major proportion of these beverages is a plant product(s), most of these offer better health protection as compared to the artificially prepared and sweetened beverages. The name of these beverages is given depending on the source from which it is derived, for example, teas are derived from the tea plant, and similarly, cocoa from cocoa beans. This section covers the composition and health benefits of some of the major plant-based beverages.

11.4.1 GREEN TEA

It is an unfermented plant-based beverage obtained from a tea plant, namely *Camellia sinensis*, a kind of evergreen laurel tree of the family Theaceae. The fermentation of tea leaves is not achieved by microorganisms; instead, it is an enzyme-based phenomenon known as "Enzymation" [89]. Therefore, the fresh leaves are steamed for 30–45 sec at 95–100 °C during the processing to deactivate the enzymes, especially polyphenol oxidase. Due to the steaming treatment, the amount of vitamins is high in green tea as compared to other fermented teas [90, 91].Therefore, fresh leaves undergoes an array of processes, such as panning or steaming (subjected to 95–100°C for 30–45 sec for enzyme activation), rolling (rupture plant cell to dstribute juice), drying/firing (pan-fired to fix juice within the leaf, reducing moisture upto 4% and thus, adding toastiness to taste) till the final product formation [89, 92]. The quality of green tea is affected by the plant growing technique and leaf harvesting time; in order to obtain superior quality, the lea leaves must be harvested in early summer seasons [93]. The major ingredients in green tea are polyphenols, theanine, caffeine, free amino acids (1–4% dry weight), and vitamins [94]. The detailed chemical composition is shown in Figure 11.2. Since ancient times, green tea has been used for medicinal purposes and as a healthful beverage. The xanthic bases, essential oils, and polyphenolic compounds are the main compounds that influence human health. Xanthic bases, especially caffeine, affect the central nervous system by decreasing fatigue, facilitating wakefulness, and association of ideas by brain [95]. Green tea has beneficial effects on human health such as vasodilator, diuretic, antibacterial, antimutagenic, anti-inflammatory, hypocholesterolemic, respiratory stimulation and antidiabetic. Various studies on animal models and cell culture support the anticancer property of green tea [96]. Various animal studies have shown that green tea inhibits carcinogenesis in the lung, skin, stomach, esophagus, oral cavity, prostate, liver, kidney, and other organs [94, 97–100]. Some studies correlate this inhibition with a decrease in cell proliferation and increase in tumor cell apoptosis [101]. Cases of breast cancer are significantly low in Asian women who have a high intake of green tea [102].

11.4.2 BLACK TEA

Black tea is the major fraction of teas produced and consumed [103]. It is obtained from the same source as the green tea, but the processing differs; in black tea, the leaves are allowed to ferment before drying, wherein polyphenol oxidase catalyze the fermentation of the leaves by oxidation. Due to the allowed fermentation time, the amount of vitamins is comparatively reduced as compared to that in green tea [91, 92]. The constituents of black tea remain the same as those of green tea and only the amount varies, except for ascorbic acid, which is absent in black tea. Black tea contains caffeine, catechins (epicatechin (EC), epigallocatechin gallate (EGCG), and epigallocatechin

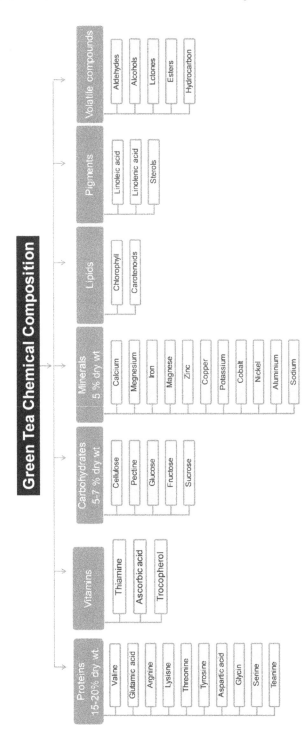

FIGURE 11.2 Chemical composition of green tea. [Source: Ref. 199]

(EGC)) [104]. Black tea was found to have a role against type 2 diabetes as it inhibits carbohydrate hydrolyzing enzyme [105], activates the biomarkers for immune system [106]. A recent study suggests that black tea does not have any antioxidant property against prostate cancer [107]. Another study by Miura [108] shows that black tea has no effect against skin cancer. In in vitro studies, black tea extract exhibited cytotoxicity against human colon carcinoma cell line and human breast carcinoma cell line [109].

11.4.3　CHAMOMILE TEA

Dried flowers of *Matricaria* species are used to produce chamomile tea; chamomile is widely used as one of the oldest medicinal plants with numerous healing applications (Astin et al., 2000) [110]. The herb belongs to the daisy family (Asteracea or Compositae). The two known varieties are Roman chamomile (*Matricaria chamomilla*) and German chamomile (*Chamaemelum nobile*) [111], and the distinguishing feature is that German chamomile has a bulging disk as compared to the Roman ones (Figure 11.3).

Chamomile contains bioactive compounds that have been used in cosmetics and medicines; of them, the main constituents are flavanoids and essential oil constituents [112]. The fresh oil can vary in color from deep green to brilliant blue, and upon storage, it turns to dark yellow but does not lose its potency. Chamomile essential oil constitutes a number of compounds in minor quantities, including matricin/chamazulene, bisaboloides, and dicycloethers; they were reported to exhibit additive effects [113]. Chamazulene and bisabolol found in German chamomile flower are unstable and can be preserved in alcoholic tincture, whereas roman chamomile has less chamazulene and contains α-pinene and farnesene and a major proportion of tiglic acid and esters of angelic acid [114]. Postpartum women when supplemented with chamomile tea showed reduction in sleep quality problems and depression [15]. Riza [116] concluded that chamomile tea protects from thyroid cancer. In Mexican women, chamomile consumption was linked with reduced mortality [117]. No growth inhibition effect of chamomile extract was observed on normal cells as compared with that on cancer cell lines [114], indicating that the effect is executed by inducing apoptosis [118]. Antiproliferative effect of epigenin (a bioactive constituent of chamomile) has been reported against skin, prostate, breast, and ovarian cancer [119, 120, 121].

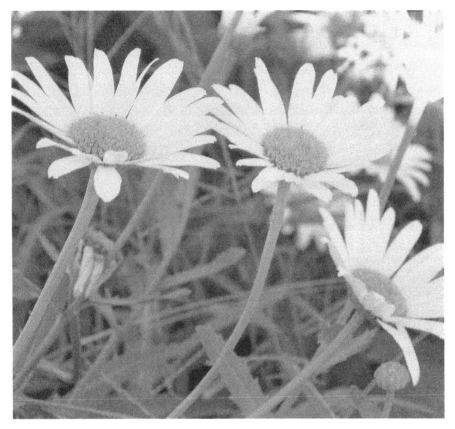

FIGURE 11.3 Chamomile tea plant.

11.4.4 COFFEE

Coffee is a widely consumed beverage and an excellent source of antioxidants [122]. Coffee contains caffeine, two specific diaterpenes known as cafestol and kahweal, polyphenols such as lignin phytoestrogen, and flavanoids [123], and chlorogenic acid. Caffeine is reported to either stimulate or suppress the tumors, depending on the phase of administration and species [124]. Diaterpenes have anticarcinogenic properties; they induce the enzymes for carcinogen detoxification [125, 126] and inhibit the enzymes for carcinogen activation [127]. Chlorogenic acid also contributes to the antioxidant property [128]. Coffee was found to inhibit prostate and breast cancer, advanced prostate cancers, postmenopausal breast cancers, and the chemopreventive effects includes DNA repair regulation, apoptosis, inhibition of oxidative damage and stress, phase II enzymatic activity, antiangiogenic effects, and antimetastatic and antiproliferative effects [129].

11.4.5 COCOA

Cocoa was first obtained from a plant named *Theobroma cacao* from the equatorial rainforest of America. Cocoa beverage is prepared from the processed cocoa beans in liquid form, which contains cocoa butter, cocoa liquor, sugar, and milk. The constituents of cocoa are described in Figure 11.4. Among flavanol-rich foods, dark chocolate is the highest flavanol containing food [130]. Cardiovascular health is improved by regular consumption of cocoa, which is achieved by reduction in insulin resistance, LDL-cholesterol [131], and blood pressure [132], thereby increasing the vascular elasticity. The other health beneficial effect of chocolate is stimulation of the kidney and treatment of anemia, fever, tuberculosis, and gout [133], helps in digestion and provides comfort to the liver [134]. Flavanoids present in cocoa protect against DNA damage caused by carcinogenic agents or by free radicals [135] and have antioxidant capacity [136]; cocoa phenols also have a synergistic effect in inducing apoptosis [137]. Cocoa was reported to be effective agains breast cancer, thyroid cancer, lung cancer, pancreatic cancer, hepatic cancer, colon cancer, and leukemia [138].

11.5 ALCOHOLIC BEVERAGES

An undistilled fermented drink or beverage containing alcohol (specifically ethanol) comes under the category of alcoholic beverages. Legend suggests that yeast from the genus *Saccharomyces* spontaneously colonized a storage jar of food sugars, fermenting them into a sweet, alcoholic beverage [139]. The history of these fermented drinks dates back to as old as 3150 BC with ancient Egyptians herbal wine, and ever since, the use of these beverages has been explored and the preparation methodology handed-down the subsequent human generations. This category contains a wide number of products with variable composition exhibiting different effects and properties.

Alcoholic beverages are ancient beverages that were produced accidentally during intentional food storage, and they are the product of anaerobic fermentation. In these beverages, the carbohydrates derived from plants are fermented by yeasts, thereby producing ethanol and carbon dioxide;

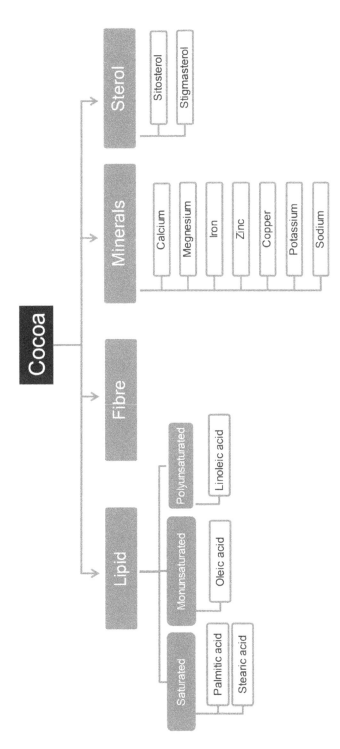

FIGURE 11.4 Cocoa and its constituents. [Source: Ref. 200]

the aroma and characteristic flavor of the beverage is also imparted by the yeast. Based on the type of raw material used, the processing methods can be divided into three categories: beer, wine, and spirits. In the following section, we have detailed the properties of widely used beer and wine.

11.5.1   BEER

In simple words, beer is any fermented drink made from cereal grains, and it is one of the oldest [140] and most widely consumed alcoholic beverage [141]. Max Nelson [142] quoted beer as the 3rd most popular drink after tea and water. Brewing is the process by which beer is made in a brewery, a building that is dedicated to the production of beer. In the process of brewing, starch is converted into the wort (sugary liquid) followed by the formation of beer by the use of yeast in a process called fermentation. The 4 major ingredients of beer are namely grain, hops, yeast, and water [143]. Water is in the largest proportion with around 95% of the beer content; grain is used for mostly malted barley, but other ingredients can also be used. Beer was also found to have macromolecules like proteins, carbohydrates, lipids, and nucleic acids in addition to 400 different compounds [144]. These compounds can be derived from the raw materials, surviving the brewing process or can be from a chemical or biochemical transformation of the raw material. The characteristics of beer are imparted by its major constituents as shown in Figure 11.5.

Two components, namely malt (70–80%) and hop (20–30%), produce phenolic compounds in the beer, which may include benzoic- and cinnamic acid derivatives; catechins; di-, tri- and oligomeric proanthocyanidins; simple phenols; coumarins; (prenylated) chalcones; and flavonoids [145]. Over the past years, sensory, medicinal, and nutritional properties of beer have made it a universally popular beverage, and many studies have reported that moderate consumption of low alcohol content beverage has many benefits on human health [146] owing to the presence of ethanol, B vitamins, protein, phenolics (antioxidants), certain minerals, dietary fibers, and prebiotic compounds [147, 148]. Beer is deficient in thiamine among B vitamins, which stimulate consumption of alcohol by interfering with glucose metabolism [149]. It has a high diuretic effect than water due to the high ratio of potassium to sodium (typically 4:1) [150]. The phenolics present in beer significantly maintains the endogenous redox balance in humans [151], and the presence of dietary

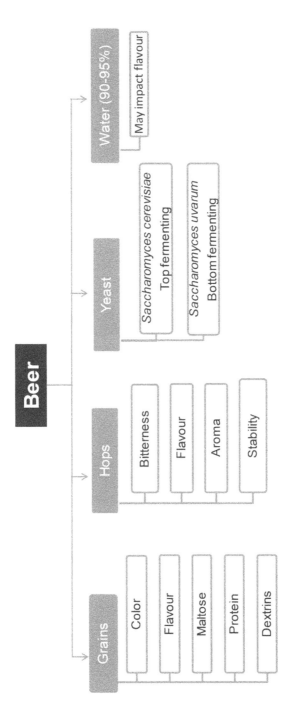

FIGURE 11.5 Properties of beer provided by its constituents. [Source: Ref. 201]

fiber aids in the prevention of colon cancer; beer consumption also inhibits the growth of pathogenic intestinal microorganisms [152]. Beer consumption is also associated with inhibition of angiogenesis (a major factor in the development of malignant tumors) thus preventing tumor growth and metastasis [153, 154]. Ethanol can increase the plasma level of high density lipoprotein (HDL), which decrease platelet aggregation and correspondingly increases blood fibrinogenesis. All these factors may contribute to low risk of coronary heart disease (CHD) [155, 156], which is known as the cardioprotective effect of beer, also lager beer (type of beer conditioned at low temperatures) consumption is associated with decreased cholesterol and triglyceride level [157]. Beer was found to stimulate nonspecific immunity in rats [158], affecting the production and secretion of cytokines [159], counteract osteoporosis [160, 161], inhibit bone resorption [162], and reduce age-induced macular degeneration [163].

11.5.2   WINE

The word "Wine" is derived from the Latin word *Vinum* meaning grapes. It is an alcoholic beverage made from fermented grapes. The earliest known evidence of wine reported from Georgia (Caucasus) dates back to 8000 years old [164]. There are two major classes of wine based on the color, namely Red wine and White wine. The color of grapes from which it is derived plays a major role in determining the class of wine; further, the flavor can vary in both the classes depending upon the variety of grapes and the processing method [165–167]. Wine is also associated with religions as ancient Egyptians relate Red wine with blood. In the making process of wine, grapes are fermented with the help of yeast, and the sugar in the fruit is converted to ethanol and carbon dioxide; there is no extra addition of acids, enzymes, water, or other nutrients. *Vitis vinifera* is the variety of grapes generally used for wine making, and different varieties of wines can be obtained using different strains of yeast and variety of grapes. Instead of grape, wine can also be prepared from fermentation of other fruits like apples and berries, which is generically called fruit wine. The chemical composition of wine is not uniform for all wines, as Red wine has varying alcohol content from 11% to 15%. Generally, wine contains 81% water, 12% alcohol, and the remaining 7% is miscellaneous products formed from fermentation. The detailed composition is summarized in Table 11.2.

TABLE 11.2 A Genearalized Composition of Constituents of Wine.

Vitamin Content of Wine	Mineral Content of Wine	Heart Healthy Nutrient Content of Wine	Other Chemical Compounds in Wine
Thiamin	Sodium	Oligomeric Proantho -cyanidins (OPC's)	Sugar
Riboflavin	Calcium	Resveratrol	Sulfites
Niacin	Iron	Flavonoids (Cat-echins,	Grape Thumatinlike
Vitamins A, B, K & G	Magnesium	Quercetin, Antho-cyanins	Proteins, Amino acids
Foliate	Phosphorus	Bioflavonoids	Gallic acid
Betaine	Potassium	Phenolic Compounds	Tartic acid
Lutein choline	Zinc	Tannins	Mallic acid
Zeakanthin	Copper		Succinic acid
	Manganese		Acetic acid
	Fluoride		Lactic acid
	Selenium		Citric acid

[Source: Ref. 22]

Red wine is rich in plant phenolics that are present in fruits and plays a major role as antioxidants [168]. Consumption of antioxidants like oligomeric proanthocyanidins, resveratrol, and flavonoids has many health benefits against cardiovascular diseases [169] and cancer [170–172]. As wine also contains ethanol, the other beneficial effects are the same as previously described in Section 11.5.2. Spirits are also derived from plant product fermentation, but the distillation recovers the fermented material with a maximum content of alcohol. This process is also used for the production of other alcoholic beverages like bourbon, gin, brandy, rum, and whisky.

11.6 OTHER BEVERAGES

There are other beverages which are neither derived from fruits nor prepared from fermentation processes. These beverages are the mixtures of several components prepared to provide refreshment, replenish ions, and provide instant energy. In preparing these beverages, certain chemicals like artificial sweetners, coloring agents, and caffeine are added, which may become a possible health concern.

11.6.1 CARBONATED DRINKS

Carbonated drinks are nonalcoholic soft drinks that contain carbonated water, a flavoring agent, and a sweetener. To distinguish them from alcoholic liquor, the term "Soft drink" was introduced; they quench thirst [173], have the ability to refresh, and are in good in taste, and hence, they are the most consumed beverage [174, 175]. Diet drinks are the other forms of carbonated drinks, viz. Pepsi®, Diet Coke®, etc. Soft drinks intake is associated with increase in body weight and energy intake. Increased soft drink intake is also associated with decreased intakes of calcium, milk, and other nutrients [176] Due to lack of calories, soft drinks are considered as a healthier alternative, but they are associated with a various health consequences as described below.

11.6.1.1 Health Effects

The adverse effect of these beverages were observed on the liver, bone, teeth, and heart vessels. Carbonated drinks are also commonly referred with different names such as soda or soda pop [177]. Over time, a number of health issues have been reported by regular consumption of soft drinks. A common ingredient of dark soft drinks and colas is caramel color, and during its manufacturing, a carcinogenic compound is produced, namely 4-methylimidazole (4-MEI); a regular intake of 4-MEI present in soft drinks may be a cause of cancer [178]. The consumption of carbonated drinks is also associated with preterm delivery in pregnant women [179]. Studies conducted by Eluwa [174] suggests that soft drinks adversely affects the cerebellum of adult female albino Wistar rats. Obesity, cardiovascular disease, dental/bone problems, diabetes mellitus, kidney stones [180, 181], and metabolic syndrome [182] are the problems associated with the usage of carbonated drinks, thereby attributing to mortality.

11.6.2 ENERGY DRINKS

Beverages containing vitamins, taurine, caffeine, sugar or sweeteners, and herbal supplements are termed as energy drinks; these drinks are supplemented to improve weight loss, athletic performance, stamina, energy, and concentration [183]. These beverages constitutes the fastest growing market in the US in 2011 [184]. They should not be confused with sports drinks or vitamin waters, as they differ in terms of their compositions and effects. Energy drinks rapidly increase energy performance and endurance by positively affecting the blood pressure, respiratory and heart rates. The constituents of energy drinks are sugar, caffeine, herbal supplements and other substances like taurine and gluconolactone. On the other hand, sports drinks contain glucose and electrolytes for rehydrating purpose, whereas vitamin water contains nutrients in addition to the rehydrating agent [185].

Additives like kola nut, guarana, cocoa, and yerba mate may also contribute to the increased amount of caffeine in energy drinks [186–188]. Guarana (Paullinia cupana) in addition to caffeine also contribute for a chronotrope (theobromine), and an inotrope (theophylline) [189, 190].

AMED is the term given when alcohol is mixed with energy drinks; such a combination is even more harmful as it reduces the sensation of intoxication, which may lead to overdrinking, impairment of judgement, decline in neurocognitive functioning, or an alcohol-related motor vehicle accident [191], Caffeine consumption in moderation can be tolerated by healthy people, but heavy consumption of caffeine can cause serious consequences. Few problems associated with high caffeine consumption are stroke, seizures, mania, and sudden death [187, 192]. Hyperactivity was observed in childrens below 2 years who had accidentally consumed energy drink [193].

11.7 IMPORTANT CONTRA-INDICATIONS

Beverages are considered as functional foods because certain beverages contains phytochemicals that promoting and maintain health. However, not all the beverages pledge for health improvement; instead, they may cause harm and are associated with various diseases. The reason for this is atributed to the presence of an artificially added coloring agent, sweeteners, and preservatives or because of the increased amount of certain constituents such as caffeine. Caffeine is the constituent of a majority of beverages such as different types of teas, cocoa drinks, energy drinks, etc. After a regular consumption of caffeine, its overdose or withdrawal can cause a variety of problems [194]. Caffeine may sometime upset stomach or cause heartburn by releasing the acid in the stomach; caffeine overdose may cause diarrhea, increased urination, and excessive thirst [195]. Nausea and vomiting are the common symptoms observed after withdrawal from caffeine. Sweeteners added to the drinks are associated with a number of health-related problems, Aspartame as a sweetener has replaced sugar in almost everything; three chemicals, namely methanol, phenylalanine, and aspartic acid, are produced from the digestion of aspartame [196]. It is highly toxic for people suffering from phenylketon-uria, as such people cannot process phenylalanine, thereby increasing their blood phenylalanine concentration. A genetically modified sweetner, namely high fructose corn syrup, is the main ingredient present in many soft drinks as it is easy to produce and inexpensive to purchase; its usage causes increase in the triglyceride levels and increase in bad cholesterol [197].

On an average, pizza and coke contains an equal concentration of salt, i.e., 55 mg; such a high concentration of salt may cause increased blood pressure, stroke, and heart diseases; dehydrate body; and cause liver over-load [198]. All these chemicals work together and contributing to today's diabetic and obesity epidemic. They are contributing to more deaths as com-pared to other nutritious causes [197].

Beverages are consumed to provide energy but at the same time contrib-ute to many obesity-related health issues. Selection of soothing and healthy beverages is therefore very much important for regular users . Because obe-sity and diabetes are very common in the population, proper medical advice is recommended for regular consumption of beverages. Use of noncalorific sweeteners has also gained importance for obese or diabetic people. Con-sidering the positive and negative effects of the beverages, caution should be taken while consuming energy drinks. Regulatory bodies must strictly monitor overambitious sales and marketing strategies and nonscientific claims.

11.8   SUMMARY

- Beverages are known as refreshment next to water since ancient era because of their health benefits, taste, and tradition.
- Their ingredients are water, salts, sugars, minerals, vitamins, and phy-tochemicals.
- Based on their ingredients and their beneficial effect, they are recom-mended in varying conditions.
- They rehydrate the body and help to regulate digestion, proper circula-tion of blood, transport of nutrients to different body parts, and main-tain the body temperature.

- Currently, many beverages are available in the market and have high demand amongst youngsters.
- The biologically active compounds in the beverages determine their nature, and accordingly, beverages are recommended in different health conditions.
- Intake of sugar-containing beverages are known to provide energy, but at the same time, contribute to many obesity-related health issues. Selection of soothing and healthy beverages is therefore very much important for regular users.
- Because obesity and diabetes are very common in the population, proper medical advice is recommended for regular consumption. Use of noncalorific sweeteners has also gained importance for obese or diabetic people.
- Considering the positive and negative effects of the beverages, caution should be taken while consuming energy drinks. Regulatory bodies must strictly monitor overambitious sales and marketing strategies and nonscientific claims.

KEYWORDS

- **anticancerous**
- **beer**
- **beverages**
- **milk**
- **wine**

REFERENCES

1. Caroli, A. M., Chessa, S., & Erhardt, G. J., (2009). Invited review: Milk protein polymorphisms in cattle: Effect on animal breeding and human nutrition. *Journal of Dairy Science.*, *92*(11), 5335–5352.
2. Kalac, P., & Samkova, E., (2010). The effects of feeding various forages on fatty acid composition of bovine milk fat: A review. *Czech Journal of Animal Science*, *55*(12), 521–537.

3. Haug, A., Hostmark, A. T., & Harstad, O. M., (2007). Bovine milk in human nutrition–a review. *Lipids in Health and Disease*, *6*(1), 1.

4. Lindmark-Mansson, H., Fonden, R., & Pettersson, H. E., (2003). Composition of Swedish dairy milk. *International Dairy Journal*, *13*(6), 409–425.

5. Severin, S., Wenshui X., (2005). Milk biologically active components as nutraceuticals: review. *Critical Reviews in Food Science and Nutrition*, *45*(7–8), 645–656.

6. Schaafsma, G., (2000). Criteria and significance of dietary protein sources in humans. *J. Nutr.*, *130*, 1865S-1867S.

7. Boye, J., Wijesinha-Bettoni, R., & Burlingame, B., (2012). Protein quality evaluation twenty years after the introduction of the protein digestibility corrected amino acid score method. *British Journal of Nutrition*, *108*(S2), S183–211.

8. Godden, S., (2008). Colostrum management for dairy calves. Veterinary Clinics of North America: *Food Animal Practice*, *24*(1), 19–39.

9. Politis, I., & Chronopoulou, R., (2008). Milk peptides and immune response in the neonate. *In Bioactive Components of Milk* (pp. 253–269). Springer, New York.

10. Holt, C., Carver, J. A., Ecroyd, H., & Thorn, D. C., (2013). Invited review: Caseins and the casein micelle: their biological functions, structures, & behavior in foods. *Journal of Dairy Science*, *96*(10), 6127–6146.

11. Shin, K., Hayasawa, H., & Lonnerdal, B., (2001). Purification and quantification of lactoperoxidase in human milk with use of immunoadsorbents with antibodies against recombinant human lactoperoxidase. *The American Journal of Clinical Nutrition*, *73*(5), 984–989.

12. Pereira, P. C., (2014). Milk nutritional composition and its role in human health. *Nutrition*, *30*(6), 619–627.

13. Ye, A., Cui, J., & Singh, H., (2010). Effect of the fat globule membrane on in vitro digestion of milk fat globules with pancreatic lipase. *International Dairy Journal*, *20*(12), 822–829.

14. Gaucheron, F., (2011). Milk and dairy products: a unique micronutrient combination. *Journal of the American College of Nutrition*, *30*(sup5), 400S-409S.

15. Miller, D. D. Welch, R. M., (2013). Food system strategies for preventing micronutrient malnutrition. *Food Policy*, *42*, 115–128.

16. Ohlsson, L., (2010). Dairy products and plasma cholesterol levels. *Food & Nutrition Research*, *19*, 54.

17. Soedamah-Muthu, S. S., Ding, E. L., Al-Delaimy, W. K., Hu, F. B., Engberink, M. F., Willett, W. C., & Geleijnse, J. M., (2011). Milk and dairy consumption and incidence of cardiovascular diseases and all-cause mortality: dose-response meta-analysis of prospective cohort studies. *The American Journal of Clinical Nutrition*, *93*(1), 158–171.

18. Huth, P. J., & Park, K. M., (2012). Influence of dairy product and milk fat consumption on cardiovascular disease risk: a review of the evidence. Advances in Nutrition: *An International Review Journal*, *3*(3), 266–285.

19. Phelan, M., Aherne, A., FitzGerald, R. J., & O'Brien, N. M., (2009). Casein-derived bioactive peptides: biological effects, industrial uses, safety aspects and regulatory status. *International Dairy Journal*, *19*(11), 643–654.

20. Politis, I., & Chronopoulou, R., (2008). Milk peptides and immune response in the neonate. *In Bioactive Components of Milk* (pp. 253–269). Springer New York.

21. Fiat, A. M., Migliore-Samour, D., Jolles, P., Drouet, L., Sollier, C. B., & Caen, J., (1993). Biologically active peptides from milk proteins with emphasis on two examples

concerning antithrombotic and immunomodulating activities. *Journal of Dairy Science*, *76*(1), 301–310.

22. Zhang, C. X., Ho, S. C., Fu, J. H., Cheng, S. Z., Chen, Y. M., & Lin, F. Y., (2011). Dairy products, calcium intake, & breast cancer risk: a case-control study in China. *Nutrition and Cancer*, *63*(1), 12–20.

23. Bessaoud, F., Daures, J. P., & Gerber, M., (2008). Dietary factors and breast cancer risk: a case control study among a population in Southern France. *Nutrition and Cancer*, *60*(2), 177–187.

24. Aune, D., Lau, R., Chan, D. S., Vieira, R., Greenwood, D. C., Kampman, E., & Norat, T., (2012). Dairy products and colorectal cancer risk: a systematic review and meta-analysis of cohort studies. *Annals of Oncology*, *23*(1), 37–45.

25. Murphy, N., Norat, T., Ferrari, P., Jenab, M., Bueno-de-Mesquita, B., Skeie, G., Olsen, A., Tjonneland, A., Dahm, C. C., Overvad, K., & Boutron-Ruault, M. C., (2013). Consumption of dairy products and colorectal cancer in the European Prospective Investigation into Cancer and Nutrition (EPIC). *PLoS One, 2, 8*(9), e72715.

26. Li, F., An, S. L., Zhou, Y., Liang, Z. K., Jiao, Z. J., Jing, Y. M., Wan, P., Shi, X. J., & Tan, W. L., (2011). Milk and dairy consumption and risk of bladder cancer: a meta-analysis. *Urology*, *78*(6), 1298–1305.

27. Huncharek, M., Muscat, J., & Kupelnick, B., (2008). Dairy products, dietary calcium and vitamin D intake as risk factors for prostate cancer: a meta-analysis of 26, *769* cases from 45 observational studies. *Nutrition and Cancer*, *60*(4), 421–441.

28. Thielen, C., Will, F., Zacharlas, J., Dietrich, H., & Jacob, H., (2004). Polyphenols in apples: Distribution of polyphenols in apple tissue and comparison of fruit and juice. *Deutsche Lebensmittel-Rundschau*, *100*(10), 389–398.

29. Łata, B., & Tomala, K., (2007). Apple peel as a contributor to whole fruit quantity of potentially healthful bioactive compounds. Cultivar and year implication. *Journal of Agricultural and Food Chemistry*, *55*(26), 10795–0802.

30. Gerhauser, C., (2008). Cancer chemopreventive potential of apples, apple juice, & apple components. *Planta Medica.*, *74*(13), 1608–1624.

31. Souci, S. W. Fachmann, W., & Kraut, H., (2005). Revised by Kirchhoff, E. *Food Composition and Nutrition Tables*, based on the 6th edition. Stuttgart: medpharm GmbH Scientific Publishers.

32. Ames, B. N. Shigenaga, M. K., & Hagen, T. M., (1993). Oxidants, antioxidants, & the degenerative diseases of aging. *Proceedings of the National Academy of Sciences*, *90*(17), 7915–7922.

33. Boyer, J., & Liu, R. H., (2004). Apple phytochemicals and their health benefits. *Nutrition Journal*, *3*(1), 1.

34. Percival, S. S., Bukowski, J. F., & Milner, J., (2008). Bioactive food components that enhance γδ T cell function may play a role in cancer prevention. *The Journal of Nutrition*, *138*(1), 1–4.

35. Feskanich, D., Ziegler, R. G., Michaud, D. S., Giovannucci, E. L., Speizer, F. E., Willett, W. C., & Colditz, G. A., (2000). Prospective study of fruit and vegetable consumption and risk of lung cancer among men and women. *Journal of the National Cancer Institute*, *92*(22), 1812–1823.

36. Ehler, S. A., (2011). Citrus and its benefits. *J. Bot.*, *5*(201207), 6.

37. Economos, C., & Clay, W. D., (1999). *Nutritional and Health Benefits of Citrus Fruits*. Energy (kcal), *62*(78), 37.

38. Craig, W. J., (1997). Phytochemicals: guardians of our health. *Journal of the American Dietetic Association*, *97*(10), S199–S204.

39. Donatus, E. O., (2008). A rich source of phytochemicals and their role in human health- a review, *International Journal of Chemical Science*, *6*(2), 451–471.

40. Benavente-García, O., Castillo, J., Marin, F. R., Ortuno, A., & Del Río, J. A., (1997). Uses and properties of citrus flavonoids. *Journal of Agricultural and Food Chemistry*, *45*(12), 4505–4515.

41. Suryawanshi, J. A., (2011). An overview of Citrus aurantium used in treatment of various diseases. *African Journal of Plant Science*, *5*(7), 390–395.

42. Gutherie, H., & Picciano, M., (1995). *Human Nutrition*, St Louis, MO, USA, Mosby.

43. Mangels, A. R. Holden, J. M. Beecher, G. R. Forman, M. R. Lanza, E., (1993). Carotenoid content of fruits and vegetables: an evaluation of analytic data. *Journal of the American Dietetic Association*, 93(3):284–296.

44. Britton, G., (1995). Structure and properties of carotenoids in relation to function. *The FASEB Journal*, *9*(15), 1551–1558.

45. Whitney, E., & Rolfes, S., (1999). *Understanding Nutrition. Eighth ed.* Belmont, Ca., USA, West/Wadsworth. (ed. W. Rolfes).

46. Vinson, J. A., Staretz, M. E., Bose, P., Kassm, H. M., & Basalyga, B. S., (1989). In vitro and in vivo reduction of erythrocyte sorbitol by ascorbic acid. *Diabetes.*, 38(8), 1036–1041.

47. Steinmetz, K. A., & Potter, J. D., (1991). Vegetables, fruits, cancer. I. Epidemiology. *Cancer Causes & Control.*, *2*(5), 325–357.

48. Okwu, D. E., & Emenike, I. N., (2007). Nutritive value and mineral content of different varieties of citrus fruits. *Journal of Food Technology*, *5*(2), 105–108.

49. Rapisarda, P., Tomaino, A., Lo Cascio, R., Bonina, F., De Pasquale, A., & Saija, A., (1999). Antioxidant effectiveness as influenced by phenolic content of fresh orange juices. *Journal of Agricultural and Food Chemistry*, *47*(11), 4718–4723.

50. Han, Y., Dong, F., Xu, J., Liu, X., Li, Y., Kong, Z., Liang, X., Liu, N., & Zheng, Y., (2014). Residue change of pyridaben in apple samples during apple cider processing. *Food Control*, *37*, 240–244.

51. Lea, A. G., (1990). Bitterness and astringency: the procyanidins of fermented apple ciders. *Developments in Food Science*.

52. Lea, A. G., & Drilleau, J. F., (2003). Cidermaking. *In Fermented Beverage Production* (pp. 59–87), Springer, US.

53. Alonso-Salces, R. M., Barranco, A., Abad, B., Berrueta, L. A., Gallo, B., & Vicente, F., (2004). Polyphenolic profiles of Basque cider apple cultivars and their technological properties. *Journal of Agricultural and Food Chemistry*, *52*(10), 2938–2952.

54. Alonso-Salces, R. M., Korta, E., Barranco, A., Berrueta, L. A., Gallo, B., & Vicente, F., (2001). Determination of polyphenolic profiles of Basque cider apple varieties using accelerated solvent extraction. *Journal of Agricultural and Food Chemistry*, *49*(8), 3761–3767.

55. Hertog, M. G., Feskens, E. J., Kromhout, D., Hollman, P. C., & Katan, M. B., (1993). Dietary antioxidant flavonoids and risk of coronary heart disease: the Zutphen Elderly Study. *The Lancet*, *342*(8878), 1007–1011.

56. Chinnici, F., Bendini, A., Gaiani, A., & Riponi, C., (2004). Radical scavenging activities of peels and pulps from cv. Golden Delicious apples as related to their phenolic composition. *Journal of Agricultural and Food Chemistry*, *52*(15), 4684–4689.

57. DuPont, M. S., Bennett, R. N., Mellon, F. A., & Williamson, G., (2002). Polyphenols from alcoholic apple cider are absorbed, metabolized and excreted by humans. *The Journal of Nutrition, 132*(2), 172–175.

58. Madrera, R. R., Lobo, A. P., & Valles, B. S., (2006). Phenolic profile of Asturian (Spain) natural cider. *Journal of Agricultural and Food Chemistry, 54*(1), 120–124.

59. Alonso-Salces, R. M., Herrero, C., Barranco, A., Lopez-Marquez, D. M., Berrueta, L. A., Gallo, B., & Vicente, F., (2006). Polyphenolic compositions of Basque natural ciders: A chemometric study. *Food Chemistry, 97*(3), 438–446.

60. Sponholz, W. R., (1993). Wine spoilage by microorganisms. *Wine Microbiology and Biotechnology*, 395–420.

61. Siebert, K. J., Carrasco, A., & Lynn, P. Y., (1996). Formation of protein-polyphenol haze in beverages. *Journal of Agricultural and Food Chemistry, 44*(8), 1997–2005.

62. Kawamoto, H., & Nakatsubo, F., (1997). Effects of environmental factors on two-stage tannin-protein co-precipitation. *Phytochemistry, 46*(3), 479–483.

63. Sairi, M. Yih, L. J., & Sarmidi, M. R., (2004). Chemical composition and sensory analysis of fresh pineapple juice and deacidified pineapple juice using electrodialysis. In *Regional Symposium on Membrane Science and Technology*, pp. 21–25.

64. Hossain, M. F., Akhtar, S., & Anwar, M., (2015). Nutritional value and medicinal benefits of pineapple. *International Journal of Nutrition and Food Sciences, 4*(1), 84.

65. Duke, J. A., (1993). *CRC Handbook of Alternative Cash Crops*. CRC press.

66. Samson, J. A., (1986). *Tropical Fruits*, 2nd ed., New York, Longman Inc.

67. Sabahel Khier, K. M., Hussain, A. S., & Ishag, K. E., (2010). Effect of maturity stage on protein fractionation, in vitro protein digestibility and anti-nutrition factors in pineapple (Ananas comosis) fruit grown in Southern Sudan. *African Journal of Food Science, 4*(8), 550–552.

68. Xie, W., Xing, D., Sun, H., Wang, W., Ding, Y., & Du, L., (2005). The effects of Ananas comosus L. leaves on diabetic-dyslipidemic rats induced by alloxan and a high-fat/high-cholesterol diet. *The American Journal of Chinese Medicine, 33*(01), 95–105.

69. Pavan, R., Jain, S., & Kumar, A., (2012). Properties and therapeutic application of bromelain: a review. *Biotechnology Research International*.

70. Cohen, A., & Goldman, J., (1964). Bromelain therapy in rheumatoid arthritis. *Pennsylvania Medical Journal, 67*, 27–30.

71. Neumayer, C., Fugl, A., Nanobashvili, J., Blumer, R., Punz, A., Gruber, H., Polterauer, P., & Huk, I., (2006). Combined enzymatic and antioxidative treatment reduces ischemia-reperfusion injury in rabbit skeletal muscle. *Journal of Surgical Research, 133*(2), 150–158.

72. Heinicke, R. M., & Gortner, W. A., (1957). Stem bromelain—a new protease preparation from pineapple plants. *Economic Botany, 11*(3), 225–234.

73. Gil, M. I., Tomas-Barberan, F. A., Hess-Pierce, B., Holcroft, D. M., & Kader, A. A., (2000). Antioxidant activity of pomegranate juice and its relationship with phenolic composition and processing. *Journal of Agricultural and Food Chemistry, 48*(10), 4581–4589.

74. Fischer, U. A., Carle, R., & Kammerer, D. R., (2013). Thermal stability of anthocyanins and colourless phenolics in pomegranate (Punica granatum L.) juices and model solutions. *Food Chemistry, 138*(2), 1800–1809.

75. Viuda-Martos, M., Fernandez-Lopez, J., Perez-Alvarez, J. A., (2010). Pomegranate and its many functional components as related to human health: a review. *Comprehensive Reviews in Food Science and Food Safety, 9*(6), 635–654.

76. Fischer, U. A., Carle, R., & Kammerer, D. R., (2011). Identification and quantification of phenolic compounds from pomegranate (Punica granatum L.) peel, mesocarp, aril and differently produced juices by HPLC-DAD–ESI/MS n. *Food Chemistry*, *127*(2), 807–821.

77. Turfan, O., Turkyılmaz, M., Yemis, O., & Ozkan, M., (2011). Anthocyanin and colour changes during processing of pomegranate (Punica granatum L., cv. Hicaznar) juice from sacs and whole fruit. *Food Chemistry*, *129*(4), 1644–1651.

78. Rajasekar, D., Akoh, C. C., Martino, K. G., & MacLean, D. D., (2012). Physico-chemical characteristics of juice extracted by blender and mechanical press from pomegranate cultivars grown in Georgia. *Food Chemistry*, *133*(4), 1383–1393.

79. Caleb, O. J., Opara, U. L., & Witthuhn, C. R., (2012). Modified atmosphere packaging of pomegranate fruit and arils: a review. *Food and Bioprocess Technology*, *5*(1), 15–30.

80. Fawole, O. A., & Opara, U. L., (2013). Effects of maturity status on biochemical content, polyphenol composition and antioxidant capacity of pomegranate fruit arils (cv.'Bhagwa'). *South African Journal of Botany*, *85*, 23–31.

81. Fawole, O. A., & Opara, U. L., (2013). Changes in physical properties, chemical and elemental composition and antioxidant capacity of pomegranate (cv. Ruby) fruit at five maturity stages. *Scientia Horticulturae*, *150*, 37–46.

82. Mphahlele, R. R., Fawole, O. A., Stander, M. A., & Opara, U. L., (2014). Preharvest and postharvest factors influencing bioactive compounds in pomegranate (Punica granatum L.)—A review. *Scientia Horticulturae*, *178*, 114–123.

83. Mphahlele, R. R., Stander, M. A., Fawole, O. A., & Opara, U. L., (2014). Effect of fruit maturity and growing location on the postharvest contents of flavonoids, phenolic acids, vitamin C and antioxidant activity of pomegranate juice (cv. Wonderful). *Scientia Horticulturae*, *179*, 36–45.

84. Miguel, M. G., Neves, M. A., & Antunes, M. D., (2010). Pomegranate (Punica granatum L.): A medicinal plant with myriad biological properties-A short review. *Journal of Medicinal Plants Research*, *4*(25), 2836–2847.

85. Cavallini, G., Dacha, M., Potenza, L., Ranieri, A., Scattino, C., Castagna, A., & Bergamini, E., (2014). Use of red blood cell membranes to evaluate the antioxidant potential of plant extracts. *Plant Foods for Human Nutrition*, *69*(2), 108–114.

86. Salgado, J. M., Ferreira, T. R., de Oliveira Biazotto, F., dos Santos Dias, C, T., (2012). Increased antioxidant content in juice enriched with dried extract of pomegranate (Punica granatum) peel. *Plant Foods for Human Nutrition*, *67*(1), 39–43.

87. Zahin, M., Ahmad, I., Gupta, R. C., & Aqil, F., (2014). Punicalagin and ellagic acid demonstrate antimutagenic activity and inhibition of benzo [a] pyrene induced DNA adducts. *Bio. Med. Research International*, *14*, 2014.

88. Les, F., Prieto, J. M., Arbones-Mainar, J. M., Valero, M. S., & Lopez, V., (2015). Bioactive properties of commercialized pomegranate (Punica granatum) juice: antioxidant, antiproliferative and enzyme inhibiting activities. *Food & Function*, *6*(6), 2049–2057.

89. Yamamoto, Takehiko, Lekh, R. J., & Mujo, K., (1997). *Chemistry and Applications of Green Tea*. CRC press.

90. Van der Stegen, G. A., (1985). A process for removing caffeine and substances that are potentially detrimental to health from coffee receptors. European Patent 0158381.

91. Adler, I. L., & Earle, E. L. Jr., (1960). Process for preparing a decaffeinated soluble coffee extract. Receptors, US. patent 2933395.

92. Zeller, B. L., Kaleda, W. W., & Saleeb, F. Z., (1985). Coffee extract decaffeination method. Receptors. US. patent 4521438.

93. Jones, G. V., Meinhold, J. F., & Musto, J. A., (1985). Non- caffeine solids recovery process. Receptors. US. patents.

94. Yamamoto, T., Hsu, S., Lewis, J., Wataha, J., Dickinson, D., Singh, B., Bollag, W. B., Lockwood, P., Ueta, E., Osaki, T., & Schuster, G., (2003). Green tea polyphenol causes differential oxidative environments in tumor versus normal epithelial cells. *Journal of Pharmacology and Experimental Therapeutics, 307*(1), 230–236.

95. Varnam, A., & Sutherland, J. M., (1994). *Beverages: technology, chemistry and microbiology.* Springer, *Science & Business Media.*

96. Erba, D., Riso P., Bordoni, A., Foti, P., Biagi, P. L., & Testolin, G., (2005). Effectiveness of moderate green tea consumption on the antioxidative status and plasma lipid profile in humans. *The Journal of Nutritional Biochemistry, 16*(3), 144–149.

97. Lambert, J. D., & Yang, C. S., (2003). Mechanisms of cancer prevention by tea constituents. *The Journal of Nutrition, 133*(10), 3262S-7S.

98. Inoue, M., Tajima, K., Hirose, K., Hamajima, N., Takezaki, T., Kuroishi, T., & Tominaga, S., (1998). Tea and coffee consumption and the risk of digestive tract cancers: data from a comparative case-referent study in Japan. *Cancer Causes & Control, 9*(2), 209–216.

99. Bianchi, G. D., Cerhan, J. R., Parker, A. S., Putnam, S. D., See, W. A., Lynch, C. F., & Cantor, K. P., (2000). Tea consumption and risk of bladder and kidney cancers in a population-based case-control study. *American Journal of Epidemiology, 151*(4), 377–383.

100. Laurie, S. A., Miller, V. A., Grant, S. C., Kris, M. G., & Ng, K. K., (2005). Phase I study of green tea extract in patients with advanced lung cancer. *Cancer Chemotherapy and Pharmacology, 55*(1), 33–38.

101. Anshumittal, M. S., & Wylie, R. C., (2004). Egcg down-regulates telomerase in human breast carcinoma MCF-7 cells, leading to suppression of cell viability and induction of apoptosis. *International Journal of Oncology, 24,* 703–710.

102. Zhou, J. R., Yu, L., Mai, Z., & Blackburn, G. L., (2004). Combined inhibition of estrogen-dependent human breast carcinoma by soy and tea bioactive components in mice. *International Journal of Cancer, 108*(1), 8–14.

103. Wu, C. D., & Wei, G. X., (2002). Tea as a functional food for oral health. *Nutrition, 18*(5), 443–444.

104. Begona Barroso, M., & Van de Werken, G., (1999). Determination of green and black tea composition by capillary electrophoresis. *Journal of High Resolution Chromatography, 22*(4), 225–230.

105. Striegel, L., Kang, B., Pilkenton, S. J., Rychlik, M., & Apostolidis, E., (2015). Effect of black tea and black tea pomace polyphenols on α-glucosidase and α-amylase inhibition, relevant to type 2 diabetes prevention. *Frontiers in Nutrition, 2,* 3.

106. Gostner, J. M., Becker, K., Croft, K. D., Woodman, R. J., Puddey, I. B., Fuchs, D., & Hodgson, J. M., (2015). Regular consumption of black tea increases circulating kynurenine concentrations: A randomized controlled trial. *BBA Clinical, 3,* 31–35.

107. Henning, S. M., Wang, P., Said, J. W., Huang, M., Grogan, T., Elashoff, D., Carpenter, C. L., Heber, D., & Aronson, W. J., (2015). Randomized clinical trial of brewed green and black tea in men with prostate cancer prior to prostatectomy. *The Prostate, 75*(5), 550–559.

108. Miura, K., Hughes, M. C., Arovah, N. I., Van der Pols, J. C., & Green, A. C., (2015). Black tea consumption and risk of skin cancer: An 11-year prospective study. *Nutrition and Cancer, 67*(7), 1049–1055.

109. Konarikova, K., Jezovicova, M., Kerestes, J., Gbelcova, H., Durackova, Z., & Zitnanova, I., (2015). Anticancer effect of black tea extract in human cancer cell lines. *Springerplus*, *4*(1), 1.

110. Astin, J. A., Pelletier, K. R., Marie, A., & Haskell, W. L., (2000). Complementary and alternative medicine use among elderly persons: one-year analysis. *J. Gerontol. Med. Sci.*, *55*, M4–9.

111. Hansen, H. V., & Christensen, K. I., (2009). The common chamomile and the scentless mayweed revisited. *Taxon.*, *58*(1), 261–264.

112. Tschiggerl, C., & Bucar, F., (2012). Guaianolides and Volatile Compounds in Chamomile Tea. *Plant Foods for Human Nutrition*, *67*(2).

113. Schilcher, H., & Die Kamille, (1987). Handbuch fur Arzte, Apotheker und andere Naturwissenschaft-ler. Stuttgart, etc.: G. Fischer Verlag.

114. Srivastava, J. K., Shankar, E., & Gupta, S., (2010). Chamomile: A herbal medicine of the past with bright future. *Molecular Medicine Reports*, *3*(6), 895.

115. Chang, S. M., & Chen, C. H., (2016). Effects of an intervention with drinking chamomile tea on sleep quality and depression in sleep disturbed postnatal women: a randomized controlled trial. *Journal of Advanced Nursing*, *72*(2), 306–315.

116. Riza, E., Linos, A., Petralias, A., de Martinis, L., Duntas, L., & Linos, D., (2015). The effect of Greek herbal tea consumption on thyroid cancer: a case-control study. *The European Journal of Public Health*, *25*(6), 1001–1005.

117. Howrey, B. T., Peek, M. K., McKee, J. M., Raji, M. A., Ottenbacher, K. J., & Markides, K. S., (2015). Chamomile Consumption and Mortality: A Prospective Study of Mexican Origin Older Adults. *The Gerontologist.*, *29*, gnv051.

118. Srivastava, J. K., & Gupta, S., (2007). Antiproliferative and apoptotic effects of chamomile extract in various human cancer cells. *Journal of Agricultural and Food Chemistry*, *55*(23), 9470–9478.

119. Birt, D. F., Mitchell, D., Gold, B., Pour, P., & Pinch, H. C., (1996). Inhibition of ultraviolet light induced skin carcinogenesis in SKH-1 mice by apigenin, a plant flavonoid. *Anticancer Research*, *17*(1A), 85–91.

120. Way, T. D., Kao, M. C., & Lin, J. K., (2004). Apigenin induces apoptosis through proteasomal degradation of HER2/neu in HER2/neu-overexpressing breast cancer cells via the phosphatidylinositol 3-kinase/Akt-dependent pathway. *Journal of Biological Chemistry.*, *279*(6), 4479–4489.

121. Patel, D., Shukla, S., & Gupta, S., (2007). Apigenin and cancer chemoprevention: progress, potential and promise (review). *International Journal of Oncology*, *30*(1), 233–246.

122. Svilaas, A., Sakhi, A. K., Andersen, L. F., Svilaas, T., Strom, E. C., Jacobs, D. R., & Ose, L., (2004). Blomhoff, R. Intakes of antioxidants in coffee, wine, & vegetables are correlated with plasma carotenoids in humans. *The Journal of Nutrition*, *134*(3), 562–567.

123. Horn-Ross, P. L., Lee, M., John, E. M., & Koo, J., (2000). Sources of phytoestrogen exposure among non-Asian women in California, USA. *Cancer Causes & Control*, *11*(4), 299–302.

124. Glade, M. J., (1999). Food, nutrition, & the prevention of cancer: a global perspective. American Institute for Cancer Research/World Cancer Research Fund, American Institute for Cancer Research, 1997. *Nutrition* (Burbank, Los Angeles County, Calif.), *15*(6), 523.

125. Huber, W. W., Scharf, G., Nagel, G., Prustomersky, S., Schulte-Hermann, R., & Kaina, B., (2003). Coffee and its chemopreventive components Kahweol and Cafestol increase the activity of O 6-methylguanine-DNA methyltransferase in rat liver—comparison

with phase II xenobiotic metabolism. *Mutation Research/Fundamental and Molecular Mechanisms of Mutagenesis*, *522*(1), 57–68.

126. Cavin, C., Holzhaeuser, D., Scharf, G., Constable, A., Huber, W. W., & Schilter, B., (2002). Cafestol and kahweol, two coffee specific diterpenes with anticarcinogenic activity. *Food and Chemical Toxicology*, *40*(8), 1155–1163.

127. Cavin, C., Marin-Kuan, M., Langouet, S., Bezencon, C., Guignard, G., Verguet, C., Piguet, D., Holzhauser, D., Cornaz, R., & Schilter, B., (2008). Induction of Nrf2-mediated cellular defenses and alteration of phase I activities as mechanisms of chemoprotective effects of coffee in the liver. *Food and Chemical Toxicology*, *46*(4), 1239–1248.

128. Rodriguez de Sotillo, D. V., & Hadley, M., (2002). Chlorogenic acid modifies plasma and liver concentrations of: cholesterol, triacylglycerol, & minerals in (fa/fa) Zucker rats. *The Journal of Nutritional Biochemistry*, *13*(12), 717–726.

129. Bohn, S. K., Blomhoff, R., & Paur, I., (2014). Coffee and cancer risk, epidemiological evidence, & molecular mechanisms. *Molecular Nutrition & Food Research*, *58*(5), 915–930.

130. Ding, E. L., Hutfless, S. M., Ding, X., & Girotra, S., (2006). Chocolate and prevention of cardiovascular disease: a systematic review. *Nutrition & Metabolism*, *3*(1), 1.

131. Hooper, L., Kay, C., Abdelhamid, A., Kroon, P. A., Cohn, J. S., Rimm, E. B., & Cassidy, A., (2012). Effects of chocolate, cocoa, & flavan-3-ols on cardiovascular health: a systematic review and meta-analysis of randomized trials. *The American Journal of Clinical Nutrition.*, *95*(3), 740–751.

132. Desch, S., Schmidt, J., Kobler, D., Sonnabend, M., Eitel, I., Sareban, M., Rahimi, K., Schuler, G., & Thiele, H., (2010). Effect of cocoa products on blood pressure: systematic review and meta-analysis. *American Journal of Hypertension*, *23*(1), 97–103.

133. Dillinger, T. L., Barriga, P., Escarcega, S., Jimenez, M., Lowe, D. S., & Grivetti, L. E., (2000). Food of the gods: cure for humanity? A cultural history of the medicinal and ritual use of chocolate. *The Journal of Nutrition*, *130*(8), 2057S–2072S.

134. Coe, S. D., & Coe, M. D., (1996). *The True History of Chocolate*. London, UK: Thames and Hudson.

135. Nakagawa, H., Hasumi, K., Woo, J. T., Nagai, K., & Wachi, M., (2004). Generation of hydrogen peroxide primarily contributes to the induction of Fe (II)-dependent apoptosis in Jurkat cells by (−)-epigallocatechin gallate. *Carcinogenesis*, *25*(9), 1567–1574.

136. Lee, K. W., Kim, Y. J., Lee, H. J., & Lee, C. Y., (2003). Cocoa has more phenolic phytochemicals and a higher antioxidant capacity than teas and red wine. *Journal of Agricultural and Food Chemistry*, *51*(25), 7292–7295.

137. Heo, H. J., & Lee, C. Y., (2005). Epicatechin and catechin in cocoa inhibit amyloid β protein induced apoptosis. *Journal of Agricultural and Food Chemistry*, *53*(5), 1445–1448.

138. Martin, M. A., Goya, L., & Ramos, S., (2013). Potential for preventive effects of cocoa and cocoa polyphenols in cancer. *Food and Chemical Toxicology*, *56*, 336–351.

139. Vaughan-Martini, A., & Martini, A., (1995). Facts, myths and legends on the prime industrial microorganism. *Journal of Industrial Microbiology*, *14*(6), 514–522.

140. Rudgley R., (1993). *The Alchemy of Culture: Intoxicants in Society*. London: British Museum Press.

141. Grigg, D., (2004). Wine, spirits and beer: world patterns of consumption. *Geography*, *1*, 99–110.

142. Nelson, M., (2005). *The Barbarian's Beverage: A History of Beer in Ancient Europe*. Routledge.

143. Nachel, M., & Steve, E., (2012). *Beer for Dummies*. John Wiley & Sons.
144. Hough, J. S., Briggs, D. E., Stevens, R., & Young, T. W., (2012). *Malting and Brewing Science: Volume II, Hopped Wort and Beer*. Springer.
145. Gerhauser, C., (2005). Beer constituents as potential cancer chemopreventive agents. *European Journal of Cancer*, 41(13), 1941–1954.
146. Sohrabvandi, S., Mortazavian, A. M., & Rezaei, K., (2012). Health-related aspects of beer: a review. *International Journal of Food Properties*, 15(2), 350–373.
147. Sohrabvandi, S., Razavi, S. H., Mousavi, S. M., & Mortazavian, A. M., (2010). Viability of probiotic bacteria in low-alcohol-and non-alcoholic beer during refrigerated storage. *Philipp. Agric. Scientist*, 93, 24–28.
148. Bokulich, N. A., & Bamforth, C. W., (2013). The microbiology of malting and brewing. *Microbiology and Molecular Biology Reviews*, 77(2), 157–172.
149. Forsander, O. A., (1998). Dietary influences on alcohol intake: a review. *Journal of Studies on Alcohol*, 59(1), 26–31.
150. Buday, A. Z., & Denis, G., (1974). *The Diuretic Effect of Beer*. Brew Dig, 49(6), 56–58.
151. Ghiselli, A., Natella, F., Guidi, A., Montanari, L., Fantozzi, P., & Scaccini, C., (2000). Beer increases plasma antioxidant capacity in humans. *The Journal of Nutritional Biochemistry*, 11(2), 76–80.
152. Bamforth, C. W., (2002). Nutritional aspects of beer—a review. *Nutrition Research*, 22(1), 227–237.
153. Boehm, T., Folkman, J., Browder, T., & O'Reilly, M. S., (1997). Antiangiogenic therapy of experimental cancer does not induce acquired drug resistance. *Nature*, 390(6658), 404–407.
154. Kim, K. J., Li, B., Winer, J., Armanini, M., Gillett, N., Pillips, H. S., & Ferrara, N., (1993). Inhibition of vascular endothelial growth factor-induced angiogenesis suppresses tumour growth in vivo. *Nature*, 362, 841–844.
155. Dimmitt, S. B., Rakic, V., Puddey, I. B., Baker, R., Oostryck, R., Adams, M. J., Chesterman, C. N., Burke, V., & Beilin, L. J., (1998). The effects of alcohol on coagulation and fibrinolytic factors: a controlled trial. *Blood Coagulation & Fibrinolysis*, 9(1), 39–46.
156. Renaud, S. C., & Ruf, J. C., (1996). Effects of alcohol on platelet functions. *Clinica Chimica Acta*, 246(1), 77–89.
157. Vinson, J. A., Mandarano, M., Hirst, M., Trevithick, J. R., & Bose, P., (2003). Phenol antioxidant quantity and quality in foods: beers and the effect of two types of beer on an animal model of atherosclerosis. *Journal of Agricultural and Food Chemistry*, 51(18), 5528–5533.
158. Autelitano, D. J., Howarth, A. E., & Pihl, E., (1984). Promoting effect of beer and ethanol on anti-tumour cytotoxicity: unaffected growth of a transplantable rat tumour. *Aus. J. Exp. Biol. Med. Sci.*, 62, 507–514.
159. Winkler, C., Wirleitner, B., Schroecksnadel, K., Schennach, H., & Fuchs, D., (2006). Beer down-regulates activated peripheral blood mononuclear cells in vitro. *International Immunopharmacology*, 6(3), 390–395.
160. Kondo, K., (2004). Beer and health: Preventive effects of beer components on lifestyle-relate disease. *Biofactors, 22*, 303–310.
161. Nozawa, H., Tazumi, K., Sato, K. Yoshida, A., Takata, J., Arimoto-Kobayashi, S., & Kondo, K., (2004). Inhibitory effects of beer on heterocyclic amine-induced mutagenesis and PhIP-induced aberrant crypt foci in rat colon. *Mutation Research/Genetic Toxicology and Environmental Mutagenesis*, 559(1), 177–187.

162. Tobe, H., Muraki, Y., Kitamura, K., Komiyama, O., Sato, Y., Sugioka, T., Maruyama, H. B., Matsuda, E., & Nagai, M., (1997). Bone resorption inhibitors from hop extract. *Bioscience, Biotechnology, & Biochemistry, 61*(1), 158–159.

163. Obisesan, T. O., Hirsch, R., Kosoko, O., Carlson, L., & Parrott, M., (1998). Moderate Wine Consumption Is Associated with Decreased Odds of Developing Age-Related Macular Degeneration in NHANES-1. *Journal of the American Geriatrics Society, 46*(1), 1–7.

164. Keys, D., (2003). Now that's what you call a real vintage: professor unearths 8, 000-year-old wine. *The Independent, 28.*

165. http://www.all-about-wine.com/types-of-red-wine.html (accessed on: 23 Nov 2016).

166. http://www.all-about-wine.com/types-of-white-wine.html (accessed on: 23 Nov 2016).

167. http://winefolly.com/review/common-types-of-wine/ (accessed on: 23 Nov 2016).

168. Lopez-Velez, M., Martinez-Martinez, F., & Del Valle-Ribes, C., (2003). "The study of phenolic compounds as natural antioxidants in wine," 233–244.

169. Willett, W. C., Sacks, F., Trichopoulou, A., Drescher, G., Ferro-Luzzi, A., Helsing, E., & Trichopoulos, D., (1995). Mediterranean diet pyramid: a cultural model for healthy eating. *The American Journal of Clinical Nutrition, 61*(6), 1402S-1406S.

170. Jang, M., & Pezzuto, J. M., (1998). Cancer chemopreventive activity of resveratrol. *Drugs Under Experimental and Clinical Research, 25*(2–3), 65–77.

171. Hertog, M. G., Kromhout, D., Aravanis, C., Blackburn, H., Buzina, R., Fidanza, F., Giampaoli, S., Jansen, A., Menotti, A., Nedeljkovic, S., & Pekkarinen, M., (1995). Flavonoid intake and long-term risk of coronary heart disease and cancer in the seven countries study. *Archives of Internal Medicine, 155*(4), 381–386.

172. Hertog, M. G., Hollman, P. C., & Venema, D. P., (1992). Optimization of a quantitative HPLC determination of potentially anticarcinogenic flavonoids in vegetables and fruits. *Journal of Agricultural and Food Chemistry, 40*(9), 1591–1598.

173. Brownell, K. D., & Horgen, K. B., (2004). *Food Fight: The Inside Story of the Food Industry,* america's obesity crisis, & what we can do about it. New York: McGraw-Hill contemporary books.

174. Eluwa, M., Inyangmme, I., Akpantah, A., Ekanem, T., Ekong, M. B., Asuquo, O., & Nwakanma, A. A., (2013). A comparative study of the effect of diet and soda carbonated drinks on the histology of the cerebellum of adult female albino Wistar rats. *African Health Sciences, 13*(3), 541–545.

175. Fahim, A., Ilyas, M. S., & Jafari, F. H., (2015). Histologic effects of carbonated drinks on rat kidney. *Journal of Rawalpindi Medical College* (JRMC), *19*(2), 165–167.

176. Vartanian, L. R., Schwartz, M. B., & Brownell, K. D., (2007). Effects of soft drink consumption on nutrition and health: a systematic review and meta-analysis. *American Journal of Public Health, 97*(4), 667–675.

177. Witzel, M. K., & Young-Witzel, G., (1998). *Soda Pop!: From Miracle Medicine to Pop Culture.* Voyageur Press.

178. Smith, T. J., Wolfson, J. A., Jiao, D., Crupain, M. J., Rangan, U., Sapkota, A., Bleich, S. N., & Nachman, K. E., (2015). Caramel color in soft drinks and exposure to 4-methylimidazole: a quantitative risk assessment. *PloS One, 10*(2), e0118138.

179. Halldorsson, T. I., Strom, M., Petersen, S. B., & Olsen, S. F., (2010). Intake of artificially sweetened soft drinks and risk of preterm delivery: a prospective cohort study of 59, 334 Danish pregnant women. *The American Journal of Clinical Nutrition, 1*:ajcn-28968.

180. Fung, T. T., Malik, V., Rexrode, K. M., Manson, J. E., Willett, W. C., & Hu, F. B., (2009). Sweetened beverage consumption and risk of coronary heart disease in women. *The American Journal of Clinical Nutrition, 89*(4), 1037–1042.

181. Palmer, J. R., Boggs, D. A., Krishnan, S. Hu, F. B., Singer, M., & Rosenberg, L., (2008). Sugar-sweetened beverages and incidence of type 2 diabetes mellitus in African American women. *Archives of Internal Medicine, 168*(14), 1487–1492.

182. Dhingra, R., Sullivan, L., Jacques, P. F., Wang, T. J., Fox, C. S., Meigs, J. B., D'Agostino, R. B., Gaziano, J. M., & Vasan, R. S., (2007). Soft drink consumption and risk of developing cardiometabolic risk factors and the metabolic syndrome in middle-aged adults in the community. *Circulation, 116*(5), 480–488.

183. Lee, J., *Energy Drinks Vs. Sports Drinks: Know thy Difference*. Available at: http://speedendurance.com/2009/07/09/energy-drinks-vs-sports-drinks-know-thydifference.

184. Press Office. New report predicts energy drink sales in the U. S. to exceed $9 billion by (2011). [press release]. www. reportbuyer.com/press/new-reportpredicts-energy-drink-sales-in-the-us-toexceed-9-billion-by-2011 (accessed Nov 23, 2016).

185. Seifert, S. M., Schaechter, J. L., Hershorin, E. R., & Lipshultz, S. E., (2011). Health effects of energy drinks on children, adolescents, & young adults. *Pediatrics, 127*(3), 511–528.

186. Brecher, E. J., (2004). Study: caffeine in sodas risky for black kids. *Miami Herald, 7E.*

187. Babu, K. M., Church, R. J., & Lewander, W., (2008). Energy drinks: the new eye-opener for adolescents. *Clinical Pediatric Emergency Medicine, 9*(1), 35–42.

188. Reissig, C. J., Strain, E. C., & Griffiths, R. R., (2009). Caffeinated energy drinks—a growing problem. *Drug and Alcohol Dependence, 99*(1), 1–0.

189. Clauson, K. A., Shields, K. M., McQueen, C. E., & Persad, N., (2008). Safety issues associated with commercially available energy drinks. *Pharmacy Today, 14*(5), 52–64.

190. O'Connor, E., (2001). A sip into dangerous territory. *Monit Psychol., 32*(6).

191. Howland, J., & Rohsenow, D. J., (2013). Risks of energy drinks mixed with alcohol. *Jama., 309*(3), 245–246.

192. Hedges, D. W., Woon, F. L., & Hoopes, S. P., (2009). Caffeine-induced psychosis. *CNS spectrums, 14*(03), 127–131.

193. Gunja, N., & Brown, J. A., (2012). Energy drinks: health risks and toxicity. *Med. J. Aust., 196*(1), 46–49.

194. Reissig, C. J., Strain, E. C., & Griffiths, R. R., (2009). Caffeinated energy drinks—a growing problem. *Drug and Alcohol Dependence, 99*(1), 1–0.

195. Shirlow, M. J., & Mathers, C. D., (1985). A study of caffeine consumption and symptoms: indigestion, palpitations, tremor, headache and insomnia. *International Journal of Epidemiology, 14*(2), 239–48.

196. Main, E., (2015). *9 Disturbing Side Effects of Soda*, Rodale organic life news, *13.*

197. Evans, R., Thien, N., Isaac, B., Olivia, B., & Mrs Newman, (2015). "*The Effects of Soda on the Human Body.*"

198. Consensus action on salt and health why is salt bad for our health?" *Why Is Salt Bad for Our Health? 24,* May 2015.

CHAPTER 12

CANCER CHEMOTHERAPY

SONAL SRIVASTAVA, SAKSHI MISHRA, JAYANT DEWANGAN,
AMAN DIVAKAR, PRABHASH KUMAR PANDEY, and
SRIKANTA KUMAR RATH

*CSIR–Central Drug Research Institute, Lucknow–226031,
Uttar Pradesh, India, E-mail: skrath@cdri.res.in*

CONTENTS

ABSTRACT

Chemotherapy is one of the most widely accepted approaches currently available for the treatment of various cancers. Enhancements in the field of drug designing and development for targeted delivery have enabled clinicians to treat cancers by using various classes of drugs. However, at present, the diversity of mechanisms in the carcinogenesis and development of tumors imposes a major challenge to the researchers involved in the development of anticancer drugs. This chapter elucidates the development of chemotherapeutic drugs, their mechanism of action, and route of administration. Cancer cells harbor a distinct population of cells, known as cancer stem cells that are responsible for the development of drug resistance in solid tumors and hematological malignancies. In order to overcome drug resistance and ameliorate the toxic effects, newer approaches such as combinatorial drug therapy are required to supplement the conventional chemotherapy for mitigation of cancer.

12.1   INTRODUCTION

Cancer is any abnormal proliferation at the cellular level that can be of two types: (1) benign, which remains localized in its original region and does not spreads and (2) malignant, which can invade the surrounding tissue and can spread to other body parts. Cancer is basically a complex process where the cell undergoes a series of alterations in DNA, causing mutations. This is a multistage process involving the initiation process of cancer development, followed by tumor promotion and progression. Cells that undergo neoplastic transformation generally express cell surface antigens, acceleration of the cell cycle, invasive growth, qualitative or quantitative chromosomal abnormalities, genomic alterations, and translocations of amplified gene sequences. Cancer may occur likely due to three factors: (1) physical carcinogens, viz, ultraviolet radiation, (2) chemical carcinogens such as aflatoxin (food-contaminating mycotoxin), pesticides, arsenic (water contaminant), inhaled asbestos, certain dioxins, and tobacco smoke, and (3) biological carcinogens, viz, viruses, bacteria, or parasites. Cancer is one of the major causes of death worldwide accounting for 8.2 million deaths in 2012. Common cancer deaths are due to mainly lung cancer (1.59 million), liver cancer (745000), stomach cancer (723000), colorectal cancer (694000), breast cancer (521000), and esophageal cancer (400000) [1].

Cancer prevention is lowering the risk of developing cancer. This may include avoiding and controlling things that can cause cancer, viz, change in lifestyle, having a healthy diet, awareness for cancer, avoiding exposure to cancerous substances and exposure to nonionizing radiation (UV) by sunlight, protection from certain viral infections (hepatitis B, human papilloma virus), and getting immunized against certain cancers.

Chemotherapy, also known as "chemo," is one the most common form for the treatment of cancer that uses one or more anticancer drugs. Chemotherapy is a drug treatment that kills the active cells and stops them from spreading by slowing their growth rate. It may harm healthy cells, which can cause side effects in other body parts. The severity of side effects depends on the type and amount of chemotherapy one gets and how the body reacts to the same. Some common side effects may include fatigue, nausea, vomiting, pain, mouth and throat sores, and hair loss. There are ways to prevent or control some side effects. Surgery and radiation therapy can remove damage or kill cancer cells in a certain area, but chemo works throughout the whole body; this means that chemotherapy can kill cancer cells that have metastasized to other parts of the body far away from the original/primary tumor.

12.2   TYPES OF CHEMOTHERAPY

There are number of strategies used for chemotherapy. It may be given with combinations of drugs, or it may aim to prolong life/reduce symptoms, also known as palliative chemotherapy. The main types of treatment for cancer are surgery, radiation therapy, and chemotherapy.

Combined modality therapy is a chemotheraphy where patient is treated with two or more treatment methods together. Different combinations are used when there are chances to cure or decrease the risk of significant complications caused by cancer by following two or three modalities instead of one. Chemoimmunotherapy, chemoradiotherapy, radioimmunotherapy, salvage therapy, and cryochemotherapy are generally used in combinations with each other and with surgery as well. Adjuvant chemotherapy is given after radiation therapy with the aim to decrease systemic micrometastases. Similarly chemo and radiation therapy are given together with particularly chosen drugs, which enhances the sensitivity of tumor cells to radiation therapy [2]. This therapy has been successfully used for treating thoracic malignancies, head and neck cancers [3], Hodgkin lymphoma [4], rectal cancer [5], and pancreatic adenocarcinoma [6].

Induction chemotherapy encompasses chemotherapy where high doses of anticancer drugs are used in initial treatment, especially in the case of advanced cancers. If the preliminary therapy is unable to give promising results or it causes severe side effects, other treatments may be used instead, making it more effective. It is also called as first line/primary therapy or primary treatment for cancer. Squamous cell carcinoma (SCC) of the head and neck at advanced stages is treated with this therapy [7]. Docetaxel along with conventional chemotherapy regimen with cisplatin and 5-fluorouracil (TPF) is now being used as the gold standard for induction chemotherapy [8].

Adjuvant chemotherapy, as the name suggest, is given in addition to the primary or main therapy to increase its effectiveness to fight cancer. Generally, it combines chemotherapy and surgery or chemotherapy and radiation, which are used together for achieving better results. For instance, in any breast cancer case, chemotherapy is usually used for removal of all the detectable and visible cancer, which have been removed surgically or with the help of radiation therapy. The purpose of adjuvant chemotherapy is to improve disease-related symptoms and overall survival of the individual [9].

Neoadjuvant chemotherapy plays an important role in the treatment of cancers. In contrast to adjuvant therapy, this is given before the main treatment where drugs are administered before surgery. For example, systemic therapy is given before the removal of a breast mainly to reduce the size of the tumor so as to facilitate more effective surgery. Phase II and III studies on breast cancer patients have demonstrated promising results for neoadjuvant chemotherapy given before radiation therapy and/or surgery [10]. Neoadjuvant chemotherapy is also showing promising results in advanced epithelial ovarian cancer [11]. Recently, neoadjuvant chemotherapy for brain tumors in infants and young children has also proved to be effective in reducing tumor vascularity and clarification of the tumor-brain interface [12].

Consolidation chemotherapy is administered once a remission has been achieved. It is more rigorous than the standard chemotherapy. The aim of this therapy is to sustain a remission. This is commonly used for the treatment of acute leukemias. The drug used can be the same for treatment and remission.

Maintenance chemotherapy is given after the preliminary cycles of initial chemotherapy to prevent cancer reoccurrence. Maintenance therapy can help in controlling advanced cancers that has improved but is not completely gone after initial cycles of chemotherapy. This therapy is given in lower doses to help in prolonging a remission. However, it is used only for certain cancer types; most commonly, it is used for acute promyelocytic leukemias and acute lymphocytic leukemias.

Intensification chemotherapy is a type of consolidation; however, the drug used in this therapy is different from the one used in consolidation chemotherapy.

First line chemotherapy is a chemotherapy regimen that has been gone through research studies and clinical trials and has been proved to have the best probability of treating a certain type of cancer. It is also known as standard therapy. First line therapy is the treatment regimen that are generally accepted by the medical clinics for treatment at the initial level for a given type and stage of cancer. It is also called primary treatment.

Second line chemotherapy is tried when the first line therapy does not work efficiently. If the first line therapy does not work or may have some limited efficacy or has produced side effects or damaged organs in the body, a break with the primary treatment is taken into account and a new regimen as a second line treatment is followed. The management of a cancer case requires regular assessment of treatment to assess its success. At times, first line therapies show progress for a limited time period, followed by a stalling or continued growth of the cancer. In some cases, it is also be referred to as salvage therapy.

Palliative chemotherapy is a type of chemotherapy that is given specifically to address symptom management without expecting to significantly reduce the cancer. It also means using medicines to reduce or control the side effects of cancer treatments so as to help someone to live longer and to live comfortably, even if they cannot be cured.

12.3   DEVELOPMENT OF CHEMOTHERAPEUTIC DRUGS

Even though chemotherapy and radiation have major side effects, they are still used as a golden standard for cancer treatment. In the last couple of decades, much research has been carried out in the development of new anticancer drugs. Development of new anticancer drugs that are selective to cancerous cells is a major challenge as majority of the drugs developed in the past are cytotoxic and may have the potential to harm the body. Cytotoxic agents may target tubulin, DNA, or cell division machinery; hence, novel compounds that can selectively target molecular pathways that are crucial for tumor survival, growth, and metastases are gaining much attention. Schwartsmann et al. noted in 1988 that of over 600,000 compounds screened by then, less than 40 agents were routinely used in the clinic [13, 14]. The recently developed molecularly targeted chemotherapeutic agents have challenged the traditionally developed pathways for anticancer drugs. Therefore, at present, there is a constant need to build up better alternative or synergistic chemotherapeutic drugs that have minimal side effects on healthy cells/on other body parts. Hence, the imperative strategy these days is to develop more effective chemotherapeutic agents that are derived from natural sources. The discovery and development of, especially cytotoxic agents, differ significantly from the drug development process. The unique challenges in the development of chemotherapeutic drugs are reflected in each stage/process. Development of new chemotherapeutic drug basically involves three steps [15] (Figure 12.1).

In the first step, drugs are discovered. Natural and synthetic compounds are screened, evaluated, and tested at various levels to discover novel drug

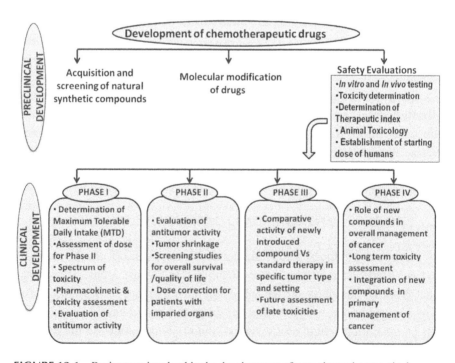

FIGURE 12.1   Basic steps involved in the development of new chemotherapeutic drugs.

molecules with useful properties. In the second step, molecular modification of the newly discovered drug is performed where an anticancer drug/molecule that shows promising properties is chemically altered in a way to produce the best properties, thus making it a more effective drug for cancer treatment. Characterization of physical properties of compounds and chemical incompatibilities and chemical combinations along with hypothesis development for the mechanism of treatment are performed. In the last step, the drug is formulated and developed into a useful pharmaceutical drug and is patented. Finally, a long process of advanced testing starts, including establishment of the starting dose, and ends up with clinical trials. Before being approved, every newly discovered chemotherapeutic drug or combination is evaluated for its safety and efficacy and is screened for its antitumor activity. Evaluation of acute and short term toxicities studies on rodent or nonrodents are conducted. Studies are performed to assess target organ toxicity; lethal dose determination; and distribution, absorption, and excretion patterns. Clinical development of chemotherapeutic drugs classically follows three main phases.

12.3.1 PHASE I TRIAL

This phase represent the first administration of a newly discovered drug or their combination to human beings and have a specific methodology. Phase I trials are conducted on patients who are suffering from cancer, have no other treatment option, and have failed to standard therapy [16]. Their primary goal is to determine the recommended maximum tolerable dose (MTD) intended for human use in phase II trials and also to collect spectrum of toxicity, pharmacokinetic, and pharmacodynamic data.

12.3.2 PHASE II TRIAL

The main purpose of phase II trial is to justify whether the compound screened has significant antitumor activity and to assess the adverse effects of new drugs. It involves screening studies aimed for identifying signals of antitumor activity in a specific group of population that have a specific tumor type and also involves correction of doses. The primary goal of phase II trials is to improve the overall survival rate [17].

12.3.3 PHASE III TRIAL

It involves critical steps before licensing any drug. This trial sets a benchmark for proving that the present drug treatment is providing better results than the available treatment. It aims to compare the efficacy of a new compound with standard therapy and also to evaluate for late toxicities. Thereafter, it can lead to regulatory approval if found positive. Phase III studies consists of extensive clinical investigation for a new treatment and are most rigorous.

12.3.4 PHASE IV TRIAL

These trials are performed once the drug is licensed. In this phase, the detailed side effects and safety of the drug is assessed within the population. Long-term risks and benefits of the chemotherapeutic drug used are assessed. Studies are also performed on how well the drug works if widely used.

12.4   IMPORTANCE OF CELL CYCLE IN CHEMOTHERAPY

All living organisms and tissues are made up of cells. The cells that are injured might be repaired or replaced by newer ones. Cell cycle is important for renewal and growth of cells in any organism. In short, the cell cycle is a life cycle of any cell. Both cancerous and normal cell follow few steps in order to grow and form new cells. Understanding the cell cycle perhaps helps in predicting about drugs that are likely to perform well together and in deciding how often doses should be administered. The cell cycle consists of five phases. The first one is the G0 phase where cells are in the resting phase. In the G1 phase, the cells prepares for the division by making more proteins and increasing its size. In the next S phase, the chromosomes containing DNA are copied so that both the new cells formed have matching strands of DNA. The G2 phase is a DNA checkpoint; here, the cell repairs if there is any damage/mutation and if it is unrepairable, then it may lead to cell death/apoptosis. In the last M phase, the cells divide into two cells. Cell cycle has a very important role as many chemotherapeutic drugs work on the active cells that are not in G0 (resting phase). Some drugs specifically target cells in a different phase of the cell cycle, i.e., in the M or S phase. Failure of cell cycle arrest responses in malignant cells can also be exploited therapeutically. Cell cycle arrest checkpoints are potential targets for chemotherapeutic drugs, as their inhibition may increase the sensitivity of tumor cells to standard chemotherapy [18]. Based on their cell cycle actions, chemotherapeutic drugs can be divided into two main classes.

Cell cycle nonspecific drugs act at several or all cell cycle phases and are active in all phases. Drugs such as antitumor antibiotics, alkylating agents, nitrosureas, noncytotoxic drugs (hormone and steroids), and miscellaneous agents like procarbazine used for cancer treatment might be effective in large tumors that have few dividing active cells at the time of dose administration. Alkylating agents act primarily by binding together to the strands of DNA, which interferes with DNA duplication and thus preventing mitosis. The effect is similar to that induced by radiation therapy, which destroys both dividing and resting cells. Chlorambucil, mitomycin, and cyclophosphamide are some examples. Similarly, antibiotics that are antitumor agents are also a class of cell cycle phase nonspecific drugs; however, some are effective during the M and S phases of the cycle. Doxorubicin and actinomycin D are few common examples of chemotherapeutic antibiotics that disrupt and inhibit DNA and RNA synthesis. Cell cycle-specific drugs are compounds that act specifically only at particular cell cycle phases. These drugs are administered in minimal amounts as the increase in dose may not increase in killing the cells. Few examples include antimetabolites that block essential enzymes necessary for DNA synthesis or may get incorporated into the DNA because of which a false message is transmitted [19]. Antimetabolites are most active during the S phase (methotrexate, 5 fluorouracil, and mercaptopurine). Derivatives from the periwinkle plant are cell cycle phase-specific compounds. They exert a cytotoxic effect by binding to microtubular proteins during the metaphase by causing mitotic arrest. The cell dies as they lose the ability to divide. However, it causes side effects known as parasthesiae as microtubular proteins are essential to nervous tissue. Examples of chemotherapeutic drugs that act in different phases of cell cycle are given in Table 12.1 [20].

The key regulators of the cell cycle are the cyclin-dependent kinases (CDKs) and their regulatory proteins called as cyclins. CDKs and cyclins are key players of cell cycle progression [21]. CDKs are activated by CDK cyclins and inhibited by their inhibitors, which break the cell cycle progression and induce cell growth arrest, thereby leading to apoptosis. Loss of

TABLE 12.1   Chemotherapeutic Drugs Targeting Different Phases of Cell Cycle

S phase-dependent	M phase-dependent	G2 phase-dependent	G1 phase-dependent
Antimetabolites- Methotrexate, Fludarabine, Cytarabine Gemcitabine Fluorouracil Floxuridine Hydroxyurea Mercaptopurine Thioguanine	Plant alkaloids and terpenoids (microtubule inhibitors) Vinca alkaloidsa, Vinblastine, Vincristine, Vinorelbine, Vindesin Taxanes Paclitaxel Docetaxel	Topoisomerase Inhibitor Irinotecan, Topotecan	Enzyme Asparaginase
Alkylating Agents Capecotabome, Procarbazine	Podophyllotoxins Etoposide, Teniposide	Antitumor Antibiotics Mitoxantrone	Hormones Corticosteroids
Antitumor Antibiotics Doxorubicin	Antitumor Antibiotics Bleomycin		
Hormones Prednisone			

[Source: Ref. 20]

cell cycle control and accumulation of mutations are hallmarks of cancer. In any cancer type, the expression and inhibition of CDKs are deregulated; therefore, in the last several years, the development of chemotherapeutic drugs that can successfully inhibit the expression of CDKs is becoming an extensively studied area for chemotherapy. Therefore, these CDKs in combination with traditional cytotoxic chemotherapy have potential to overcome drug resistance and to improve cytotoxic efficacy. Chemotherapeutic drugs that inhibit different CDKs are listed in Table 12.2 [22].

12.5   CLASSIFICATION OF CHEMOTHERAPEUTIC DRUGS

The various classes of chemotherapeutic drugs based on their mechanism of action are categorized as follows (Figure 12.2).

TABLE 12.2 List of Chemotherapeutic Drugs Inhibiting Different Cyclin-Dependent Kinases

Drug	COMPANY	Mode of Administration	Target
Palbociclib = PD-0332991	Pfizer	Oral	CDK4/6
Abemaciclib = LY2835219	Eli LIlly	Oral	CDK4/6
LEE-011	Novartis/Astex	Oral	CDK4/6
Alvocidib = Flavo-piridol	Sanofi-Aventis	Intravenous	CDK1/4/9
Milciclib = PHA-848125	Nerviano	Oral	CDK2, TrKA
MM-D37K	MetaMax	Intravenous	CDK4
AZD5438	AstraZeneca	Oral	CDK1/2/5/9
G1T28-1 = GZ38-1 G-1	G-1 Therapeutics	Intravenous	CDK4/6
AT-7519	Astex (NCIC)	Intravenous	CDK2/5/9
Roniciclib = BAY-1000394	Bayer	Oral	CDK1/2/4/7/9
RGB-286638	Agennix	Intravenous	CDK1/2/3/4/5/6/7 /9
TG-02 = SB-1317 = EX45	Tragara Pharmaceuticals	Oral	CDK1/2/3/5/7/9
TG02/SG1317	S*BIO/Tragara	Oral	CDK1/2/3/5/9
Dinaciclib = SCH-727965 = MK-7965	Merck(NCI)	Intravenous	CDK1/2/5/9
Seliciclib = R-Roscovitine = CY-202	Cyclacel	Oral	CDK1/2/5/7/9 AT-7519
ZK-304709	Bayer/Schering	Oral	CDK1/2/9
AG-024322	Pfizer	Intravenous	CDK1/2/4
Riviciclib = P276-00	Piramal	Intravenous	CDK1/4/9
R547 = RO-4584820	Hoffmann-LA Roche Inc	Intravenous	CDK1/2/4
PHA-793887	Nerviano	Intravenous	CDK2/5/7 CDK1/4/9, GSK3b
P1446A-05	Piramal	Oral	CDK4
BMS-387032 = SNS-032	Sunesis/BMS	Intravenous	CDK2/7/9
EM-1421	Erimos	Intravenous	CDK1

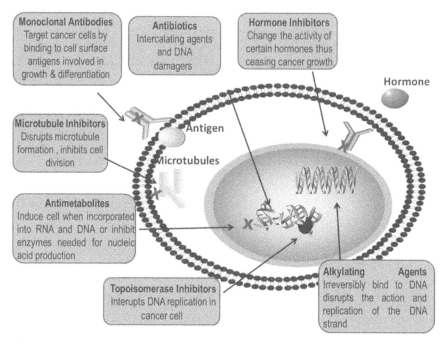

FIGURE 12.2 Chemotherapeutic drugs-targets and mechanism.

12.5.1 ALKYLATING AGENTS

Alkylating drugs are the oldest class of antineoplastic drugs that have been effectively used in the treatment of several types of cancers [23]. These are most useful in treating cancers that grow slowly, like solid tumors and leukemia. Alkylating agents react chemically with DNA by directly modifying DNA bases, intercalating between DNA bases, or by forming crosslinks in DNA on opposite strands of the double helix (interstrand crosslinks) [24]. Simple methylating agents form adducts at the N- and O-atoms in DNA bases.

DNA integrity is crucial for proliferation and normal functioning of the cellular machinery, and the DNA lesions if not repaired properly, may result in cell death. Cell cycle checkpoint proteins detect high levels of DNA damage upon activation causing cell cycle arrest and thereby preventing transmission of damaged DNA during mitotic cell division. Cancer cells are more susceptible to DNA damage as they have a comparatively less stringent DNA damage sensing/repair potential and are able to ignore cell-cycle checkpoints, allowing the cells to attain high proliferation rates. The replication of damaged DNA increases the likelihood of cell death induction; therefore, the concept of targeting DNA inspired the development of numerous alkylating agents as anticancer compounds.

The five major classes of alkylating agents are nitrogen mustards, alkyl sulfonates, nitrosoureas, ethylenimines, and triazine [25]. These work by the same chemical mechanism. The most popular drugs in each category have been described below.

12.5.1.1 Nitrogen Mustards

Alkylation of the purine bases on the DNA by derivatives of nitrogen mustards stalls the progression.

of the replication fork and subsequently leads to cell death via apoptosis. Nitrogen mustards react referentially with guanine N7 and adenine N3 positions, resulting in the formation of monoadducts, as well as intrastrand and interstrand crosslinks in DNA *in vitro* [26, 27]. Cyclophosphamide mechlorethamine, chlorambucil, bendamustine, and melphalan are among the currently used nitrogen mustards in clinical therapeutics. Bendamustine and melphalan kill myeloma cells by generating reactive oxygen species and activating the p53 pathway [28]. However, these derivatives target the DNA of tumor cells with low specificity and eventually lose their activity due to cellular DNA repair mechanisms.

12.5.1.2 Alkyl Sulfonates

Among the dimethanesulfonates, busulfan and its hydrophilic analog treosulfan are used in high-dose chemotherapy in combination with other alkylating drugs [29]. Busulphan is a bifunctional alkylating agent that drastically alters cell replication, DNA repair, and gene transcription by cross-linking DNA--DNA and DNA--protein. The ability to form DNA interstrands by reacting with guanines (N7) is correlated with in vitro cytotoxicity [30]. It also induces binding between DNA and cysteine 114 of histone H3 [31]. The diepoxide derivative of treosulphan (S,S)-DEB acts as a monofunctional alkylating agent, leading to miscoding DNA, strand breakage, and depurination and causing slight cytotoxicity. In contrast, its monoepoxide derivative (S,S)-EBDM acts as a bifunctional alkylating agent and leads to interstand cross-linking within the DNA helix and inhibits mitosis and transcription [32].

12.5.1.3   Nitroureas

2-Chloroethyl carbonium ion is generated upon the chemical degradation of nitrosoureas and is responsible for its alkylating activity [33]. Carbamoylation of cellular proteins modifies DNA and RNA polymerization enzymes, which leads to the inhibition of DNA synthesis, RNA synthesis, and RNA processing. The ability of nitrosoureas to cross the blood-brain barrier make them suitable for the treatment of brain tumors [34]. Some of the commonly used nitrourea drugs include estramustine, carmustine, lomustine, and fotemustine.

12.5.1.4   Ethylenimines

Thiotepa, an ethylenimine alkylating agent, is used for the treatment of Hodgkin's disease, non-Hodgkin's lymphoma, and breast cancer. Altretamine, also called hexamethylmelamine or HMM, is used to treat ovarian cancer.

12.5.1.5   Triazines

The highly reactive derivative, methyldiazonium ion is responsible for the activity of triazenes. This class of drug includes dacarbazine (DTIC) and temozolomide (TMZ). Both drugs are cell cycle nonspecific, i.e., they are active in all phases of the cell cycle. Metabolism in the liver is required for the activation of DTIC. The methylated species frequently alkylate at the N7 position of guanine; however, methylation at the O^6-guanine generates incorrect base pairing is mainly responsible for the cytotoxic effect of DTIC [35].

TMZ is spontaneously converted into active metabolite and is completely bioavailable when administered orally. Treatment of TMZ leads to inhibition of DNA, RNA, and protein synthesis but without cross-linking DNA strands. It forms DNA adducts by methylating the purines in the DNA helix at various positions like O6-guanine, N7-guanine, and N3-adenine. TMZ is used for the treatment of aggressive type astrocytoma, known as glioblastoma multiforme [36].

12.5.2 ANTHRACYCLINES

Anthracyclines are antitumor antibiotics that are active in all phases of the cell cycle. These drugs inhibit production of free radicals and mitochondrial oxidative phosphorylation. They interfere with DNA polymerases, RNA polymerases, and DNA repair enzymes. High doses of these drugs lead to the development of myocardial damage that limits its lifetime dose. Daunorubicin and doxorubicin display a large spectrum of antitumor activity against leukemias and various solid tumors. Other well-categorized anthracycliuns include epirubicin, idarubicin, mitoxantrone, and valrubicin [37].

12.5.3 CYTOSKELETAL DISRUPTORS

Rapid microtubule dynamics during mitosis has a critical role at the metaphase. Mitotic inhibitors are derivatives of natural products, mostly plant alkaloids, which disrupt spindle function by suppressing microtubule dynamics, thus blocking cell cycle progression at the metaphase to anaphase transition. Persistent mitotic block causes cells to exit mitosis and undergo apoptosis [38]. They are used to treat various types of cancer, including breast cancer, lung cancer, myelomas, lymphomas, and leukemias. These drugs can be divided into the following two categories: (i) microtubule-stabilizing agents, and (ii) microtubule-destabilizing agents.

12.5.3.1 Microtubule-Stabilizing Agents

These agents stabilize microtubules by binding to polymeric tubulin thus preventing disassembly.

Taxanes are microtubule-stabilizing agents that include paclitaxel and docetaxel.Paclitaxel allows microtubule attachment but alters tension across kinetochore, thereby suppressing spindle microtubule dynamics in mitosis. Docetaxel disrupts centrosome organization, resulting in accumulation of cells in the G2M phase and subsequent cell death.

Epothilones cause disruption of microtubule dynamics targeting the cell for G2/M phase arrest, thereby resulting in apoptosis. It can also disrupt the dynamic equilibrium between the intracellular pool of basic tubulin components and the microtubule polymer, thereby inducing apoptosis without arresting the cell cycle. Patupilone (epothilone B), ixabepilone, BMS 310705, sagopilone, epothilone D, and KOS-1584 are few epothilones that have been studied [39].

Discodermolide is a polyhydroxylated lactone isolated from the marine sponge *Discodermia dissoluta*. It also acts as a tubulin polymerizer.

12.5.3.2 Microtubule-Destabilizing Agents

These agents destabilize microtubules by preventing the attachment of microtubules to the kinetochores, thus inhibiting microtubule assembly.

Vinca alkaloids like vinblastine, vincristine, and vinorelbine bind to high affinity sites on tubulin, causing destabilization of spindle microtubules and mitotic arrest. Other drugs in this category include colchicines, podophyllotoxin, and nocodazole [40].

12.5.4   *HISTONE DEACETYLASE INHIBITORS*

Histone deacetylase (HDAC) activity removes acetyl groups from the histones, causing compaction of the DNA/histone complex. Removal of acetylation marks is associated with gene repression as DNA compaction makes part of the genome inaccessible, thereby blocking gene transcription and inhibiting differentiation. HDAC inhibitors cause decompaction of the histone/DNA complex, resulting in elevated gene transcription; they also affect acetylation status and function of nonhistone proteins. HDAC inhibitors promote growth arrest, induce differentiation and/or apoptosis, and inhibit proliferation of tumor cells. Vorinostat, a HDAC inhibitor, has been approved by the US Food and Drug Administration for the treatment of cutaneous T-cell lymphoma [41].

12.5.5   *INHIBITORS OF TOPOISOMERASES*

Various DNA processes like replication, recombination, repair, and transcription requires the assembly of proteins onto the DNA; therefore, targeting protein DNA complexes is also an approach to disrupt normal DNA functions. Topoisomerases are a class of enzymes that function to release the torsional strain of the DNA double helix so that it can be copied during the S phase. Topoisomerase inhibitor blocks the progression of the replication fork by binding the DNA-enzyme complex, which prevents the religation of the break and also causes toxic double-stranded breaks. This class of drugs are used in the treatment of certains leukemias and solid malignancies like lung, ovarian, and gastrointestinal tumors. Topoisomerase inhibitors are grouped according to the type of enzyme they affect.

12.5.5.1   Inhibitors of Topoisomerase I

Topoisomerase I creates a transient single-strand break in the complementary strand of the double helix and allows the passage of a single DNA strand through it. Camptothecin, a plant product, was found to be a topoisomerase I inhibitor that binds to the DNA-topoisomerase complex to inhibit strand religation [42]. 9-Dimethylaminomethyl-10-hydroxycamptothecin (topotecan) and a prodrug, 7-ethyl-10-[4-(l-piperidino)-l-piperidino]-carbonyloxy-camptothecin (Irinotecan), are water-soluble analogs of camptothecin that have been approved by the US Food and Drug Administration for relapsed/refractory ovarian cancer and small cell lung cancer [43, 44].

12.5.5.2   Inhibitors of Topoisomerase II

Topoisomerase II unwinds the supercoiled DNA by cutting both strands of the double helix and allowing the passage of an intact helix through it. Plant analogs such as etoposide and teniposide have shown antineoplastic effects. A study reported that DNA strand breaks caused by etoposide were unable to form when etoposide was incubated with purified DNA [45]. Chen et al. found that etoposide binds to the topoisomerase II-DNA complex [46]. Higher cellular levels of topoisomerase II leads to greater efficacy of etoposide as a cytotoxic agent, and this correlation can be employed in designing topoisomerase II-mediated chemotherapy [47].

12.5.6   *KINASE INHIBITORS*

The epidermal growth factor receptor (EGFR) plays a pivotal role in mediating cancer cell proliferation, metastasis, invasion, and apoptotic inhibition. Tyrosine kinases phosphorylate the ligands that bind to this receptor, thereby activating the downstream pathways. Therefore, blocking the activity of these tyrosine kinases will disable the activation of EFGR. Regression of human tumors that overexpress EGFR is possible upon treatment with kinase inhibitors such as bortezomib, erlotinib, gefitinib, imatinib, vemurafenib, and vandetanib. In a randomized trial, the efficacy of gefitinib has been shown in symptomatic patients with nonsmall cell lung cancer (NSCLC) [48]. Crizotinib, a potent anaplastic lymphoma kinase (*ALK*) inhibitor, has shown significant in vitro mesenchymal-epithelial transition (MET) inhibitory activity in NSCLC [49].

12.5.7   mTOR INHIBITORS

The mammalian target of rapamycin (mTOR) is crucial in regulation of cellular metabolism, growth, and proliferation. The frequent hyperactivation of mTOR signaling makes it a promising therapeutic target for cancer management and has driven the development of a number of mTOR inhibitors [50]. The efficacy of everolimus was demonstrated in a phase III, randomized trial in patients with metastatic renal cell carcinoma [51].

12.5.8   PLATINUM-BASED AGENTS

The platinum-based drugs are coordination complexes of platinum. Cisplatin, carboplatin, and oxaliplatin are platinum-based antineoplastic agents that are widely used in cancer chemotherapy. DNA is the primary biological target of these drugs. The platinum atom in these drugs forms covalent bond to the N7 position of the purines and result in monoadduct, interstrand crosslinks or intrastrand crosslinks. The crosslinking inhibits DNA repair and/or DNA synthesis in cancer cells, while the resultant DNA adducts activate many cellular processes that are responsible for the cytotoxic potential of this drug [52]. A phase II study established the safety and efficacy of oxaliplatin monotherapy in previously untreated metastatic colorectal carcinoma [53]. In a meta-analysis, the response rate and prolonged survival effects generated in patients with advanced-stage NSCLC by cisplatin-based chemotherapy were found to be superior to carboplatin-based chemotherapy without an increase in severe toxic effects [54].

12.5.9 ANTIMETABOLITES

The antimetabolite drugs mimic the cellular molecules involved in the normal metabolic processes within the cells but differ enough so that they interfere with normal cell function. This class of drug interferes with the synthesis of DNA and RNA by replacing the normal building blocks of these nucleic acids or by blocking nucleotide metabolism pathways. They are commonly used for the treatment of leukemias and cancers of the breast, ovary, and the intestinal tract.

12.5.9.1 Folic Acid Analogs

Folates are essential one-carbon donors required for the production of nucleotides. Antifolates are structural analogs of folates that inhibit key enzymes in folate metabolism, namely dihydrofolate reductase (DHFR), β-glycinamide ribonucleotide transformylase (GARFT), 5'-amino-4'-imidazolecarboxamide ribonucleotide transformylase (AICARFT), and thymidylate synthetase_(TYMS). Methotrexate, aminopterin, and pemetrexed inhibit DHFR, thereby depleting the intracellular pools of reduced folates and blocking the synthesis of purines and pyrimidines. Lometrexol is a selective inhibitor of GARFT, which results in depletion of intracellular purine levels. Another antifolate, ralitrexed, is an analog of tetrahydrofolate and selectively inhibits TYMS [55].

12.5.9.2 Nucleotide Analogs

Pyrimidine and purine bases are the building blocks in the synthesis of DNA and RNA nucleotides. The incorporation of purine and pyrimidine structural analogs into DNA during the S phase of the cell cycle leads to faulty nucleotide base incorporation, causing DNA replication to fail.

Some of the commonly used purine analogs include cladribine, fludarabine, thioguanine, 6-mercaptopurine, and 8-azaguanine. Cladribine is a purine analog commonly used to treat hairy cell leukemia and B-cell chronic lymphocytic leukemia, which targets the lymphocytes thereby suppressing the immune system [56]. Fludarabine is one of the most effective drugs used for the treatment of chronic lymphocytic leukemia. It destroys cancerous cells through inhibition of DNA synthesis by acting on ribonucleotide reductase, DNA polymerase alpha, and DNA primase [57].

Pyrimidine analogs include 5-flurouracil, cytarabine, cytarabine (Ara-C), azacitidine, gemcitabine, capecitabine, and floxuridine. 5-FU can be incorporated into DNA and RNA in the place of thymine or uracil, respectively. 5-FU contains a fluoride atom at the 5'-carbon position on the ring, which prevents the addition of a subsequent nucleotide on the strand, leading to termination of chain elongation and induction of apoptosis [58].

12.5.10 IMMUNOTHERAPY

Different types of immunotherapy are used for the treatment of cancer. Active immunotherapy stimulates the immune system of the patient to attack the cancer cells, whereas passive immunotherapy enriches it by providing man-made immune system proteins for a better response. The main types of immunotherapy now being used to treat cancer include the following.

12.5.10.1 Monoclonal Antibodies (mAbs)

Antibodies can be very useful in targeting cancer cells as they can be specifically designed to attack a definite protein in the cancer cell. These can be naked or conjugated with radioactive probes or tagged with another drug. A study reported that alemtuzumab induced significant response in relapsed or refractory B-cell chronic lymphocytic leukemia patients who have failed fludarabine therapy [59]. Ibritumomab tiuxetan (Zevalin), a yttrium-90 (^{90}Y)-labeled anti-CD20 antibody showed high rate of tumor response in B-cell non-Hodgkin's lymphoma patients [60].

12.5.10.2 Immune Checkpoint Inhibitors

These drugs target the molecules on certain immune cells whose activation or inactivation is required to generate an immune response. Cancer cells are able to evade these checkpoints; therefore, the development of drugs that target these checkpoints is crucial and promising. Preliminary results from a Phase Ib study showed that pembrolizumab, an inhibitor of programmed death-1 (PD-1) checkpoint protein on T cells, was associated with clinical benefit in patients with heavily pretreated Classical Hodgkin lymphoma [61].

12.5.10.3   Cancer Vaccines

Vaccines may help to prevent or treat cancer. Some strains of the human papilloma virus (HPV) have been linked to cervical, anal, throat, and some other cancers. Vaccines against HPV may help protect against some of these cancers. Sipuleucel-T (PROVENGE) was the first cancer vaccine for the treatment of advanced prostate cancer that was approved by the US Food and Drug Administration[62].

12.5.10.4   Nonspecific Immunotherapies and Adjuvants

These include cytokines, Bacille Calmette-Guérin, and immunomodulatory drugs like thalidomide, lenalidomide, and pomalidomide that are able to boost the immune response. Herr et al. conducted a randomized trial in patients with superficial bladder cancer and found that intravesical therapy with BCG was able to delay the progression of the tumor[63].

12.5.11   HORMONE THERAPY

This class of drugs includes sex hormones, or hormone analogs, that modify the action or production of sex hormones. They are used to decrease the growth rate of breast, endometrial (uterine) and prostate cancers, which physiologically respond to sex hormones naturally produced in the body. Their mode of action differs from the standard chemotherapy as they either prevent the production of these hormones in the body or prevent the cancer cells to use the hormone that are essential for their growth. Antiandrogens such as bicalutamide (Casodex), flutamide (Eulexin), and nilutamide (Nilandron) are used in the treatment of prostate cancer [64]. Tamoxifen was shown to be effective in the treatment of patients with advanced breast cancer, provided the tumors express estrogen receptors or those that have responded to previous hormonal treatments [65].

12.6   ROUTES OF DELIVERY

Chemotherapeutic drugs can be administered through a variety of routes depending on the type, stage of cancer, type of chemotherapy, and dosage.

Dosage of chemotherapy can be difficult to determine because if the dose is too low, it can be ineffective against the tumor, whereas, at excessive doses, the drug might exert toxic effect and can be intolerable to the patients. Administration of drugs along with the doses is determined after rigorous clinical trials. Specificity of administration depends on how the drug is being absorbed in the body and how it works.

Oral chemotherapy medications can be swallowed (pills, tablets, capsules, and liquid), which are absorbed by the stomach, or placed under the tongue (sublingual). After oral administration, the digestive juices in the stomach break down the cased protective coating of the drug. The stomach acids dissolve the coating, releasing the medication, which is then absorbed through the lining of the stomach. Many drugs cannot be given orally as the stomach acids may destroy them or might not be absorbed into the patient's body. If unabsorbed, it may pass through the stool or urine, thus becoming ineffective. Other medications may be harsh and could cause damage to the stomach lining after digestion by the stomach juices. Hence, intravenous chemotherapy may be given if found to have better anticancer effects. Drugs administered through the intravenous route allow for rapid entry of drug into the blood stream and is carried throughout the body. This is the most common method of chemotherapy administration, because this administration offers the most rapid absorption time amongst all currently available methods. Some medications are administered as an intramuscular injection that is deeper than subcutaneous and into the muscle. Intramuscular is much rapid than the oral form but slower than sublingual, subcutaneous, and intravenous administration. Topical chemotherapies are used to treat some cases of nonmelanoma skin cancer where drugs are applied topically on skin. Intraventricular/Intrathecal chemotherapy is used when drugs are required to be administered in the cerebrospinal fluid, which is present in the brain and spinal cord as the blood-brain barrier of the body does not allow many chemotherapeutic drugs given systemically to reach the cerebrospinal fluid. The chemotherapy can be given to the CSF via two routes, namely intrathecal and intraventrical. In the intrathecal route, the drug is administered through lumbar puncture to the cerebrospinal fluid, while in the intraventrical route, a catheter is placed in the lateral ventricle of the brain. Intraperitoneal chemotherapy is given inside the abdominal cavity. A catheter is placed inside the peritoneal cavity that surrounds the organs. The chemotherapeutic drug is administered inside the peritoneal cavity and is drained out after given hours. In intra-arterial chemotherapy, a drug is infused inside the artery that is directly supplying blood to the tumor. The purpose of this kind of administration is to reduce other organ toxicity by chemotherapeutic agents as it directly targets the cancer cells. Intrapleural chemotherapy is given inside the pleural cavity so as to prevent the malignant pleural infusions.

12.7   CHEMORESISTANCE

Drug resistance is the major phenomenon by which cancer cells evade the chemotherapy drugs, thereby limiting the efficacy of chemotherapy. Cancer cells of both blood cancers and solid tumors can have the intrinsic property of resistance prior to chemotherapy or it can acquire resistance during the course of chemotherapy regimen [66]. The drug-resistant cells that escape chemotherapy are responsible for the relapse of cancer. P-glycoprotein and the multidrug resistance-associated protein (MRP) are the two molecular pumps in the tumor cell membranes that confer chemoresistance in cancer by expelling the chemotherapy drugs from the interior [67]. Increased drug efflux; drug activation and inactivation; alteration in drug target; DNA methylation; processing of drug-induced damage; and evasion of apoptosis are the numerous factors that promote drug inhibition and degradation.

12.7.1   DRUG EFFLUX

Reduction of drug accumulation by enhancing drug efflux is one of the mechanisms of cancer drug resistance. ABC transporters are transmembrane proteins having a highly conserved nucleotide binding domain and a variable transmembrane domain [68]. When the substrate binds the transmembrane domain, ATP hydrolysis at the nucleotide binding site changes the protein conformation that pushes the substrate out of the cell [69]. Enhanced expression of members of the ATP-binding cassette (ABC) transporter family proteins enables the efflux of drug [70]. Multidrug resistance protein 1 (MDR1), multidrug resistance-associated protein 1 (MRP1), and breast cancer resistance protein (BCRP) are mainly implicated in drug-resistant cancers.

Overexpression of P glycoprotein (Pgp) has been reported in many drug-resistant cell lines as well as in a number of solid tumors; therefore, its inhibition can reverse multidrug resistance [71]. Cyclosporine A, a first generation Pgp inhibitor, showed success in the treatment of retinoblastoma patients in combination with chemotherapy; however, it exhibited unacceptable toxicity [72, 73]. The second generation Pgp inhibitor valspodar was shown to be less toxic and more potent than cyclosporine in numerous clinical trials, but its use was limited as it targeted other ABC transporter proteins and had erratic pharmacokinetic interactions [74–75]. A third generation of Pgp inhibitors, tariquidar, binds with high affinity to the Pgp transporter and inhibits its activity [76]. It is specific and does not alter the levels of co-administered cytotoxic agents. Similarly, the expression of BCRP was reported in small cell lung cancer patient and its inhibition can decrease drug efflux. Gefitinib, a tyrosine kinase inhibitor, blocks the transporter function of BCRP, thereby reversing drug resistance [77]. Thus, the inhibition of these transcripts can sensitize cancer cells to pharmaceutical treatments.

12.7.2 DRUG INACTIVATION

Interaction of the drug with several proteins can induce modification or degradation of the drug, ultimately leading to its activation. Metabolic activation of the drug may also be required for it to gain efficacy. Inactivation of drug can decrease the quantity of free drug available to bind its cellular target, therefore, it fails to generate clinical response. However, cancer cells can develop resistance to treatments and the mechanisms that decrease drug activation play a critical role in drug resistance.

- Platinum drugs such as cisplatin are applied postoperatively in the treatment of ovarian cancers. These drugs are inactivated upon formation of conjugates with thiol glutathione (GSH) and thiol metallothionein (MT) and become a substrate for ABC transporter proteins. Increased levels of GSH have been reported in platinum drug-resistant tumors [78, 79]. Glutathione-S-transferase (GST) catalyzes the conjugation of GSH with platinum drugs, and its increased expression has been correlated with resistance to cisplatin in ovarian cancer cells and tumors [80].
- Irinotecan, a topoisomerase I inhibitor, is inactivated by glucuronidation catalyzed by uridine diphosphogluronysl transferase 1A1 (UG-T1A1) [81]. This process metabolizes these drugs to more water-soluble compounds and later are excreted into the urine or bile. Increased glucuronidation may lead to irinotecan resistance [82].
- Cytarabine (Ara-C), a nucleoside drug is converted to active form Ara-

C-triphosphate by multiple phosphorylation events [83]. Acute myelogenous leukemia cells can gain Ara-C resistance if this pathway is
downregulated or mutated.

12.7.3   ALTERATIONS OF DRUG TARGETS

The maximal effectiveness of a drug is influenced by its molecular targets.
Mutations or modifications in expression levels of these drug targets can
alter the drug response and lead to drug resistance. A few alterations have
been discussed below:

- Modification of enzyme expression levels: Fluorodeoxyuridine monophosphate (FdUMP), the active metabolite of 5-flurouracil, inhibits thymidylate synthase (TS). In the unbound state, TS inhibits the
  translation of its own mRNA by binding it but is unable to suppress its
  translation when bound to FdUMP. The expression of the TS protein
  is increased and is a key determinant of 5FU response. Some of the de
  novo synthesized TS protein remains unbound by FdUMP and may
  lead to 5-FU resistance [84].
- Genetic alterations: Mutations in β-tubulin lead to resistance to paclitaxel and other taxanes in ovarian cancer [85].
- Alterations in signal transduction pathways: Transtuzumab, a monoclonal antibody, is used for the treatment of HER2-positive breast cancer tumors. It is highly effective in combination with chemotherapy;
  however, its efficacy is limited as a single agent. Trastuzumab-resistant
  cell line exhibit significant expression of insulin-like growth factor 1
  receptor (IGF1R) in comparison to the nonresistant parental cell line.
  Therefore, dual targeting of IGF1R and HER2 and IGF1R can improve
  response in HER2-positive tumors [86].

12.7.4   DNA MISMATCH REPAIR

Many chemotherapeutic drugs used for the treatment of established tumors
have been associated with loss of DNA mismatch repair (MMR), cell cycle
arrest, and cell death. The MMR system is crucial for maintaining the stability of the genome by scanning the newly synthesized DNA, excising

single-base mismatches and insertion-deletion loops. MMR deficiency not only predisposes the cells to gain oncogenicity but also make them drug resistant by impairing their ability of DNA damage detection, causing inhibition of apoptosis induction. This also leads to an increased rate of mutation throughout the genome [87]. Loss of MMR activity has been associated with resistance to DNA-damaging agents, including platinum drugs [88].

- Hypermethylation of the promoter region of the hMLH1 gene makes the MMR system faulty, and this has been associated with cisplatin resistance [89]. It has been observed that cell lines that have MMR defects are resistant to cisplatin but remain sensitive to oxaliplatin. This has been accredited to the differences in the structure of their respective DNA adducts as the MMR system fails to recognize the bulky oxaliplatin DNA adducts [90].
- Homologous recombination and nucleotide excision repair are attributed to cause platinum-based drug resistance as they repair the harmful DNA crosslinks and inhibit the activation of apoptosis. Thus, the inhibition of repair pathways can increase the efficacy of DNA-damaging cytotoxic drugs [91].
- The overexpression of O6-methylguanine DNA methyltransferase (MGMT) in many tumors converts the nucleotides alkylated by the various alkylating chemotherapeutic drugs back to guanine before mismatch can occur, thereby rendering them resistant to these alkylating agents [92].

12.7.5   DNA METHYLATION

DNA methylation occurs by the addition of a methyl group at a 5' carbon group, usually at cytosine-guanosine dinucleotides (CpGs), resulting in gene silencing and transcription inhibition [93]. The inactivation of key tumor suppressor genes is known to undergo this epigenetic modification, which may consequently lead to drug resistance.

- The cisplatin-resistant ovarian cancer cell line exhibits hypermethylation of the promoters of both hMLH1 alleles, resulting in loss of hMLH1 expression. Treatment of the resistant cell line with the methylation inhibitor 5-azacytidine leads to re-expression of hMLH1 and increased sensitivity to cisplatin, hinting toward the probable mechanism of drug resistance [94].

- Promoter hypermethylation of the caspase 8 gene was reported in various death receptor-resistant solid brain tumor cell lines and in primary tumor samples with decreased caspase 8 protein expression. Pre-treatment with the demethylating agent 5-aza-2'-deoxycytidine not only made them death ligand sensitive but also enhanced their response to various chemotherapies [95].
- Promoter hypermethylation of the MGMT gene functions as a favorable prognostic marker in glioblastoma patients undergoing chemotherapy involving an alkylating agent. Methylation of the DNA repair enzyme MGMT has been reported in both cell lines and xenografts from gliomas and in 40% of grade III or IV gliomas, which was parallel with the response to the alkylating agent carmustine [92]. In a phase II study, 68% of glioblastomas analyzed exhibited methylation of the MGMT promoter, and this correlated with a longer overall survival when treated with the alkylating agent temozolomide [96].

12.7.6   CELL DEATH INHIBITION

Autophagy and apoptosis are the two major regulatory events contributing to cell death. The antiapoptotic BCL-2 family proteins are highly expressed in various types of cancers, contributing to resistance to chemotherapy and radiotherapy. Inhibitors of the BCL-2 family protein are useful in inducing apoptosis in cancer cells, but prolonged use can lead to development of resistance. Use of antisense techniques to downregulate BCL-2 and Bcl-XL help in sensitizing cells to chemotherapy, whereas an increased resistance is reported upon loss of Bax expression [97].

Altered expression of cellular inhibitors of apoptosis proteins (cIAPs) family members such as cIAP1, XIAP, and survivin have been reported in several types of cancers. They inhibit chemotherapy-induced cell death by binding to active caspases like caspase 3, 7, and 9. Silencing of these proteins in thyroid cancer cells by RNA interference has shown to increase their sensitivity to chemotherapeutic drugs [98]. Therefore, the use of one drug that alters the expression of cell death pathway members along with another cytotoxic drug that kills these cells in their vulnerable state is a better strategy to treat drug-resistant cancer cells.

Autophagy is the catabolic process of phagolytic death upon lysosomal acidification, which is temporarily used as a survival mechanism by the cells under stressed conditions. Drugs such as chloroquine and its derivatives prevent autophagy by raising the pH to inactivate digestive enzymes in lysosomes [99]. Therefore, they can be advantageous in sensitizing cancer cells to chemotherapeutic drugs and inhibiting autophagy-dependent resistance to chemotherapy. Sasaki et al. suggested the combination therapy of chloroquine and 5-FU as an effective approach for the treatment of colorectal cancer [100]. Derivatives of chloroquine, such as hydroxychloroquine, have been shown to inhibit autophagy in ER-positive cancer cells and restore their sensitivity to tamoxifen [101].

12.7.7   TUMOR HETEROGENEITY

Enrichment of a small fraction of drug-resistant cells having stem cell-like properties residing in the heterogeneous cancer cell population of the tumor may lead to the development of drug resistance. A small fraction of adult cancer cells may also be drug resistant. Both cancer cells in circulation as well as in solid tumors possess heterogeneous cell populations due to aberrant DNA repair mechanisms, accumulating mutations and epigenetic alterations that lead to defects in their ability to differentiate and in their control of proliferation. Some of these resistant cancers cells may be in the circulation and can form tumors in distant organs. MCF-7 human breast cancer cells cultured in the presence of an antiestrogen or in the absence of estrogen develop resistance against rapamycin by acquiring changes in the ploidy status and proliferation rates [102].

All forms of cancers have clonal subpopulations that differ in drug sensitivity and resistant characteristics [103]. Relapse or reoccurrence of cancer in patients after successful therapy may be a result of cancer cell growth from the drug-resistant clone. A study on acute myeloid leukemia (AML) demonstrates the presence of two coexisting dominant clones in the clinical samples of which one was chemotherapy sensitive and one was resistant. Partial eradication of AML founder clones underlies AML relapse and persistence upon induction chemotherapy [104]. Therefore, the development of better therapies is required to reduce the relapse of cancers.

12.7.8   METASTASIS

The epithelial to mesenchymal transition (EMT) is a mechanism by which cells in the solid tumors become metastatic by detaching themselves from other cells upon reduced expression of cell adhesion receptors like integrins and cadherins, and gaining cell motility, leading to increased survival and development of drug resistance [105]. Signaling processes of differentiation during EMT may also contribute to resistance toward chemotherapeutic drugs. For instance, during EMT, the expression of transforming growth factor β (TGFβ) is regulated by increase in integrin αvβ1 expression that subsequently leads to survival of colon cancer cells [106]. Laubli and co-workers demonstrated the role of stromal cells in drug resistance that participate in EMT by interacting with the extracellular matrix via selectin and other cell adhesion receptors [107]. Further, Straussman et al. co-cultured melanoma and fibroblast cells and found that the stromal cell influenced the innate resistance of 45 cancer cell lines when screened against B-Raf inhibitor drugs [108, 109].

12.8   TOXIC EFFECTS OF CHEMOTHERAPY

A drug having maximum therapeutic index, i.e., higher therapeutic effects and least toxicity, are preferred for anticancer treatment, but the clinical use of chemotherapeutic drugs is limited by the toxic effects that they produce on normal cells. The side effects associated with these drugs can be short term that are usually encountered during the therapy or long term that arise as a result of the complications after the therapy. The side effect profile varies across individuals and may also depend on the dose used and the duration of treatment.

The risk of gastrointestinal toxicity is one of the profound effects of chemotherapeutic drugs. At the time of onset of systemic chemotherapy, nausea and vomiting have been reported as a common consequence whose severity and duration vary with the drug regimen. Drugs like dactinomycin, methotrexate, vinca alkaloids and 5-FU have been associated with mucositis. Treatment with 5-FU sometimes also leads to bloody diarrhea and high mortality [110]. A study conducted by Holland et al. reported the presence of constipation in one-third of patients treated with vincristine, where severity and frequency were found to be dose dependent [111].

Cardiovascular toxicities that increase cardiovascular risk in cancer patients are also a consequence of modern chemotherapies. Hypertension, heart failure, thrombosis, cardiomyopathy, and arrhythmias are fatal effects caused by chemotherapeutic agents drugs such as alkylating agents, antimetabolites, and anticancer antibiotics. Antiangiogenic drugs that inhibit vascular endothelial growth factor signaling are also associated with cardiovascular pathology, especially hypertension, thromboembolism, myocardial infarction, and proteinuria [112]. 5-FU can exert direct toxic effects on vascular endothelium to reduce endothelial NO synthase activity and provoke coronary artery vasospasm and endothelium-independent vasoconstriction via protein kinase C [113].

The use of cisplatin for treatment has been associated with adverse nephrotoxic effects, leading to reduction in renal function. Higher blood pressure levels and development of microalbuminuria have also been indicated with the use of this drug [114].

Few chemotherapy regimens may also lead to the depletion of sperm count often to azoospermic levels, which may persist for several years or could be permanent. Semen analyses of non-Hodgkin's lymphoma patients treated with cyclophosphamide, doxorubicin, vincristine, prednisone, and bleomycin chemotherapy was associated with a high risk of permanent sterility[115].

Chemotherapeutic agents show several signs and symptoms of neurotoxicity, amongst which the most common are headache and seizures. Other CNS toxicity includes asceptic meningitis; acute, subacute or chronic encephalopathy; cerebellar dysfunction; and movement disorders [116]. Patients treated with the chemotherapeutic agent oxaliplatin in a phase II study were reported to have experienced ptosis, jaw and eye pain, leg cramps, and signs of hyperexcitability in motor nerves in nerve conduction studies [117]. 5-FU may cause encephalopathy and coma in patients who are deficient in the rate-limiting enzyme dihydropyrimidine dehydrogenase, which is responsible for metabolic clearance [118].

Hepatotoxic insult caused by chemotherapeutic agents includes necrosis, cholestasis, steatosis, fibrosis, and vascular injury [119]. Plicamycin (mithramycin) was reported to be the most hepatotoxic drug used for treating tumor hypercalcemia, which is refractory to other therapies. Plicamycin was able to block the synthesis of many intercellular enxymes crucial for normal functioning of the liver by binding the DNA and inhibiting RNA transcription [120].

12.9 CONCLUSION

Chemotherapeutic drugs are not very specific to any cancer type because they are multiple etiological factors/variation for carcinogenesis. The success rate of chemotherapy varies amongst different cancer types. For some, it is quite low and for some, its considerably very high. Few cancers respond very well to chemotherapy, where others do not, and also for some cancers, chemotherapy is not even suggested. At present, hematological cancers respond very well to chemotherapy. For example, 80% success rate has been observed in the case of acute promyelocytic leukemia with all-trans-retinoic acid (a form of vitamin A). Further, it is 90% for metastasized choriocarcinoma when treated with methotrexate alone/methotrexate combined with other chemotherapeutic drug. According to the 2016 report of The American Cancer Society, the 5-year relative survival rate for all cancers diagnosed during the years 2005–2011 was 69%, which increased from 49% during 1975–1977 [121]. Survival rates may vary greatly by cancer type and stage at diagnosis. Improvements in the survival rate can only be achieved when certain cancers can be diagnosed in their early stages as well as in the improvements in treatment schedule. Among all types of cancers, one-third cancer cases are preventable. Prevention of cancer is the most cost-effective and long-term suggested strategy. At present, herbal chemotherapy and their nano-formulations have gained considerable attention in the last few decades. Various herbal nano-formulations are in different stages of trials with some available for use, such as nano-curcumin. These help in reaching specific targets, thereby killing only the cancer cells and having reduced toxicity on normal cells.

Although there is growing research on the use and formulations of chemotherapeutic drugs, the main debate still lies on the funding, availability, and impact upon quality of life it makes, which raises a serious concern. In summary, a rigorous re-evaluation of the impact of chemotherapy on quality of life and their financial cost-effectiveness should be undertaken primarily.

12.10 SUMMARY

- Chemotherapy is the most common treatment of cancer that uses one or more anticancer drugs that kill or retard the growth of active cells.

- Development of a new chemotherapeutic drug involves three steps: screening of natural and synthetic compounds to identify novel drug molecules, chemical alteration of the anticancer drug/molecule to enhance its efficacy, and formulating it into a useful pharmaceutical drug that gets patented.
- Cell cycle plays an important role in the activity of many chemotherapeutic drugs as they target active cells that are not in G0 (resting phase). Cell cycle nonspecific drugs, act at several or all cell cycle phases, whereas cell cycle-specific drugs act specifically only at particular cell cycle phases.
- Chemotherapy drugs are usually classified based on their chemical structure, source, and how they act on cancer cells.
- Increased drug efflux, drug activation and inactivation, alteration in drug target, DNA methylation, processing of drug-induced damage, and evasion of apoptosis are the numerous factors that assist cancer cells to acquire drug resistance and evade chemotherapy.
- The clinical use of chemotherapeutic drugs is limited by the toxic effects that they produce on normal cells, which may include gastrointestinal toxicity, hepatotoxicity, cardiovascular toxicity, neurotoxicity, and nephrotoxicity.
- In order to overcome drug resistance and ameliorate the toxic effects, newer approaches such as combinatorial drug therapy are required to supplement the conventional chemotherapy for mitigation of cancer.

ACKNOWLEDGMENTS

S. S is thankful to Indian Council of Medical Research for the award of Senior Research Fellowship. S.M. is thankful to Department of Science and Technology (DST) for providing financial assistance (SR/WOS-A/LS-1290/2015. J.D is thankful to UGC for the award of Senior Research Fellowship. A.D is thankful to DBT for the award of Junior Research Fellowship. One of us (P.K.P) (PDF/2015/000033) is thankful to Department of Science and Technology (DST) for providing financial assistance. This work was supported by Council of Scientific and Industrial Research network project BSC0103.The CDRI communication No. for this manuscript is 9471.

KEYWORDS

- cancer
- chemoresistance
- chemotherapy
- neoadjuvant therapy
- toxicity

REFERENCES

1. *World Cancer Report*, 2014.
2. Mierzwa, M. L., Nyati, M. K., Morgan, M. A., & Lawrence, T. S., (2010). Recent advances in combined modality therapy. *The Oncologist, 15*, 372–381.
3. Franco, P., Fiorentino, A., Dionisi, F., Fiore, M., Chiesa, S., Vagge, S., Cellini, F., Caravatta, L., Tombolini, M., De Rose, F., Meattini, I., Mortellaro, G., Apicella, G., Marino, L., & Greto, D., (2016). Combined modality therapy for thoracic and head and neck cancers: a review of updated literature based on a consensus meeting. *Tumori, 102*, 459–471.
4. Narang, A. K., & Terezakis, S. A., (2015). Contemporary radiation therapy in combined modality therapy for Hodgkin lymphoma. *Journal of the National Comprehensive Cancer Network : JNCCN, 13*, 597–605.
5. Patel, S. A., Ryan, D. P., & Hong, T. S., (2016). Combined modality therapy for rectal cancer. *Cancer Journal, 22*, 211–217.
6. Cavalcante, L., Kelsen, D. P., & Yu, K. H., (2014). Combined modality therapy in pancreatic adenocarcinoma: review and updates on a controversial issue. *Current Pharmaceutical Design, 20*, 6697–6701.
7. Argiris, A., (2013). Current status and future directions in induction chemotherapy for head and neck cancer. *Critical Reviews in Oncology/Hematology, 88*, 57–74.
8. Driessen, C. M., de Boer, J. P., Gelderblom, H., Rasch, C. R., de Jong, M. A., Verbist, B. M., Melchers, W. J., Tesselaar, M. E., van der Graaf, W. T., Kaanders, J. H., & Van Herpen, C. M., (2016). Induction chemotherapy with docetaxel/cisplatin/5-fluorouracil followed by randomization to two cisplatin-based concomitant chemoradiotherapy schedules in patients with locally advanced head and neck cancer (CONDOR study) (Dutch Head and Neck Society 08–01): A randomized phase II study. *European Journal of Cancer, 52*, 77–84.
9. Schultz, J., Bran, G., Anders, C., Sadick, H., Faber, A., Hormann, K., & Sauter, A., (2010). Induction chemotherapy with TPF (Docetaxel, carboplatin and fluorouracil) in the treatment of locally advanced squamous cell carcinoma of the head and neck. *Oncology Reports, 24*, 1213.
10. Trimble, E., Ungerleider, R., Abrams, J., Kaplan, R., Feigal, E., Smith, M., Carter, C., & Friedman, M., (1993). Neoadjuvant therapy in cancer treatment. *Cancer, 72*, 3515–3524.

11. Hall, T. R., & Dizon, D. S., (2016). Neoadjuvant chemotherapy for advanced epithelial ovarian cancer. *Clinical Advances in Hematology & Oncology: H& 14*, 262–268.

12. Iwama, J., Ogiwara, H., Kiyotani, C., Terashima, K., Matsuoka, K., Iwafuchi, H., & Morota, N., (2015). Neoadjuvant chemotherapy for brain tumors in infants and young children. *Journal of neurosurgery. Pediatrics, 15*, 488–492.

13. Van Schaik, R. H., (2005). Cancer treatment and pharmacogenetics of cytochrome P450 enzymes. *Investigational New Drugs, 23*, 513–522.

14. Schwartsmann, G., Winograd, B., & Pinedo, H., (1988). The main steps in the development of anticancer agents. *Radiotherapy and Oncology, 12*, 301–313.

15. Umscheid, C. A., Margolis, D. J., & Grossman, C. E., (2011). Key concepts of clinical trials: a narrative review. *Postgraduate Medicine, 123*, 194–204.

16. Manji, A., Brana, I., Amir, E., Tomlinson, G., Tannock, I. F., Bedard, P. L., Oza, A., Siu, L. L., & Razak, A. R., (2013). Evolution of clinical trial design in early drug development: systematic review of expansion cohort use in single-agent phase I cancer trials. *Journal of Clinical Oncology : Official Journal of the American Society of Clinical Oncolog, 31*, 4260–4267.

17. Wang, M., Dignam, J. J., Zhang, Q. E., DeGroot, J. F., Mehta, M. P., & Hunsberger, S., (2012). Integrated phase II/III clinical trials in oncology: a case study. *Clinical Trials (London, England), 9*, 741–747.

18. Hartwell, L. H., & Kastan, M. B., (1994). Cell cycle control and cancer. *Science (New York) 266*, 1821.

19. Peters, G. J., (2014). Novel developments in the use of antimetabolites. *Nucleosides, Nucleotides & Nucleic acid, 33*, 358–374.

20. Morgan, G., (2003). Chemotherapy and the cell cycle. *Cancer Nursing Practic, 21*, 27–30.

21. Schwartz, G. K., & Dickson, M., (2009). Development of cell cycle inhibitors for cancer therapy. *Current Oncology, 16*, 36–43.

22. Sanchez-Martínez, C., Gelbert, L. M., Lallena, M. J., & De Dios, A., (2015). Cyclin dependent kinase (CDK) inhibitors as anticancer drugs. *Bioorganic & Medicinal Chemistry Letters, 25*, 3420–3435.

23. Chaney, S. G., & Sancar, A., (1996). DNA repair: enzymatic mechanisms and relevance to drug response. *Journal of the National Cancer Institute, 88*, 1346–1360.

24. Fischhaber, P. L., Gall, A. S., Duncan, J. A., & Hopkins, P. B., (1999). Direct demonstration in synthetic oligonucleotides that N, N'-bis(2-chloroethyl)-nitrosourea cross links N1 of deoxyguanosine to N3 of deoxycytidine on opposite strands of duplex DNA. *Cancer Research, 59*, 4363–4368.

25. Puyo, S., Montaudon, D., & Pourquier, P., (2014). From old alkylating agents to new minor groove binders. *Critical Reviews in Oncology/Hematology, 89*, 43–61.

26. Hemminki, K., & Kallama, S., (1986). Reactions of nitrogen mustards with DNA. *IARC Scientific Publications, 78*, 55–70.

27. Peng Wang, G. B. B., Richard, A. O., Bennett, L., & Povirk, L. F., (1991). Thermolabile adenine adducts and A.cntdot. T base pair substitutions induced by nitrogen mustard analogs in an SV40-based shuttle plasmid. *Biochemistry, 30*, 11515–11521.

28. Surget, S., Lemieux-Blanchard, E., Maiga, S., Descamps, G., Le Gouill, S., Moreau, P., Amiot, M., & Pellat-Deceunynck, C., (2014). Bendamustine and melphalan kill myeloma cells similarly through reactive oxygen species production and activation of the p53 pathway and do not overcome resistance to each other. *Leukemia & Lymphoma, 55*, 2165–2173.

29. Galaup, A., & Paci, A., (2013). Pharmacology of dimethanesulfonate alkylating agents: busulfan and treosulfan. *Expert Opinion on Drug Metabolism & Toxicology, 9*, 333–347.

30. Tong, W. P., & Ludlum, D. B., (1980). Crosslinking of DNA by busulfan. Formation of diguanyl derivatives. *Biochimica et Biophysica Acta, 608*, 174–181.

31. Hartley, J. A., & Fox, B. W., (1986). Cross-linking between histones and DNA following treatment with a series of dimethane sulphonate esters. *Cancer Chemotherapy and Pharmacology, 17*, 56–62.

32. Hartley, J. A., O'Hare, C. C., & Baumgart, J., (1999). DNA alkylation and interstrand cross-linking by treosulfan. *British Journal of Cance, 79*, 264–266.

33. Chuang, R. Y., Laszlo, J., & Keller, P., (1976). Effects of nitrosoureas on human DNA polymerase activities from acute and chronic granulocytic leukemia cells. *Biochimica et Biophysica Acta, 425*, 463–468.

34. Brandes, A. A., Bartolotti, M., Tosoni, A., & Franceschi, E., (2016). Nitrosoureas in the Management of Malignant Gliomas. *Current Neurology and Neuroscience Reports, 16*, 13.

35. Moody, C. L., & Wheelhouse, R. T., (2014). The medicinal chemistry of imidazotetrazine prodrugs. *Pharmaceuticals (Basel, Switzerland), 7*, 797–838.

36. Marchesi, F., Turriziani, M., Tortorelli, G., Avvisati, G., Torino, F., & De Vecchis, L., (2007). Triazene compounds: mechanism of action and related DNA repair systems. *Pharmacological Research, 56*, 275–287.

37. Booser, D. J., & Hortobagyi, G. N., (1994). Anthracycline antibiotics in cancer therapy. Focus on drug resistance. *Drugs, 47*, 223–258.

38. Jordan, M. A., & Wilson, L., (1998). Microtubules and actin filaments: dynamic targets for cancer chemotherapy. *Current Opinion in Cell Biology, 10*, 123–130.

39. Cheng, K. L., Bradley, T., & Budman, D. R., (2008). Novel microtubule-targeting agents - the epothilones. *Biologics: Targets & Therapy, 2*, 789–811.

40. Jordan, M. A., Thrower, D., & Wilson, L., (1991). Mechanism of inhibition of cell proliferation by Vinca alkaloids. *Cancer Research, 51*, 2212–2222.

41. Lane, A. A., & Chabner, B. A., (2009). Histone deacetylase inhibitors in cancer therapy. *Journal of Clinical Oncology : Official Journal of the American Society of Clinical Oncology 27*, 5459–5468.

42. Hsiang, Y. H., Hertzberg, R., Hecht, S., & Liu, L. F., (1985). Camptothecin induces protein-linked DNA breaks via mammalian DNA topoisomerase I. *Journal of Biological Chemistry 260*, 14873–14878.

43. Aktas, G., Kus, T., Kalender, M. E., Sevinc, A., Camci, C., & Kul, S., (2016). Survival analysis in second-line and third-line chemotherapy with irinotecan followed by topotecan or topotecan followed by irinotecan for extensive-stage small-cell lung cancer patients: a single-center retrospective study. *OncoTargets and Therapy, 9*, 1921.

44. Houghton, P. J., Cheshire, P. J., Hallman II, J. D., Lutz, L., Friedman, H. S., Danks, M. K., & Houghton, J. A., (1995). Efficacy of topoisomerase I inhibitors, topotecan and irinotecan, administered at low dose levels in protracted schedules to mice bearing xenografts of human tumors. *Cancer Chemotherapy and Pharmacology, 36*, 393–403.

45. Wozniak, A. J., & Ross, W. E., (1983). DNA damage as a basis for 4'-demethylepipodophyllotoxin-9-(4, 6-O-ethylidene-β-d-glucopyranoside)(etoposide) cytotoxicity. *Cancer Research, 43*, 120–124.

46. Chen, G. L., Yang, L., Rowe, T., Halligan, B. D., Tewey, K. M., & Liu, L. F., (1984). Nonintercalative antitumor drugs interfere with the breakage-reunion reaction of mammalian DNA topoisomerase II. *Journal of Biological Chemistry, 259*, 13560–13566.

47. Burgess, D. J., Doles, J., Zender, L., Xue, W., Ma, B., McCombie, W. R., Hannon, G. J., Lowe, S. W., & Hemann, M. T., (2008). Topoisomerase levels determine chemotherapy response in vitro and in vivo. *Proceedings of the National Academy of Sciences, 105*, 9053–9058.

48. Kris, M. G., Natale, R. B., Herbst, R. S., Lynch Jr, T. J., Prager, D., Belani, C. P., Schiller, J. H., Kelly, K., Spiridonidis, H., & Sandler, A., (2003). Efficacy of gefitinib, an inhibitor of the epidermal growth factor receptor tyrosine kinase, in symptomatic patients with non–small cell lung cancer: a randomized trial. *Jama., 290*, 2149–2158.

49. Ou, S. H. I., Kwak, E. L., Siwak-Tapp, C., Dy, J., Bergethon, K., Clark, J. W., Camidge, D. R., Solomon, B. J., Maki, R. G., & Bang, Y. J., (2011). Activity of crizotinib (PF02341066), a dual mesenchymal-epithelial transition (MET) and anaplastic lymphoma kinase (ALK) inhibitor, in a non-small cell lung cancer patient with de novo MET amplification. *Journal of Thoracic Oncology, 6*, 942–946.

50. Zaytseva, Y. Y., Valentino, J. D., Gulhati, P., & Evers, B. M., (2012). mTOR inhibitors in cancer therapy. *Cancer Letters, 319*, 1–7.

51. Motzer, R. J., Escudier, B., Oudard, S., Hutson, T. E., Porta, C., Bracarda, S., Grünwald, V., Thompson, J. A., Figlin, R. A., & Hollaender, N., (2008). Efficacy of everolimus in advanced renal cell carcinoma: a double-blind, randomised, placebo-controlled phase III trial. *The Lancet, 372*, 449–456.

52. Robillard, M. S., & Reedijk, J., (2005). Platinum-Based Anticancer Drugs. *Encyclopedia of Inorganic and Bioinorganic Chemistry*.

53. Becouarn, Y., Ychou, M., Ducreux, M., Borel, C., Bertheault-Cvitkovic, F., Seitz, J., Nasca, S., Nguyen, T., Paillot, B., & Raoul, J., (1998). Phase II trial of oxaliplatin as first-line chemotherapy in metastatic colorectal cancer patients. Digestive Group of French Federation of Cancer Centers. *Journal of Clinical Oncology, 16*, 2739–2744.

54. Ardizzoni, A., Boni, L., Tiseo, M., Fossella, F. V., Schiller, J. H., Paesmans, M., Radosavljevic, D., Paccagnella, A., Zatloukal, P., & Mazzanti, P., (2007). Cisplatin-versus carboplatin-based chemotherapy in first-line treatment of advanced non–small-cell lung cancer: an individual patient data meta-analysis. *Journal of the National Cancer Institute, 99*, 847–857.

55. Hagner, N., & Joerger, M., (2010). Cancer chemotherapy: targeting folic acid synthesis. *Cancer Management and Research, 2*, 293–301.

56. Maevis, V., Mey, U., Schmidt-Wolf, G., & Schmidt-Wolf, I., (2014). Hairy cell leukemia: short review, today's recommendations and outlook. *Blood Cancer Journal, 4*, e184.

57. Ricci, F., Tedeschi, A., Morra, E., & Montillo, M., (2009). Fludarabine in the treatment of chronic lymphocytic leukemia: a review. *Therapeutics and Clinical Risk Management, 5*, 187.

58. Parker, W. B., & Cheng, Y. C., (1990). Metabolism and mechanism of action of 5-fluorouracil. *Pharmacology & Therapeutics, 48*, 381–395.

59. Keating, M. J., Flinn, I., Jain, V., Binet, J.-L., Hillmen, P., Byrd, J., Albitar, M., Brettman, L., Santabarbara, P., & Wacker, B., (2002). Therapeutic role of alemtuzumab (Campath-1H) in patients who have failed fludarabine: results of a large international study. *Blood, 99*, 3554–3561.

60. Witzig, T. E., White, C. A., Gordon, L. I., Wiseman, G. A., Emmanouilides, C., Murray, J. L., Lister, J., & Multani, P. S., (2003). Safety of yttrium-90 ibritumomab tiuxetan radioimmunotherapy for relapsed low-grade, follicular, or transformed non-Hodgkin's lymphoma. *Journal of Clinical Oncology, 21,* 1263–1270.

61. Moskowitz, C. H., Ribrag, V., Michot, J.-M., Martinelli, G., Zinzani, P. L., Gutierrez, M., De Maeyer, G., Jacob, A. G., Giallella, K., & Anderson, J. W., (2014). PD-1 blockade with the monoclonal antibody pembrolizumab (MK-3475) in patients with classical Hodgkin lymphoma after brentuximab vedotin failure: preliminary results from a phase 1b study (KEYNOTE-013). *Blood, 124,* 290–290.

62. Cheever, M. A., & Higano, C. S., (2011). PROVENGE (Sipuleucel-T) in prostate cancer: the first FDA-approved therapeutic cancer vaccine. *Clinical Cancer Research, 17,* 3520–3526.

63. Herr, H. W., Schwalb, D. M., Zhang, Z.-F., Sogani, P. C., Fair, W. R., Whitmore, W., & Oettgen, H. F., (1995). Intravesical bacillus Calmette-Guérin therapy prevents tumor progression and death from superficial bladder cancer: ten-year follow-up of a prospective randomized trial. *Journal of Clinical Oncology, 13,* 1404–1408.

64. Trump, D. L., Waldstreicher, J. A., Kolvenbag, G., Wissel, P. S., & Neubauer, B. L., (2001). Androgen antagonists: potential role in prostate cancer prevention. *Urology, 57,* 64–67.

65. Kiang, D. T., & Kennedy, B., (1977). Tamoxifen (antiestrogen) therapy in advanced breast cancer. *Annals of Internal Medicine, 87,* 687–690.

66. Kerbel, R. S., Kobayashi, H., & Graham, C. H., (1994). Intrinsic or acquired drug resistance and metastasis: are they linked phenotypes? *Journal of Cellular Biochemistry, 56,* 37–47.

67. Li, W., Zhang, H., Assaraf, Y. G., Zhao, K., Xu, X., Xie, J., Yang, D. H., & Chen, Z. S., (2016). Overcoming ABC transporter-mediated multidrug resistance: Molecular mechanisms and novel therapeutic drug strategies. *Drug Resistance Updates : Reviews and Commentaries in Antimicrobial and Anticancer Chemotherapy, 27,* 14–29.

68. Borst, P., & Elferink, R. O., (2002). Mammalian ABC transporters in health and disease. *Annual Review of Biochemistry, 71,* 537–592.

69. Sauna, Z. E., & Ambudkar, S. V., (2001). Characterization of the catalytic cycle of ATP hydrolysis by human P-glycoprotein. The two ATP hydrolysis events in a single catalytic cycle are kinetically similar but affect different functional outcomes. *The Journal of Biological Chemistry, 276,* 11653–11661.

70. Gottesman, M. M., Fojo, T., & Bates, S. E., (2002). Multidrug resistance in cancer: role of ATP-dependent transporters. *Nature Reviews. Cancer, 2,* 48–58.

71. Thomas, H., & Coley, H. M., (2003). Overcoming multidrug resistance in cancer: an update on the clinical strategy of inhibiting p-glycoprotein. *Cancer Control : Journal of the Moffitt Cancer Center, 10,* 159–165.

72. Chan, H. S., DeBoer, G., Thiessen, J. J., Budning, A., Kingston, J. E., O'Brien, J. M., Koren, G., Giesbrecht, E., Haddad, G., Verjee, Z., Hungerford, J. L., Ling, V., & Gallie, B. L., (1996). Combining cyclosporin with chemotherapy controls intraocular retinoblastoma without requiring radiation. *Clinical Cancer Research : An Official Journal of the American Association for Cancer Research, 2,* 1499–1508.

73. Theis, J. G., Chan, H. S., Greenberg, M. L., Malkin, D., Karaskov, V., Moncica, I., Koren, G., & Doyle, J., (2000). Assessment of systemic toxicity in children receiving chemotherapy with cyclosporine for sarcoma. *Medical and Pediatric Oncology, 34,* 242–249.

74. Advani, R., Fisher, G. A., Lum, B. L., Hausdorff, J., Halsey, J., Litchman, M., & Sikic, B. I., (2001). A phase I trial of doxorubicin, paclitaxel, & valspodar (PSC 833), a modulator of multidrug resistance. *Clinical Cancer Research : An Official Journal of the American Association for Cancer Research, 7,* 1221–1229.

75. Dorr, R., Karanes, C., Spier, C., Grogan, T., Greer, J., Moore, J., Weinberger, B., Schiller, G., Pearce, T., Litchman, M., Dalton, W., Roe, D., & List, A. F., (2001). Phase I/II study of the P-glycoprotein modulator PSC *833* in patients with acute myeloid leukemia. *Journal of Clinical Oncology : Official Journal of the American Society of Clinical Oncology, 19,* 1589–1599.

76. Pusztai, L., Wagner, P., Ibrahim, N., Rivera, E., Theriault, R., Booser, D., Symmans, F. W., Wong, F., Blumenschein, G., Fleming, D. R., Rouzier, R., Boniface, G., & Hortobagyi, G. N., (2005). Phase II study of tariquidar, a selective P-glycoprotein inhibitor, in patients with chemotherapy-resistant, advanced breast carcinoma. *Cancer, 104,* 682–691.

77. Yanase, K., Tsukahara, S., Asada, S., Ishikawa, E., Imai, Y., & Sugimoto, Y., (2004). Gefitinib reverses breast cancer resistance protein-mediated drug resistance. *Molecular Cancer Therapeutics, 3,* 1119–1125.

78. Meijer, C., Mulder, N. H., Timmer-Bosscha, H., Sluiter, W. J., Meersma, G. J., & De Vries, E. G., (1992). Relationship of cellular glutathione to the cytotoxicity and resistance of seven platinum compounds. *Cancer Research, 52,* 6885–6889.

79. Kelley, S. L., Basu, A., Teicher, B. A., Hacker, M. P., Hamer, D. H., & Lazo, J. S., (1988). Overexpression of metallothionein confers resistance to anticancer drugs. *Science (New York) 241,* 1813–1815.

80. Green, J. A., Robertson, L. J., & Clark, A. H., (1993). Glutathione S-transferase expression in benign and malignant ovarian tumours. *British Journal of Cancer, 68,* 235–239.

81. Xu, Y., & Villalona-Calero, M. A., (2002). Irinotecan: mechanisms of tumor resistance and novel strategies for modulating its activity. *Annals of Oncology : Official Journal of the European Society for Medical Oncology / ESMO, 13,* 1841–1851.

82. Cummings, J., Boyd, G., Ethell, B. T., Macpherson, J. S., Burchell, B., Smyth, J. F., & Jodrell, D. I., (2002). Enhanced clearance of topoisomerase I inhibitors from human colon cancer cells by glucuronidation. *Biochemical Pharmacology, 63,* 607–613.

83. Sampath, D., Cortes, J., Estrov, Z., Du, M., Shi, Z., Andreeff, M., Gandhi, V., & Plunkett, W., (2006). Pharmacodynamics of cytarabine alone and in combination with 7-hydroxystaurosporine (UCN-01) in AML blasts in vitro and during a clinical trial. *Blood, 107,* 2517–2524.

84. Zhang, N., Yin, Y., Xu, S. J., & Chen, W. S., (2008). 5-Fluorouracil: mechanisms of resistance and reversal strategies. *Molecules, 13,* 1551–1569.

85. Wang, Y., O'Brate, A., Zhou, W., & Giannakakou, P., (2005). Resistance to microtubule-stabilizing drugs involves two events: beta-tubulin mutation in one allele followed by loss of the second allele. *Cell Cycle (Georgetown, Tex.), 4*(12), 1847–1853.

86. Browne, B. C., Crown, J., Venkatesan, N., Duffy, M. J., Clynes, M., Slamon, D., O'Donovan, N., (2011). Inhibition of IGF1R activity enhances response to trastuzumab in HER-2-positive breast cancer cells. *Annals of Oncology : Official Journal of the European Society for Medical Oncology / ESMO, 22,* 68–73.

87. Fink, D., Aebi, S., & Howell, S. B., (1998). The role of DNA mismatch repair in drug resistance. *Clinical Cancer Research, 4,* 1–6.

88. Fink, D., Nebel, S., Aebi, S., Zheng, H., Cenni, B., Nehmé, A., Christen, R. D., & Howell, S. B., (1996). The role of DNA mismatch repair in platinum drug resistance. *Cancer Research 56,* 4881–4886.

89. Plumb, J. A., Strathdee, G., Sludden, J., Kaye, S. B., & Brown, R., (2000). Reversal of drug resistance in human tumor xenografts by 2'-deoxy-5-azacytidine-induced demethylation of the hMLH1 gene promoter. *Cancer Research, 60*, 6039–6044.

90. Chaney, S. G., Campbell, S. L., Temple, B., Bassett, E., Wu, Y., & Faldu, M., (2004). Protein interactions with platinum–DNA adducts: from structure to function. *Journal of Inorganic Biochemistry, 98*, 1551–1559.

91. Selvakumaran, M., Pisarcik, D. A., Bao, R., Yeung, A. T., & Hamilton, T. C., (2003). Enhanced cisplatin cytotoxicity by disturbing the nucleotide excision repair pathway in ovarian cancer cell lines. *Cancer Research, 63*, 1311–1316.

92. Esteller, M., Garcia-Foncillas, J., Andion, E., Goodman, S. N., Hidalgo, O. F., Vanaclocha, V., Baylin, S. B., & Herman, J. G., (2000). Inactivation of the DNA-repair gene MGMT and the clinical response of gliomas to alkylating agents. *New England Journal of Medicine, 343*, 1350–1354.

93. Clark, S. J., & Melki, J., (2002). DNA methylation and gene silencing in cancer: which is the guilty party? *Oncogene, 21*, 5380–5387.

94. Strathdee, G., MacKean, M., Illand, M., & Brown, R., (1999). A role for methylation of the hMLH1 promoter in loss of hMLH1 expression and drug resistance in ovarian cancer. *Oncogene, 18*.

95. Fulda, S., Kufer, M., Meyer, E., van Valen, F., Dockhorn-Dworniczak, B., Debatin, K.-M., (2001). Sensitization for death receptor-or drug-induced apoptosis by re-expression of caspase-8 through demethylation or gene transfer. *Oncogene 20*, 5865–5877.

96. Hegi, M. E., Diserens, A.-C., Godard, S., Dietrich, P.-Y., Regli, L., Ostermann, S., Otten, P., Van Melle, G., de Tribolet, N., & Stupp, R., (2004). Clinical trial substantiates the predictive value of O-6-methylguanine-DNA methyltransferase promoter methylation in glioblastoma patients treated with temozolomide. *Clinical Cancer Research, 10*, 1871–1874.

97. Frenzel, A., Grespi, F., Chmelewskij, W., & Villunger, A., (2009). Bcl2 family proteins in carcinogenesis and the treatment of cancer. *Apoptosis, 14*, 584–596.

98. Tirrò, E., Consoli, M. L., Massimino, M., Manzella, L., Frasca, F., Sciacca, L., Vicari, L., Stassi, G., Messina, L., & Messina, A., (2006). Altered expression of c-IAP1, survivin, & Smac contributes to chemotherapy resistance in thyroid cancer cells. *Cancer Research, 66*, 4263–4272.

99. Kimura, T., Takabatake, Y., Takahashi, A., & Isaka, Y., (2013). Chloroquine in cancer therapy: a double-edged sword of autophagy. *Cancer Research, 73*, 3–7.

100. Sasaki, K., Tsuno, N. H., Sunami, E., Kawai, K., Hongo, K., Hiyoshi, M., Kaneko, M., Murono, K., Tada, N., & Nirei, T., (2012). Resistance of colon cancer to 5-fluorouracil may be overcome by combination with chloroquine, an in vivo study. *Anti-Cancer Drugs, 23*, 675–682.

101. Solomon, V. R., & Lee, H., (2009). Chloroquine and its analogs: a new promise of an old drug for effective and safe cancer therapies. *European Journal of Pharmacology, 625*, 220–233.

102. Leung, E., Kannan, N., Krissansen, G. W., Findlay, M. P., & Baguley, B. C., (2010). MCF-7 breast cancer cells selected for tamoxifen resistance acquire new phenotypes differing in DNA content, phospho-HER2 and PAX2 expression, & rapamycin sensitivity. *Cancer Biology & Therapy, 9*, 717–724.

103. Navin, N., Krasnitz, A., Rodgers, L., Cook, K., Meth, J., Kendall, J., Riggs, M., Eberling, Y., Troge, J., & Grubor, V., (2010). Inferring tumor progression from genomic heterogeneity. *Genome Research, 20*, 68–80.

104. Parkin, B., Ouillette, P., Li, Y., Keller, J., Lam, C., Roulston, D., Li, C., Shedden, K., & Malek, S. N., (2012). Clonal evolution and devolution following chemotherapy in adult acute myelogenous leukemia. *Blood, blood-2012*–04–427039.
105. Voulgari, A., & Pintzas, A., (2009)., Epithelial–mesenchymal transition in cancer metastasis: mechanisms, markers and strategies to overcome drug resistance in the clinic. *Biochimica et Biophysica Acta (BBA)-Reviews on Cancer, 1796,* 75–90.
106. Bates, R. C., & Mercurio, A., (2005). The epithelial-mesenchymal transition (EMT) and colorectal cancer progression. *Cancer Biology & Therapy, 4,* 371–376.
107. Läubli, H., & Borsig, L., (2010). In Selectins promote tumor metastasis, *Seminars in Cancer Biology,* Elsevier, pp. 169–177.
108. Straussman, R., Morikawa, T., Shee, K., Barzily-Rokni, M., Qian, Z. R., Du, J., Davis, A., Mongare, M. M., Gould, J., & Frederick, D. T., (2012). Tumour micro-environment elicits innate resistance to RAF inhibitors through HGF secretion. *Nature, 487,* 500–504.
109. Housman, G., Byler, S., Heerboth, S., Lapinska, K., Longacre, M., Snyder, N., & Sarkar, S., (2014). Drug resistance in cancer: an overview. *Cancers, 6,* 1769–1792.
110. Mitchell, E. P., (2006). In Gastrointestinal toxicity of chemotherapeutic agents, *Seminars in Oncology,* Elsevier, pp. 106–120.
111. Holland, J. F., Scharlau, C., Gailani, S., Krant, M. J., Olson, K. B., Horton, J., Shnider, B. I., Lynch, J. J., Owens, A., & Carbone, P. P., (1973). Vincristine treatment of advanced cancer: a cooperative study of *392* cases. *Cancer Research, 33,* 1258–1264.
112. Cameron, A. C., Touyz, R. M., & Lang, N. N., (2015). Vascular complications of cancer chemotherapy. *Canadian Journal of Cardiology.*
113. Alter, P., Herzum, M., Soufi, M., Schaefer, J., & Maisch, B., (2006). Cardiotoxicity of 5-fluorouracil. *Cardiovascular & Hematological Agents in Medicinal Chemistry (Formerly Current Medicinal Chemistry-Cardiovascular & Hematological Agents), 4,* 1–5.
114. Miller, R. P., Tadagavadi, R. K., Ramesh, G., & Reeves, W. B., (2010). Mechanisms of cisplatin nephrotoxicity. *Toxins, 2,* 2490–2518.
115. Pryzant, R. M., Meistrich, M. L., Wilson, G., Brown, B., & McLaughlin, P., (1993). Long-term reduction in sperm count after chemotherapy with and without radiation therapy for non-Hodgkin's lymphomas. *Journal of Clinical Oncology, 11,* 239–247.
116. Kalita, J., & Misra, U., (2013). Neurotoxicity of Chemotherapeutic Agents. *ECAB Reviews in Neurology, 2014,* 71.
117. Wilson, R. H., Lehky, T., Thomas, R. R., Quinn, M. G., Floeter, M. K., & Grem, J. L., (2002). Acute oxaliplatin-induced peripheral nerve hyperexcitability. *Journal of Clinical Oncology, 20,* 1767–1774.
118. Takimoto, C. H., Lu, Z.-H., Zhang, R., Liang, M. D., Larson, L. V., Cantilena, L. R., Grem, J. L., Allegra, C. J., Diasio, R. B., & Chu, E., (1996). Severe neurotoxicity following 5-fluorouracil-based chemotherapy in a patient with dihydropyrimidine dehydrogenase deficiency. *Clinical Cancer Research, 2,* 477–481.
119. King, P. D., & Perry, M. C., (2001). Hepatotoxicity of chemotherapy. *The Oncologist, 6,* 162–176.
120. Kennedy, B., (1970). Metabolic and toxic effects of mithramycin during tumor therapy. *The American Journal of Medicine, 49,* 494–503.
121. American Cancer Society. Cancer Facts & Figures 2016. Atlanta: American Cancer Society; 2016.

PART IV

NOVEL THERAPEUTIC APPROACHES FOR CANCER

CHAPTER 13

NON-CODING RNAS: THE NEW REINS IN MALIGNANCIES

DEBA PRASAD MANDAL

Department of Zoology, West Bengal State University, Berunanpukuria, Malikapur, North-24 Parganas, Barasat, Kolkata–700126, West Bengal, India, E-mail: dpmandal1972@gmail. com

CONTENTS

ABSTRACT

It is well accepted that out of the so called "junk DNAs," a new set of RNAs has emerged that do not code for any protein but control and contribute to various cellular process. The coding genome accounts for less than 2% of all sequences, and various studies on cancer-associated mutations indicate extensive functional mutations within the noncoding genome. These RNAs that do not code for a definite protein but have proven biologically significant function are collectively referred to as noncoding RNAs (ncRNAs). ncRNA's are broadly subdivided into small ncRNAs (less than 200 bp) and long ncRNAs (greater than 200 bps). These broad heads are further divided into a variety of ncRNAs whose functions are varied and complex. Transcription of ncRNA many involve any of the three RNA polymerases, viz., RNA polymerases I (RNA Pol I), RNA polymerases II (RNA Pol II), or RNA polymerases III (RNA Pol III). These ncRNAs have been implicated in cancer progression. Their varied complex functions stretch from DNA methylation to acting as "sponges" for other RNAs. Being safe from degradation in body fluids, ncRNAs serve as good contenders in molecular diagnosis, and their variously modified expression in malignant cells endow upon them the promise to pose as therapeutic targets in cancer treatment. This chapter, however, does not aim to name all the ncRNAs or to elaborate all their functions, but aims to give an understanding of the capabilities and importance of these RNAs in cancer biology, which are truly holding the reigns of cancer.

13.1   RNA IN THE POST RNA WORLD

It is well accepted that after the ribonucleic acid (RNA) world, came the era of the more stable form of nucleic acid, the deoxyribonucleic acid (DNA). Soon, scientist concentrated on this new genetic material as it was the considered the "blueprint" of cellular information. Pioneering works of Gregor Mendel (1865) and later the structure of DNA by Rosalind Franklin, James Watson, and Francis Harry Compton Crick (1953) triggered scientist to speculate DNA as the ultimate hardware of cellular identity and function. Crick's "central dogma," which equivocated the mono-directional process involving the two principal steps, viz., transcription and translation, through which genetic information is converted to biologically active forms, i.e., proteins, DNA → RNA → protein, restricted RNA to be visualized as a harbinger of DNA. It was in 2001 that John Craig Venter and the International Human Genome Sequencing Consortium concluded the human genome project, revealing that only about 1–2% of the 3 billion (approximately) base pairs of human genome dictate translational entity. The notion of "central dogma" so dominated the scientific scenario that the majority of scientists dismissed the nonprotein sequencing parts as "junk DNA." Recent research shows that out of these "junks," a new set of RNA has emerged that do not code for any protein but control and contributes various cellular process. Such RNAs, now referred to as noncoding RNA (ncRNA), has gained much attention in recent research. It seems like the rise of the Phoenix, the neo era of the RNA world has yet again begun. Very interestingly, RNAs are no longer considered to be mere harbingers of DNA, as they exert epigenetic control over cellular function. These "reins"/control not only appear in signaling modification or modification of enzymatic function but also extend to gene silencing and DNA regulation by formation of heterochromatin, modification of histone proteins, and targeted DNA methylation. This and much more incites us to speculate if at all the RNA gave up their dominance in post RNA world or rather only stabilized its code as DNA while keeping the "reins" of cellular control in their own domain.

13.2   NONCODING RNAS

An ncRNA are RNA molecules that, after its transcription from DNA, is not translated into a protein. Such RNAs are also referred to as nonmessenger RNA (nmRNA), nonprotein-coding RNA (npcRNA), or functional RNA (fRNA). The RNA gene is referred to that segment of DNA from which such a functional ncRNA is transcribed.

13.2.1   HISTORY AND DISCOVERY

Friedrich Miescher first discovered nucleic acids in 1868, but it took another seven decades for it to get implicated in protein synthesis in 1939. It was in 1965 that the first ncRNA, tRNA for alanine (tRNA^{Ala}), was characterized and its structure elucidated. The credit goes to Robert W. Holley and his colleagues who had purified 1 g of this 80-nucleotide tRNA using140 kg of commercial baker's yeast. They had to primarily digest the baker's yeast with pancreatic ribonuclease (producing fragments ending in cytosine or uridine), followed by chromatographic separation. Ultimately, the identification of the 5' and 3' ends helped arrange the fragments to establish the RNA sequence. Though initially three structures of tRNA were proposed, the "cloverleaf" structure was eventually accepted as it was independently proposed by several independent publications. X-ray crystallography analysis of the cloverleaf secondary structure by two independent research groups in 1974 finalized its present day structure.

Ribosomal RNA followed by URNA was subsequently discovered in the early 1980s. Slowly, ncRNAs like sXist, noRNAs, and CRISPR made headlines in scientific journals. Notable path-breaking discoveries include that of riboswitches and miRNA. In fact, it was the RNAi mechanism associated with miRNA that earned Craig C. Mello and Andrew Fire the Nobel Prize in Physiology or Medicine in 2006.

13.2.2 TYPES OF NONCODING RNAS

ncRNAs are not limited to the vastly found and functionally dominating RNAs such as transfer RNAs (tRNAs) and ribosomal RNAs (rRNAs), but include as well microRNAs (miRNAs), small nucleolar RNAs (snoRNAs), short interfering RNAs (siRNAs), piwi-associated RNAs (piRNAs), small Cajal body-specific RNAs (scaRNAs), small nuclear RNAs (snRNAs), and long ncRNAs. siRNAs occur naturally in plants and lower animals, but their natural occurrence in mammals is unknown/under question. The exact number of ncRNAs encoded within the cellular DNA is not yet deciphered. However, scientists speculate the existence of thousands of ncRNAs, and with advancing transcriptomic and bioinformatic explorations, the number seems quite staggering. These findings are just a beginning as the functions of many of the newly identified ncRNAs are yet to be specified. It is also speculated that many ncRNAs are products of spurious transcription and are nonfunctional (junk RNA).

ncRNAs are broadly divided into two principal categories based on the stretch of nucleotides, viz., small ncRNAs that are less than 200 bp and long ncRNAs that are greater than 200 bp [1]. Apart from these two principal divisions, sometimes another division under the name of housekeeping RNAs is kept to include ribosomal RNA (rRNA), transfer RNA (tRNA), and small nuclear RNAs. Both small and long ncRNA are further subdivided into various subgroups. Keeping in view with the developments, a chart has been attempted to categorize ncRNAs; however, this table is based on present knowledge and gathered keeping in view of acceptability and sustainability of data (Figure 13.1).

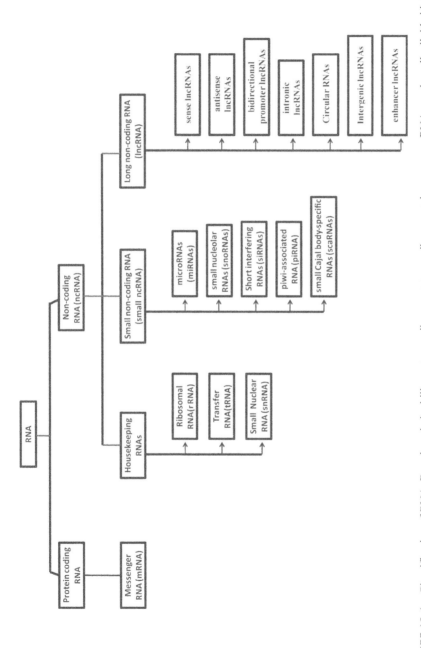

FIGURE 13.1 Classification of RNA. Based on their ability to transcribe or not transcribe a protein sequence, RNAs are broadly divided into two groups, viz., protein-coding RNA and noncoding RNAs. Noncoding RNAs are further divided into two classes based on size, viz., long or small noncoding RNAs. Further subgroups are based on genomic positions, structures, or functions.

13.2.3 NONCODING RNA AND CANCER

Cancer is fundamentally a disease arising from alterations of genetic information flow that modifies cellular homeostasis and promotes uncontrolled growth [2]. These changes/alterations of genetic flow occur principally due to mutations or changes in the DNA, which results in altered function. Such mutations are random and stabilize when more than one function is altered irreparably [3]. However, the coding genome accounts for less than 2% of all sequences, and if mutations (that too stable) were to occur exclusively in these regions to initiate cancer, the disease would be far less in occurrence than its present threat implies! Interestingly, in the neo genomics era of biology, scientists have found extensive transcription of RNA from nonprotein-coding regions of the genome [4]. Moreover, it has become apparent that mutations within these noncoding regions are responsible for many important cancer phenotypes [1]. It is now acknowledged that mutations within the noncoding genome are major determinants of not only cancer but also of other human diseases [5].

The last two decades brought to light a great diversity of neo ncRNAs, thereby strengthening the overall conceptual understanding of ncRNAs. Transcription of ncRNA many involve any of the three RNA polymerases, RNA polymerases I (RNA Pol I), RNA polymerases II (RNA Pol II), or RNA polymerases III (RNA Pol III), and this choice largely depends on the type of ncRNA. The importance and biological relevance of ncRNAs have gained considerably with the scientific advancements in the last two decades. However, scientists are still a bit confused about the functional elements associated with the primary sequence of noncoding genes that determine their role as RNA molecules as its varies within the different groups of ncRNAs and also from those of protein-coding sequences. Protein-coding genes follow an established language with a defined grammar stating specific three nucleotide sequences for an established amino acid [6]. Changes in sequence (mutation) can be traced in terms of altered amino acid sequence in the protein, which in turn can be associated with structural and/or functional alterations. The changes in functional attributes can be associated with disease manifestations that occur due to change in structure. On the contrary, our limited knowledge about the functional and biochemical (e.g., sequences or structural motifs) aspect of the ncRNA or as may be also referred as "the ncRNA alphabet," it becomes difficult to predict/ascertain changes in diseases. Interestingly, recent multidirectional scientific endeavor has fueled colossal information that indicates/proves the involvement/contribution of several ncRNAs as the crucial functional importance for normal development, functional physiology, and occurrence/progression of disease [7]. Of these varieties of ncRNA that have been linked with cancer or other diseases, the most extensively studied to date are the microRNAs (miRNAs) [8, 9]. Convincing studies have shown that epigenetic and genetic defects/altered expression in miRNAs and their maturation process are a familiar hallmark of disease, especially cancer [10–13]. It should be kept in mind that miRNAs are just the beginning and the long tale of ncRNAs extend much beyond to other variants such as snoRNAs, piRNAs, large intergenic noncoding RNAs (lincRNAs) and, overall, the diverse group of lncRNAs, all of which have been shown to contribute to diseases like cancer. It must be noted that with the volume of information presently available, a separate book can be written on each of the variants' link with cancer and to bundle it all up in a single book chapter will naturally mean to skip various details. In this chapter, we will try to present an overall picture of the major classes of short and long ncRNAs and their relevance to cancer, hoping the reader gets a holistic view of the subject.

13.3 SMALL NONCODING RNAS

13.3.1 MICRORNA

13.3.1.1 Early Discovery

MicroRNAs (miRNAs) are a subgroup of short noncoding RNAs, consisting of 20 to 24 nucleotides that has the potentiality to play crucial roles in practically all cellular pathways in multicellular organisms including mammals [14]. Lin-4 was the first miRNA to be discovered by Ambros and colleagues, in 1993, while studying development in *Caenorhabditis elegans* (*C. elegans*) [15]. They labeled it as a small ncRNA controlling a protein, lin-14. It took 7 more years, in 2000, for the discovery of the second miRNA, let-7, yet again in *C. elegans* by Reinhart and coworkers. This time, the epigenetic control induced by miRNA came to the limelight; let-7 was found to negatively regulate the expression of the heterochronic gene lin-41 using sequence-specific RNA–RNA interactions at the 3'-untranslated segment of its mRNA [15].

This created snowball effect on the discoveries of miRNAs, and by 2001, independent workers reported this class of ncRNA to be copious in both invertebrates and vertebrates. Some of the miRNAs were found to be highly conserved, which suggested that miRNA-mediated posttranscriptional regulation as a universal and evolutionarily conserved regulatory function across various species. The diversity and quantity of miRNA has propelled the creation of a website "mirBase" (http://www.mirbase.org) which was hosted by Wellcome Trust Sanger Institute. Currently, the custodians of the website are Griffiths-Jones lab at the Faculty of Life Sciences, University of Manchester with funding from the BBSRC (for details, visit http://www.bbsrc.ac.uk). Presently, there are about 1872 specific human miRNA precursor genes that are matured into roughly 2578 miRNA sequences. Functions of many of these miRNAs are yet to be elucidated [15].

13.3.1.2   miRNA and Cancer

The first miRNA to be indicted with human cancer was from a work by Dr Croce's group (2002), who were experimenting in order to unravel tumor suppressor genes at chromosome 13q14 region in B-cell chronic lymphocytic leukemia. It was found that this particular chromosome region was commonly deleted in the particular malignancy [15]. Their studies revealed that these deleted regions contained two miRNA genes, viz., miR-15a and miR-16-1; furthermore, both these genes were either deleted or downregulated in the majority of clinical manifestation of B-cell chronic lymphocytic leukemia. Detailed molecular studies confirmed that both these miRNAs function as tumor suppressors by inducing apoptosis by downregulating Bcl-2, which is an anti-apoptotic protein and is overexpressed in malignant non-dividing B cells and many other solid cancers [15]. Since then, miRNA has become the central attention of ncRNA-related cancer, and fruitful studies have successfully established the importance of miRNAs in cancer. Studies in cancer biology have revealed that microRNAs act by targeting their sequence-specific mRNAs and influence the various aspects of malignancies, viz., tumor growth, invasion, angiogenesis, and immune evasion [16, 17]. The various hallmarks established by Hanahan and Weinberg [18] have been found to be influenced miRNAs. Moreover, miRNA profile of cancer patients (body fluid or cancer tissue biopsy) can be used to detect cancer (act as biomarkers), specify cancer subtypes, and predict prognosis [19–21].

13.3.1.3   miRNA: Biogenesis and Mechanism

microRNAs primarily bind to the complementary sequences in the 3' untranslated region (UTR) of target messenger RNAs (mRNAs) and regulate protein translation [22]. miRNA biogenesis follows well-defined and conserved processing mechanisms. miRNAs are programmed in the DNA in multiple styles. RNA pol II is usually responsible for miRNA transcription. Transcription may occur from intronic as well as intergenic regions and may encode a single or multiple (clusters) hairpin miRNA precursors [23]. Post trimming of the primary transcriptional entity occurs by a microprocessor complex consisting of Drosha (RNase III enzyme) in the nucleus; this hairpin pre-miRNA is then transported to the cytoplasm by exportin 5 (XPO5) [14]. A protein complex comprising DICER (endoribonuclease Dicer or helicase with RNase motif) and TRBP (TAR RNA-binding protein) further shapes the pre-miRNA hairpin to ultimately produce the mature miRNA that is single-stranded. The mature single-stranded miRNA associates with Argonaute 2 (AGO2) protein of the RNA-induced silencing complex (RISC). It then binds to the 3'UTRs of target mRNAs, either to reduce translation or to deadenylate and degrade the target mRNA (see Figure 13.2). A single miRNA may target up to several hundreds of target mRNAs; so, aberrant/altered miRNA expression may modify myriad of transcripts participating in various cancer signaling pathways [14].

13.3.1.4   MicroRNAs and Cancer: Mechanisms

Hayes and co-authors [23] rightly categorizes microRNA functions into two broad, apparently opposite or encompassing all, principal groups based on function: (i) homeostatic regulation of gene expression, which works by regulating the process of translation in accordance to requirements of the cell and (ii) robustness in cellular responses, a function that dictates major cellular activity and/or cellular destiny decisions in which a number of miRNAs acting as in groups determine the cellular differentiation state, by performing "locks" to maintain cellular identity; this usually encompasses multifarious reciprocal negative-feedback loops [24]. In case of cancer, the second function predominates, for example, miRNA linked with terminal differentiation is downregulated to ensure uncontrolled proliferation [23]. Examples of feedback mechanisms may be exemplified by the role of miR-

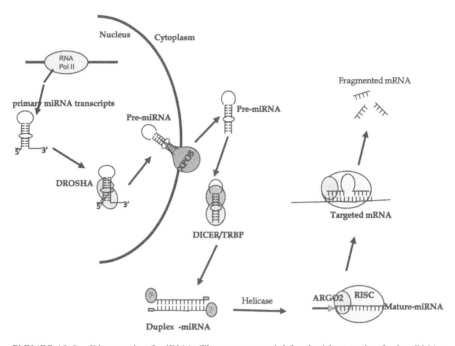

FIGURE 13.2 Biogenesis of miRNA: The current model for the biogenesis of microRNAs – MicroRNAs are generally transcribed by RNA polymerase II (RNA Pol II) to yield primary miRNAs (pri-miRNA) transcripts are first processed into ~70 nucleotide pre-miRNAs by the RNase III enzyme Drosha inside the nucleus. Pre-miRNAs are transported to the cytoplasm by Exportin 5 (XPO5) and are processed into miRNAs by a protein complex comprising DICER (endoribonuclease Dicer or helicase with RNase motif) and TRBP (TAR RNA-binding protein). Only one strand of the miRNA duplex is preferentially assembled into the RNA-induced silencing complex (RISC). The mature single-stranded miRNA, associates with Argonaute 2 (AGO2) in RISC, which subsequently acts on its target by translational repression as it binds to the 3'UTRs of target mRNAs, resulting in either reduced translation or deadenylation and degradation of the mRNA.

451 in glioblastoma. In glioblastoma, low concentrations of glucose result in downregulation of miR-451, a prerequisite for AMP-activated protein kinase (AMPK) pathway activation and cell survival. Reversely, when glucose levels are adequate, upregulation of miR-451 act to curb AMPK signaling and uphold mammalian target of rapamycin (mTOR) activation-induced cell proliferation [25]. The capacity of a single miRNA to influence cellular identity/destiny has been substantiated with overexpression studies [14]. Using a single miRNA transfection in HeLa cells, leading to overexpression of miR-124, produced the expression profile similar to that of the brain, where miR-124 is naturally overexpressed [14]. To sum it up, the role of

miRNA extends from that of differentiation to construction of cellular identity and regulation of the translation process, and perturbation in miRNA expression may push the cell toward increased plasticity, de-differentiation, and a higher predisposition for malignant transformation [14].

Induced pluripotent stem cells (iPSC) are those stem cells that originate from skin or blood cells and have been modified to endow upon them an embryonic-like pluripotent state. miRNA is known to uphold the key features of stem cell function and differentiation [26]. Interestingly, in induced pluripotency, a single miRNA cluster, miR-302, has been established to be capable of producing iPSC from fibroblasts of both human and mouse origin [14].

It is predicted that more than 60% of the overall mRNA in a cell is under the control of miRNAs. However, understanding the regulation is an uphill process due to various complexities [27]. Primarily, a particular miRNA targets a huge number of mRNAs; so, the phenotypic response is highly unprobable to be mediated by a single targeted mRNA. Often multiple mRNAs residing in the same pathway are targeted by a single miRNA. Secondly, many miRNAs exist in groups/families with identical seed sequences, which complicates the analysis of many investigational experimentations. Again, the scenario becomes more complicated as different miRNAs with similar seed sequences may co-repress the same target [14]. Moreover, a definite miRNA that may be upregulated in certain forms of cancer may act as tumor suppressors in a different type of cancer [14]. An interesting example may be found with miR-29, which functions as a tumor suppressor in lung cancers but changes its role to pro-oncogenic functions in breast cancer [14]. This raises the question of cellular context and other factors illusive to us.

13.3.1.5 Cancerous Conditions are Generally Associated with Downregulation of miRNAs

A huge amount of data suggests that miRNAs are generally downregulated in cancer. Reduction may be an outcome of alterations in the miRNA processing machinery or overall reduction of miRNA expression in cancer cells as compared to the normal tissue (23). Mutations have also been reported to cause deficiency in the microRNA processing machinery, thereby affecting the levels of mature miRNA. Trapping of the miRNA in the nucleus has been associated with microsatellite instability or mutations in XPO5 have been reported in various cancers [23]. Reduced expression of Dicer was correlated to drug resistivity and poor prognosis of ovarian cancer [28]. Alteration by mutations, SNPs, deletions, and duplications leading to inefficient processing of miRNAs are associated with initiation of carcinogenesis [29]. Such initiation processes exemplified the need for the formation of proper loop structures in pre-microRNA sequences [29], which is associated with the secondary structure of the pre-microRNA. Indirect evidence from experiments involving radiation and/or chemotherapy-induced DNA damage in HCT116 cells show increased nuclear export of pre-microRNAs [30].

Deregulation/decreased miRNA can also occur in altered processing. For example, specific sequence within the primary transcripts that certify/determine the hairpin for processing allows the association of specific proteins such as SRp20 [31]. Alternatively, binding of BCDIN3D (bicoid-interacting 3, domain-containing) lead to imprecise processing [32]. Such improper binding leads to O-methylation of the 50 monophosphate, which is required for efficient cleavage by Dicer, leading to decreased functional miRNA [32].

During post-transcriptional editing, base pairing with cytidine, a nucleoside formed by β-N1-glycosidic bond formation between cytosine and ribose ring, may change target recognition [23]. Such reactions involving conversion of adenine to inosine are enacted by enzymes known as ADARs, adenosine deaminases that act on RNA, influences miRNA action [23]. Examples include the deterioration of prognosis in advanced stages of glioma following changes in the passenger strand of miR-376 [31]. Studies further suggest that the ratio between Dicer–ADAR1 complexes and ADAR1–ADAR1 homodimers determines the extent of editing and processing of microRNA in the cell [33].

Competing endogenous RNAs (ceRNAs, also refer as miRNA sponges) are RNA sequences consisting of several miRNA binding sites. ceRNAs include a variety of genera of RNA including long noncoding RNAs (lncRNAs), pseudogenes, circular RNAs, and even at times protein-coding mRNAs. ceRNAs redirect the RISC complex by competing with the miRNA and preventing miRNA-target RNA interaction. Cancer cells regulate levels of phosphatase and tensin homolog (PTEN) by using several ceRNAs to neutralize the action of miRNAs that targets PTEN [23]. Lung cancer progression is influenced by a circular RNA, CDR1 (cerebellar degeneration related protein 1), containing more than 60 binding sites for miR-7 [34], which enacts it tumor suppressing role by targeting various oncogenic transcripts [35]. Another miRNA encoding HMGA2 (high mobility group AT-hook 2) behaves like ceRNA for the entire family of let-7.

13.3.1.6   miRNA Networks in Cancer

miRNA networks are complex and diverse. The fact that a number of miR-NAs can target a particular mRNA coupled by the fact a single miRNA can have multiple mRNA targets makes it difficult to understand/assign any specific function to any miRNA. The situation gets even more complicated with the presence of ceRNAs and multiple sequences that may interfere with microRNA activity. Moreover, imperfect match due to comparatively short 6–8 base pair seed sequence, which is typical for miRNA–mRNA interactions, prevents biologists from being able to design effective models for understanding miRNA function/interaction. These increasing baffling scenarios have prompted scientists to use bioinformatic prediction algorithms to get a probable clearer picture of any miRNA interactive network [23]. Once bioinformatically targets are established/predicted, further experimental relevance and validity can be performed biologically. This flowchart of experimentations has been successful in establishing various function/interaction of miRNAs not only accurately but also economically with respect to time. It must be kept in mind that targeting a miRNA interaction for a single mRNA or function may lead to biased interpretations. To circumvent this issue, global approaches has been employed for better understanding of interactions. Such global approaches include proteomics, gene expression arrays, and RNA cross-linking/AGO2 pull-down approaches, including methods such as HITS-CLIP (high-throughput sequencing of RNA isolated by crosslinking immunoprecipitation) that is used to assess miRNA–target binding within a cellular environment [36, 37].

miRNA may also function in networks, which includes sponge interactions and feedback loops that build up affinity-based competitive binding of miRNAs and their target mRNA(s). miRNA may also work in interconnected groups or clusters, which generally have clubbed expression coupled with cooperative action. Examples of miRNA cluster can be traced to that of miR-17~92 family, where three extremely conserved yet related polycistronic miRNA genes are known to transcribe as many as miRNAs [38]. In a B-cell-specific transgenic mouse model, miR-17~92 cluster of miRNAs has been reported to induce lymphoma [39]. Interestingly, three miRNAs of this family/cluster, viz., miR-19b, miR-20a, and miR-92 in combination with miR-26a and miR-223 initiate acute lymphoblastic leukemia (ALL) in murine models [23].

In early stage colorectal cancer (CRC), cell-fate determinants are located at either opposed poles during cell division, culminating in asymmetric cell division producing one self-renewing and one differentiating daughter. This asymmetric cell division is orchestrated by miR-146a acting in tandem with the Snail–Numb–β-catenin axis [40]. Here, Snail-dependent β-catenin and TCF induces miR-146a, and mi-146a then decreases Numb. Decreased Numb reduces its β-catenin degradation activity, thereby promoting Wnt signaling [23]. For cancer cells, epithelial to mesenchymal transition (EMT) is of utmost importance as it is a prerequisite for metastasis (spread of transformed cells from its point of origin to organs). Any blockade/perturbation in this transition will render cancer from being nothing more than a benign form as it will be restricted to a particular site. Cellular epithelial state is promoted and maintained by miR-200 family and miR-34a. At the time of EMT, these miRNAs are downregulated, which promotes mesenchymal transitional targets ZEB1 (zinc finger E-box binding homeobox 1) and ZEB2 [41]. In a feedback loop effect, ZEB1 inhibits the miR-34a family, ensuring a stronger push toward the mesenchymal fate [23]. Sometimes, antimetastatic effects of miRNAs are countersilenced by other miRNAs. For example, in malignant breast tissues, antimetastatic miR-200 is inhibited by miR-22 [23]. miR-22 interacts with the ten eleven translocation (TET) family of methylcytosine dioxygenases, thereby inhibiting miR-200 [23]. miR-138 positively regulates the mesenchymal transition by inhibition of ZEB2, which represses vimentin and also by modulation of epigenetic regulation of EZH2 (enhancer of zeste homolog 2) [23]. In another study, miR-155 inhibited mesenchymal transition by downregulating repress transforming growth factor-β (TGF-β) activity [23].

13.3.1.7   MicroRNAs in Prognosis and Drug Resistivity

With the better understanding of the disease in terms of molecular alterations, newer and more accurate diagnosis and prognosis are now possible. The concept of personalized treatment has further incited the better understanding of such molecular analysis. miRNA is now increasing becoming an important player in such molecular endeavors. It is due to both greater stability and substantial expression in clinical samples that gives miRNAs greater utility than mRNAs as prognostic indicators [23]. This information has propelled scientists to consider their use, and many clinical trials are under progress. For example, the variations in the amount of miR-10b are considered suitable biomarkers of tumor grading, prediction of patient survival, and marker for genotypic variation in case of glioma. Again, miR-29b being stable in clinical tissues, blood and saliva are considered as prognostic markers for oral squamous cell carcinoma. miRNA profiling from nipple aspirate fluid is being explored as potential biomarker identification for breast cancers. miR-29 family in head and neck squamous cell carcinoma is being evaluated as markers for Twist1-mediated cancer metastasis [23].

In recent times, next-generation sequencing (NGS) has proved to be a more lucrative option in terms of accuracy and cost as compared to conventional qRT-PCR and microarray-based techniques [23]. NGS is massively parallel or deep sequencing platform capable of analyzing millions of small fragments of DNA in tandem. This has revolutionized genomic research, and it is assumed if NGS was used to sequence the entire human genome, it would have been completed within a single day as compared to Sanger sequencing technology, which took a little more than a decade to decipher the human genome! In NGS, each of the billions of bases present in the human genome is sequenced multiple times, delivering greater depth to analysis, prompting more accurate data and a comparable insight into unexpected DNA variation. Finally, bioinformatics analyses using statistical procedure for combining data from multiple studies (meta-analysis) are used to put together these small data by mapping the individual readings with reference to that of human genome. Such a meta-analysis from 43 studies involving 20 types of cancers brought to the limelight the variability in microRNA signatures, which may arise due to various reasons such as sample preparation, assay methodology, and patient characteristics revealed some interesting facts [23]. Amongst the thousands of miRNA identified to date, miR-21 (increased level) and let-7 (decreased level) are the most frequent miRNAs involved in cancer patient outcome [23]. miR-21 is considered as an oncogenic miRNA as it was found to be overexpressed in various cancers, such as breast, liver, lung, brain, stomach, colorectal, and prostate cancers [23]. It has been adjudged that miR-21 promotes a pro-malignant environment by interacting with various tumor suppressor genes that are involved in/with apoptosis, invasion, and proliferation [23], making it a novel molecular target in cancer therapy.

miRNAs can act as predictors of drug efficacy. Various investigations have associated miRNAs with conventional or established biomarkers for the judgment for the choice of therapy. Studies indicate that in case of

chronic myeloid leukemia (CML), miR-451 levels inversely correlate with
BCR-ABL levels both at the time of detection and also during progression
of treatment. Interestingly, imatinib treatment leads to decrease in BCR-
ABL, which is the characteristic feature of the disease [42]. In another study
involving 100 metastatic CRC cancer patients, it was found that the LCS6
polymorphism in the let-7 binding site of the 3'UTR of KRAS can be used
to predict the response to treatment with anti-EGFR molecules [43]. Moreover, it has been found that sensitivity to chemotherapy in ovarian cancers is
influenced by improper targeting of miR-191 in the 3'UTR of MDM4 due to
the involvement of SNP34091 [44].

   miRNA polymorphisms are also molecular markers for predisposition
to the development of cancer. Apart from its contribution to drug resistivity,
various SNPs in miRNA binding sites are involved in risk for development
of cancer and are considered to be markers for genetic susceptibility, leading to the progression of certain types of cancers [23]. Such SNPs may be
associated with miRNA binding sequences of the target or in the miRNA
sequence itself or in some way associated with the development of the said
miRNA. Such polymorphisms are being speculated to be used as markers to
predict poor prognosis or lack of treatment response [23].

13.3.1.8   miRNAs as Noninvasive Biomarkers

miRNAs secreted by tumor cells are usually incorporated into microvesicles
in which they are stabilized. This renders not only immunity from degradation from circulating enzymes in the blood but also chemical integrity during
repetitive freeze-thaw cycles and prolonged stability even at room temperature [23, 45]. This and coupled with their presence and chemical integrity
in other body fluids like urine and saliva make these circulating miRNAs
attractive molecules for use as markers in different cancers [23]. A study
involving 391 nonsmall cell lung cancer (NSCLC) patients revealed 35 frequently expressed miRNAs that were postulated to have attachment sites
with one of the 11 genes involved in the TGFβ signaling axis. Interestingly,
these 35 miRNAs were inversely frequent at the either ends of the survival
limits. Again, 17 of them strongly correlated with patient survival and could
be scaled in accordance to varying prognosis [23]. Isolation of exosomes
from serum of patients suffering from glioblastoma revealed a definite pattern of expression of two miRNAs along with another small ncRNA variant

[23]. However, one must keep in mind that quantification of these miRNAs in serum is challenging and debatable as endogenous controls for miRNA are under question because most mRNA and rRNA variants are unstable in circulating fluids due to the presence of RNases [23]. Furthermore, differences in circulating miRNAs may also be due to viral infections, food habits, and other variables, thereby contributing to more background interferences for these assays. Patterns and levels of miRNA changes very rapidly, even to traumatic venipuncture [23]. All these factors and many more have been the reason for contradiction and disparity in reports even when related cancer types have been studied [23]. Despite these pitfalls and difficulties, it is clear that identification and quantitative evaluation of specific miRNAs in the body fluids are definitely an option for noninvasive detection of cancer and estimation of prognosis.

13.3.1.9   miRNA-Based Therapeutics and Clinical Trials

In the previous section, we have explored miRNAs as potential biomarkers for cancer. Drawing a corollary to the findings, it can be postulated that such specificity can be used to target cancer cells. miRNA constructs and anti-miRNA constructs are being investigated as possible therapeutic agents for cancer. However, the stiffness of this process involves the delivery of such entities in cancer cells. MRX34 was the first synthetic miRNA prototype to enter clinical trials in cancer therapeutics; it was designed to deliver a functional sense of the biologically occurring tumor suppressor miRNA, miR-34. miR-34 is reported to be downregulated in most cancers. The first phase multicenter study to validate the safety, pharmacokinetics, and pharmacodynamics of MRX34 is underway to treat hepatic cancer and liver metastases. Local and systemic administration of miR-34a using a lipophylic delivery system in animal models with lung cancers exhibited encouraging response coupled with a bioavailability half-life of more than 7 hours in blood. miRNA may be directly used to treat cancer cells or to indirectly boost an existing therapeutic modality. In this context, miR-100, in case of lung cancer, may have a positive role in overcoming drug resistivity. Similarly, ovarian cancer that is otherwise resistant to chemotherapy may be reversed to the chemosensitive form by silencing of miR-199b-5p. The exploration in the use of miRNA in cancer therapeutics is still in its experimental stages as both eminent and long-term side effects need to be explored properly.

13.3.2 SMALL NUCLEOLAR RNAS

SnoRNAs are small ncRNAs ranging in size from 60–300 nucleotides. To date, about 200 snoRNAs have been identified; however, the list is ever increasing. According to their structure and function, they are categorized into two types: C/D snoRNAs or Box H/ACA snoRNAs (Figure 13.3). Both these types are transcribed by RNA pol II as snoRNAs are mostly situated within introns of genes. Interestingly, snoRNAs may also arise from introns of lncRNA, for example, nine (snoRNDs74-81) C/D box snoRNAs are transcribed from an lncRNA named GAS5. After being released from introns, snoRNAs are processed by deleting unwanted nucleotides from both ends by using exonuclease activity. snoRNA usually serve to initiate and direct chemical modifications of other RNA species, chiefly rRNAs, tRNAs, and snRNAs. Activity-specific sequences are lodged within the snoRNAs centered at boxes C and D or H and ACA, which directs binding of protein-interacting partners that represent the functional snoRNP complex [46].

13.3.2.1 SnoRNAs: Structure and Function

The structure functional analysis principally divides snoRNAs into two basic action mechanisms: 2′-O-methylation and pseudouridylation. The box

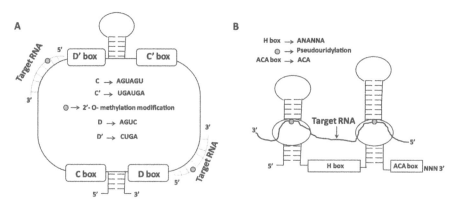

FIGURE 13.3   Schematic structures of the (A) C/D-box and (B) H/ACA-box snoRNAs. n 2′-O-methylation guide snoRNAs; the box C and D motifs and a short 5′, 3′-terminal stem constitute a kink-turn (K-turn) structural motif that is specifically recognized by the snoRNP protein. The C′ and D′ boxes represent internal, frequently imperfect copies of the C and D boxes (A). The pseudouridylation guide snoRNAs fold into a "hairpin-hinge-hairpin-tail" structure and contain the H and ACA boxes (B).

C/D snoRNA family that orchestrates 2'-O-methylation is composed of two small motifs, namely C and D (Figure 13.3). C' and D' boxes are their complimentary components. The 4–5 nucleotides at either ends of the snoRNA constitute the terminal stem-box, which is a requisite for snoRNA biosynthesis and localization in the nucleolus. The C, C', D and D' box are conserved elements and situated in the middle of the snoRNA structure. This serves as the RNA-protein interface that directs the appropriate congregation of the bioactive ribonucleoprotein complexes. The complementary specific site for rRNA binding is situated upstream of the D or D' box. There may be one or two such antisense motifs. These sequences propel correct alignment and methylation of the targeted nucleotide. Small nucleolar RNA-protein complexes, called snoRNPs, are guided by the snoRNA component to the target rRNA nucleotide, and subsequently methyltransferase and fibrillarin catalyze the methylation modification. The H/ACA box snoRNAs family is responsible for pseudouridylation and consists of dual hairpins motifs, forming a hairpin-hinge-hairpin-tail secondary structure. Connecting the two hairpin structure is a hinge region where the H box is situated, and the terminal region harbors the ACA motif. The guide sequences, which are responsible for proper rRNA sequence (along with the specific point of action), are situated in the hairpin domains. The target RNA may link with either one or both of the hairpin loops. The substrate rRNA uridine locates at the base of the upper stem of the loop (Figure 13.3). The pseudouridine synthase, dyskerin, is situated at 14–16 nt distance between the box motifs [46].

13.3.2.2 snoRNA and Cancer

It was in 2002 that Chang and his colleagues first linked snoRNA with cancer. They found h5sn2, a box H/ACA snoRNA, to be repressed in human meningiomas in contrast to their population in normal brain tissues [46]. It took the next 6 years to identify the next snoRNA link with cancer; this time, Donsante and coworkers unraveled something very motivating. They found that on introduction of β-glucuronidase-expressing adenovirus (AAV) vector, both neonatal normal mice and mice with mucopolysaccharidosis VII develop liver cancers. Rolling back, the vector was derived from a 6-kb region of chromosome 12 of malignant tissue specimens. This region of the chromosome was a locus that encoded several snoRNA transcripts. This locus included the *Rian* gene, which also encoded for nine snoRNAs and miRNAs. The findings implicated snoRNAs with the development of hepatocellular carcinoma (HCC). Dong et al. attempted to identify the prostate cancer gene associated with chromosome 6q14-q22, the deletion of which is frequent in a variety of human carcinomas. They managed to concentrate their findings to a deletion of 2.5-Mb interval at 6q14-15. Finally, of the 11 genes located in this minimal deletion region, only snoRNA U50 was discovered to be mutated in prostate cancer cells [47]. Further studies revealed homozygous 2 bp (TT) deletion in the snoRNA U50 to be consistent in prostate cancer cell lines/xenografts and breast cancer cell lines [46]. Corroborating the result with clinical samples revealed similar deletions in 9 of 89 clinical prostate cancers samples [46]. Furthermore, chromosome 6q14-15, home for snoRNA U50, was determined as the breakpoint for the chromosomal translocation t(3;6)(q27;q15) in human B-cell lymphoma. A long ncRNA, GAS5, was found to have growth arrest-specific motif and was significantly downregulated in breast cancer. GAS5 is known to harbor nine C/D snoRNAs in its introns. Slowly, evidence pointed chromosomal translations or breakages as these points of GAS5, leading to the development of certain human lymphomas due to the altered expressions of the snoRNAs. ncRNA expression signatures of 22 NSCLC tissues versus nonmalignant tissues from lungs revealed six snoRNAs that exhibited higher expression levels in malignant forms than in nonmalignant counterparts [46]. Five of the six snoRNAs displaying dysregulations in lung tumor specimens were also found to be associated with other solid human cancers as amplified regions in the altered genome. Notably, another snoRNA situated at chromosome 19, SNORD33 is also considered to have oncogenic properties as it is associated with the development of pulmonary malignancies [46]. Amplification in the chromosomal regions 3q27.1 and 1q25.1 are common in many human malignancies of solid tissue. Studies have revealed the presence of two snoRNAs namely, SNORD66 and SNORD76, to be situated in the same chromosomal region. snoRNAs, namely RNU44, RNU48, RNU43, and RNU6B, are associated with both breast and head and neck squamous cell carcinomas. Their association was so strong that Gee et al. used them as check controls to associate miRNAs with these types of cancers [48]. Analysis also revealed poor prognosis in malignant situations is linked with low expression of the aforesaid snoRNAs.

snoRNAs' basic function includes modification and structural orientation of rRNAs to ensure proper and specific functional ribosomes. On this tune, the involvement of snoRNAs in cancer initiation, maintenance, and progression can be casually linked as deregulated ribosome biosynthesis and ribosomopathies are associated with cancer [46]. Furthermore, loss of chromosomal stability, another correlative feature of cancer initiation, maintenance, and progression, is also a fall out of deregulated ribosome biosynthesis [46]. The gene associated with retinoid-interferon-induced mortality-1 (GRIM-1) downregulates and inhibits the H/ACA box snoRNA, because of which rRNA maturation and expression are stalled. GRIM-1 exerts this activity by interacting with NAF1, which instruments the loss of box H/ACA, thereby restricting the bioactive rRNA levels. In prostate cancer, GRIM-1 expression is suppressed to ensure abundant supply of functionally active ribosomes to enable synthesis of proteins required for aggressive cell division [46].

Some snoRNAs have been found to promote cellular pathways that lead to cancers. snoRA42, an ongogenic H/ACA snoRNA, is most frequently overexpressed as compared to other snoRNAs in malignancies of the lungs [46]. Another snoRA42 located in the genomic sequence of human 1q22 has been frequently found to be amplified in various solid cancer tissues, including NSCLC. Shutting down of snoRA42 in NSCLC cells inhibits malignant phenotype in both in vitro and murine models. On the contrary, its overexpression in pulmonary cell lines exhibited tumor-like phenotype [46]. It was documented that this snoRNA, if repressed, initiated apoptosis though a caspase 3-dependent pathway. Apart from its cancer-promoting properties, some snoRNAs have been shown to play tumor suppressor roles. An analysis of deletion mapping of 30 prostate tumors revealed that the snoRNA U50 was consistently mutated. The wild-type snoRNA U50 exhibited anti-tumorigenic activity such as prevention of cellular multiplication or colony forming ability, and this activity was obliterated on mutation of the specific gene [46].

All the above and many more recent findings have proven beyond doubt a positive link of certain snoRNAs with cancer.

13.3.2.3   snoRNAs in Diagnosis and Prognosis of Cancer

Just like miRNAs, snoRNAs are not degraded in body fluids and can be quantified from samples like sera, sputum, and urine, thus making them potential fluid-based biomarkers for cancers. Mannoor et al. [46] explored three snoRNAs (SNORD33, SNORD66, and SNORD76) from isolated blood samples and found them to be both highly specific and extremely accurate in distinguishing between normal individuals and those suffering from lung diseases. Furthermore, the same team investigated clinical significance and prognosis evaluation of altered expression of SNORA42 from cryopreserved pulmonary tissues from people in preliminary stages of NSCLC. They found high SNORA42 expression was a negative predictive marker that signified shorter survival time. Gee et al. reported expression levels of C/D box SnoRNAs RNU44 and RNU43 to be linked with low survivability in head and neck squamous cell carcinomas and breast cancers. These are a few examples to illustrate the role of snoRNA as prognosis markers, and more work is underway revealing diverse possibilities in using snoRNAs for detecting and predicting the clinical outcome in various malignancies.

13.3.3 PIWI-INTERACTING RNAS

P-element-induced wimpy testis (PIWI)-interacting RNAs (piRNAs) are the largest family amongst the ncRNAs found in the eukaryotic system. Conservative estimates put the total number of piRNAs equal to protein-coding genes, that is approximately 20,000, which is roughly ten times that of miRNA [49]. Though initially dubbed as "repeat associated small interfering RNAs" (rasiRNAs), they were universally rechristened with the name piRNAs due to their involvement with the PIWI subfamily of Argonaute proteins [49]. The name Argonaute is derived from the Greek mythology; it basically refers to a crew amongst a group of sailors/adventurers who voyaged in a ship called Argo, with Jason to Colchis (the kingdom in which the golden fleece was kept) to retrieve the golden fleece. PIWI proteins were extensively studied in germ line cells and stem cells as it was discovered primarily in *Drosophila melanogaster* to better understand the germline stem cell self-renewal/maintenance. The unique ability of PIWI-binding proteins is to associate itself with the 2'-*O*-methylated RNAs–a characteristic attribute harbored by 3'end of the piRNAs [50]. This association of the said nucleic acid recognition sequence and the specific protein belonging to Argonaute class is highly conserved [49]. Interestingly, Argonauts proteins are also known to interact with another set of ncRNAs involving gene silencing, viz., the siRNAs and miRNA. Argonaute proteins are subdivided into two principal subfamilies, Ago and PIWI proteins. Ago interacts with siRNAs or miRNAs, while the PIWI proteins interact with piRNAs. The piRNA/PIWI complex primarily functions by silencing genes of target proteins through epigenetic control rather than neutralizing transcripts of target proteins as seen in the functioning of siRNA and miRNA [49].

Histone H3K9 can turn genes on by acetylation, but can silence them just as easily by methylation. H3K9 methylation is the mark of heterochromatin, the condensed, transcriptionally inactive state of chromatin. Methylation can produce mono (H3K9me1), di (H3K9me2), and tri (H3K9me3) forms of H3K9, and each of these have distinct distribution patterns. H3K9me1 is enriched at the transcriptional start site of active genes, while H3K9me2/3 are found more often in silenced genes [51]. H3K9me3 associates with heterochromatin protein 1 (HP1) at point of heterochromatinization. HP1 acts as an agent for both inhibition of transcription and stabilization of heterochromatin [51]. The PIWI proteins works at the transcriptional level and thus localizes itself with the nuclear membrane. The PIWI protein establishes a repressed chromatin state by enabling transcriptional alteration, leading to increased association of H3K9me3 and HP1 in the heterochromatin regions. During mitosis, the Lys-9 residue of H3 is methylated by Su(var)3–9 (suppressor of variegation 3-9). Su(var)3–9 accomplishes this feat using its SET domain (acronym for **S**u(var)3-9, **E**nhancer-of-zeste and **T**rithorax as was first identified in *Drosophila*) situated in the C terminal. Overexpression of piRNA results in employment of PIWI, HP1, and Su(var)3–9, along with downregulation of RNA pol II, and the enrichment of H3K9me2/3.

piRNAs forms a silencing complex by associating with the PIWI members of the Argonaute protein family, and this association is capable of recognizing and silencing complementary sequences. The other distinguishable feat that is established with this association is the protection of the genomic sequence from the onslaughts of the *transposable element* (TE or transposon) that threatens to perturb the DNA sequences. This silencing is accomplished at both transcriptional and posttranscriptional levels. Looking back at its origin of discovery (in *Drosophila*), the PIWI proteins Aubergine (Aub) and Argonaute 3 (Ago3) localize to the cytoplasm and repress transposons at the posttranscriptional level [49]. Furthermore, in *Drosophila*, Ago3 was found to be involved in tailoring of RNA, leading to the development of antisense piRNAs that target specific RNAs for PIWI protein-mediated silencing at the transcriptional level. This and more evidence point to the dual existence of piRNAs in the cytoplasm and nucleus [49].

13.3.3.1 Functional Roles of piRNAs in Cancer

piRNAs after being associated with genomic maintenance and gene silencing, their role/implication in human disease like cancer came to the forefront. Having understood the association of PIWI proteins with malignancies, the existence and importance of the piRNA/PIWI complex in tumorigenesis became quite evident. It could be postulated that over or repressed expression of those piRNAs that target mRNA, especially those related to the maintenance of genomic integrity (for example, those piRNAs involved with restriction of transposon or methylation), could also a play an important function in both inhibition or progression of malignancies. Normally, one would guess that if piRNAs were perturbed, it would lead to lesser control of the TE activity and ultimately lead to the stability of mutagenic retrotranspositions that could interfere with the DNA (genomic) sequence integrity and enhance the initiation/maintenance of malignancies. Contrary to this notion, it has been found that ectopic expression of piRNA/PIWI leads to enhanced aggressive malignant forms. This fact is further fortified by the fact that genomic DNA hypo/hypermethylation along with histone modifications is profoundly associated with both initiation and progression of malignancies [49]. Studies have led to understanding and speculation that the upregulation of piRNA/PIWI protein association possibly would promote tumorigenesis due to anomalous DNA methylation in regions close to their binding sites, thereby inducing genomic silencing (of tumor suppression genes) and enhancing the "stem-like" phenotype/genotype and preventing differentiation and securing the undifferentiated state [49]. Genomic studies involving malignancies of lymphatic origin or that related to the breast have revealed that specific piRNA-mediated DNA methylation at particular genomic sequences was caused by improper binding near targeted CpGs, which were not associated with TE. Enhanced migratory property in cancer cells of the breast could be achieved when transfected with specific piRNAs. Further studies revealed that hypomethylation at targeted CpG sites was responsible for the enhanced phenotype. piRNAs have also been found to be able to enhance gene expression by enhancement of the euchromatin state. This usually involves dual mechanisms: one involving upregulation of H3K4me3, while the other involves the inhibition of H3K27me3 associated with the subtelomeric heterochromatin. H3K4 methylation coupled with H3K27 demethylation results in activation of TRAIL at the transcriptional level, which ultimately contributes to inhibition of malignant growth [49].

There are also reports which show that depletion of certain piRNAs also have tumorigenic implications. Examples include repression of piRNA piR-L-163 in human bronchial epithelium (HBE) cell lines that was associated with increased DNA synthesis and accumulation at G2-M, coupled with aggressive migratory capabilities.

13.3.3.2 Altered Expression of piRNAs in Cancers

The major hindrance in understanding the role of piRNA/PIWI association in cancer is principally due to the fact that the function of piRNA is yet to be properly elucidated in normal conditions and normal phenotypes. However, these early pictures do link anomalous expression of the piRNA/PIWI or their association with clinical features in malignant tissues, indicating their association with cancer. Strikingly, a very minimal percent of the entire piRNAs encoded in the human genome is constantly available in either non-malignant or malignant tissues. Adding to both the difficulty and complexity of the situation is the fact that piRNA signature expression is highly variable and differs dramatically depending on the origin/type of tissue [52]. The variation is not only in types but also in their combination patterns along with expression levels (quantity) that are found in different tissues. Deep sequencing and RT-PCR revealed piRNAs, namely piR-4987, piR-20365, piR-20485, and piR-20582, which are upregulated in breast cancer tumors when compared to their normal counterparts [53].

In a study, sequencing for identification of small ncRNA from commercial available breast cancer cells and clinical tumor samples revealed 30 piRNAs that were differentially available in malignant and non-malignant mammary epithelial cells. Interestingly these piRNAs were related to cell cycle progression and/or estrogen receptor β. Amongst these, piR-932, piR-34736, piR-36249, piR-35407, piR-36318, piR-34377, piR-36743, piR-36026, and piR-31106 were mapped to regions related to the expression of various cancer phenotypes [49]. Another study revealed upregulation of PIWIL2 in stem cells found in malignancies of the breast. PIWIL2 not only induced EMT following TGF-β1 treatment but also formed complexes with piR-932 [49]. Detailed studies revealed that piR-932/PIWIL2 association promoted hypermethylation of an EMT-inducer, Latexin [54]. Using xenograft mouse models with inhibited expression of piR-823 resulted in decreased tumor growth, signifying the piRNA's role in tumor progression [55].

Differential expression of novel piRNA-like (piRNAL) sncRNAs was identified in a comparison between 8 nonsmall cell lung cancers (NSCLC) and 3 normal counterparts [49]. The most commonly downregulated piRNA in NSCLC was piR-L-163. Its function was related to negative control of cell cycle progression as silencing its expression positively influenced cell survival and proliferation.

In vitro and in vivo studies implicated piR-823 and piR-651 with cancer proliferation [49]. Corroborating with the previous statement was a study on gastrointestinal malignancies, which revealed that piR-823 expression was considerably lower in malignant tissue than in their normal counterparts. In fact, overexpression of the said piRNA inhibited cellular proliferation [56]. piR-651 was found to upregulated in samples of malignancies of the liver; mesothelioma; and malignancies of the cervix, breast, and lung [49]. piR-59056, piR-32105, and piR-58099 were also found to be overexpressed in clinical gastric cancer tissues when compared with their normal counterparts [49].

Deep sequencing of the renal cancer tissue revealed differential expression of 19 piRNAs when benign and malignant renal tissues were compared, while 46 piRNAs differed in their expression depending on the degree of metastasis. piR-32051, piR-39894, and piR-43607, transcribed within chromosome 17 belong to the same cluster. All the aforesaid piRNAs were upregulated in renal cancer cell lines as compared with noncancerous cells [49]. Interestingly, downregulated piR-38756, piR-57125, and piR-30924 in nonmetastatic primary tumors were upregulated upon bone metastasis [57].

Deep sequencing of hepatic cancers revealed upregulation of a novel piRNA, piR-Hep1. Interestingly, PIWIL2 expression, unlike PIWIL4 expression, was linked to the development of hepatocellular carcinoma. Further studies revealed that PIWIL2 associates with piR-Hep1 to promote tumorigenesis. piR-Hep1/PIWIL2 complexes were found to enhance survival through the phosphorylated Akt pathway [49].

Pancreatic cancer involved downregulation of piR-017061, while piR-823 overexpression was found in clinical manifestations of multiple myeloma.

13.3.3.3   Diagnostic and Prognostic Utility of piRNAs

Stability in plasma and differential expressions of various identified piR-NAs make them an attractive biomarker of specific cancers [49]. Countering the miRNA specificity as cancer biomarkers, a recent study in gastric cancers revealed piRNAs to have greater sensitivity and specificity than the former. piRNA signature of piR-59056, piR-54878, and piR-62701 could be used as a correlative marker for the relapse of gastric cancer. Both piR-823 and piR-65 were found to be effective biomarkers in blood for gastric cancer, along with the advantage of staging the tumor and predicting distant metastasis. Similarly, piR-4987 upregulation in breast ductal carcinoma showed a correlation with cancer cell migration in the lymph. The only problem is the variation found in normal tissue in both piRNAs and miRNAs that pose the biggest problem in using them as potential markers [49].

Recent studies also demonstrate that piRNA has the potential of being used as a therapeutic tool. Simulated piRNA was produced by injecting transgene cassettes into fertilized eggs. Such cassettes produced using both sense and antisense expression were effective to provoke specified epigenetic gene silencing. A detailed study is underway to explore such possibilities.

13.4   LONG NONCODING RNAS

lncRNAs are ncRNAs that have a sequence string with more than of 200 nt, and their transcription corresponds to those of other protein-coding genes, which is mediated by RNA pol II [58]. Functional Annotation of Mammalian cDNA 5 (FANTOM5), a complementary DNA (cDNA) sequencing project, was able to identify 27,919 long ncRNAs from various human sources [59]. However, lncRNAs demonstrate ~10-fold lower abundance than mRNAs in cells, exhibiting higher cell-to-cell variation in expression levels than that for protein-coding genes [60]. Approximately 78% of lncRNAs are characterized as tissue-specific, as opposed to about 19% in case of mRNAs [60]. lncRNAs' functional roles are largely unknown [61].

lncRNAs are commonly grouped depending on their genomic loci with respect to protein-coding genes [61] (Figure 13.4). In light of the previous statement, lncRNAs are differentiated as follows [61]:

a) sense lncRNAs – they usually span and are shared with a protein-coding sequence;

b) antisense lncRNA – they are encoded in antisense region of a protein-coding sequence;

c) bidirectional promoter lncRNAs – they are situated in the antisense region of a protein-coding sequence, starting about 1 kb from a promoter sequence region;

d) intronic lncRNAs – they are encoded in an intronic region of a protein-coding gene;

e) intergenic lncRNAs – they are encoded in a region that lies between protein-coding genes;

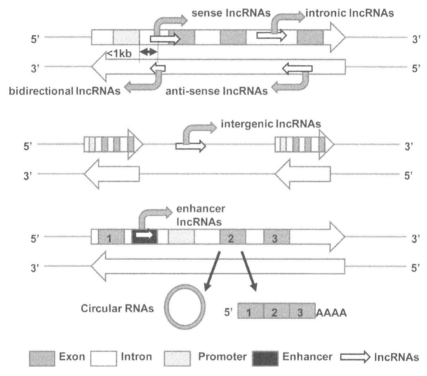

FIGURE 13.4 Schematic representation of genomic locations/categories of lncRNAs. According to their genomic location relative to protein-encoding transcripts, lncRNAs can be classified as follows: sense lncRNAs, antisense lncRNA, bidirectional promoter lncRNAs, intronic lncRNAs, intergenic lncRNAs, enhancer lncRNAs, and circular RNAs. Intragenic transcripts are transcribed from the sense, antisense, intronic, or gene regulatory regions such as promoters and enhancers and accordingly derive their names. Bidirectional transcripts share the same promoter with protein-coding genes but are transcribed in the opposite direction, while intergenic transcripts (also known as lincRNAs) are located in the genomic interval between two protein-coding genes. Circular RNAs are characterized by a circular structure in which the 3'- and 5'-ends are covalently linked. Arrows indicate the direction of transcription.

f) enhancer lncRNAs – they are encoded in the enhancer region of a protein-coding gene;

g) circular RNAs – these ncRNAs are distinctly recognizable by their circular configuration in which the 3'- and 5'-ends are covalently associated.

Most lncRNA are 5' capped, polyadenylated, and spliced, and they usually contain lesser number of exons than mRNAs. Unlike mRNAs, lncRNA have much lesser quantity/presence in various tissue types [62, 60]. Usually, it is framed that RNA transcripts with less than 100-nucleotide non-conserved open reading frame (ORF), having no similarity in amino acid/peptide sequences or match to known/identified components when screened with mass spectrometry, is labeled as noncoding [63]. lncRNA too shares the stated characteristics and has an ORF. Interestingly, even though non-coding for any peptides or not bearing the universal 3-nucleotide code for specified amino acids in an ORF format, a major chunk of the lncRNAs associate themselves with ribosomes. Moreover, despite such association, no meaningful oligopeptides are synthesized from lncRNAs [64-66]. There are examples of alternative splicing-induced protein-coding and noncoding transcripts from the same genes, but these are few and usually have no functional role [67]. RNA secondary structures may be created by looping to form double-stranded motifs, single-stranded loops, and protruding lariat-like structures, which again can further form three-dimensional structures. Thus, RNA molecules have the capacity to form highly structured macromolecules [68]. It must also be kept in mind that chemical analysis, and by postulating the probability of base pairing of single-stranded RNA by various RNases, has the potentiality of predicting the secondary structures, leaving the possibility of tertiary (3D) structure unexplored [68]. By using computational predictions potentiated by advanced techniques with the combination of high-throughput sequencing, such as SHAPE-MaP and icSHAPE, scientists are now able to provide reliable data about probable tertiary (3D) structure [68].

Irrespective of the fact whether the lncRNA is derived from its own promoter or from an enhancer, both mRNA-encoding and lncRNA genes usually have transcriptional start site marked by the H3K4me3 histone modification and the transcribed region by theH3K36me3mark [68]. Distinctiveness arises from the fact that these histone modifications are lowly significant in lncRNA as compared to mRNAs and H3K4me1, the hallmark enhancer region, appears to be more pronounced at places harboring lncRNAs [68]. Promoter regions of lncRNA are also characterized by DNaseI hypersensitive sites [68].

As already stated previously, the greatly diverse lncRNAs are categorized in accordance with their location with respect to protein-coding genes [68]. LncRNAs may be transcribed in different directions within the ORF of a protein-coding gene (pancRNAs) or between two protein-coding genes as in case of lincRNAs. Promoter-associated lncRNAs (plncRNAs) are transcribed from a promoter having higher H3K4me3 than H3K4me1. Enhancer-associated lncRNAs (elncRNAs) are synthesized from enhancers and are transcribed in a single direction from a promoter having higher H3K4me3 than H3K4me1. Bidirectional promoter lncRNAs are transcribed in both directions. Sense lncRNAs are overlapping with a protein-coding sequence, while antisense lncRNAs are transcribed from the antisense region of protein-coding sequence [68]. lncRNAs may also be produced by reverse splicing of introns of mRNAs or other lncRNAs forming a circular structure and are referred to as circular RNAs (circRNAs). lncRNAs occur/act in both nuclear and cytosolic regions. In fact, the subcellular localization serves as an excellent suggestion of the presumed role of the particular lncRNA as lncRNAs can readily carry on its assigned job even when the process of its transcription is occurring. Interestingly, chromatin withholding lncRNAs coregulate both its synthesis and the chromatin structure using the proximity of their transcriptional site [68].

13.4.1 LNCRNAS IN CANCER BIOLOGY

H19 was probably the pioneering lncRNAs to be associated with cancer in 1995, and its role exemplified its capabilities in controlling gene expression. Molecular understanding of the role of lncRNA in cancer may have been best documented with the discovery of the function of the *HOX* locus lncRNA *HOTAIR* in malignancies of the breast. The 6,232-bp HOTAIR gene encodes for 2.2-kb lncRNA. This lncRNA was the pioneering example of trans-chromosomal transcription regulator. Metastatic breast cancer tissues usually overexpress *HOTAIR*, and this initiates the former to recruit polycomb repressive complex 2 (PRC2) by using its 5' end to various chromatin sites to initiate epigenetic silencing, a prerequisite for cancer development [58]. HOTAIR recruits histone demethylase LSD1 with its 3' end, leading to methylation of H3K27 (H3K27me) and increase in cellular metastatic potential. Researches revealed the numerous roles of lncRNAs in recruiting complexes capable of epigenetic modifications, like PRC2 (24% of all lncRNAs), PRC1, H3K4me3 demethylase *SMCX,* H3K17 methylase *CoREST*, and histone methyltransferase *MLL1* [58]. Epigenetic regulation has been the predominant and basic mechanism by which lncRNAs affect cellular processes, especially oncogenic signaling. LINC00913 also referred to as *SChLAP1* (second chromosome locus associated with prostate-1) recruits the nucleosome positioning complex SWI/SNF by using *SNF5* (*SMARCB1*), leading to targeted positioning of SWI/SNF. These complex associations ultimately regulate a large number of genes that are involved in increasing the migratory potential of cancer cells [58].

LincRNA researchers Felix Y. Feng and Arul M. Chinnaiyan, both hold US patents on the use of specific RNAs, together with Joseph R. Evans categorized the myriad classical cancer biology pathways by which lncRNAs are linked with cancer [58]. This section will follow their categorizations using signaling pathways.

13.4.1.1 p53 Pathway

TP53 mRNA directly binds to the E3 ubiquitin ligase MDM2 and inhibits it, thus stabilizing and enhancing p53 function. Interestingly, mutations in the sequences used by TP53 to recruit MDM2 have been identified in various clinical tumor tissues, which dampens p53 availability. Moreover, in a previous study, it was found that 16 lncRNAs that form a network target the p53 gene. In another study, lncRNA LED was found to be associated with the enhancer sequence of the CDKN1A gene, inhibiting its transcription. CDKN1A functions as a p53-dependent cell cycle repressor. Knocking down lncRNA LED releases the restriction on CDKN1A and enables the latter to restrict cell cycle progression upon p53 induction. The lncRNA *MEG3* was found to be downregulated in various cancers. Interestingly, this lncRNA is known to downregulate *MDM2*, thereby increasing p53-dependent repression of cell cycle and induction of programmed cell death as well as modulation of autophagy. The lncRNA *loc285194* is regulated by p53 and restricts cellular multiplication by inhibiting proliferation inducing miR-211. lncRNA p21-associated ncRNA DNA damage activation (*PANDA*), a tumor-suppressor locus in *CDKN1AI*, extends its resistance to p53-induced apoptosis by dampening the presence of death inducers by acting at the transcriptional level. *Linc-p21* recruits the heterogeneous nuclear ribonucleoprotein K (hnRNP-K) at relevant genomic sequences, thus enhancing p53-mediated suppression of targeted genetic expression. Silencing *linc-p21* decreases doxorubicin-induced apoptosis [58].

13.4.1.2   Hypoxia Signaling and EMT

Cancer cells utilize low oxygen environment (hypoxic environment)-induced signal transduction mechanisms to establish/enhance their existence in the host as well as for conferring themselves both metastatic properties and drug resistivity in both normoxic and hypoxic conditions. *lncRNA-LET* promotes disintegration of nuclear factor 90, a protein crucial for signal transduction in hypoxic environment. Cancer cells are capable of expressing hypoxia-inducible histone deacetylase 3 (HDAC3), which induces promoter deacetylation of *lncRNA-LET*, thereby decreasing its expression and allowing hypoxia-induced signaling to proceed. EMT, a prerequisite for cancer cell migration, is stimulated by hypoxia signaling. lncRNA HOTTIP (HOXA transcript at the distal tip) is capable of triggering Wnt/β-catenin signal transduction cascade, leading to E-cadherin (*CDH1*) downregulation, an important step in EMT induction. The EMT regulator Snail1 upregulates the *Zeb2* gene. The transcribed *Zeb2* gene further acts as a transcriptional inhibitor for epithelial phenotype marker E-cadherin, stimulating mesenchymal transition. Interestingly, Zeb2 translation is promoted by an antisense lncRNA situated at the initial intronic region of *Zeb2* itself. Further, this lncRNA preserves 5′-UTR intron that reserves within itself an internal ribosomal entry site (IRES), which assists in translation of the *Zeb2* gene [58].

13.4.1.3   Telomere Maintenance

Telomere maintenance has been linked with lncRNA *TERC* and *TERRA*, which belong to the large heterogeneous ncRNA group. Telomerase RNA component, also known as TERC, component of telomerase, provides the template for synthesis of telomeric repeats by using the reverse transcriptase activity of telomerase. Telomerase reverse transcriptase (TERT or hTERT in humans) is a subunit of telomerase and is responsible for the latter's catalytic activity. Telomeres synthesize *TERRA* that counters TERT-induced catalysis by associating with both telomeres and TERT. In malignancies, the gene associated with TERRA synthesis is highly methylated and thus can bypass the *TERRA*-mediated TERT inhibition [58].

13.4.1.4 Hormone Receptor Signaling

lncRNAs have also been reported to be associated with nuclear hormone receptors for androgens (AR) and estrogens (ER). This association further links these lncRNAs in playing a vital role in hormone-dependent malignancies arising in prostate and breast tissues. The lncRNA *PCGEM1* is overexpressed in prostate cancer and has been seen to confer resistance to apoptosis by using the AR-mediated signaling cascades. Delineating the mechanism revealed the involvement of another lncRNA, *PRNCR1*. *PRNCR1* assists recruitment of *PCGEM1* in the N terminal of AR by associating itself and a histone H3 methyltransferase DOT1L in the C-terminal end of AR. The associated complex promotes the transcriptional capabilities of AR by activating its association with other factors and targeting enhancers of specific genes. Increased synthesis of *PRNCR1* and *PCGEM1* continues to promote AR signaling even in castrated conditions in prostrate malignancies. The antisense lncRNA *CTBP1-AS* is capable of inhibiting the synthesis of AR signaling inhibitor *CTBP1*. This repression not only inhibits a number of genes responsible for countering the process of AR-induced tumorigenesis but also accelerates cellular proliferation. The lncRNA *NEAT1* transcription is upregulated by ERα; such upregulations are linked with reduced prognosis [58].

ER dominates the regulation for almost a quarter of genome transcription in malignancies of the breast. This encompasses more than 1,500 sequences harbored in intergenic regions and antisense regions and also other divergent transcriptions. The abovementioned sequences encompass many lncRNAs. HOTAIR, being the most widely studied lncRNA in malignancies of the breast, is best documented with procancer capabilities and is transcriptionally upregulated by estrogen. This lncRNA supports proliferation and suppresses apoptosis [58].

13.4.1.5 Competitive Endogenous RNA

Studies have indicated lncRNAs and miRNAs to complement each other in the expression of a particular cellular phenotypic expression as well as regulating their mutual expressions. It has been postulated that miRNA binding regulates lncRNAs. In this context, it has been demonstrated the *PTEN* pseudogene *PTENP1* counters miRNAs that are specific for *PTEN*, leading to *PTEN*'s elimination. Such lncRNAs are sometimes referred to as competitive endogenous RNAs (ceRNAs) [58]. *KRAS* and its pseudogene *KRAS1P* show similar activity; both share affinity toward miRNA *let-7*. The genomic region encoding for *KRAS1P* has been found to be amplified in various malignant situations. Thus, the ceRNA function of lncRNAs modulates miRNA function and has an important role in cancer biology.

A nonprotein-coding pseudo gene BRAFP1 has been found to have molecular (sequence specific) and/or expression aberrations similar to its protein-coding counterpart BRAF in multiple malignancies. Studies also showed Braf-rs1 (the murine homologue of BRAFP1) targeted miRNA specific for Braf RNAs (molecular sponge), thereby stabilizing and upregulating Braf. Here, the role of Braf-rs1 resembles that of a ceRNA [68].

13.4.1.6   RNA Processing

MALAT-1 (metastasis-associated lung adenocarcinoma transcript 1), sometimes referred to as NEAT2 (noncoding nuclear-enriched abundant transcript 2), belongs to the family of infrequently spliced lncRNA. Early studies related this lncRNA with the control of genes related to cellular migration in pulmonary malignancies. Increased expression of MALAT1 in tumor tissues proved to be an indicator of low survival amongst patients suffering from various malignancies. Detailed studies revealed MALAT1 to be associated with various genome-modulating processes, leading to tumor formation. These processes include alternative splicing, nuclear re-organization, and epigenetic modulation. Though its relevance started with lung cancer, MALAT-1's role has been established in development of various other malignancies such as those of the colorectal region and prostate.

13.4.2   *LNCRNA DEREGULATION IN CANCER*

Intense and extensive research is underway to understand how lncRNAs contribute to cancer initiation, maintenance, and progression. High output experiments coupled with intricate statistical analysis revealed differences in the state of the promoter region of protein-coding sequences as compared to those transcribable nonprotein components. Such differences included both nature of chromatinization as well as that of association of components in the specified sites. As in the case of protein-coding sequences, the number of repeats (copy number) of a lncRNA in a particular tissue varies depending on the cellular state and type, viz., malignant and benign. *FAL1,* a lncRNA, was found to be overexpressed by CNAs (copy number alterations), and such increased presence determined the clinical manifestations of ovarian cancers. The association of *FAL1* with BMI1 involves the latter's PRC1 portion. The association in question is able to modulate a number of genetic sequences, including downregulation of *CDKN1A*. The lncRNA *PVT1* is present on the amplicon of the *MYC* gene. Interestingly, *PVT1* amplification is essential for malignant manifestation arising from amplification of MYC [58].

13.4.2.1   lncRNAs in cancer risk and SNP studies

Genome-wide association study (GWA study or GWAS) and whole genome association study (WGA study or WGAS) explored the variations occurring in a particular segment of the genome (gene) in a population and linked them with phenotypic alterations, if any. GWAS enlisted 301 single nucleotide polymorphisms (SNPs) that were linked with greater probability of cancer occurrence. Amazingly, of the total variations listed for polymorphism to be linked with altered phenotype, protein-coding entities contributed to only 12 (3.3%). Further finding and analysis point to the proposition that indicates the nonlinked SNPs mainly contributed to those noncoding sequences for which the exact phenotype was not determined. The deletion allele of SNP rs10680577 associates itself with greater probability of occurrence of HCC. The 14q13.3 lncRNA *PTCSC3* is downregulated by the presence of the SNP rs944289 risk allele in papillary thyroid cancer [58].

13.4.3   LNCRNAS AS DIAGNOSTIC AND PROGNOSTIC BIOMARKERS

Research has led to more accurate cancer diagnosis and prognostics markers. Detection, classification, and prognosis have improved the landscape of the disease. Molecular heterogeneity and prevalence studies are still underway to improve the understanding and delineation of the disease. Further subclassification of the disease for better understanding has also been a concern, and this requires more accurate and prominent biomarker development. Scientists have unraveled nearly 8,000 cancer- and/or lineage-specific lncRNAs that have a promising future for biomarker studies. Coupled with specificity is the advantage of detection in noninvasive body fluid tests, which promotes lncRNAs' candidature. *SChLAP1* has been nominated and categorized as a marker for the spread of malignancies [58]. Interestingly, *PCA3* and *TMPRSS2-ERG* fusion detected from urine tests can be used to detect prostate cancer better than conventional markers [58]. For nonsmall cell pulmonary malignancies, the lncRNA *MALAT-1,* isolated and quantified from blood samples, serves as a marker for the disease and has high sensitivity and specificity [58]. Similarly, *HULC* from patient plasma can be used to detect HCC and *H19* can be used in gastric cancer patients. Interestingly, several lncRNAs from patients' saliva can be used for the detection of oral cavity squamous cell carcinoma [58].

13.4.4   LNCRNAS AS THERAPEUTIC TARGETS

lncRNAs are variously expressed in cancer cells and this variation is distinct from their normal counterparts. ncRNAs hold promise to pose as therapeutic targets in cancer treatment. However, it must be kept in mind that the proposed lncRNA to be used as a target should not have regular housekeeping activities. Thus, the side effects and toxicity issues can be lowered. The lncRNA *MALAT-1* holds promise in these aspects. Interestingly, *MALAT-1*-knockout mice, though resistant to carcinogenesis, show a minimal phenotype, indicating that *MALAT-1* depletion would otherwise show no serious toxicity. Antisense oligonucleotides (ASOs) for *MALAT-1* demonstrated antitumorigenic potential in animal models for malignancies of the breast but are yet to receive US FDA approval [58].

siRNA-based therapeutics and hammerhead ribozymes, which possess nucleolytic activity and great fidelity in sequence detection, store promises for future cancer therapy. Artificial RNAs/small RNAs-directed change in chromatin state for specific segments can also be utilized for altering the nature of genome expression. AntagoNAT, a modified oligonucleotide that hybridizes with a natural antisense transcript (NAT), could be used to target lncRNAs. An alternative strategy could be targeting the specific lncRNA regulatory elements. One such is BC-819; its plasmid harbors the toxin-related genetic sequence isolated from *Diphtheria* but under the direct influence of the *H19* promoter. BC-819 treatment yielded exciting results in terms of tumor reduction for malignancies of the bladder, ovary, and pancreas. Improvising the molecular relationship between mTOR and *GAS5* expression for androgen-dependent malignancies of the prostrate, repression of mTOR led to rise in *GAS5* transcripts, yielding reduction in tumor proliferation [58]. Though the leads are interesting and promising, extensive research and understanding of lncRNA is needed to enable more therapeutic options for cancer treatment.

13.5 CONCLUSION

The strings that control the various aspects of carcinogenesis were in oblivion as the scientists' engaged their attention on protein-coding sequences. The advent of ncRNAs has unveiled a new horizon in medical research, especially in cancer. Noncoding RNAs have helped scientist unravel various quizzes of cancer. Currently, better and more comprehensive approach can be taken in understanding of the disease. ncRNAs have taken the central stage in cancer research. Their varied nature and functions pose a challenge to researchers in solving their network. The amazing variety of ncRNAs control the various cellular processes in myriad ways. They may simply act at the mRNA level, protein level, or DNA level. Starting from mRNA interaction to DNA methylation, from transcription to translation, or even in the signaling pathways, ncRNAs seem to have their reign on every cellular process. They may even act as "sponges" for other ncRNAs, thus keeping homeostasis, or in a very different path, induce carcinogenesis. Being safe from degradation in body fluids, they serve as good contenders in molecular diagnosis and their variously modified expression in malignant cells endows upon them the promise to pose as therapeutic targets in cancer treatment.

This chapter, however, does not aim to name all the ncRNAs or elaborate all their functions, as each class of ncRNAs have enough information for a book compilation. The simple aim of the chapter is to introduce readers to the concept of ncRNAs and give a broad overview of the participation in the process of carcinogenesis. In short, an understanding of the capabilities and importance of these RNAs in cancer biology is required. Truly, these ncRNAs hold the reigns of cancer.

13.6 SUMMARY

- Friedrich Miescher first discovered nucleic acids in 1868, but it took another seven decades for it to get implicated in protein synthesis in 1939. Characterization of noncoding RNA began with the pioneering work with a tRNA for alanine (tRNA[Ala]), which was isolated from baker's yeast. Finally, the structure of this tRNA was reported in 1965.
- Craig C. Mello and Andrew Fire were awarded the Nobel Prize for medicine in 2006 for the delineation of the RNAi mechanism associated with miRNA.
- ncRNAs are expressed in high amounts and are crucial in contributing to cellular homeostasis. ncRNAs are broadly divided within two groups, viz., small ncRNAs that are within 200 base pair and long ncRNA that are beyond the 200 bp mark.
- MicroRNAs are 20- to 24-bp in length with the potentiality to participate/modulate various cellular events/pathways in practically all living systems. Lin-4 was the first miRNA to be discovered by Ambros and colleagues in 1993.
- The first miRNA to be indicted with human cancer was from a work by Dr. Croce and coworkers (2002), who were studying the genes related with repression of tumorigenic activities at chromosome 13q14 region from samples of B-cell-mediated leukemia.
- SnoRNAs are small ncRNAs ranging in size from 60–300 nucleotides. To date, about 200 snoRNA have been identified; however, the list is ever increasing. They are categorized according to structure and function into two types: C/D or Box H/ACA snoRNAs.
- P- element-induced wimpy testis (PIWI)-interacting RNA or piRNA constitutes the biggest subgroup of small ncRNA consisting of approximately 20,000 variants.
- Approximately 78% of the 27,919 long ncRNAs (lncRNAs) are characterized as tissue-specific, as opposed to about 19% in case of mRNAs.
- lncRNAs can be categorized as follows: sense lncRNAs, antisense lncRNA, bidirectional promoter lncRNAs, intronic lncRNAs, intergenic lncRNAs, enhancer lncRNAs, and circular RNAs
- Being safe from degradation in body fluids, ncRNAs serve as good contenders in molecular diagnosis, and their variously modified expression in malignant cells endows upon them the promise to pose as therapeutic targets in cancer treatment.

KEYWORDS

- **antisense lncRNA**
- **bidirectional promoter lncRNAs**
- **cancer**
- **circular RNAs**
- **enhancer lncRNAs**
- **intergenic lncRNAs**
- **intronic lncRNAs**
- **long non-coding RNA**
- **microRNAs**
- **molecular markers**
- **non-codingRNAs**
- **PIWI-interacting RNAs**
- **sense lncRNAs**
- **small neclolar RNA**
- **small non-coding RNA**
- **therapeutic targets**

REFERENCES

1. Kapranov, P., Cheng, J., Dike, S., Nix, D. A., Duttagupta, R., Willingham, A. T., Stadler, P. F., Hertel, J., Hackermüller, J., Hofacker, I. L., Bell, I., Cheung, E., Drenkow, J., Dumais, E., Patel, S., Helt, G., Ganesh, M., Ghosh, S., Piccolboni, A., Sementchenko, V., Tammana, H., & Gingeras, T. R., (2007). RNA maps reveal new RNA classes and a possible function for pervasive transcription. *Science, 316,* 1484–1488.
2. Schmitt, A. M., & Chang, H. Y., (2016). Long noncoding RNAs in cancer pathways. *Cancer Cell, 29,* 452–463.
3. Hanahan, D., & Weinberg, R. A., (2011). Hallmarks of cancer: The next generation. *Cell, 144,* 646–674.
4. Morris, K. V., & Mattick, J. S., (2014). The rise of regulatory RNA. *Nat. Rev. Genet, 15,* 423–437.
5. Maurano, M. T., Humbert, R., Rynes, E., Thurman, R. E., Haugen, E., Wang, H., Reynolds, A. P., Sandstrom, R., Qu, H., Brody, J., Shafer, A., Neri, F., Lee, K., Kutyavin, T., Stehling-Sun, S., Johnson, A. K., Canfield, T. K., Giste, E., Diegel, M., Bates, D., Hansen, R. S., Neph, S., Sabo, P. J., Heimfeld, S., Raubitschek, A., Ziegler, S., Cotsapas, C., Sotoodehnia, N., Glass, I., Sunyaev, S. R., Kaul, R., & Stamatoyannopoulos, J. A., (2012). Systematic localization of common disease-associated variation in regulatory DNA. *Science, 337,* 1190–1195.

6. Crick, F. H., Barnett, L., Brenner, S., & Watts-Tobin, R. J., (1961). General nature of the genetic code for proteins. *Nature, 192,* 1227–1232.

7. Mercer, T. R., Dinger, M. E., & Mattick, J. S., (2009). Long non-coding RNAs insight into functions. *Nat. Rev. Genet, 10,* 155–159.

8. He, L., & Hannon, G. J., (2004). MicroRNAs: small RNAs with a big role in gene regulation. *Nature Rev. Genet, 5,* 522–531.

9. Mendell, J. T., (2005). MicroRNAs: critical regulators of development, cellular physiology and malignancy. *Cell Cycle, 4,* 1179–1184.

10. Esquela-Kerscher, A., & Slack, F. J., (2006). OncomiRs-microRNAs with a role in cancer. *Nature Rev. Cancer, 6,* 259–269.

11. Hammond, S. M., (2007). MicroRNAs as tumor suppressors. *Nature Genet, 39,* 582–583.

12. Croce, C. M., (2009). Causes and consequences of microRNA dysregulation in cancer. *Nature Rev. Genet, 10,* 704–714.

13. Nicoloso, M. S., Spizzo, R., Shimizu, M., Rossi, S., & Calin, G. A., (2009). MicroRNAs — the micro steering wheel of tumour metastases. *Nature Rev. Cancer, 9,* 293–302.

14. Jansson, M. D., & Lund, A. H., (2012). MicroRNA and cancer. *Mol. Oncol., 6,* 590–610.

15. Peng, Y., & Croce, C. M., (2016). The role of MicroRNAs in human cancer. *Signal Transduct. Target Ther.* [Online], *1,* 15004 https://www.nature.com/articles/sigtrans20154.pdf.

16. Kasinski, A. L., & Slack, F. J., (2011). Epigenetics and genetics. MicroRNAs en route to the clinic: progress in validating and targeting microRNAs for cancer therapy. *Nat. Rev. Cancer, 11,* 849–864.

17. Stahlhut, C., & Slack, F. J., (2013). MicroRNAs and the cancer phenotype: profiling, signatures and clinical implications. *Genome Med.* [Online], *5, 111* https://genomemedicine.biomedcentral.com /articles / 10. 1186/gm516.

18. Hanahan, D., & Weinberg, R. A., (2011). Hallmarks of cancer: the next generation. *Cell, 144,* 646–674.

19. Dvinge, H., Git, A., Graf, S., Salmon-Divon, M., Curtis, C., Sottoriva, A., Zhao, Y. Hirst, M., Armisen, J., Miska, E. A., Chin, S. F., Provenzano, E., Turashvili, G., Green, A., Ellis, I., Aparicio, S., & Caldas, C., (2013). The shaping and functional consequences of the microRNA landscape in breast cancer. *Nature, 497,* 378–382.

20. Kim, T. M., Huang, W., Park, R., Park, P. J., & Johnson, M. D., (2011). A developmental taxonomy of glioblastoma defined and maintained by MicroRNAs. *Cancer Res., 71,* 3387–3399.

21. Manterola, L., Guruceaga, E., Gallego Perez-Larraya, J., Gonzalez-Huarriz, M., Jauregui, P., Tejada, S., Diez-Valle, R., Segura, V., Sampron, N., Barrena, C., Ruiz, I., Agirre, A., Ayuso, A., Rodriguez, J., Gonzalez, A., Xipell, E., Matheu, A., Lopez de Munain, A., Tunon, T., Zazpe, I., Garcia-Foncillas, J., Paris, S., Delattre, J. Y., & Alonso, M. M., (2014). A small noncoding RNA signature found in exosomes of GBM patient serum as a diagnostic tool. *Neuro. Oncol., 16,* 520–527.

22. Krol, J., Loedige, I., & Filipowicz, W., (2010). The widespread regulation of microRNA biogenesis, function and decay. *Nat. Rev. Genet., 11,* 597–610.

23. Hayes, J., Peruzzi, P. P., & Lawler, S., (2014). MicroRNAs in cancer: biomarkers, functions and therapy. *Trends Mol. Med., 20,* 460–469.

24. Ebert, M. S., & Sharp, P. A., (2012). Roles for microRNAs in conferring robustness to biological processes. *Cell, 149,* 515–524.

25. Godlewski, J., Bronisz, A., Nowicki, M. O., Chiocca, E. A., & Lawler, S., (2010). mi-croRNA-451: A conditional switch controlling glioma cell proliferation and migration. *Cell Cycle, 9*, 2742–2748.

26. Heinrich, E. M., & Dimmeler, S., (2012). MicroRNAs and stem cells:control of pluripotency, reprogramming, & lineage commitment. *Circ. Res., 110*, 1014e1022 http://circres.ahajournals.org /content/110/7/1014.long.

27. Bartel, D. P., (2009). MicroRNAs: target recognition and regulatory functions. *Cell, 136*, 215–233.

28. Kuang, Y., Cai, J., Li, D., Han, Q., Cao, J., & Wang, Z., (2013). Repression of dicer is associated with invasive phenotype and chemoresistance in ovarian cancer. *Oncol. Lett., 5*, 1149–1154.

29. Gu, S., Jin, L., Zhang, Y., Huang, Y., Zhang, F., Valdmanis, P. N., & Kay, M. A., (2012). The loop position of shRNAs and pre-miRNAs is critical for the accuracy of dicer processing in vivo. *Cell.,151*, 900–911.

30. Wan, G., Zhang, X, Langley, R. R., Liu, Y., Hu, X., Han, C., Peng, G., Ellis, L. M., Jones, S. N., & Lu, X., (2013). DNA-damage-induced nuclear export of precursor mi-croRNAs is regulated by the ATM-Akt pathway. *Cell Rep., 3*, 2100–2112.

31. Choudhury, Y., Tay, F. C., Lam, D. H., Sandanaraj, E., Tang, C., Ang, B. T., & Wang, S., (2012). Attenuated adenosine-to-inosine editing of microRNA-376a* promotes invasiveness of glioblastoma cells. *J. Clin. Invest., 122*, 4059–4076.

32. Xhemalce, B., Robson, S. C., & Kouzarides, T., (2012). Human RNA methyltransferase BCDIN3D regulates microRNA processing. *Cell, 151*, 278–288.

33. Ota, H., Sakurai, M., Gupta, R., Valente, L., Wulff, B. E., Ariyoshi, K., Iizasa, H., Da-vuluri, R. V., & Nishikura, K., (2013). ADAR1 forms a complex with Dicer to promote microRNA processing and RNA-induced gene silencing. *Cell, 153*, 575–589.

34. Memczak, S., Jens, M., Elefsinioti, A., Torti, F., Krueger, J, Rybak, A., Maier, L., Mack-owiak, S. D., Gregersen, L. H., Munschauer, M., Loewer, A., Ziebold, U., Landthaler, M., Kocks, C., le Noble, F., & Rajewsky, N., (2014). Circular RNAs are a large class of animal RNAs with regulatory potency. *Nature, 495*, 333–338.

35. Hansen, T. B., Kjems, J., & Damgaard, C. K., (2013). Circular RNA and miR-7 in Cancer. *Cancer Res., 73*, 5609–5612 .

36. Boudreau, R. L., Jiang, P., Gilmore, B. L., Spengler, R. M., Tirabassi, R., Nelson, J. A., Ross, C. A., Xing, Y., & Davidson, B. L., (2014). Transcriptome-wide discovery of microRNA binding sites in human brain. *Neuron, 81*, 294–305.

37. Hu, C. W., Tseng, C. W., Chien, C. W., Huang, H. C., Ku, W. C., Lee, S. J., Chen, Y. J., & Juan, H. F., (2013). Quantitative proteomics reveals diverse roles of miR-148a from gastric cancer progression to neurological development. *J. Proteome Res., 12*, 3993–4004 .

38. Concepcion, C. P., Bonetti, C., & Ventura, A., (2012). The microRNA-17–92 family of microRNA clusters in development and disease. *Cancer J., 18*, 262–267.

39. Sandhu, S. K., Fassan, M., Volinia, S., Lovat, F., Balatti, V., Pekarsky, Y., & Croce, C. M., (2013). B-cell malignancies in microRNA Emu-miR- 17_92 transgenic mice. *Proc. Natl. Acad. Sci. USA, 110*, 18208–18213.

40. Lerner, R. G., & Petritsch, C., (2014). A microRNA-operated switch of asymmetric-to-symmetric cancer stem cell divisions. *Nat. Cell Biol., 16*, 212–214 .

41. Hao, J., Zhang, Y., Deng, M., Ye, R., Zhao, S., Wang, Y., Li, J., & Zhao, Z., (2014). MicroRNA control of epithelial-mesenchymal transition in cancer stem cells. *Int. J. Cancer., 135*, 1019–1027.

42. Scholl, V., Hassan, R., & Zalcberg, I. R., (2012). miRNA-451: A putative predictor marker of Imatinib therapy response in chronic myeloid leukemia. *Leukemia Res., 36,* 119–121.

43. Sebio, A., Pare, L., Paez, D., Salazar, J., Gonzalez, A., Sala, N, del Rio, E., Martin-Richard, M.l, Tobena, M., Barnadas, A., & Baiget, M., (2013). The LCS6 polymorphism in the binding site of let- 7 microRNA to the KRAS 30-untranslated region: its role in the efficacy of anti-EGFR-based therapy in metastatic colorectal cancer patients. *Pharmacogenet Genomics, 23,* 142–147.

44. Wynendaele, J., Böhnke, A., Leucci, E., Nielsen, S. J., Lambertz, I., Hammer, S., Sbrzesny, N., Kubitza, D., Wolf, A., Gradhand, E., Balschun, K., Braicu, I., Sehouli, J., Darb-Esfahani, S., Denkert, C., Thomssen, C., Hauptmann, S., Lund, A., Marine, J. C., & Bartel, F., (2010). An illegitimate microRNA target site within the 30 UTR of MDM4 affects ovarian cancer progression and chemosensitivity. *Cancer Res., 70,* 9641–9649.

45. Schwarzenbach, H., Nishida, N., Calin, G. A., & Pantel, K., (2014). Clinical relevance of circulating cell-free microRNAs in cancer. *Nat. Rev. Clin. Oncol., 11,* 145–156.

46. Mannoor, K., Liao, J., & Jiang, F., (2012). Small nucleolar RNAs in cancer. *Biochim. Biophys. Acta, 1826.* 121–128.

47. Dong, X. Y., Rodriguez, C., Guo, P., Sun, X., Talbot, J. T., Zhou, W., Petros, J., Li, Q., Vessella, R. L., Kibel, A. S., Stevens, V. L., Calle, E. E., & Dong, J. T., (2008). SnoRNA U50 is a candidate tumor-suppressor gene at 6q14. 3 with a mutation associated with clinically significant prostate cancer. *Hum. Mol. Genet., 17,* 1031–1042.

48. Gee, H. E., Buffa, F. M., Camps, C., Ramachandran, A., Leek, R., Taylor, M., Patil, M., Sheldon, H., Betts, G., Homer, J., West, C., Ragoussis, J., & Harris, A. L., (2011). The small-nucleolar RNAs commonly used for microRNA normalisation correlate with tumour pathology and prognosis. *Br. J. Cancer, 104,* 1168–1177.

49. Ng, K. W., Anderson, C., Marshall, E. A., Minatel, B. C., Enfield, K. S., Saprunoff, H. L., Lam, W., & Martinez, V. D., (2016). Piwi-interacting RNAs in cancer: emerging functions and clinical utility. *Mol. Cancer* [Online], *15,* 5 https://molecular-cancer. biomedcentral.com /articles /10. 1186. /s12943–016–0491–0499.

50. Juliano, C., Wang, J., & Lin, H., (2011). Uniting germline and stem cells: the function of Piwi proteins and the piRNA pathway in diverse organisms. *Annu. Rev. Genet., 45,* 447–469.

51. http://epigenie.com/key-epigenetic-players/histone-proteins-and-modifications/histone-h3k9/.

52. Martinez, V. D., Vucic, E. A., Thu, K. L., Hubaux, R., Enfield, K. S., Pikor, L. A., Becker-Santos, D. D., Brown, C. J., Lam, S., & Lam, W. L., (2015). Unique somatic and malignant expression patterns implicate PIWI-interacting RNAs in cancer-type specific biology. *Sci. Rep. [Online], 5,* 10423 https://www.nature.com/articles/srep10423.

53. Huang, G., Hu, H., Xue, X., Shen, S., Gao, E., Guo, G., Shen, X., & Zhang, X., (2013). Altered expression of piRNAs and their relation with clinicopathologic features of breast cancer. *Clin. Transl. Oncol., 15,* 563–568.

54. Zhang, H., Ren, Y., Xu, H., Pang, D., Duan, C., & Liu, C., (2013). The expression of stem cell protein Piwil2 and piR-932 in breast cancer. *Surg. Oncol., 22,* 217–223.

55. Yan, H., Wu, Q. L., Sun, C. Y., Ai, L. S., Deng, J., Zhang, L., Chen, L., Chu, Z. B., Tang, B., Wang, K., Wu, X. F., Xu, J., & Hu, Y., (2015). piRNA-823 contributes to tumorigenesis by regulating de novo DNA methylation and angiogenesis in multiple myeloma. *Leukemia, 29,* 196–206.

56. Cheng, J., Deng, H., Xiao, B., Zhou, H., Zhou, F., Shen, Z., & Guo, J., (2012). piR-823, a novel non-coding small RNA, demonstrates in vitro and in vivo tumor suppressive activity in human gastric cancer cells. *Cancer Lett., 315*, 12–17.

57. Busch, J., Ralla, B., Jung, M., Wotschofsky, Z., Trujillo-Arribas, E., Schwabe, P., Kilic, E., Fendler, A., & Jung, K., (2015). Piwi-interacting RNAs as novel prognostic markers in clear cell renal cell carcinomas. *J. Exp. Clin. Cancer Res.* [Online], *34*, 61 https://jeccr.biomedcentral.com /articles/10. 1186/s13046–015–0180–0183.

58. Evans, J. R., Feng, F. Y., & Chinnaiyan, A. M., (2016). The bright side of dark matter: lncRNAs in cancer. *J. Clin. Invest., 126*, 2775–2782.

59. Hon, C. C., Ramilowski, J. A., Harshbarger, J., Bertin, N., Rackham, O. J., Gough, J., Denisenko, E., Schmeier, S., Poulsen, T. M., Severin, J., Lizio, M., Kawaji, H., Kasukawa, T., Itoh, M., Burroughs, A. M., Noma, S., Djebali, S., Alam, T., Medvedeva, Y. A., Testa, A. C., Lipovich, L., Yip, C. W., Abugessaisa, I., Mendez, M., Hasegawa, A., Tang, D., Lassmann, T., Heutink, P., Babina, M., Wells, C. A., Kojima, S., Nakamura, Y., Suzuki, H., Daub, C. O., de Hoon, M. J., Arner, E., Hayashizaki, Y., Carninci, P., & Forrest, A. R., (2017). An atlas of human long non-coding RNAs with accurate 5' ends. *Nature, 543*, 199–204.

60. Cabili, M. N., Trapnell, C., Goff, L., Koziol, M., Tazon-Vega, B., Regev, A., & Rinn, J. L., (2011). Integrative annotation of human large intergenic noncoding RNAs reveals global properties and specific subclasses. *Genes & Development, 25*, 1915–1927.

61. Lorenzen, J. M., & Thum, T., (2016). Long noncoding RNAs in kidney and cardiovascular diseases. *Nat. Rev. Nephrol., 12*, 360–373.

62. Derrien, T., Johnson, R., Bussotti, G., Tanzer, A., Djebali, S., Tilgner, H., Guernec, G., Martin, D., Merkel, A., Knowles, D. G., Lagarde, J., Veeravalli, L., Ruan, X., Ruan, Y., Lassmann, T., Carninci, P., Brown, J. B., Lipovich, L., Gonzalez, J. M., Thomas, M., Davis, C. A., Shiekhattar, R., Gingeras, T. R., Hubbard, T. J., Notredame, C., Harrow, J., & Guigó, R., (2012). The GENCODE v7 catalog of human long noncoding RNAs: analysis of their gene structure, evolution, & expression. *Genome Res., 22*, 1775–1789.

63. Harrow, J., Frankish, A., Gonzalez, J. M., Tapanari, E., Diekhans, M., Kokocinski, F., Aken, B. L., Barrell, D., Zadissa, A., Searle, S., Barnes, I., Bignell, A., Boychenko, V., Hunt, T., Kay, M., Mukherjee, G., Rajan, J., Despacio-Reyes, G., Saunders, G., Steward, C., Harte, R., Lin, M., Howald, C., Tanzer, A., Derrien, T., Chrast, J., Walters, N., Balasubramanian, S., Pei, B., Tress, M., Rodriguez, J. M., Ezkurdia, I., van Baren, J., Brent, M., Haussler, D., Kellis, M., Valencia, A., Reymond, A., Gerstein, M., Guigó, R., & Hubbard, T. J., (2012). GENCODE: the reference human genome annotation for The ENCODE Project. *Genome. Res., 22*, 1760–1774.

64. Frith, M. C., Forrest, A. R., Nourbakhsh, E., Pang, K. C., Kai, C., Kawai, J., Carninci, P., Hayashizaki, Y., Bailey, T. L., & Grimmond, S. M., (2006). The abundance of short proteins in the mammalian proteome. *PLoS Genet., 2*, e52. http://journals.plos.org/plosgenetics /article?id=10. 1371/journal.pgen. 0020052 .

65. Anderson, D. M., Anderson, K. M., Chang, C. L., Makarewich, C. A., Nelson, B. R., McAnally, J. R., Kasaragod, P., Shelton, J. M., Liou, J., Bassel-Duby, R., & Olson, E. N., (2015). A micropeptide encoded by a putative long noncoding RNA regulates muscle performance. *Cell, 160*, 595–606.

66. Pauli, A., Norris, M. L., Valen, E., Chew, G. L., Gagnon, J. A., Zimmerman, S., Mitchell, A., Ma, J., Dubrulle, J., Reyon, D., Tsai, S. Q., Joung, J. K., Saghatelian, A., & Schier, A. F., (2014). Toddler: an embryonic signal that promotes cell movement via Apelin receptors. *Science, 343*, 1248636.

67. Yan, Y., Cooper, C., Hamedani, M. K., Guppy, B., Xu, W., Tsuyuki, D., Zhang, C., Nugent, Z., Blanchard, A., Davie, J. R., McManus, K., Murphy, L. C., Myal, Y., & Leygue, E., (2015). The steroid receptor RNA activator protein (SRAP) controls cancer cell migration/motility. *FEBS Lett, 589*, 4010–4018.

68. Schmitz, S. U., Grote, P., & Herrmann, B. G., (2016). Mechanisms of long noncoding RNA function in development and disease. *Cell Mol. Life. Sci., 73*, 2491–2509.

CHAPTER 14

EPIGENETICS IN CANCER PREVENTION AND THERAPY: ROLE OF PHYTOCHEMICALS

SAJID KHAN,[1] SAMRIDDHI SHUKLA,[1] and
SYED MUSTHAPA MEERAN[2]

[1]Laboratory of Cancer Epigenetics, Division of Endocrinology, CSIR-Central Drug Research Institute, Lucknow–226 031, India

[2]Laboratory of Cancer Epigenetics, Department of Biochemistry, CSIR-Central Food Technological Research Institute, Mysore, India, E-mail: s.musthapa@cftri.res.in

CONTENTS

ABSTRACT

Cancer is a heterogeneous disease and the major cause of mortality worldwide. Epigenetic changes including DNA methylation, chromatin remodeling, and miRNA-mediated gene regulation play a crucial role in the initiation, promotion, and progression of cancer. Epigenetic dysregulation alters several cellular functions in cancer by the downregulation of tumor suppressor genes (TSGs) and upregulation of oncogenes. Hence, targeting these epigenetic aberrations could be of tremendous value for both prevention and treatment of cancer. Some of the drugs targeting epigenetic alterations, including inhibitors of DNA methyltransferases (DNMTs) and histone deacetylases (HDACs), are approved for the treatment of hematological malignancies and are under clinical development against solid tumors. The reversible nature of epigenetic changes has encouraged many investigators to investigate the chemopreventive and therapeutic efficacy of dietary phytochemicals such as green tea polyphenols, genistein, curcumin, resveratrol, and sulforaphane in several cancers. These phytochemicals have shown promising chemopreventive potential against various cancer types by interfering with epigenetic events. In this chapter, we summarize the key epigenetic mechanisms and their role in the regulation of tumor-regulated genes in different cancers. We have also discussed extensively the available therapeutic and chemopreventive compounds possessing epigenetic modulatory activities and their use in cancer prevention and therapy.

14.1   INTRODUCTION

Cancer is a multistep process encompassing three critical steps, i.e., initiation, promotion, and progression. Previously, it was believed that tumor initiation is caused by a mutation in a single cell followed by tumor promotion by the clonal amplification of that mutated cell. However, in the rapidly evolving field of cancer biology, it has now been well established that epigenetic modifications alter the gene expression without changing the DNA sequence and play a significant role in the process of carcinogenesis [1]. Due to their reversible nature, epigenetic modifications have become the promising therapeutic targets for cancer prevention and therapy.

The epigenetic alterations include changes in the DNA methylation patterns, post-translational histone tail modifications, and miRNA-mediated gene regulation. These epigenetic alterations may contribute to the process of carcinogenesis through their myriad roles in several biological processes including cell proliferation, survival, differentiation, and senescence [2]. In the subsequent sections, we have comprehensively discussed the role of epigenetics in the silencing of key tumor suppressor genes (TSGs) and activation of oncogenes. Further, we have discussed the clinical value of available epigenetic drugs as well as the role of dietary and bioactive phytochemicals in altering different epigenetic marks and their significance in cancer prevention and therapy.

14.2 EPIGENETIC MODIFICATIONS

14.2.1 *DNA METHYLATION*

DNA methylation involves the covalent addition of a methyl group ($-CH_3$) from the universal methyl donor S-adenosyl-L-methionine (SAM) to the 5'-carbon of the pyrimidine ring of cytosine, leading to its conversion to 5-methylcytosine. The DNA methylation is primarily catalyzed by a group of enzymes known as DNA methyltransferases (DNMTs). There are mainly three DNMTs: DNMT1, DNMT3a, and DNMT3b that are involved in carrying out the process of DNA methylation. DNMT1 has a major role in maintaining the methylation patterns in the hemimethylated DNA, while DNMT3a and 3b methylate previously unmethylated DNA sequences, thereby acting as *de novo* methyltransferases. Most of the dispersed CpG dinucleotide sequences are methylated in mammals, and unmethylated CpGs are found in clusters known as "CpG islands" that are present in the 5'-regulatory regions of approximately 50% of genes. The hypermethylated promoters at CpG islands are, in general, inaccessible to the transcription factors and transcriptional coactivators [3]. DNA hypermethylation has been known to silence the expression of endogenous repeats and retrotransposons in order to protect normal gene expression. The classical examples of DNA hypermethylation-induced gene silencing are X-chromosome inactivation in women and genomic imprinting, where one gene is expressed depending upon its maternal or paternal origin and the repression of a set of germ cell-specific genes in somatic cells [4]. The constitutively expressed genes usually display lower promoter methylation. On the other hand, genes with regulative expression maintain higher promoter methylation. This indicates the important regulatory role of this epigenetic mechanism in the maintenance of cellular homeostasis. Any alteration in the DNA methylation patterns of a healthy cell, therefore, might result in the loss of the cellular dynamics.

14.2.1.1   DNA Hypermethylation in Cancer

Hypermethylation of CpG sequences within gene promoters leads to the transcriptional silencing of TSGs [3]. Overexpression of DNMTs is commonly associated with the gene-specific DNA hypermethylation observed in cancer cells. DNA hypermethylation at promoters influences gene transcription in dual manner. First, DNA methylation prevents the binding of transcriptional regulators that normally require unmethylated DNA within their binding sites in the gene promoter. Second, methylated DNA is bound by methyl-CpG binding domain (MBD) proteins that recruit additional proteins like histone deacetylases (HDACs) and other chromatin remodeling complexes, leading to the transcriptional repression [5]. A large number of genes involved in various cellular processes such as cell growth and regulation, DNA repair, apoptosis, angiogenesis, and metastasis have been reported to be hypermethylated in different types of cancers. DNA hypermethylation at gene promoters may serve as a biomarker and also result in poor prognosis in cancers. For example, aberrant methylation at the promoter of $p16^{INK4a}$ has been considered to be an early biomarker for lung cancer [6]. In addition, hypermethylation at the promoters of *estrogen receptor-α* (*ERα*) is responsible for the loss of ER expression in breast cancer cells, due to which these tumors do not respond to anti-estrogenic therapy, resulting into poor prognosis. Furthermore, hypermethylation at the promoters of *breast cancer susceptibility gene-1* (*BRCA1*) leads to its repression, which is the major cause of hereditary breast cancer [7, 8]. There are certain crucial genes involved in cell growth and development, which are commonly hypermethylated in specific cancer types and predict disease progression and prognosis. For example, the hypermethylation of mismatch repair gene *human mutL homolog 1 (MLH1)* is quite common in the case of colorectal cancer, whereas the *glutathione s-transferase π-1* (*GSTP1*) gene is methylated in more than 90% cases of prostate cancer [4, 9]. In addition to its crucial role in suppressing TSGs, DNA hypermethylation may also indirectly contribute to carcinogenesis by silencing endogenous inhibitors of oncogenes. For example, the silencing of the secreted frizzled-related protein (SFRP) family of genes leads to the activation of the Wnt pathway in colorectal cancer [4].

14.2.1.2   DNA Hypomethylation in Cancer

The first epigenetic alteration observed in cancer was global genomic hypomethylation, which is in contrast to the gene-specific hypermethylation, in particular to the TSGs. The inhibition of global hypomethylation in skin cancer model has been shown to protect against UVB-induced photocarcinogenesis [10]. The global DNA hypomethylation in cancer affects both repetitive elements such as LINE1 and Alu as well as specific gene promoters. Global hypomethylation leads to genomic instability, which may partially occur through reactivation of mobile elements. Global hypomethylation correlates with a higher rate of chromosomal aberrations in cancer and is responsible for poor prognosis. In other instances, DNA hypomethylation has been associated with the reactivation of normally silenced proto-oncogenes, which leads to the activation of several tumorigenic pathways [4]. For example, promoter hypomethylation of numerous proto-oncogenes involved in uncontrolled proliferation and metastasis (e.g., *synuclein γ* and *urokinase*) and development of drug resistance (e.g., *N-cadherin, ID4, β-catenin, annexin A4*, and *WNT11*) are common in breast cancer. Moreover, the mutations in *BRCA1* have been shown to be associated with the aberrant regulation of DNMTs, leading to global hypomethylation and increased expression of various proto-oncogenes such as *c-Fos, Ha-Ras*, and *c-Myc* [11]. Furthermore, promoter hypomethylation may also lead to the reactivation of certain oncogenic-miRNAs (onco-miRs), thereby causing the translational inhibition of its target tumor suppressor mRNA transcripts [4].

14.2.2   HISTONE MODIFICATIONS

Other epigenetic alterations commonly observed in human malignancies are posttranslational histone modifications. These are reversible covalent modifications including acetylation at lysine residues, methylation at lysine and arginine, phosphorylation at serine and threonine, ubiquitination at lysine, and poly-ADP ribosylation and sumoylation [12]. The most important histone modifications implicated in carcinogenesis are histone acetylation/deacetylation and histone methylation/demethylation. These modifications are catalyzed by the specialized sets of enzymes. Histone acetyltransferases (HATs) and histone deacetylases (HDACs) catalyze the processes of histone acetylation and deacetylation, respectively, while histone methyltransferases (HMTs) and histone demethylases (HDMs) catalyze histone methylation and demethylation, respectively. Acetylation of histones, in general, causes chromatin relaxation (euchromatin) leading to gene expression, whereas deacetylation causes chromatin condensation (heterochromatin) leading to gene repression (Figure 14.1). The increased activity of HDACs can be linked with the repression of TSGs in several human cancers [2, 13]. In contrast to the acetylation, histone methylation can both be active or repressive depending upon the degree and site of methylation. For example, trimethylation of lysine 4 on histone H3 (H3K4me3) is associated with gene activation, whereas trimethylation of lysine 9 on histone H3 (H3K9me3) and trimethylation of lysine 27 on histone H3 (H3K27me3) are responsible for transcriptional repression during carcinogenesis [14]. The shifting in the balance of HATs/HDACs or HMTs/HDMs can occur in cancer through their altered expression or activities. For example, the overexpression of polycomb group (PcG) protein, Enhancer of Zeste homolog 2 (EZH2), that

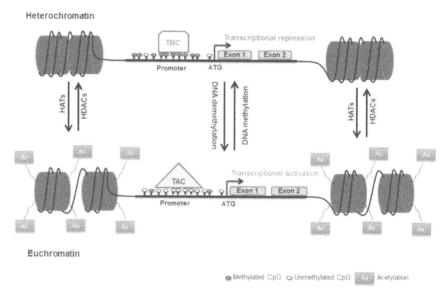

FIGURE 14.1   Role of epigenetic modulations in transcriptional gene regulations. HDACs remove the acetyl moieties from lysine residues of histones, which enables attraction between negatively charged DNA and positively charged histones, leading to chromatin compaction called as heterochromatin. Heterochromatin, in general, is considered as a transcriptionally repressed state of chromatin due to hypoacetylation and is accessible to the transcriptional activator complex (TAC). Hypermethylation at CpG sites allows the binding of the transcriptional repressor complex (TRC) such as DNMT1/Rb/E2F1/HDAC1 that represses transcription from E2F-responsive promoters. On the other hand, histone acetylation by the action of HATs lead to chromatin relaxation through repulsion between negatively charged DNA and histones; this is called as euchromatin. Further, DNA demethylation removes TRC and enables the recruitment of TAC consisting of general transcription factors and coactivator HATs that lead to transcriptional activation of genes involved in tumor suppression.

catalyzes the trimethylation of H3K27, promotes tumor growth in several cancers such as melanomas, lymphomas, and prostate and breast cancers. EZH2 expression has been correlated with aberrant H3K27 trimethylation in prostate cancer and affects potential TSGs. Alternatively, H3K27 repressive methylation mark can also be enriched through the inactivation of a specific H3K27 demethylase, i.e., *UTX*. SUV39H1 is a specific H3K9 methyltransferase that plays a key role in tumor initiation and progression [4].

14.2.3   MICRORNA (miRNA) DEREGULATION

Currently, an emerging epigenetic process, miRNA-mediated gene regulation has been proven to have a greater impact on carcinogenesis. miRNAs are transcribed by RNA polymerase II as long primary miRNA molecules (pri-miRNAs), which are then processed into short hairpin RNAs of ~70 nucleotides (pre-miRNA) by the action of Drosha and DGCR8. Pre-miRNAs are then transported into the cytoplasm by Exportin-5 to be cleaved by the Dicer enzyme releasing a ~22-nucleotide-long miRNA duplex. After that, one of the strands is incorporated into RNA-induced silencing complex (RISC), which directs miRNA binding to the 3'-UTRs of target mRNAs, resulting in target cleavage or degradation and ultimately leads to translational inhibition [15]. However, recent reports have suggested that miRNAs can also bind to other regions such as 5'-UTR or coding sequences [16, 17]. These miRNAs can function as both tumor suppressor or oncogenic, depending upon their target sequences. For example, if a miRNA targets a TSG, it functions as an oncogenic miRNA, whereas if it targets a proto-oncogene transcript, it functions as a tumor suppressor. A single miRNA molecule can target several genes depending upon its sequence complementarity. The miRNA expression might be altered either through the hypermethylation in the miRNA-encoding gene promoters or through copy number variations. Alteration in the miRNA processing machinery might also cause deregulated miRNA expression. miRNA dysregulation has been found to be involved in various processes of carcinogenesis such as cell differentiation, proliferation, apoptosis, autophagy, metastasis, and drug resistance in almost all human cancers [18–23]. Genome-wide studies revealed that miRNAs are globally downregulated in cancer and are associated with diverse cellular phenotypes. For example, the depletion of let-7 family of miRNAs promotes the tumorigenicity of breast, lung, and colon cancers, whereas the overexpression of miR-21 provides increased invasion capacities of breast cancer and confers lung metastatic abilities [2]. Due to their important regulatory role in the processes of cancer promotion and progression and their therapeutic value, these miRNAs can serve as prognostic markers as well as potential therapeutic targets in cancer [24].

14.3   TARGETING EPIGENETIC REGULATORS IN CANCER

14.3.1   SYNTHETIC EPIGENETIC DRUGS

In recent years, studies have largely focused on the role of epigenetic modifications in cancer prevention and therapy [25-27]. As an outset, several epigenetic drugs are under different stages of preclinical and clinical trials for the treatment of various cancers (Table 14.1).

Targeted molecular strategies by utilizing DNMTs and HDACs as epigenetic targets are becoming popular due to the fact that the inhibitors of these epigenetic enzymes reverse the hypermethylation and deacetylation patterns of TSGs, respectively, and contribute to their upregulation. The best studied synthetic DNMT inhibitor, 5-azacytidine (5-aza-C; also known as azacitidine) and 5-aza-2'-deoxycytidine (5-aza-dC; also known as decitabine) have been widely used for the treatment of hematological malignancies [28]. Zebularine, a nucleoside analog of cytidine, is another DNMT inhibitor that is more stable than azacitidine or decitabine and has been reported to be effective in the growth inhibition of several cancers such as breast, colorectal, lung, and head and neck cancers [29–32]. Two pan-HDAC inhibitors, vorinostat (also known as SAHA) and romidepsin, have shown promising results in clinical trials and have been approved for the clinical use in patients with cutaneous T cell lymphoma (CTCL), but the efficacy of these drugs in other cancers is still lacking [28]. Belinostat has been approved by US-FDA for the treatment of peripheral T-cell lymphoma (PTCL) in USA, but it has not been approved in the European countries [34]. Another HDAC inhibitor, panobinostat, is in phase III clinical trial for multiple myeloma [36]. Vorinostat and other HDAC inhibitors such as entinostat and pivanex are in the initial phases of clinical development for the treatment of nonsmall cell lung cancer (NSCLC) [39, 40]. The HDAC inhibitor LAQ824 either alone or in combination with other drugs has been shown to be effective against multiple cancers [38]. Two inhibitors of bromodomain-

TABLE 14.1 List of Synthetic Epigenetic Drugs/Compounds for Cancer Treatment

Drug name	Target	Highest phase of development	References
5-azacytidine	DNMT inhibitor	FDA approved for the treatment of MDS and AML	[28]
5-aza-2'-deoxycytidine	DNMT inhibitor	FDA approved for the treatment of MDS and AML	[28]
SGI 110	DNMT inhibitor	HCC (phase II); MDS (phase I/II); AML (phase I/II); ovarian cancer (phase I/II)	[28]
Zebularine	DNMT inhibitor	Preclinical phase	[29-32]
RG-108	DNMT inhibitor	Preclinical phase	[33]
Vorinostat (SAHA)	HDAC inhibitor	FDA approved for clinical use in CTCL patients; Brain cancer (phase I); NSCLC (phase I)	[28]
Romidepsin	HDAC inhibitor	FDA approved for clinical use in CTCL and PTCL patients	[28]
Belinostat	HDAC inhibitor	Approved in USA for the treatment of PTCL	[34]
LBH-589 (panobinostat)	HDAC inhibitor	AML and MDS (phase I/II); multiple myeloma (phase III)	[35,36]
Pracinostat	HDAC inhibitor	AML (phase III); MDS (phase II)	[37]
Resminostat	HDAC inhibitor	Phase II clinical trial in liver cancer	[37]
LAQ824 (Dacinostat)	HDAC inhibitor	Phase I clinical trial	[38]
MS-275 (entinostat)	Class I HDAC inhibitor	Phase II clinical trial for NSCLC, breast cancer, CRC, AML and Hodgkin's lymphoma	[28]
Mocetinostat	Class I HDAC inhibitor	Phase II clinical trial for diffuse large B cell lymphoma and follicular lymphoma	[28]
Pivanex	HDAC inhibitor	Phase I clinical trial for NSCLC	[39,40]
Valproic acid (VPA)	HDAC inhibitor	Phase I/II clinical trial	[41]

TABLE 14.1 (Continued)

Drug name	Target	Highest phase of development	References
CI-994 (Tacedinaline)	HDAC inhibitor	Phase II clinical trial for treating multiple myeloma patients	clinicaltrials.gov Identifier: NCT00005624 NCT00005624
ACY 1215 (ricolinostat)	HDAC6 inhibitor	Phase I/II clinical trial for multiple myeloma	[28]
ACY 1215 (ricolinostat)	HDAC6 inhibitor	Phase I/II clinical trial for multiple myeloma	[28]
Trichostatin A (TSA)	HDAC inhibitor	Preclinical	[34]
GSK 525762	Bromodomain-containing protein inhibitor	Phase I clinical trial for carcinoma	[28]
OTX015	Bromodomain-containing protein inhibitor	Phase I clinical trial against haematological malignancies	[28]
EPZ-5676	Histone methyltransferase inhibitor	Phase I clinical trial for mixed lineage rearranged leukaemia	[28]

containing proteins (GSK525762 and OTX015) are in phase I clinical trial for the treatment of multiple carcinomas and hematological malignancies, respectively. The rationale and empirical testing of HDAC inhibitors with available chemotherapeutic and targeted drugs have shown varying degree of success (Table 14.2).

For example, the combination of vorinostat with paclitaxel (a chemo-therapeutic agent) and bevacizumab (VEGF-A inhibitor) is in phase II clinical trial against metastatic breast cancer. A phase II trial of the combination of vorinostat with idarubicin and cytarabine in patients with acute myelog-enous leukemia (AML) and myelodysplastic syndrome (MDS) resulted in an overall significant response rate of 85% [42]. The rationally designed combination of vorinostat and the proteasome inhibitor bortezomib has been tested in phase I clinical trials against relapsing and/or refractory multiple myeloma with overall response rates of 42% and 27%, respectively [43, 44]. It has recently been shown that the combinatorial use of DNMT and HDAC inhibitors could provide better therapeutic outcome than individual inhibi-tors [46]. The treatment of ERα-negative breast tumors with the combina-tion of DNMT and HDAC inhibitors resulted in the reactivation of ERα expression, making hormonal-refractory breast tumors responsive to estro-gen antagonists [47–49]. In one of these studies, the synergistic action of trichostatin A (TSA) and 5-aza-dC led to the reactivation of ERα expression in ERα-negative breast cancer cells [47]. The chemical structures of FDA approved and/or clinically tested DNMT and HDAC inhibitors against can-cer are presented in Figures 14.2 and 14.3, respectively.

14.3.2 DIETARY PHYTOCHEMICALS WITH EPIGENETIC MODULATORY EFFECTS

Dietary phytochemicals are of great importance in cancer prevention and therapy due to their ability to alter epigenetic marks. Several studies have provided strong evidences on the potential use of dietary phytochemicals to reverse epigenetic changes in cancer cells. These phytochemicals possess the ability to alter most of the epigenetic processes, including DNA meth-ylation, histone modifications, and miRNA expression [3, 13, 25, 50, 51]. The importance of the use of dietary phytochemicals in cancer prevention and therapy lies in the facts that a) they are abundant in nature; b) they are endowed with lesser side effects than synthetic drugs; and c) they can be

TABLE 14.2 Clinical Development of the Combination of Synthetic Epigenetic Drugs with Available Anticancer Drugs

Drug combination	Class of drug/s	Highest phase of development	References
Vorinostat in combination with paclitaxel and bevacizumab	HDAC inhibitor + chemotherapeutic agent and angiogenesis inhibitor	Phase II clinical trial for metastatic breast cancer	clinicaltrials.gov Identifier:NCT00368875
Vorinostat in combination with idarubicin and cytarabine	HDAC inhibitor + DNA damaging chemotherapeutics	Phase II clinical trial against AML and MDS	[42]
Vorinostat in combination with bortezomib	HDAC inhibitor + proteasome inhibitor	Phase I clinical trial against relapsing and refractory multiple myeloma	[43,44]
Entinostat in combination with trastazumab	HDAC inhibitor + HER-2 inhibitor	Phase I clinical trial for metastatic HER-2 positive breast cancer	clinicaltrials.gov Identifier: NCT01434303
Panobinostat in combination with trastazumab	HDAC inhibitor + HER-2 inhibitor	Phase I clinical trial for metastatic HER-2 positive breast cancer	clinicaltrials.gov Identifier: NCT00567879
CI-994 in combination with Gemcitabine	HDAC inhibitor + chemotherapeutic agent	Phase III clinical trial for treating advanced NSCLC	[42]
Entinostat in combination with 5-azacitidine	HDAC inhibitor +DNMT inhibitor	Phase II clinical trial in patients with hormonal-refractory or triple-negative breast cancer	clinicaltrials.gov Identifier: NCT01349959
Panobinostat in combination with 5-aza-2′-deoxycytidine	HDAC inhibitor +DNMT inhibitor	Phase I/II clinical trial for triple nega-tive breast cancer	[45]

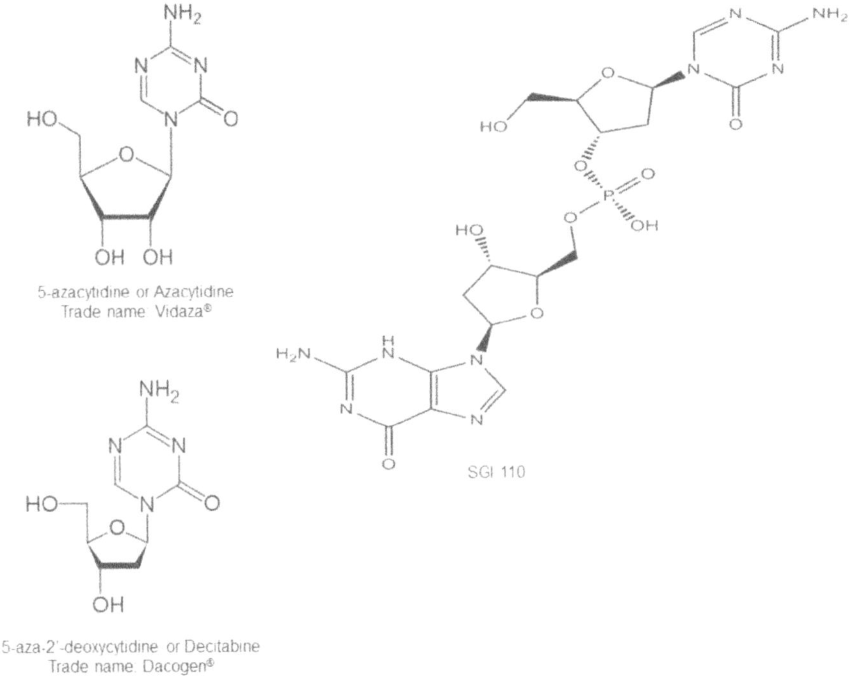

FIGURE 14.2 Chemical structures of FDA-approved and other clinically tested DNMT inhibitors in cancer. The cytidine analogs, 5-azacytidine and 5-aza-2'-deoxycytidine, are approved for the treatment of hematological cancers. The second generation DNA hypomethylating agent SGI 110 (a deoxyguanosine) is in phase II clinical trial against multiple cancers.

easily obtained in the routine diet. The epigenetic mechanisms of actions of some of the selected dietary phytochemicals in different cancer types are detailed in the following subsections.

14.3.2.1 Green Tea Polyphenols

Green tea polyphenols (GTPs) are the active components present in green tea, which include (–)-epigallocatechin gallate (EGCG), (–)-epicatechin gallate (ECG), (–)- epigallocatechin (EGC), and (–)-epicatechin (EC). EGCG, an active ingredient of GTPs, has been shown to have anticancer effects through various mechanisms including epigenetic alterations of key genes involved in cancer progressions [52–54]. Notably, for the first time, Fang et al. [55] have demonstrated that the EGCG-induced gene-specific demeth-

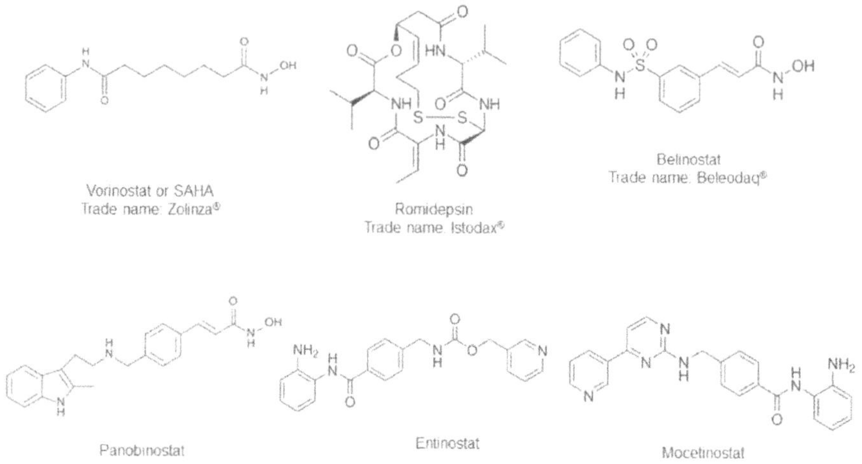

FIGURE 14.3   Chemical structures of FDA-approved and other clinically tested HDAC inhibitors in cancer. The hydroxamate-type HDAC inhibitors, Vorinostat and Belinostat, and Romidepsin (a thiol) are approved for hematological malignancies. Entinostat and Mocetinostat (both are benzamides), and Panobinostat (a hydroxamate) are under different stages of clinical trials against various cancers.

ylation at the promoters of key TSGs leads to their transcriptional reactivation, which might be due to the direct inhibition of DNMT1 in cancer cell lines. Thereafter, several other research groups have shown DNA demethylating activity of EGCG in different cancer cells [56, 57]. Studies have also demonstrated that the treatment of cancer cells with EGCG not only reactivates TSGs, but also leads to the downregulation of tumor promoter gene *human telomerase reverse transcriptase* (*hTERT*). EGCG-mediated downregulation of *hTERT* was further attributed to its demethylating activity, which was correlated well with the findings that demethylation of the *hTERT* promoter is generally associated with its transcriptional repression instead of activation [58, 59]. Demethylation of the *hTERT* promoter recruits methylation-sensitive transcriptional repressors such as MAD1 and CTCF, which led to the transcriptional repression of *hTERT*. In an *in vitro* study, treatment of NSCLC cells with EGCG led to the promoter demethylation and restoration of Wnt inhibitory factor 1 (WIF-1). WIF-1 is an antagonist of *Wnt* proto-oncogene, an extracellular stimulus of Wnt/β-catenin pathway, which is involved in several tumorigenesis functions of cancer cells [60].

GTPs either alone or in combinational therapy have been shown to reactivate the expression of hormonal receptors in hormonal-refractory breast cancer cells, making them responsive to available hormonal therapy. For example, Li et al. [47] demonstrated that the GTPs in combination with HDAC inhibitor, Trichostatin A (TSA), reactivate ERα expression in ER-negative human breast cancer cells. Recently, we have also demonstrated that GTPs in combination with other bioactive supplements reactivate ERα expression through epigenetic modifications in hormonal refractory breast cancer cells, thus making these cells responsive to tamoxifen therapy [49, 61]. The limited chemical stability of EGCG under normal physiological conditions is of great concern for its translational relevance in humans. In an attempt to deal with this limitation, synthetic analogs of EGCG have been generated with stronger anticancer activities and more stability and efficacy [62, 63]. Two such analogs of EGCG have been demonstrated to be more efficacious than EGCG in breast cancer cells by inducing DNA hypomethylation and promoter deacetylation [64]. EGCG has also shown to modulate the expression of oncogenic and tumor suppressor miRNAs in cancer cells, thus contributing to its anticancer activity. EGCG was first reported to modulate the expression of 61 miRNAs in human hepatocellular carcinoma HepG2 cells. One of the significantly upregulated miRNA was discovered to be miR-16, which targets the antiapoptotic gene *Bcl-2* [65]. Since then, other reports have also shown modulations of miRNA profiles by EGCG in cancer cells both in vitro and in vivo. For example, EGCG treatment in human and mouse lung cancer cells led to the upregulation of miR-210, resulting in reduced cellular proliferation [66]. Further, the administration of 0.4% EGCG-containing diet to cigarette smoke-condensate (NNK)-induced lung cancer model resulted in an alteration of 21 different tumor-related miRNAs, from which 13 miRNAs were upregulated including miR-210 and 8 miRNAs were downregulated. Most of these miRNAs have targets that are involved in molecular pathways modulated by EGCG in vivo [67]. EGCG treatment in human malignant neuroblastoma cell lines downregulated the expression of onco-miRs and upregulated the expression of tumor suppressor-miRs leading to cellular apoptosis [68].

GTPs have emerged as promising chemopreventive agents against cancer, as many of their effects observed in vitro can be reproducible in animal studies. Henning et al. [69] demonstrated that drinking green tea leads to the inhibition of DNMT1 protein expression and reduced tumor growth in prostate cancer xenografts. Further, Volate et al. [70] demonstrated that the administration of green tea solution (containing 0.6% of GTPs) to Apc(Min/−) mice significantly increased the transcriptional and translational levels of retinoid X receptor-α (RXRα) through promoter demethylation in colon tissue samples. In another study, the topical application of EGCG in a hydrophilic cream led to global DNA demethylation indicated by decreased levels of 5-methylcytosine, which contributed to the anticancer activity of EGCG in UVB-exposed SKH-1 hairless mice [10]. There are only few human studies demonstrating the effect of GTPs on cancer prevention and therapy. In a clinical study, the authors examined the methylation status of six genes in 106 patients with primary gastric carcinomas. In this study, high consumption of green tea (seven cups or more per day compared with six cups or less) was inversely related to the methylation status of caudal type homeobox 2 (CDX2) and bone morphogenetic protein 2 (BMP-2), but not p16[INK4a], calcium channel voltage-dependent alpha 2/delta subunit 3 (CACNA2D3), GTA-5, and *ER* [71]. Hence, EGCG, a key component of GTPs, has been demonstrated to have anticancer activity largely by epigenetic modifications of key genes involved in carcinogenesis, leading to their altered expression.

14.3.2.2   Curcumin

Curcumin is the major active ingredient of turmeric, and it has been reported to affect multiple signaling pathways involved in several carcinogenic processes such as proliferation, survival, apoptosis, invasion, and inflammation [3]. Previously, curcumin was shown to be a direct inhibitor of DNMT1 and caused global DNA demethylation in leukemia cells, without alterations in gene-specific methylation patterns [72]. Later, curcumin has been reported to reactivate the expression of epigenetically silenced gene *nuclear factor erythroid 2-related factor 2 (Nrf2)*, a master regulator of cellular antioxidant defense mechanism, through promoter demethylation in murine prostate cancer TRAMP C1 cells. The reactivation of *Nrf2* further led to enhanced expression of a major downstream target gene, *NQO1* that encodes an antioxidative enzyme [73]. Curcumin has been shown to alter the HDACs expression and decrease the enrichment of H3K27me3 levels at the promoter region of another epigenetically silenced gene, *Neurog1,* leading to its reactivation in prostate cancer cells [74]. Furthermore, curcumin treatment of the human cervical cancer HeLa cells caused promoter demethylation-mediated reactivation of *RARβ2,* a retinoic acid-regulated TSG [75].

In addition to its potent demethylating activity, curcumin also alters histone modification marks attributed to its HAT and HDAC modulatory activities [76, 77]. Curcumin was reported to inhibit the expression levels of class I HDACs and increase histone H4 acetylation in Burkitt's lymphoma and Raji cells [78]. Curcumin treatment of highly invasive human breast cancer MDA-MB-435 cells led to the downregulation of EZH2, leading to the inhibition of cellular proliferation [79].

Treatment with curcumin in different types of cancer cells has also shown to modulate the miRNA expression profiling. For example, treatment of human breast cancer MCF-7 cells with curcumin led to increased expression of miR-15a and miR-16 and caused the downregulation of the antiapoptotic protein Bcl-2, leading to cellular apoptosis [80]. Curcumin treatment of human pancreatic carcinoma BxPC-3 cells altered the expression of 29 different miRNAs including the upregulation of miR-22, leading to the downregulation of its target genes, *Sp1* and *ERα* [81]. Treatment of curcumin also decreased the expression of miR-186 in multidrug-resistant human lung carcinoma A549/DDP cells and induced cellular apoptosis [82]. Curcumin treatment led to reduced promoter activity and expression of miR-21 attributed to decreased binding of AP-1 to the promoter and induction of programmed cell death protein 4 (Pdcd4), a tumor suppressor, in human colorectal cancer HCT116 cells [83].

14.3.2.3   Genistein

Genistein is an isoflavone found in soy and other legumes, and it exerts various anticancer effects such as cell cycle arrest, induction of apoptosis, and suppression of angiogenesis and metastasis. Genistein alters the DNA methylation and histone modification patterns on tumor-related genes and regulates their expression [84]. A genome-wide methylation profiling of genistein-treated DU-145 and LNCaP prostate cancer cells showed an altered methylation profile of 58 genes involved in cell proliferation, growth, and differentiation [85]. Genistein treatment of three prostate cancer cell lines (LNCaP, LAPC-4, and PC-3) significantly reduced *ERβ* promoter methylation, leading to an increase in ERβ expression in LNCaP and LAPC-4 but not in PC-3 cells. Further, genistein treatment induced phosphorylation, nuclear translocation, and transcriptional activity of ERβ in all three cell lines. In the same study, the authors have concluded that genistein-mediated promoter demethylation and reactivation of ERβ may be attributed to cancer preventive actions of genistein in prostate cancer cells [86]. Treatment of human breast

cancer MDA-MB-231 and MCF-7 cells with genistein was shown to reactivate the expression of *BRCA1* and *BRCA2* through promoter demethylation
[87]. In a study by Xie et al., the authors reported that treatment of MCF-7
and MDA-MB-231 cells with genistein induced global demethylation, and
reduced expression as well as activity of DNMTs, particularly DNMT1. The
molecular docking results showed that genistein might directly interact with
the catalytic domain of DNMT1[88]. In an in vivo model of neuroblastoma,
genistein treatment was shown to reduce the tumor growth through promoter hypomethylation and upregulation of CHD5 and p53 tumor suppressors [89]. Genistein treatment significantly induced the mRNA expression
of *Protocadherin 17* (*PCDH17*) through promoter demethylation in a gastric
cancer AGS cell line, leading to cell cycle arrest [90]. In an in vitro study,
genistein has been shown to decrease the enrichment of trimethylated markers (e.g., H3K27me3, H3K9me3, and H3K4me3) and increased the acetylat-
ing markers (e.g., H4K8ac and H3K4ac) at the promoters of six different
key genes involved in cell proliferation, motility, and differentiation [91].
Genistein treatment of breast cancer cells increased the expression levels
of TSGs including $p21^{WAF1\ CIP1}$ and $p16^{INK4a}$ and decreased the expression of
tumor promoter genes (TPGs) including *BMI1* and *c-Myc* through histone
modifications. Genistein-mediated upregulation of TSGs and downregulation of TPGs led to the suppression of breast tumorigenesis both in vitro and
in vivo [92, 93].

In addition to altering DNA methylation and histone modifications,
genistein has been shown to increase the expression of tumor suppressor
miR-34a, leading to downregulation of its target gene, *HOX transcript antisense RNA* (*HOTAIR*). The inhibition of *HOTAIR* decreased the cell proliferation, migration, and invasion, and induced cellular apoptosis and cell
cycle arrest [94]. Genistein also upregulated the expression of miR-574-3p,
leading to inhibited cell proliferation, migration, and invasion, and induction
of apoptosis both in vitro and in vivo [95]. Further, the treatment of PC-3
cells with genistein upregulated miR-1296 and suppressed the expression
of its target gene, i.e., *minichromosome maintenance-2* (*MCM2*) that is frequently found to be upregulated in various cancers including prostate cancer
[96]. Genistein treatment downregulated the expression of onco-miRs such
as miR-221 and miR-222 in PC-3 cells leading to upregulation of *aplysia
ras homolog I* (*ARH1*), which is a putative target of these miRNAs. Genis-
tein-induced overexpression of *ARH1* led to inhibition of cell proliferation
and invasion [97]. Genistein treatment of prostate cancer cells significantly

downregulated the expression of onco-MiR-1260b and induced the expression of *SFRP1* and *Smad4* via direct regulation. Genistein also increased the expression of these two genes via promoter hypomethylation and histone modifications, leading to inhibition of cellular proliferation, invasion, and induction of apoptosis [98]. In addition, genistein treatment has shown to inhibit the expression of miR-27a in uveal melanoma, ovarian cancer, and pancreatic cancer cells. The downregulation of miR-27a led to the upregulation of *zinc finger and BTB domain containing 10* (*ZBTB10*) and *Sprouty2* and suppressed proliferation, migration, and invasion and induced apoptosis in these cells [15].

14.3.2.4   Resveratrol

Resveratrol is a dietary polyphenol found mostly in grapes, but also found in other plant sources like berries and peanuts. Resveratrol has shown to exert anticancer activities through various mechanisms, including epigenetic modulations against different cancers. Resveratrol treatment was previously reported to restore aromatic hydrocarbon receptor (AHR)-mediated enrichment of monomethylated-H3K9, DNMT1, and MBD2 at the *BRCA-1* promoter, leading to its reactivation in human breast cancer MCF-7 cells [99]. Resveratrol treatment of MCF-7 cells also decreased methylation at the promoter region of phosphatase and tensin homolog (PTEN), which led to the induction of PTEN expression and resulting in inhibition of cellular proliferation. Furthermore, resveratrol treatment downregulated the expression of DNMTs and unregulated p21$^{WAF1/CIP1}$ expression in these cells [100]. The acetylation of oncogenic transcription factor, STAT3, helps in maintaining methylation at the promoters of TSGs through interaction between acetylated-STAT3 and DNMT1.

The treatment of triple-negative breast cancer cells with resveratrol reduced the levels of acetylated-STAT3 and led to demethylation and activation of *ERα*, thereby sensitizing these cells to antiestrogens [101]. In an *in vivo* study, resveratrol treatment decreased the expression of DMNT3b in mammary tumor tissues, whereas the expression was increased in normal mammary tissue. Furthermore, resveratrol treatment significantly increased the expression of miR-21, miR-129, miR-204, and miR-489 in tumors and decreased their expression in the normal tissue. In the same study, the authors provide evidence for an inverse association between DNMT3b and miR129, miR-204, and miR-489 in normal and tumor tissues [102]. Resveratrol treatment inhibited estradiol (E2)-mediated alterations in promoter methylation of *Nrf2*, leading to its induction well as downregulation of miR-93, which led to suppression of breast carcinogenesis in vivo [103].

Several studies have shown that resveratrol treatment activates SIRT1 expression in both in vitro and in vivo models [104, 105]. On the contrary, resveratrol treatment of Hodgkin lymphoma (HL)-derived L-428 cells decreases the expression and activity of SIRT1 and led to a marked increase in acetylated-p53 and -FOXO3a, leading to cellular apoptosis [106]. Considering the dual function of SIRT1 as tumor promoter and/or tumor suppressor, both the activation and inhibition of SIRT1 in cancer cells might be beneficial [107]. Wang et al. [108] found that bioactive dietary components including resveratrol induce BRCA1 expression by altering H3 acetylation. Resveratrol treatment of prostate cancer cells causes downregulation of the MTA1 protein, resulting in the destabilization of MTA1/NuRD chromatin remodeling complex, which led to p53 acetylation/activation and induction of cellular apoptosis in these cells [109]. Resveratrol treatment of hepatocellular carcinoma HepG2 cells showed specific inhibition of HDACs, leading to histone hyperacetylation and decreased cellular proliferation [110]. Furthermore, resveratrol treatment was shown to promote acetylation and reactivation of PTEN via inhibition of the MTA1/HDAC complex, which results in the inhibition of the Akt pathway and decreased proliferative index of prostate cancer cells both in vitro and in vivo [111].

14.3.2.5   Sulforaphane

Sulforaphane is an isothiocyanate found in cruciferous vegetables such as broccoli sprouts, cauliflower, and cabbage. Sulforaphane has shown to exert anticancer activities against different cancers through regulating several carcinogenic processes including cell cycle arrest and induction of cellular apoptosis. The epigenetic modulatory activity of sulforaphane is mostly attributed to its HDAC inhibitory effects [2, 13, 49, 112]. In addition to its HDAC-inhibitory activity, sulforaphane also downregulates the expression of DNMTs that led to downregulation of *hTERT* through promoter demethylation-induced binding of the CTCF repressor protein. The downregulation of *hTERT* further led to the inhibition of cellular proliferation and induction of apoptosis in human breast cancer cells [113]. Recently, sulforaphane treatment has also shown to inhibit the telomerase activity in prostate cancer cells through acetylation of H3K18 and di-methylation of H3K4, and enrichment of methyl-CpG binding protein 2 (MeCP2) at the *hTERT* promoter [114]. Sulforaphane treatment also decreases the expression of DNMT1 and DNMT3b in prostate cancer cells, which was associated with the promoter demethylation of *cyclin D2* and exerts antiproliferative effect [115]. Sulforaphane-mediated demethylation of *Nrf2* promoter enhances the expression of its target genes in 12-Otetradecanoylphorbol-13-acetate (TPA)-stimulated mouse skin epidermal JB6 (JB6 P+) cells [116]. Treatment of colon cancer cells with sulforaphane causes loss of HDAC3, HDAC6, and SIRT6, and subsequently enhanced the acetylation and degradation of critical repair proteins including CtIP [117]. Sulforaphane treatment stimulated the ubiquitination and acetylation of SUV39H1 in highly metastatic prostate cancer PC3 cells, and thus led to a decrease in H3K9me3 levels [118]. Further, the combination of sulforaphane with GTPs has shown to reactivate the expression of key TSGs (*p21^{CIP1 WAF1}* and *KLOTHO*) in ERα-negative human breast cancer cells [61].

The role of sulforaphane in modulating miRNA expressions in cancer cells is limited and has been extensively reviewed recently [119]. Sulforaphane has been shown to downregulate the expression of miR-21 through Wnt/β-catenin signaling. This effect of sulforaphane was shown to enhance temozolomide (TMZ)-induced apoptosis in TMZ-resistant glioblastoma cells [120]. Sulforaphane treatment in ERα-negative ductal carcinoma in situ (DCIS) model of early breast cancer restored the expression of downregulated miR-140 and decreased stemness markers, SOX9 and ALDH1, resulting in reduced tumor growth [121].

14.3.2.6 Other Dietary Phytochemicals

In addition to the abovementioned compounds, some other dietary phytochemicals have also shown potential epigenetic modulatory activities against certain cancers. For example, lycopene, a tomato-derived dietary agent, has shown to demethylate the promoter of *GSTP1*, leading to its reactivation in human breast cancer MDA-MB-468 cells [122]. Lycopene treatment significantly decreased the promoter methylation of *GSTP1* and increased the expression of the GSTP1 protein in androgen-independent prostate cancer PC-3 cells, but not in androgen-dependent LNCaP cells. Further, lycopene treatment decreases DNMT3A expression in PC-3 cells [123].

Quercetin is another dietary polyphenol found in many fruits, vegetables, and grains. Quercetin treatment of human colon cancer RKO cells diminished the promoter hypermethylation of $p16^{INK4a}$, thereby inhibiting cellular proliferation [124]. Quercetin has been shown to decrease the methylation of EGCG (which is 50% of total EGCG found in prostate tissue and is less bioactive), thereby increasing the antiproliferative activity of EGCG in prostate cancer cells [125]. Quercetin treatment of human leukemia cells causes histone hyperacetylation contributing to its anticancer activity through induction of apoptotic cell death [126]. Treatment of human leukemia HL-60 cells with quercetin increased histone H3 acetylation and the upregulation of FasL, an inducer of extrinsic apoptotic pathway. Furthermore, quercetin led to the activation of HATs and the inhibition of HDACs, which contributed to quercetin-induced histone acetylation [127].

Allyl derivatives derived from garlic including allyl mercaptan, diallyl disulfide, S-allylcysteine, S-allylmercaptocysteine, and allicin have been shown to inhibit HDAC activities in human cancer cells. Amongst them, allyl mercaptan was found to be the most potent HDAC inhibitor and enhanced sp3 binding at the promoter of $p21^{CIP1/WAF1}$, leading to G0/G1 phase cell cycle arrest in colon cancer cells [128]. In addition, grape seed proanthocyanidins (GSPs) show inhibition of DNA methylation and induce histone modifications, leading to the activation of TSGs in skin cancer A431 and SCC13 cells [129]. Overall, most of the bioactive supplements possess epigenetic modulatory potential which plays a significant role in cancer prevention and therapy (Figure 14.4).

14.4 CONCLUSION AND FUTURE PERSPECTIVES

It is well accepted from the abovementioned studies that epigenetic modifications play a significant role in the process of carcinogenesis and might serve as therapeutic targets. DNMTs and HDACs are the well-known epigenetic targets, which have been already targeted with drugs successfully in certain types of cancers particularly hematological malignancies. However, the efficacy of these drugs in solid tumors is still lacking, and better strategies are required to optimize the use of such inhibitors in multiple cancer types. Moreover, rapid development of drugs against novel and emerging epigenetic targets is needed. The usage of dietary phytochemicals in cancer prevention and therapy is highly encouraged due to their wide availabil-

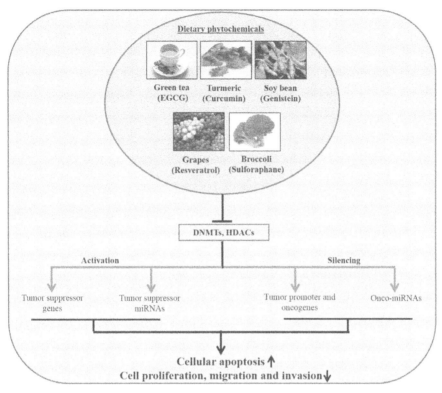

FIGURE 14.4 Epigenetic modulatory effects of various dietary phytochemicals in cancer prevention and therapy. Different phytochemicals and their active constituents mentioned within the parenthesis are endowed with several epigenetic modulatory activities. The inhibition of DNMTs and HDACs by dietary phytochemicals leads to the activation of TSGs and tumor suppressor miRNAs, and silencing of oncogenes and onco-miRNAs. These epigenetic alterations ultimately lead to cancer-specific effects through induction of cellular apoptosis and inhibition of cell proliferation, migration, and invasion.

ity and negligible side effects compared with synthetic drugs. The reports mentioned in this chapter clearly demonstrate that these dietary components target different epigenetic markers and execute anticancer effects. Recent studies have also shown that dietary phytochemicals in combination with available chemotherapeutic agents exert synergistic anticancer effects by overcoming chemotherapy resistance and increasing sensitivity. More preclinical studies are required for better understanding of the epigenetic modulatory activities of these dietary phytochemicals to further enhance the efficacy of these compounds. Further, preclinical studies are of great need to optimize the dosage, route of administration, tissue distribution, and bioavailability of these compounds to push them into clinical phases. Additionally, the exploration of more dietary compounds with epigenetic modulatory activities and promising strategies for their use in cancer prevention and therapy is warranted.

14.5 SUMMARY

- The epigenetically induced silencing of TSGs and overexpression of oncogenes paves the way for epigenetic manipulations in cancer prevention and therapy.
- Enzymes catalyzing DNA methylation, i.e., DNMTs, and histone deacetylation, i.e., HDACs, are well-studied epigenetic targets in cancer.
- MicroRNA-mediated gene silencing is an emerging epigenetic phenomenon targeting several tumor suppressors and oncogenes.
- The inhibitors of DNMTs and HDACs are approved for the treatment of hematological malignancies and are undergoing clinical development against solid tumors.
- As diet has greater impact on altering epigenetic patterns, dietary phytochemicals are proven to be of great importance in cancer prevention and therapy.
- The added advantages with dietary phytochemicals are lesser side effects and easy accessibility compared with synthetic drugs.

KEYWORDS

- **dietary phytochemicals**
- **DNA methylation**
- **DNA methyltransferase**
- **histone deacetylase**
- **histone modifications**
- **microRNA**
- **oncogenes**
- **tumor suppressor genes**

REFERENCES

1. Tsai, H. C., & Baylin, S. B., (2011). Cancer epigenetics: linking basic biology to clinical medicine. *Cell Res., 21*(3), 502–517.
2. Khan, S., Shukla, S., Sinha, S., & Meeran, S. M., (2016). Epigenetic targets in cancer and aging: dietary and therapeutic interventions. *Expert Opin. Ther. Targets,* 1–15.
3. Thakur, V. S., Deb, G., Babcook, M. A., & Gupta, S., (2014). Plant phytochemicals as epigenetic modulators: role in cancer chemoprevention. *AAPS J., 16*(1), 151–163.
4. Taby, R., & Issa, J. P., (2010). Cancer epigenetics. *CA Cancer J. Clin., 60*(6), 376–392.
5. Meeran, S. M., Ahmed, A., & Tollefsbol, T. O., (2010). Epigenetic targets of bioactive dietary components for cancer prevention and therapy. *Clin. Epigenetics, 1*(3–4), 101–116.
6. Belinsky, S. A., Nikula, K. J., Palmisano, W. A., Michels, R., Saccomanno, G., Gabrielson, E., Baylin, S. B., & Herman, J. G., (1998). Aberrant methylation of p16(INK4a) is an early event in lung cancer and a potential biomarker for early diagnosis. *Proc. Natl. Acad. Sci. USA, 95*(20), 11891–11896.
7. Weigel, R. J., & deConinck, E. C., (1993). Transcriptional control of estrogen receptor in estrogen receptor-negative breast carcinoma. *Cancer Res. 53*(15), 3472–3474.
8. Tapia, T., Smalley, S. V., Kohen, P., Muñoz, A., Solis, L. M., Corvalan, A., Faundez, P., Devoto, L., Camus, M., Alvarez, M., & Carvallo, P., (2008). Promoter hypermethylation of BRCA1 correlates with absence of expression in hereditary breast cancer tumors. *Epigenetics, 3*(3), 157–163.
9. Kanwal, R., & Gupta, S., (2010). Epigenetics and cancer. *J. Appl. Physiol., 109*(2), 598–605.
10. Mittal, A., Piyathilake, C., Hara, Y., & Katiyar, S. K., (2003). Exceptionally high protection of photocarcinogenesis by topical application of (--)-epigallocatechin-3-gallate in hydrophilic cream in SKH-1 hairless mouse model: relationship to inhibition of UVB-induced global DNA hypomethylation. *Neoplasia, 5*(6), 555–565.
11. Shukla, S., & Meeran, S. M., (2013). Epigenetic factors in breast cancer progression, in: Ahmad A. (Ed.), *Breast Cancer Metastasis and Drug Resistance*, Springer Publications, New York, 341–365.
12. Shukla, S., Khan, S., Tollefsbol, T. O., & Meeran, S. M., (2013). Genetics and epigenetics of lung cancer: mechanisms and future perspectives. *Curr. Cancer Ther. Rev., 9*, 97–110.
13. Shukla, S., Meeran, S. M., & Katiyar, S. K., (2014). Epigenetic regulation by selected dietary phytochemicals in cancer chemoprevention. *Cancer Lett., 355*(1), 9–17.
14. Dawson, M. A., & Kouzarides, T., (2012). Cancer epigenetics: from mechanism to therapy. *Cell, 150*(1), 12–27.
15. Phuah, N. H., & Nagoor, N. H., (2014). Regulation of microRNAs by natural agents: new strategies in cancer therapies. *Biomed. Res. Int.,* 804510.
16. Winter, J., Jung, S., Keller, S., Gregory, R. I., & Diederichs, S., (2009). Many roads to maturity: microRNA biogenesis pathways and their regulation. *Nat. Cell Biol., 11*(3), 228–234.
17. Hammond, S. M., Bernstein, E., Beach, D., & Hannon, G. J., (2000). An RNA-directed nuclease mediates post-transcriptional gene silencing in Drosophila cells. *Nature, 404*(6775), 293–296.
18. Calin, G. A., & Croce, C. M., (2006). MicroRNA signatures in human cancers. *Nat. Rev. Cancer, 6*(11), 857–866.

19. Wiemer, E. A., (2007). The role of microRNAs in cancer: no small matter. *Eur. J. Cancer, 43*(10), 1529–1544.

20. Palanichamy, J. K., & Rao, D. S., (2014). miRNA dysregulation in cancer: towards a mechanistic understanding. *Front. Genet, 5*, 54.

21. Di Leva, G., Garofalo, M., & Croce, C. M., (2014). MicroRNAs in cancer. *Annu. Rev. Pathol., 9*, 287–314.

22. Ling, H., Fabbri, M., & Calin, G. A., (2013). MicroRNAs and other non-coding RNAs as targets for anticancer drug development. *Nat. Rev. Drug Discov., 12*(11), 847–865.

23. Titone, R., Morani, F., Follo, C., Vidoni, C., Mezzanzanica, D., & Isidoro, C., (2014). Epigenetic control of autophagy by microRNAs in ovarian cancer. *Biomed. Res. Int., 343*–542.

24. Tan, S., Wu, Y., Zhang, C. Y., & Li, J., (2013). Potential microRNA targets for cancer chemotherapy. *Curr. Med. Chem., 20*(29), 3574–3581.

25. Tollefsbol, T. O., (2014). Dietary epigenetics in cancer and aging. *Cancer Treat. Res., 159*, 257–267.

26. Ayissi, V. B., Ebrahimi, A., & Schluesenner, H., (2014). Epigenetic effects of natural polyphenols: a focus on SIRT1-mediated mechanisms. *Mol. Nutr. Food Res., 58*(1), 22–32.

27. Provinciali, M., Cardelli, M., Marchegiani, F., & Pierpaoli, E., (2013). Impact of cellular senescence in aging and cancer. *Curr. Pharm. Des., 19*(9), 1699–1709.

28. DeWoskin, V. A., & Million, R. P., (2013). The epigenetics pipeline. *Nat. Rev. Drug Discov., 12*(9), 661–662.

29. Chen, M., Shabashvili, D., Nawab, A., Yang, S. X., Dyer, L. M., Brown, K. D., Hollingshead, M., Hunter, K. W., Kaye, F. J., Hochwald, S. N., Marquez, V. E., Steeg, P., & Zajac-Kaye, M., (2012). DNA methyltransferase inhibitor, zebularine, delays tumor growth and induces apoptosis in a genetically engineered mouse model of breast cancer. *Mol. Cancer Ther., 11*(2), 370–382.

30. Yang, P. M., Lin, Y. T., Shun, C. T., Lin, S. H., Wei, T. T., Chuang, S. H., Wu, M. S., & Chen, C. C., (2013). Zebularine inhibits tumorigenesis and stemness of colorectal cancer via p53-dependent endoplasmic reticulum stress. *Sci. Rep., 3*, 3219.

31. You, B. R., & Park, W. H., (2014). Zebularine inhibits the growth of A549 lung cancer cells via cell cycle arrest and apoptosis. *Mol. Carcinog., 53*(11), 847–857.

32. Napso, T., & Fares, F., (2014). Zebularine induces prolonged apoptosis effects via the caspase-3/PARP pathway in head and neck cancer cells. *Int. J. Oncol., 44*(6), 1971–1979.

33. Graça, I., Sousa, E. J., Baptista, T., Almeida, M., Ramalho-Carvalho, J., Palmeira, C., Henrique, R., & Jerónimo, C., (2014). Anti-tumoral effect of the non-nucleoside DNMT inhibitor RG108 in human prostate cancer cells. *Curr. Pharm. Des., 20*(11), 1803–1811.

34. Falkenberg, K. J., & Johnstone, R. W., (2014). Histone deacetylases and their inhibitors in cancer, neurological diseases and immune disorders. *Nat. Rev. Drug Discov., 13*(9), 673–691.

35. Tan, P., Wei, A., Mithraprabhu, S., Cummings, N., Liu, H. B., Perugini, M., Reed, K., Avery, S., Patil, S., Walker, P., Mollee, P., Grigg, A., D'Andrea, R., Dear, A., & Spencer, A., (2014). Dual epigenetic targeting with panobinostat and azacitidine in acute myeloid leukemia and high-risk myelodysplastic syndrome. *Blood Cancer J., 4*, e170.

36. San-Miguel, J. F., Hungria, V. T., Yoon, S. S., Beksac, M., Dimopoulos, M. A., Elghandour, A., Jedrzejczak, W. W., Günther, A., Nakorn, T. N., Siritanaratkul, N., Corradini,

P., Chuncharunee, S., Lee, J. J., Schlossman, R. L., Shelekhova, T., Yong, K., Tan, D., Numbenjapon, T., Cavenagh, J. D., Hou, J., LeBlanc, R., Nahi, H., Qiu, L., Salwender, H., Pulini, S., Moreau, P., Warzocha, K., White, D., Bladé, J., Chen, W., de la Rubia, J., Gimsing, P., Lonial, S., Kaufman, J. L., Ocio, E. M., Veskovski, L., Sohn, S. K., Wang, M. C., Lee, J. H., Einsele, H., Sopala, M., Corrado, C., Bengoudifa, B. R., Binlich, F., & Richardson, P. G., (2014). Panobinostat plus bortezomib and dexamethasone versus placebo plus bortezomib and dexamethasone in patients with relapsed or relapsed and refractory multiple myeloma: a multicentre, randomised, double-blind phase 3 trial. *Lancet. Oncol., 15*(11), 1195–1206.

37. Guha, M., (2015). HDAC inhibitors still need a home run, despite recent approval. *Nat. Rev. Drug Discov., 14*(4), 225–226.

38. Jovanovic, J., Rønneberg, J. A., Tost, J., & Kristensen, V., (2010). The epigenetics of breast cancer. *Mol. Oncol., 4*(3), 242–254.

39. Witta, S., (2012). Histone deacetylase inhibitors in non-small-cell lung cancer. *J. Thorac. Oncol., 7*(16 Suppl 5), S404–406.

40. Gridelli, C., Rossi, A., & Maione, P., (2008). The potential role of histone deacetylase inhibitors in the treatment of non-small-cell lung cancer. *Crit. Rev. Oncol. Hematol., 68*(1), 29–36.

41. Lo, P. K., & Sukumar, S., (2008). Epigenomics and breast cancer. *Pharmacogenomics, 9*(12), 1879–1902.

42. Garcia-Manero, G., Tambaro, F. P., Bekele, N. B., Yang, H., Ravandi, F., Jabbour, E., Borthakur, G., Kadia, T. M., Konopleva, M. Y., Faderl, S., Cortes, J. E., Brandt, M., Hu, Y., McCue, D., Newsome, W. M., Pierce, S. R., De Lima, M., & Kantarjian, H. M., (2012). Phase II trial of vorinostat with idarubicin and cytarabine for patients with newly diagnosed acute myelogenous leukemia or myelodysplastic syndrome. *J. Clin. Oncol., 30*(18), 2204–2210.

43. Badros, A., Burger, A. M., Philip, S., Niesvizky, R., Kolla, S. S., Goloubeva, O., Harris, C., Zwiebel, J., Wright, J. J., Espinoza-Delgado, I., Baer, M. R., Holleran, J. L., Egorin, M. J., & Grant, S., (2009). Phase I study of vorinostat in combination with bortezomib for relapsed and refractory multiple myeloma. *Clin. Cancer Res., 15*(16), 5250–5257.

44. Weber, D. M., Graef, T., Hussein, M., Sobecks, R. M., Schiller, G. J., Lupinacci, L., Hardwick, J. S., & Jagannath, S., (2012). Phase I trial of vorinostat combined with bortezomib for the treatment of relapsing and/or refractory multiple myeloma. *Clin. Lymphoma. Myeloma. Leuk., 12*(5), 319–324.

45. Fenaux, P., & Ades, L., (2009). Review of azacitidine trials in Intermediate-2-and High-risk myelodysplastic syndromes. *Leuk. Res., 33, Suppl 2*, S7–11.

46. Gore, S. D., (2011). New ways to use DNA methyltransferase inhibitors for the treatment of myelodysplastic syndrome. *Hematology Am. Soc. Hematol. Educ. Program.*, 550–555.

47. Li, Y., Yuan, Y. Y., Meeran, S. M., & Tollefsbol, T. O., (2010). Synergistic epigenetic re-activation of estrogen receptor-α (ERα) by combined green tea polyphenol and histone deacetylase inhibitor in ERα-negative breast cancer cells. *Mol. Cancer, 9*, 274.

48. Saxena, N. K., & Sharma, D., (2010). Epigenetic reactivation of estrogen receptor: Promising tools for restoring response to endocrine therapy. *Mol. Cell Pharmacol., 2*(5), 191–202.

49. Meeran, S. M., Patel, S. N., Li, Y., Shukla, S., & Tollefsbol, T. O., (2012). Bioactive dietary supplements reactivate ER expression in ER-negative breast cancer cells by active chromatin modifications. *PLoS One, 7*(5), e37748.

50. Pudenz, M., Roth, K., & Gerhauser, C., (2014). Impact of soy isoflavones on the epigenome in cancer prevention. *Nutrients, 6*(10), 4218–4272.

51. Chang, L. C., & Yu, Y. L., (2016). Dietary components as epigenetic-regulating agents against cancer. *Biomedicine (Taipei), 6*(1), 2.

52. Shirakami, Y., Shimizu, M., & Moriwaki, H., (2012)., Cancer chemoprevention with green tea catechins: from bench to bed. *Curr. Drug Targets, 13*(14), 1842–1857.

53. Henning, S. M., Wang, P., Carpenter, C. L., & Heber, D., (2013). Epigenetic effects of green tea polyphenols in cancer. *Epigenomics, 5*(6), 729–741.

54. Gao, Y., & Tollefsbol, T. O., (2015). Impact of Epigenetic Dietary Components on Cancer through Histone Modifications. *Curr. Med. Chem., 22*(17), 2051–2064.

55. Fang, M. Z., Wang, Y., Ai, N., Hou, Z., Sun, Y., Lu, H., Welsh, W., & Yang, C. S., (2003). Tea polyphenol (-)-epigallocatechin-3-gallate inhibits DNA methyltransferase and reactivates methylation-silenced genes in cancer cell lines. *Cancer Res., 63*(22), 7563–7570.

56. Nandakumar, V., Vaid, M., & Katiyar, S. K., (2011). (-)-Epigallocatechin-3-gallate reactivates silenced tumor suppressor genes, Cip1/p21 and p16INK4a, by reducing DNA methylation and increasing histones acetylation in human skin cancer cells. *Carcinogenesis, 32*(4), 537–544.

57. Montenegro, M. F., Sáez-Ayala, M., Piñero-Madrona, A., Cabezas-Herrera, J., & Rodríguez-López, J. N., (2012). Reactivation of the tumour suppressor RASSF1A in breast cancer by simultaneous targeting of DNA and E2F1 methylation. *PLoS One, 7*(12), e52231.

58. Mittal, A., Pate, M. S., Wylie, R. C., Tollefsbol, T. O., & Katiyar, S. K., (2004). EGCG down-regulates telomerase in human breast carcinoma MCF-7 cells, leading to suppression of cell viability and induction of apoptosis. *Int. J. Oncol., 24*(3), 703–710.

59. Berletch, J. B., Liu, C., Love, W. K., Andrews, L. G., Katiyar, S. K., & Tollefsbol, T. O., (2008). Epigenetic and genetic mechanisms contribute to telomerase inhibition by EGCG *J. Cell Biochem., 103*(2), 509–519.

60. Gao, Z., Xu, Z., Hung, M. S., Lin, Y. C., Wang, T., Gong, M., Zhi, X., Jablon, D. M., & You, L., (2009). Promoter demethylation of WIF-1 by epigallocatechin-3-gallate in lung cancer cells. *Anticancer. Res., 29*(6), 2025–2030.

61. Sinha, S, Shukla, S., Khan, S., Tollefsbol, T. O., & Meeran, S. M., (2015). Epigenetic reactivation of p21CIP1/WAF1 and KLOTHO by a combination of bioactive dietary supplements is partially ERα-dependent in ERα-negative human breast cancer cells. *Mol. Cell Endocrinol., 406*, 102–114.

62. Lambert, J. D., Sang, S., Hong, J., Kwon, S. J., Lee, M. J., Ho, C. T., & Yang, C. S., (2006). Peracetylation as a means of enhancing in vitro bioactivity and bioavailability of epigallocatechin-3-gallate. *Drug Metab. Dispos., 34*(12), 2111–2116.

63. Landis-Piwowar, K. R., Huo, C., Chen, D., Milacic, V., Shi, G., Chan, T. H., & Dou, Q. P., (2007). A novel prodrug of the green tea polyphenol (-)-epigallocatechin-3-gallate as a potential anticancer agent. *Cancer Res., 67*(9), 4303–4310.

64. Meeran, S. M., Patel, S. N., Chan, T. H., & Tollefsbol, T. O., (2011). A novel prodrug of epigallocatechin-3-gallate: differential epigenetic hTERT repression in human breast cancer cells. *Cancer Prev. Res. (Phila), 4*(8), 1243–1254.

65. Tsang, W. P., & Kwok, T. T., (2010). Epigallocatechin gallate up-regulation of miR-16 and induction of apoptosis in human cancer cells. *J. Nutr. Biochem., 21*(2), 140–146.

66. Wang, H., Bian, S., & Yang, C. S., (2011). Green tea polyphenol EGCG suppresses lung cancer cell growth through upregulating miR-210 expression caused by stabilizing HIF-1α. *Carcinogenesis, 32*(12), 1881–1889.

67. Zhou, H., Chen, J. X., Yang, C. S., Yang, M. Q., Deng, Y., & Wang, H., (2014). Gene regulation mediated by microRNAs in response to green tea polyphenol EGCG in mouse lung cancer. *BMC Genomics, 15 Suppl., 11*, S3.

68. Chakrabarti, M., Ai, W., Banik, N. L., & Ray, S. K., (2013). Overexpression of miR-7–1 increases efficacy of green tea polyphenols for induction of apoptosis in human malignant neuroblastoma SH-SY5Y and SK-N-DZ cells. *Neurochem. Res., 38*(2), 420–432.

69. Henning, S. M., Wang, P., Said, J., Magyar, C., Castor, B., Doan, N., Tosity, C., Moro, A., Gao, K., Li, L., & Heber, D., (2012). Polyphenols in brewed green tea inhibit prostate tumor xenograft growth by localizing to the tumor and decreasing oxidative stress and angiogenesis. *J. Nutr. Biochem., 23*(11), 1537–1542.

70. Volate, S. R., Muga, S. J., Issa, A. Y., Nitcheva, D., Smith, T., & Wargovich, M. J., (2009). Epigenetic modulation of the retinoid X receptor alpha by green tea in the azoxymethane-Apc Min/+ mouse model of intestinal cancer. *Mol. Carcinog., 48*(10), 920–933.

71. Yuasa, Y., Nagasaki, H., Akiyama, Y., Hashimoto, Y., Takizawa, T., Kojima, K., Kawano, T., Sugihara, K., Imai, K., & Nakachi, K., (2009). DNA methylation status is inversely correlated with green tea intake and physical activity in gastric cancer patients. *Int. J. Cancer 124*(11), 2677–2682.

72. Liu, Z., Xie, Z., Jones, W., Pavlovicz, R. E., Liu, S., Yu, J., Li, P. K., Lin, J., Fuchs, J. R., Marcucci, G., Li, C., & Chan, K. K., (2009). Curcumin is a potent DNA hypomethylation agent. *Bioorg. Med. Chem. Lett., 19*(3), 706–709.

73. Khor, T. O., Huang, Y., Wu, T. Y., Shu, L., Lee, J., & Kong, A. N., (2011). Pharmacodynamics of curcumin as DNA hypomethylation agent in restoring the expression of Nrf2 via promoter CpGs demethylation. *Biochem. Pharmacol., 82*(9), 1073–1078.

74. Shu, L., Khor, T. O., Lee, J. H., Boyanapalli, S. S., Huang, Y., Wu, T. Y., Saw, C. L., Cheung, K. L., & Kong, A. N., (2011). Epigenetic CpG demethylation of the promoter and reactivation of the expression of Neurog1 by curcumin in prostate LNCaP cells. *AAPS J., 13*(4), 606–614.

75. Jha, A. K., Nikbakht, M., Parashar, G., Shrivastava, A., Capalash, N., & Kaur, J., (2010). Reversal of hypermethylation and reactivation of the RARβ2 gene by natural compounds in cervical cancer cell lines. *Folia. Biol. (Praha), 56*(5), 195–200.

76. Marcu, M. G., Jung, Y. J., Lee, S., Chung, E. J., Lee, M. J., Trepel, J., & Neckers, L., (2006). Curcumin is an inhibitor of p300 histone acetylatransferase. *Med. Chem., 2*(2), 169–174.

77. Balasubramanyam, K., Varier, R. A., Altaf, M., Swaminathan, V., Siddappa, N. B., Ranga, U., & Kundu, T. K., (2004). Curcumin, a novel p300/CREB-binding protein-specific inhibitor of acetyltransferase, represses the acetylation of histone/nonhistone proteins and histone acetyltransferase-dependent chromatin transcription. *J. Biol. Chem., 279*(49), 51163–51171.

78. Liu, H. L., Chen, Y., Cui, G. H., & Zhou, J. F., (2005). Curcumin, a potent anti-tumor reagent, is a novel histone deacetylase inhibitor regulating B-NHL cell line Raji proliferation. *Acta. Pharmacol. Sin., 26*(5), 603–609.

79. Hua, W. F., Fu, Y. S., Liao, Y. J., Xia, W. J., Chen, Y. C., Zeng, Y. X., Kung, H. F., & Xie, D., (2010). Curcumin induces down-regulation of EZH2 expression through the MAPK pathway in MDA-MB-435 human breast cancer cells. *Eur. J. Pharmacol., 637*(1–3), 16–21.

80. Yang, J., Cao, Y., Sun, J., & Zhang, Y., (2010). Curcumin reduces the expression of Bcl-2 by upregulating miR-15a and miR-16 in MCF-7 cells. *Med. Oncol., 27*(4), 1114–1118.

81. Sun, M., Estrov, Z., Ji, Y., Coombes, K. R., Harris, D. H., & Kurzrock, R., (2008). Curcumin (diferuloylmethane) alters the expression profiles of microRNAs in human pancreatic cancer cells. *Mol. Cancer Ther., 7*(3), 464–473.

82. Zhang, J., Zhang, T., Ti, X., Shi, J., Wu, C., Ren, X., & Yin, H., (2010). Curcumin promotes apoptosis in A549/DDP multidrug-resistant human lung adenocarcinoma cells through an miRNA signaling pathway. *Biochem. Biophys. Res. Commun., 399*(1), 1–6.

83. Mudduluru, G., George-William, J. N., Muppala, S., Asangani, I. A., Kumarswamy, R., Nelson, L. D., & Allgayer, H., (2011). Curcumin regulates miR-21 expression and inhibits invasion and metastasis in colorectal cancer. *Biosci. Rep., 31*(3), 185–197.

84. Karsli-Ceppioglu, S., Ngollo, M., Judes, G., Penault-LLorca, F., Bignon, Y. J., Guy, L., & Bernard-Gallon, D., (2015). The Role of Soy Phytoestrogens on Genetic and Epigenetic Mechanisms of Prostate Cancer. *Enzymes, 37*, 193–221.

85. Karsli-Ceppioglu, S., Ngollo, M., Adjakly, M., Dagdemir, A., Judes, G., Lebert, A., Boiteux, J. P., Penault-LLorca, F., Bignon, Y. J., Guy, L., & Bernard-Gallon, D., (2015). Genome-wide DNA methylation modified by soy phytoestrogens: role for epigenetic therapeutics in prostate cancer? *OMICS, 19*(4), 209–219.

86. Mahmoud, A. M., Al-Alem, U., Ali, M. M., & Bosland, M. C., (2015). Genistein increases estrogen receptor beta expression in prostate cancer via reducing its promoter methylation. *J. Steroid. Biochem. Mol. Biol., 152*, 62–75.

87. Bosviel, R., Dumollard, E., Dechelotte, P., Bignon, Y. J., & Bernard-Gallon, D., (2012). Can soy phytoestrogens decrease DNA methylation in BRCA1 and BRCA2 oncosuppressor genes in breast cancer? *OMICS, 16*(5), 235–244.

88. Xie, Q., Bai, Q., Zou, L. Y., Zhang, Q. Y., Zhou, Y., Chang, H., Yi, L., Zhu, J. D., & Mi, M. T., (2014). Genistein inhibits DNA methylation and increases expression of tumor suppressor genes in human breast cancer cells. *Genes Chromosomes Cancer,53*(5), 422–431.

89. Li, H., Xu, W., Huang, Y., Huang, X., Xu, L., & Lv, Z., (2012). Genistein demethylates the promoter of CHD5 and inhibits neuroblastoma growth in vivo. *Int. J. Mol. Med., 30*(5), 1081–1086.

90. Yang, Y., Liu, J., Li, X., & Li, J. C., (2012). PCDH17 gene promoter demethylation and cell cycle arrest by genistein in gastric cancer. *Histol. Histopathol., 27*(2), 217–224.

91. Dagdemir, A., Durif, J., Ngollo, M., Bignon, Y. J., & Bernard-Gallon, D., (2013). Histone lysine trimethylation or acetylation can be modulated by phytoestrogen, estrogen or anti-HDAC in breast cancer cell lines. *Epigenomics, 5*(1), 51–63.

92. Li, Y., Chen, H., Hardy, T. M., & Tollefsbol, T. O., (2013). Epigenetic regulation of multiple tumor-related genes leads to suppression of breast tumorigenesis by dietary genistein. *PLoS One, 8*(1), e54369.

93. Wang, H., Li, Q., & Chen, H., (2012). Genistein affects histone modifications on Dickkopf-related protein 1 (DKK1) gene in SW480 human colon cancer cell line. *PLoS One, 7*(7), e40955.

94. Chiyomaru, T., Yamamura, S., Fukuhara, S., Yoshino, H., Kinoshita, T., Majid, S., Saini, S., Chang, I., Tanaka, Y., Enokida, H., Seki, N., Nakagawa, M., & Dahiya, R., (2013). Genistein inhibits prostate cancer cell growth by targeting miR-34a and oncogenic HOTAIR. *PLoS One, 8*(8), e70372.

95. Chiyomaru, T., Yamamura, S., Fukuhara, S., Hidaka, H., Majid, S., Saini, S., Arora, S., Deng, G., Shahryari, V., Chang, I., Tanaka, Y., Tabatabai, Z. L., Enokida, H., Seki, N., Nakagawa, M., & Dahiya, R., (2013). Genistein up-regulates tumor suppressor microRNA-574–3p in prostate cancer. *PLoS One, 8*(3), e58929.

96. Majid, S., Dar, A. A., Saini, S., Chen, Y., Shahryari, V., Liu, J., Zaman, M. S., Hirata, H., Yamamura, S., Ueno, K., Tanaka, Y., & Dahiya, R., (2010). Regulation of minichromosome maintenance gene family by microRNA-1296 and genistein in prostate cancer. *Cancer Res., 70*(7), 2809–2818.

97. Chen, Y., Zaman, M. S., Deng, G., Majid, S., Saini, S., Liu, J., Tanaka, Y., & Dahiya, R., (2011). MicroRNAs 221/222 and genistein-mediated regulation of ARHI tumor suppressor gene in prostate cancer. *Cancer Prev. Res., (Phila), 4*(1), 76–86.

98. Hirata, H., Hinoda, Y., Shahryari, V., Deng, G., Tanaka, Y., Tabatabai, Z. L., & Dahiya, R., (2014). Genistein downregulates onco-miR-1260b and upregulates sFRP1 and Smad4 via demethylation and histone modification in prostate cancer cells. *Br. J. Cancer, 110*(6), 1645–1654.

99. Papoutsis, A. J., Lamore, S. D., Wondrak, G. T., Selmin, O. I., & Romagnolo, D. F., (2010). Resveratrol prevents epigenetic silencing of BRCA-1 by the aromatic hydrocarbon receptor in human breast cancer cells. *J. Nutr., 140*(9), 1607–1614.

100. Stefanska, B., Salamé, P., Bednarek, A., & Fabianowska-Majewska, K., (2012). Comparative effects of retinoic acid, vitamin D and resveratrol alone and in combination with adenosine analogues on methylation and expression of phosphatase and tensin homologue tumour suppressor gene in breast cancer cells. *Br. J. Nutr., 107*(6), 781–790.

101. Lee, H., Zhang, P., Herrmann, A., Yang, C., Xin, H., Wang, Z., Hoon, D. S., Forman, S. J., Jove, R., Riggs, A. D., & Yu, H., (2012). Acetylated STAT3 is crucial for methylation of tumor-suppressor gene promoters and inhibition by resveratrol results in demethylation. *Proc. Natl. Acad. Sci. USA, 109*(20), 7765–7769.

102. Qin, W., Zhang, K., Clarke, K., Weiland, T., & Sauter, E. R., (2014). Methylation and miRNA effects of resveratrol on mammary tumors vs. normal tissue. *Nutr. Cancer, 66*(2), 270–277.

103. Singh, B., Shoulson, R., Chatterjee, A., Ronghe, A., Bhat, N. K., Dim, D. C., & Bhat, H. K., (2014). Resveratrol inhibits estrogen-induced breast carcinogenesis through induction of NRF2-mediated protective pathways. *Carcinogenesis, 35*(8), 1872–1880.

104. Borra, M. T., Smith, B. C., & Denu, J. M., (2005). Mechanism of human SIRT1 activation by resveratrol. *J. Biol. Chem., 280*(17), 17187–17195.

105. De Boer, V. C., de Goffau, M. C., Arts, I. C., Hollman, P. C., & Keijer, J., (2006). SIRT1 stimulation by polyphenols is affected by their stability and metabolism. *Mech. Ageing. Dev., 127*(7), 618–627.

106. Frazzi, R., Valli, R., Tamagnini, I., Casali, B., Latruffe, N., & Merli, F., (2013). Resveratrol-mediated apoptosis of hodgkin lymphoma cells involves SIRT1 inhibition and FOXO3a hyperacetylation. *Int. J. Cancer, 132*(5), 1013–1021.

107. Morris, B. J., (2013). Seven sirtuins for seven deadly diseases of aging. *Free Radic. Biol. Med., 56*, 133–171.

108. Wang, R. H., Zheng, Y., Kim, H. S., Xu, X., Cao, L., Luhasen, T., Lee, M. H., Xiao, C., Vassilopoulos, A., Chen, W., Gardner, K., Man, Y. G., Hung, M. C., Finkel, T., &

Deng, C. X., (2008). Interplay among BRCA1, SIRT1, & Survivin during BRCA1-associated tumorigenesis. *Mol. Cell, 32*(1), 11–20.

109. Kai, L., Samuel, S. K., & Levenson, A. S., (2010). Resveratrol enhances p53 acetylation and apoptosis in prostate cancer by inhibiting MTA1/NuRD complex. *Int. J. Cancer, 126*(7), 1538–1548.

110. Venturelli, S., Berger, A., Böcker, A., Busch, C., Weiland, T., Noor, S., Leischner, C., Schleicher, S., Mayer, M., Weiss, T. S., Bischoff, S. C., Lauer, U. M., & Bitzer, M., (2013). Resveratrol as a pan-HDAC inhibitor alters the acetylation status of histone [corrected] proteins in human-derived hepatoblastoma cells. *PLoS One, 8*(8), e73097.

111. Dhar, S., Kumar, A., Li, K., Tzivion, G., & Levenson, A. S., (2015). Resveratrol regulates PTEN/Akt pathway through inhibition of MTA1/HDAC unit of the NuRD complex in prostate cancer. *Biochim. Biophys. Acta., 1853*(2), 265–275.

112. Myzak, M. C., Karplus, P. A., Chung, F. L., & Dashwood, R. H., (2004). A novel mechanism of chemoprotection by sulforaphane: inhibition of histone deacetylase. *Cancer Res., 64*(16), 5767–5774.

113. Meeran, S. M., Patel, S. N., & Tollefsbol, T. O., (2010). Sulforaphane causes epigenetic repression of hTERT expression in human breast cancer cell lines. *PLoS One, 5*(7), e11457.

114. Abbas, A., Hall, J. A., Patterson, W. L., Ho, E., Hsu, A., Al-Mulla, F., & Georgel, P. T., (2016). Sulforaphane modulates telomerase activity via epigenetic regulation in prostate cancer cell lines. *Biochem. Cell Biol., 94*(1), 71–81.

115. Hsu, A., Wong, C. P., Yu, Z., Williams, D. E., Dashwood, R. H., & Ho, E., (2011). Promoter de-methylation of cyclin D2 by sulforaphane in prostate cancer cells. *Clin. Epigenetics., 3*, 3.

116. Su, Z. Y., Zhang, C., Lee, J. H., Shu, L., Wu, T. Y., Khor, T. O., Conney, A. H., Lu, Y. P., & Kong, A. N., (2014). Requirement and epigenetics reprogramming of Nrf2 in suppression of tumor promoter TPA-induced mouse skin cell transformation by sulforaphane. *Cancer Prev. Res. (Phila), 7*(3), 319–329.

117. Rajendran, P., Kidane, A. I., Yu, T. W., Dashwood, W. M., Bisson, W. H., Löhr, C. V., Ho, E., Williams, D. E., & Dashwood, R. H., (2013). HDAC turnover, CtIP acetylation and dysregulated DNA damage signaling in colon cancer cells treated with sulforaphane and related dietary isothiocyanates. *Epigenetics, 8*(6), 612–623.

118. Watson, G. W., Wickramasekara, S., Palomera-Sanchez, Z., Black, C., Maier, C. S., Williams, D. E., Dashwood, R. H., & Ho, E., (2014). SUV39H1/H3K9me3 attenuates sulforaphane-induced apoptotic signaling in PC3 prostate cancer cells. *Oncogenesis, 3*, e131.

119. Tortorella, S. M., Royce, S. G., Licciardi, P. V., & Karagiannis, T. C., (2015). Dietary Sulforaphane in Cancer Chemoprevention: The Role of Epigenetic Regulation and HDAC Inhibition. *Antioxid. Redox Signal, 22*(16), 1382–1424.

120. Lan, F., Pan, Q., Yu, H., & Yue, X., (2015). Sulforaphane enhances temozolomide-induced apoptosis because of down-regulation of miR-21 via Wnt/β-catenin signaling in glioblastoma. *J. Neurochem., 134*(5), 811–818.

121. Li, Q., Yao, Y., Eades, G., Liu, Z., Zhang, Y., & Zhou, Q., (2014). Downregulation of miR-140 promotes cancer stem cell formation in basal-like early stage breast cancer. *Oncogene, 33*(20), 2589–2600.

122. King-Batoon, A., Leszczynska, J. M., & Klein, C. B., (2008). Modulation of gene methylation by genistein or lycopene in breast cancer cells. *Environ. Mol. Mutagen., 49*(1), 36–45.

123. Fu, L. J., Ding, Y. B., Wu, L. X., Wen, C. J., Qu, Q., Zhang, X., & Zhou, H. H., (2014)., The Effects of Lycopene on the Methylation of the GSTP1 Promoter and Global Methylation in Prostatic Cancer Cell Lines PC3 and LNCaP. *Int. J. Endocrinol.*, 1–9.

124. Tan, S., Wang, C., Lu, C., Zhao, B., Cui, Y., Shi, X., & Ma, X., (2009). Quercetin is able to demethylate the p16INK4a gene promoter. *Chemotherapy, 55*(1), 6–10.

125. Wang, P., Heber, D., & Henning, S. M., (2012). Quercetin increased the antiproliferative activity of green tea polyphenol (-)-epigallocatechin gallate in prostate cancer cells. *Nutr. Cancer, 64*(4), 580–587.

126. Jia, J., & Chen, J., (2008). Histone hyperacetylation is involved in the quercetin-induced human leukemia cell death. *Pharmazie, 63*(5), 379–383.

127. Lee, W. J., Chen, Y. R., & Tseng, T. H., (2011). Quercetin induces FasL-related apoptosis, in part, through promotion of histone H3 acetylation in human leukemia HL-60 cells. *Oncol. Rep., 25*(2), 583–591.

128. Nian, H., Delage, B., Pinto, J. T., & Dashwood, R. H., (2008). Allyl mercaptan, a garlic-derived organosulfur compound, inhibits histone deacetylase and enhances Sp3 binding on the P21WAF1 promoter. *Carcinogenesis, 29*(9), 1816–1824.

129. Vaid, M., Prasad, R., Singh, T., Jones, V., & Katiyar, S. K., (2012). Grape seed proanthocyanidins reactivate silenced tumor suppressor genes in human skin cancer cells by targeting epigenetic regulators. *Toxicol. Appl. Pharmacol., 263*(1), 122–130.

CHAPTER 15

CANCER STEM CELL: CURRENT UNDERSTANDING AND FUTURE PERSPECTIVES

SONAL SRIVASTAVA, JAYANT DEWANGAN, DIVYA TANDON, and SRIKANTA KUMAR RATH

CSIR-Central Drug Research Institute, Lucknow-226031, India, E-mail: skrath@cdri.res.in

CONTENTS

ABSTRACT

Over the years, advances in stem cell biology have provided new perception in cancer biology. Not all the cancerous cells are equal, as these cells show marked heterogeneity in their morphology, proliferation, genetic injury, and therapeutic response. Thus, cellular and molecular heterogeneity in tumor cells casts a major problem for cancer researchers. Cancer stem cells (CSCs) are "stem-like" cells with exclusive capacity to regenerate tumors and are also referred to as tumorigenic cells. The cancer stem cell hypothesis provides a useful framework for investigating the mechanisms of cancer initiation, progression, and treatment. CSCs share many characteristics with normal stem cells, including self-renewal and differentiation. CSCs can evade the chemopreventive strategies for cancer treatment, and hence, it is necessary to develop therapies that selectively target this population. This chapter will focus on cancer stem cells, their microenvironment, and self-renewal pathways that play a role in cancer propagation and the current therapies that target these cells.

15.1   INTRODUCTION

It was believed that a tumor was a homogenous mass of dysregulated cells, but this concept has now largely been replaced by the view that within a malignant tumor or among the circulating cells of leukemia, there can be a subset of cells with stem cell-like properties. These cells have the properties of self-renewal and of producing progeny that can differentiate into various cell types like the normal stem cells [1]. The normal stem cells help our organs and tissue to renew and sustain. Similarly, the cancer stem cells (CSCs) can reproduce themselves and sustain cancer. CSCs play a central role in tumor progression and recurrence by developing resistance to chemotherapy and radiation [2]. This possibly occurs due to the few stem cells that are left behind after apparently successful chemotherapy that lead to regrowth of the tumor (Figure 15.1). Molecular and genetic analysis of CSCs is the key to understand how these cells differ from other cells of the same tumor type and from normal stem cells. Thus, therapies are needed to effectively and selectively target this population of cells for the cure and management of the tumor.

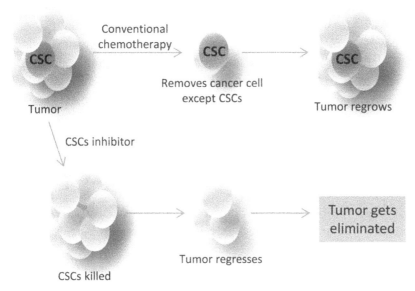

FIGURE 15.1   Selectively targeting CSCs prevents recurrence of tumor after therapy.

15.2   EVIDENCE FOR CANCER STEM CELLS

The first evidence demonstrating the presence of a small subset of cancer cells that were capable of extensive proliferation was documented in leukemia and multiple myeloma. Park and McCulloch et al. separated mouse myeloma cells from mouse ascites, obtained from normal hematopoietic cells. When these cells were subjected to clonal in vitro colony-forming assays, only 1 in 10,000 normal hematopoietic cells to 1 in 100 cancer cells was able to form colonies [3]. These assays implicated that either all leukemia cells had a low probability of extensive proliferation or most leukemia cells were not capable of proliferating extensively and only a subset of cells was consistently clonogenic. Studies of acute myelogenous leukemia (AML) in humans helped in the identification of cells exhibiting CD34+ CD38⁻ cell-surface antigen marker phenotypes comparable with the normal human hematopoietic progenitor cells. These cells represented a small but variable proportion of AML cells and were found to be capable of regenerating human AML cell populations when transplanted in irradiated nonobese diabetic (NOD)/severe combined immunodeficient (SCID) mice [4]. This eliminated the first possibility that all AML cells had a similar clonogenic capacity. Identification of the subset from the different classes of leukemia cells that was capable of proliferating and transferring the disease and was highly enriched for clonogenic capacity proved the second possibility.

Cells within solid tumors are less accessible, thereby limiting the development of functional assays for their detection and quantification. Therefore, it was difficult to substantiate the existence of CSCs. Phenotypically, heterogeneous population of cells are found in solid tumors, out of which only a small proportion is clonogenic in culture and in vivo [5]. Only 1 in 1,000 to 1 in 5,000, lung cancer, ovarian cancer or neuroblastoma cells formed colonies on soft agar [6]. Cells isolated from human medulloblastomas and glioblastomas were able to produce serially transplantable brain tumors in NOD/SCID mice. These cells expressed CD133+, a normal neural stem cell marker. Transplanting a few hundred CD133+ expressing tumor cells was sufficient to initiate the formation of a tumor in the recipient animal, whereas none of the mice injected with the negative population developed brain tumors [7]. Similarly, serial transplantations of CD44+ CD24⁻ cells isolated from human breast tumors were able to develop breast cancer in NOD/SCID mice. These studies implicate that a small subset of tumorigenic cells is capable of tumor formation in such transplant assays, and these cells were considered as CSCs.

15.3 MODELS OF CANCER PROPAGATION

The various models that have been proposed to explain how established tumors propagate themselves are described herein. These models explain that phenotypically and functionally heterogeneous cells exist in tumors just like they exist in normal organs.

15.3.1 THE CSC MODEL

This model refers to the means by which established tumors propagate themselves [8]. The fundamental of the CSC model is that subpopulations of tumorigenic cells existing within a tumor have the ability to divide asymmetrically, yielding a daughter cell that remain as CSC and another daughter cell that differentiates into a non-tumorigenic cell, leading to the formation of the bulk of the tumor. This parallels the development of differentiated cells from normal stem cells in development and homeostasis [9]. In order to make the CSC model useful and testable, it is important to separate tumorigenic cells from nontumorigenic and evaluate them independently. The possibility that a particular cancer follows the CSC model will facilitate understanding of the mechanisms of progression of these cancers, as these rare "stem cell" like populations are different from the bulk population of irreversible nontumorigenic cells and can be studied by identification and separation [10].

15.3.2   THE CLONAL EVOLUTION MODEL

Intratumoral genetic heterogeneity has been observed in several cancers [11]. This model of cancer propagation predicts that genetic instability and epigenetic differences confer tumorigenic potential to some cancer cells [12]. Carcinogenic mutations lead to heterogeneity in phenotype and function of these cells. Mutations cause erroneous activation of normal stem cell self-renewal pathways or it blocks the epigenetic programs that underlie differentiation. These cells may also acquire additional genetic mutation, forming genetically divergent clones that are capable of independently maintaining the malignant potential. Thus, clonal evolution provides a basis for understanding cancer proliferation in cancers that are not hierarchically organized and their response to therapy [13].

15.3.3   THE INTERCONVERSION MODEL

The ability of tumorigenic cancer cells to interconvert between less and more proliferative/malignant states is the basis of this model [14]. A cell that is nontumorigenic in one perspective is capable of becoming tumorigenic in another perspective and has not lost its tumorigenic potential. This suggests that tumorigenicity at a particular point in time is reversible and milieu dependent. The model does not consider the likelihood of two-way interconversion between tumorigenic and non-tumorigenic cells as it is only focused on the intrinsic potential of cancer cells to form tumors [15].

15.4   CANCER STEM CELL: AN OVERVIEW

The American Association for Cancer Research (AACR) has defined CSCs as cells within a tumor that "possess the capacity for self-renewal and to cause the heterogeneous lineages of cancer cells that complete the tumor" [16]. CSCs or tumor-initiating cells or tumorigenic cells are a small subset of cancer cells that display characteristics similar to normal stem cells. CSCs are multipotent and are capable of self-renewal and proliferation, which facilitates tumor maintenance. These cells develop resistance to chemotherapy and radiation primarily due to their ability to regenerate, accumulate mutations, and differentiate into chemoresistant cells and secondly because of their quiescent behavior, which protects them from cytotoxic therapy that targets rapidly dividing cells. Therefore, CSCs are primarily responsible for relapse and poor survival in various cancers [17].

A single asymmetric self-renewing mitotic division results in one progeny that remains quiescent and retains stem cell identity, and the other more differentiated progenitor cell that divides actively and undergoes multiple rounds of divisions before entering a post-mitotic fully differentiated state. This ensures the production of large numbers of differentiated progeny, while maintaining a relatively small pool of long-lived CSCs [18].

During development or, in the adult, after tissue injuries, the stem cells expand in number. As this cannot be accounted by asymmetric divisions, another concept was proposed that stem cells undergo rounds of symmetric self-renewing divisions, whereby each stem cell produces two daughter cells that have similar ability to replicate and generate differentiated cell lineages as the parental cell. However, this can lead to depletion of the CSC population. Thus, promoting this form of division can be an alternative strategy of inducing cell death to treat cancer.

15.5   NORMAL STEM CELL VERSUS CANCER STEM CELL

Although the normal stem cells and tumorigenic cancer cells conceptually share the same functional ability of extensive proliferation, the two cell types are basically different in some ways. Normal stem cells are remarkable for controlled proliferation rate due to which their genomic integrity in maintained. Cancer cells are commonly marked by their loss of controlled cell division. Identification of both mutual and distinctive mechanisms that control normal stem cell proliferation and tumor development will assist to disclose targets for better treatment opportunities of cancer patients. Indeed, the self-renewal property of normal stem cells also often mediates carcinogenesis. These concepts gain support from interpretations that tumorigenic cancer cells not only possess self-renewal property, but they can also produce cell population that is nontumorigenic in nature.

15.5.1   GENOMIC INTEGRITY IN NORMAL STEM CELLS AND TUMORIGENIC CELLS

Normal stem cells have carefully regulated mechanisms to maintain genomic integrity as it is critical to their function. If normal stem cells could easily acquire genetic mutations, then it will be passed in the next generation of cells, possibly interfering with normal organ function and reporting malignant transformation in long time. Individuals exposed to high level of radiation acquire genetic mutations in long-lived tissue-specific stem cells, causing high incidence of cancer [19]. In contrast, at least some tumorigenic cells have the ability to acquire and retain additional genetic mutations. This ability leads to the formation of malignant clones that can acclimatize to changing environmental circumstances and possess an inevitable tendency to progressively malignant behavior [20] (Figure 15.2).

15.5.2   INTERCONVERSION IN NORMAL STEM CELLS AND TUMORIGENIC CELLS

A cell labeling study suggests that expression of CD34 increased in murine hematopoietic stem cells (HSCs) during the activated state under condi-

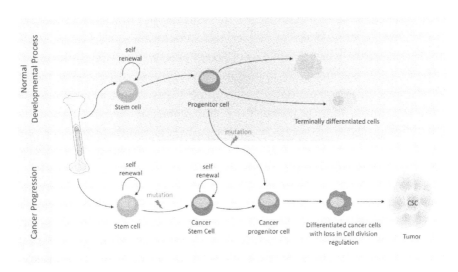

FIGURE 15.2   Genetic mutations disrupts normal stem cell development pathway, leading to the formation of cancer stem cells.

tions of hematopoietic stress and reduced after the resumption of the steady state. Phenotypic interconversion causes functional changes in stem cells [21]. In the skin, the hair follicle (HF) is maintained primarily by HF stem cell populations, and the interfollicular integrity of the epidermis is retained primarily by interfollicular epidermal stem cells [22]. However, HF stem cells temporarily contribute to repair of the interfollicular epidermis during healing of epidermal wounds, and interfollicular epidermal stem cells help in hair follicle neogenesis in newly repaired skin [23]. These studies indicate that environmental cues may alter the proliferative and differentiation fate of normal cells. Interconversion of at least some normal cells is useful in homeostatic maintenance.

Presence of heterogeneously quiescent cell populations in cell cycle studies of leukemogenic human chronic myeloid leukemia (CML) cells suggests that tumorigenic cells are capable of interconversion between different malignant fates and even different states of sensitivity to therapy. By adopting reversible quiescent states, leukemogenic cells escape cytotoxic-induced death [24].

Microenvironment also plays a vital role in maintaining tumorigenic cell proliferation and providing drug resistance. Certain antibodies inhibit tumor microenvironment homing of leukemogenic cells by targeting adhesion molecules VLA-4 and CD44, thereby reducing disease engraftment in transplantation models [25]. Some cellular mechanisms lead to chemotherapeutic drug resistance in cancer cells. Epithelial to mesenchymal transitions (EMT) were induced in breast cancer cells by knockdown to E-cadherin. This caused increase in paclitaxel resistance and salinomycin sensitivity, suggesting that cancer cells acclimatize to different morphological and functional destinies that are associated with intrinsically varied sensitivity to therapies [26]. Moreover, pharmacologically inhibition of histone modification leads to therapy resistance in lung cancer cell subpopulations, showing epigenetic basis of drug resistance in some cancer cells [27]. Consequently, by this interconversion mechanism, CSCs gain properties to become phenotypically heterogeneous and resistant to chemotherapies.

15.5.3 SELF-RENEWAL IN NORMAL STEM CELLS AND TUMORIGENIC CELLS

The CSC model cites that self-renewal is an attribute of tumorigenic cells. Self-renewal in normal tissue stem cells faces technical limitations due to which it has only been evaluated in a limited number of organs [28, 29]. Clonal *in vivo* expression of self-renewal and multilineage differentiation in primary transplants of stem cells are required to test self-renewal property. Similar properties should be demonstrated in serial transplants of the same cells [30]. There is a limit to the ability of tissue-specific stem cell to be serially transplanted. Exhaustion has been demonstrated in HSCs [31] and mammary stem cells [32]. Therefore, some tissues-specific stem cell progenies do not resemble their parental cells after self-renewal.

Polyclonal tumors show serial transplantability and similar phenotypic heterogeneity in parental and daughter tumors. This property is required to evaluate self-renewal in tumorigenic cancer cells. There are several limitations in testing self-renewal properties in CSCs. Firstly, the tumorigenic cells that possess a high potential for non-self-renewing proliferations may not undergo self-renewal in serial transplantations. Secondly, phenotypic changes in the tumor progeny are limited to very few markers. Thus, the demonstration of self-renewal in CSCs is far more challenging compared to normal tissue-specific stem cells [33].

There are two types of cancer cell population, first one is self-renewing and the other one is non-self-renewing. Non-self-renewing population is also important because it helps in larger cell proliferation and increase metastatic capacity. Tumorigenic cell progeny may augment malignant behavior via acquiring additional mutations, even though self-renewal did not occur. Furthermore, a large number of non-tumorigenic population comes from the non-self-renewed tumorigenic cells that follow CSC model. Self-renewal provides malignant potential to cancer stem cells for disease propagation and makes it important from clinical perspective.

15.5.4 MARKER EXPRESSION IN NORMAL STEM CELLS AND TUMORIGENIC CELLS

Cell surface markers (immunophenotype) help in phenotypically distinguishing stem cells from their differentiated progeny. Different pattern of cell surface markers are expressed in CSCs of different tumor type (Table 15.1). Methods for identifying CSCs include analysis of surface cell adhesion molecules (CAM) expression profiles using fluorescence activated cell sorting (FACS) [34], and immunofluorescent detection by confocal microscopy [35]. These techniques allow stem cells to be isolated and studied

TABLE 15.1   Cell Surface Markers Expressed by Cancer Stem Cells in Various Tumors

Tumor	Csc Cell Surface Markers	References
Leukemia	CD34+, CD38-	[135]
Breast cancer	EPCAM(ESA)+, CD44+, CD24-, ALDH1+	[136]
Colon cancer	CD133+, CD44+, ALDH1+, CD26+	[137,138]
Head and neck squmous cell carcinoma	CD44+, ALDH1+	[139]
Neuroblastoma	CD133+, CD15+	[140]
Small cell and non-small cell lung cancer	CD133+	[141]
Pancreas adenocarcinoma	CD133+, CD44+, CD24+, ESA+	[142, 143]
Hepatocellular carcinoma	CD90+, CD45−	[144]
Prostate Cancer	CD133+, CD44+, $\alpha_2\beta_1^{high}$	[145]
Ovarian Cancer	CD133+, CD44+, CD117+, CD24+	[146]
Melonoma	CD20+, CD271+	[147]
Renal Carcinoma	CD133+	[146]

separately from their progeny. Normal stem cells and tumorigenic cancer cells do not express an exclusive pattern of markers. The use of the same surface markers to identify stem cell populations from two different tissues or tumor types is misleading. Even cells arising from the same tissues need not express the same markers. Therefore, these markers cannot be described as stemness markers.

- Sca-1 is used for the identification of murine blood stem cells, but it is not expressed by murine mammary duct stem cells.
- Brain tumor stem cell marker CD133 is also present on normal brain stem cells and on many non-stem cells in various tumors and tissues [36].
- Human AML stem cells and normal human HSCs are enriched in the CD34+CD38− fraction of bone marrow [37]

The occurrence of cells in the SP (side population) fraction that is characterized by the efflux of Hoechst dye is also a phenotype that is used to differentiate cells [38]. Possession of this phenotype is not a universal property of stem cells as it has been seen that the SP fraction isolated from some tissues does not contain the stem cells. The ability to generate mammary glands in cleared fat pads helped in the identification of normal breast stem cells, but the majority of these cells were not included within the SP fraction. Therefore, other methods are first employed to isolate stem cells and then their occurrence within the SP fraction is checked.

Identification of stem cells also can be done through label retention or bromodeoxyuridine incorporation. The labeling method assumes that normal stem cells or CSCs go through a process of "immortal stand" DNA replication and consequently preserve the labeled state for a prolonged period [39]. Nevertheless, all CSCs do not hold label nor all the label-holding cells are CSCs. Thus, to consider any marker as a CSC marker, the label-holding cells must express tumor regeneration property *in vivo.*

Tumorsphere culture [40], detection of enzymatic activity of aldehyde dehydrogenase 1 (ALDH1) (e.g., Aldefluor assay) [41], serial colony-forming unit assays [42], and migration assays [43] are few other techniques that are used to isolate and characterize cancer stem/progenitor cells.

One cannot be sure of that tumorigenic cells are CSCs on the basis of cancer cell phenotype alone. Hence, in vivo models are required to confirm tumorigenicity [10]. Although there are some markers that stably express on normal stem cells, some functional assays need to be utilized to confirm stemness property of normal as well as CSCs.

15.6   THE MICROENVIRONMENT AND THE CSC NICHE

A remarkable difference between normal stem cells and tumorigenic cells is their measure of dependence on the specialized niche in which these cells reside, called "microenvironment" [44]. The stem cell niche comprises a group of cells in a special location that anchors the stem cells by generating extrinsic factors that control stem cell number, proliferation, and fate determination. This niche has been characterized by cell–cell contacts, pro-inflammatory signals, extracellular matrix adhesion molecules and factors secreted by the stromal microenvironment such as Hedgehog, Wnt, transforming growth factor (TGF), and vascular endothelial growth factor (VEGF). CSCs may arise from deregulation or alteration of the niche by dominant proliferation-promoting signals. The niche protects the stem cells either by physically sequestering them away from differentiation signals by enhancing the survival signaling or by the maintaining them in a quiescent state. Understanding the interaction of the molecules implicated in activation and mobilization of stem cells from the niche and homing to the niche will delineate the possible targets for cancer development and metastasis [45].

In adult somatic tissue, this niche suppresses tumorigenesis by providing inhibitory signals for stem cell proliferation and differentiation [46]. The niche supports ongoing tissue regeneration by providing transient signals for stem cell division. The disruption of the balance between proliferation-inhibiting and proliferation-promoting signals results in tumorigenesis. Studies demonstrate that the disruption of stem cell niche in the mammary gland leads to abnormal expression of TFFα, resulting in the development of breast cancer [47].

HSCs are primarily located in the osteoblastic niche on the bone surface [48] but are found adjacent to the sinusoid endothelial cells upon mobilization. The osteoblastic niche provides a quiescent microenvironment, and the vascular niche favors proliferation and further differentiation [49]. Thus, a gradient of osteoblastic niche to vascular niche exists in bone marrow.

15.6.1 HYPOXIA

Hypoxia creates a specialized CSC microenvironment that favors poorly differentiated tumor cells [50]. It shifts the cells toward pro-survival pathways by promoting a stress response that is regulated by hypoxia inducible factor (HIF) proteins. In vitro exposure to hypoxic conditions increases the SP fraction in several solid tumors to a considerable extent [51]. Furthermore, the SP cells migrated toward the hypoxic zones in the injured conditioned medium model derived from hypoxic bone marrow stromal cells, suggesting the contribution of hypoxia to the CSC niche [52]. Numerous studies establish that hypoxia and HIF pathways contribute to neuroblastoma progression. Exposure to hypoxia led to the upregulation of hypoxia-induced genes (HIF-1 and HIF-2), and neural crest marker genes including c-kit and Notch-1 in neuroblastoma [53]. HIF-2 has been associated with the regulation of several stem cell-associated genes and correlated with advanced clinical stage and worse prognosis in neuroblastoma [54]. The knockdown of HIF-2 caused partial sympathetic neural differentiation of neuroblastoma stem cells [55], thereby helping in the maintenance of immature stem like tumor cells.

15.6.2   CANCER-ASSOCIATED FIBROBLASTS AND THE EXTRACELLULAR MATRIX

Cancer-associated fibroblasts (CAFs) are activated fibroblasts arising from fibroblasts or other progenitor cells like bone marrow-derived cells, endothelial cells, and epithelial cells via mesenchymal transition [56]. CAFs remain in an activated state and do not return to a normal phenotype or undergo apoptosis unlike the normal fibroblasts [57]. They produce extracellular matrix (ECM), chemokines, cytokines, proteinases, and growth factors. They play an important role in promoting tumor growth, invasion, and angiogenesis.

Matrix metalloproteinases (MMPs) are zinc-containing endopeptidases that are required for proteolysis of the extracellular matrix components in order to convert the stem cell factor from a membrane-bound form to a free form, thereby promoting proliferation and mobilization of stem cells. It remodels the ECM and plays a role in cancer cell metastasis and tumor growth and invasion [58]. MMPs are frequently overexpressed by CAFs [59]. Fibronectin and collagen are cleaved products of MMPs that serve as chemotactic factors for inflammatory cells. When neuroblastoma tumor cells were implanted into MMP-9-deficient mice, the tumor vasculature was inhibited. MMP-9 is involved in recruiting bone marrow-derived leukocytes into the tumor microenvironment [60].

15.6.3   INFLAMMATORY AND IMMUNE CELLS OF THE MICROENVIRONMENT

Inflammatory and immune cells include T cells, B cells, and natural killer (NK) cells, which are cells of the lymphoid lineage, and macrophages, neutrophils and myeloid-derived suppressor cells (MDSCs), which are of the myeloid lineage [61]. They either promote or inhibit tumorigenesis and may also contribute to a metastatic phenotype. After transformation, the tumor cells redirect the immune cells to assume an immunosuppressive state, leading to the suppression of the antitumor capabilities of immune cells [62]. Tumor-associated macrophage (TAM) secretes factors such as IL-6 that activate the JAK (Janus kinase)–STAT (signal transducer and activator of transcription) pathway within the cancer cells, thus imparting stem cell like properties that enhance their tumorigenicity and resistance to che-motherapy [63].

Natural killer (NK) cells and natural killer T (NKT) cells are potent anti-tumor cells [64] that have the ability to attack human tumor cells. They dis-play strong cytotoxic activity against neuroblastoma both *in vitro* [65] and *in vivo* [66]. NK-cell-based immunotherapies are under study for cancer treat-ment [67, 68]. MDSCs comprise another population of tumor-infiltrating immune cells that secrete cytokines and growth factors, thereby creating an immunosuppressive microenvironment enabling carcinoma cells to acquire and maintain stemness. Inhibition of MDSCs in mouse models of neuroblas-toma which were immunocompetent, but not immunodeficient, resulted in inhibition of tumor growth [69].

15.6.4 CYTOKINES AND CHEMOKINES

CSCs use the same homing and mobilization machinery of normal stem cells to metastasize [70]. Cytokines influence tumor progression, whereas chemo-kines recruit specific types of lymphoid and myeloid cells [71]. CXCR4 is a chemokine receptor that is highly expressed on tumor cells and upon activa-tion directly stimulates cancer cell proliferation [72]. Both the receptor and its ligand, stromal cell-derived factor-1 (SDF-1), also known as CXCL12, play a role in tumor metastasis. CSCs expressing CXCR4 metastasize to organs like bone, lung, lymph nodes and liver, which have a high expression of the ligand CXCL12 [71].

15.6.5 CELL ADHESION MOLECULES

Cadherins are a large family of transmembrane glycoproteins, which form adherent complex composed of regulatory proteins, including β-catenin and α-catenin, which in turn mediates cell to cell adhesion. Different forms of β-catenin interact with different protein complexes. Non-Wnt signals phos-phorylate the COOH terminus of β-catenin, thereby regulating its conver-sion between the heterodimeric and monomer forms [73]. β-Catenin is a key molecule that links the two states of stem cells [44]: The heterodimeric form of β-catenin binds with membrane-bound cadherin and is responsible for the state of arrest of the stem cell in which they remain attached to the niche [74]. The monomeric form that interacts with Tcf and is nuclearly localized is responsible for the activated state of the stem cells, thereby turning on cell cycle-related genes, including cyclin D1 and c-Myc [75]. Defining the signals that regulate the conformational change of β-catenin will help in understanding stem cell activation. It has been observed in breast cancer that a mutation in E-cadherin leads to nuclearly localized β-catenin, thereby suggesting the involvement of Wnt signaling, which primarily prevents β-catenin from degradation, to fully activate stem cells [76].

15.7   SELF-RENEWAL PATHWAYS OF CANCER STEM CELLS

CSCs help in tumor maintenance and propagation through continuous self-renewal and differentiation. Similar signaling pathways that occur in normal stem cells regulate the self-renewal process in CSCs. The major pathways that play pivotal roles in CSC self-renewal and in regulating lineage fate in different systems have been summarized in Figure 15.3 and are described in detail below. Understanding the mechanisms that trigger the self-renewal behavior of CSCs is important for developing anticancer drugs targeting CSCs.

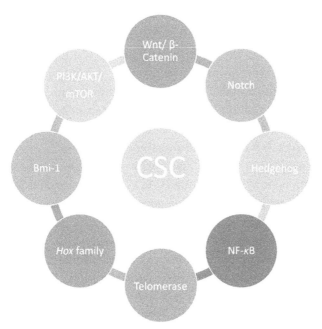

FIGURE 15.3   Signaling molecules involved in self renewal mechanism of cancer stem cells.

15.7.1   WNT/β-CATENIN PATHWAY

The Wnt family of secreted glycoproteins is highly conserved and regulates many biological processes. In the embryonic development, appropriate activation of Wnt/β-catenin signaling regulates cell proliferation, cell differentiation, and determination of cell fate, whereas its inappropriate activation is implicated in the maintenance of self-renewal in CSCs of leukemia [77], melanoma [78], breast [79], colon [80], liver [81], and lung [82] cancers.

β-Catenin is the mediator of canonical Wnt signaling. Depending on its cellular localization, it performs two discrete functions. In the nonpathological state, membrane-localized β-catenin is sequestered by the epithelial cell-cell adhesion protein E-cadherin to maintain cell-cell adhesion [83]. Wnt/β-catenin signaling is initiated on binding of Wnt to Frizzled receptor, resulting in accumulation of β-catenin in the cytoplasm and its subsequent nuclear translocation. This is preceded by interaction with the transcription factors T-cell factor/lymphoid enhancer factor (TCF/LEF) as a transcription activator, which leads to the activation of downstream target genes of Wnt such as c-Myc, c-Jun, cyclin D1, and fibronectin [84].

In the absence of Wnt signaling, β-catenin forms a multiprotein complex with glycogen synthase kinase 3β (GSK3β), casein kinase 1α, adenomatous polyposis coli, and axin [85]. GSK3β plays a central role in controlling the activity of the WNT/β-catenin pathway by regulating β-catenin stability and degradation. Phosphorylation of β-catenin at Ser33/Ser37/Thr41 by GSK3β subjects it to ubiquitin-proteasome degradation, thereby restricting its nuclear translocation [86]. Thus, GSK3β acts as a tumor suppressor by curbing canonical WNT/β-catenin signaling.

The Wnt/GSK3β/β-catenin signaling axis has been linked with self-renewal of both normal stem cells and CSCs. Suppression of GSK3β activity was shown to be critical for the maintenance of murine pluripotent stem cells [87]. Inactivating mutations of GSK3β have been associated with faulty CSC development programs in Breakpoint Cluster Region-Abelson (BCR–ABL) CM), thus corroborating earlier findings that associated nuclear accumulation of β-catenin in BCR–ABL CSCs with the progression of the disease. Mouse xenografts of pre-leukemic and leukemic stem cells of mixed lineage myeloid leukemia (MML) exhibited differential Wnt/GSK3β/β-catenin signaling including elevation of β-catenin levels in the tumorigenic CSCs that resulted in enhanced self-renewal, higher tumor relapse rates, and poorer survival outcomes than MLL pre-leukemic CSCs. Yang et al. demonstrated that the introduction of constitutively active β-catenin in tumorigenic hepatocellular carcinoma cells imparted cisplatin chemoresistance and promoted expansion of the hepatic progenitor cell population, whereas loss of β-catenin nearly reduced the chemoresistant cell population endowed with progenitor-like characteristics [81].

15.7.2   HEDGEHOG PATHWAY

The Hedgehog family of signaling molecules play a role in tissue development by regulating cellular differentiation and proliferation. When secreted, hedgehog ligands bind to the transmembrane receptor Patched (Ptch), and Smoothened (Smo) is released. This leads to transcription of various genes such as cyclin D, cyclin E, Myc, and elements of the EGF pathway by triggering the dissociation of the transcription factors Gli1, Gli2, and Gli3 from Fused (Fu) and suppressor of Fused (SuFu) [88]. When the hedgehog ligands are absent, Ptch binds with Smo thereby blocking its function [89].

Dysregulation of the Hedgehog pathway is reported in a wide variety of cancer types and is also known to be involved in stem cell self-renewal [90]. Although several Hedgehog inhibitory drugs are approved or presently under clinical development, it has been reported that these drugs may actually promote drug-resistant tumors, potentially due to CSC selection [91].

The Hedgehog pathway has been shown to play a pivotal role in self-renewal regulation of normal and malignant human mammary stem cells in both in vitro and mouse model system. Hedgehog-Gli signaling controls the self-renewal behavior of human glioma CSCs and tumorigenicity [92].

Sonic hedgehog pathway is also linked to transcription factor NF-κB signaling. NF-κB activates overexpression of sonic hedgehog in pancreatic cancer and accelerates pancreatic cancer cell proliferation [93]. Kasperczyk et al. characterized sonic hedgehog as a novel NF-κB target gene and mapped minimal NF-κB consensus site to position +139 of sonic hedgehog promoter [94]. The transcription factor NF-κB is a downstream factor activated by the Sonic Hedgehog (Shh) pathway in pancreatic cancers [93]. In human leukemia, CD34+ sub-population exhibits the preponderance of Hedgehog signaling. Su et al. examined the role of Shh in survival and growth of CML progenitor cells [95]. CML bone marrow stromal cells expressed low level of the Shh protein. This was associated with CD34+ progenitor cells that were less sensitive to exogenous Shh peptide, but more sensitive to cyclopamine than CD34− cells. This implies that the activation of Shh signaling can occur autonomously in progenitor cells. Cyclopamine treatment was able to downregulate the expression of stemness markers *NANOG, POU5F1, CD-44,* and *EpCAM,* sonic hedgehog downstream genes, and EMT markers on HCT-116 spheres [96]. Estradiol (E2) increases the cell growth of estrogen receptor (ER)-positive breast cancer cells as well as its CSC proportion. GANT61, a non-canonical Hh inhibitor was able to decrease both the cell growth and SC proportion increased by E2 signaling [97]. Similarly, curcumin exhibited its interventional effect on lung CSCs by reducing the number of CD133-positive cells, decreasing the expression levels of lung CSC markers (CD133, CD44, ALDHA1, Nanog and Oct4), and inhibiting Wnt/β-catenin and Sonic Hedgehog pathways [98].

15.7.3   NOTCH PATHWAY

Notch signaling is a highly evolutionarily conserved component that controls cell proliferation and apoptosis, thereby modulating the development of many organs [99]. It is involved in the maintenance of cell diversity and stem-cell self-renewal [100]. Four known Notch proteins, Notch1 to Notch 4, express as transmembrane receptors in various stem and progenitor cells. The activation of Notch signaling occurs *via* binding of Delta-like and Jagged surface ligands, which triggers cleavage of the Notch proteins by A Disintegrin and Metalloproteinase (ADAM) protease family and γ-secretase proteolytic enzymes. The Notch intracellular domain is released and translocated into the nucleus, where it acts as a transcription co-activator of recombination signal sequence-binding protein Jκ (RBP-J) and activates various genes that promote proliferation, including *c-Myc*, NF-κB, cyclin D1, and *p21* [101].

The Notch-activated genes and pathways drive the growth of tumor through the expansion of CSCs [102]. The Notch pathway has been shown to play an important role in the self-renewal function of malignant breast cancer CSCs [103]. Functional cross-talk between the Notch and NF-κB pathways was demonstrated in hyperproliferative colon cancer. Cross-talk between Notch1 and NF-κB has been reported in diverse cellular situations [104]. Notch-1 is specifically required for the expression of several NF-κB subunits and stimulation of NF-κB promoter activity [105].

NumbL, or Numb-like, is a tumor suppressor that inhibits the Notch pathway and regulates the CSC pool [106]. MAP17 (PDZKIP1), a small cargo protein overexpressed in tumors, interacts with NUMB through the PDZ-binding domain, thereby downregulating NumbL and inducing activation of the Notch pathway. Increase in epithelial-mesenchymal transitions (EMT) and CSC-related gene transcripts and CSC-like phenotypes, including an increase in the CSC-like pool, was also demonstrated [107].

15.7.4 PI3K/Akt/mTOR AND CROSSTALK

The PI3K/Akt/mTOR axis is a central intracellular signaling pathway regulating cellular apoptotic function. PI3K/Akt/mTOR plays a key role in many cancers owing to the high frequency of mutation in the tumor suppressor gene phosphatase and tensin homolog (PTEN), which regulates PI3K signaling. Unrepressed PI3K signaling results in constitutive activation of the downstream pathway components that include the Akt and mTOR kinases and drive a host of cellular pro-survival adaptations [108]. PTEN loss has been shown to mediate Akt activation and increase stemness properties of CSC populations in prostate cancer [109]. Furthermore, crosstalk between PI3K/Akt and other pro-survival as well as mitogenic pathways has been shown to drive cancer growth [110]. Inactivation of GSK3β by Akt may result in downregulation of the WNT, Hedgehog, and Notch signaling pathways [111]. Korkaya et al. demonstrated the link between Wnt/β-catenin and PI3K/Akt pathway in mammary stem cells. Activated Akt (i.e., phospho-Akt Ser473) was shown to phosphorylate Ser9 on GSK3β, which decreased the activity of GSK3β, thereby stabilizing β-catenin and promoting β-catenin downstream events [112]. Crosstalk between tyrosine kinase receptors, GSK3β, and Bone Morphogenetic Protein 2 (BMP2) signaling during osteoblastic differentiation of human mesenchymal stem cells was observed [113]. It was suggested that PI3K signaling together with nuclear accumulation of β-catenin is necessary to fully activate canonical WNT signaling in colon cancer and is correlated with a high risk of distant metastasis in patients with colon cancer [114].

15.8   THERAPY

CSCs are integral to the development and maintenance of human cancers. Resistance to anticancer treatments like chemotherapy, radiation therapy, and molecularly targeted therapy is a consequence of the development of tumor cell heterogeneity. There exist a number of intrinsic drug-resistance mechanisms in CSCs that can inactivate cytotoxic (CT) drugs, resulting in tumor recurrence. Most CT drugs mediate apoptotic response in differentiated tumor cells, thereby conferring CSCs with a survival advantage with even greater proliferative potential [115].

The result is that tumor cells repopulate with lineage-dependent genotypic and phenotypic alterations, including multidrug resistance (MDR), that render CT drugs ineffective and lead to more rapid disease progression and poorer prognoses. Furthermore, hypoxic stability of CSCs enables them to survive in poorly vascularised microenvironments that challenge drug accessibility to niche networks and contributes to MDR. Current cancer therapies do not target the CSCs specifically and effectively. Developing CSC-specific drugs is complicated by the genotypic variability of CSCs and genomic instability of hyperplastic progeny that makes karyotyping of tumor cell populations enormously challenging [116].

Mitotic inhibitors like paclitaxel selectively kill cells during the M phase of the cell cycle, whereas antimetabolite drugs like 6-mercaptopurine and 5-fluorouracil destroy cancer cells during the S phase. However, the anticancer effects are exhibited only when tumor cells are undergoing proliferation. In contrast, CSCs are able to evade such conventional anticancer drugs as they become quiescent and stay in the G0 phase of the cell cycle. Therefore, drugs that target "normal" rapidly dividing tumor tissue are not active against CSCs. Tumors may re-grow from a few stem cells that escape the therapy; thus, it is important to develop drugs to target these cells. Endogenous cyclin-dependent kinase inhibitors like p57 and Fbw7 determine the cell cycle status of CSCs and are responsible for its delay or arrest [117]. Fbw7 is a component of E3 ubiquitin ligase that targets a network of substrates for degradation, including some key human oncoproteins. Most of these substrates function as transcription factors (TFs) that allow Fbw7 to regulate various pathways with oncogenic potential. Thus, Fbw7 inactivation leads to arousal of dormant CSCs in niche and is a novel target for CSCs elimination.

The self-renewal potential of gliomas is enhanced by repeated irradiation. This is mediated by an increase in IGF-1 secretion and upregulation of IGF-1 receptor expression [118]. Chronic receptor activation leads to slowing of the cell cycle by inhibiting the PI3K-Akt signaling pathway, which in turn activates the transcription factor FoxO3a. Acute irradiation of the slow-cycling CSCs induces rapid activation of IGF1–Akt survival signaling and promotes radioprotection [119]. These studies suggest that if we block the aberrant IGF signaling, this will be a potential novel therapeutic strategy to selectively attack quiescent CSCs of glioma.

Imatinib is the drug of choice for treating CML, and CML stem cells develop resistance to imatinib due to their dormant stage and are responsible for minimal residual disease (MRD) [120] . Patients with MRD show a high level of Fbw7, which results in degradation of c-Myc. The anticancer effect of this drug in imatinib-resistant CML cells was significantly enhanced in vivo by eroding Fbw7. This also led to molecular stabilization of c-Myc, thereby inducing cell proliferation [121]. Thus, a therapeutic strategy combining Fbw7 inhibition with conventional anticancer drugs to target CSCs in dormant stage is thus effective for overcoming the less susceptibility of CSCs to anticancer drugs.

The polyether antibiotic salinomycin (SAL) has recently been demonstrated to be an inhibitor of CSCs in various cancer types. SAL treatment on colorectal cancer cells decreased cancer stemness and telomerase activity by inhibiting IL-6 and TNF-α induced STAT3 and STAT1, suggesting a novel targeted-therapy for metastatic colorectal cancer [122]. Codelivery of salinomycin and doxorubicin using nanoliposomes were able to target both liver cancer cells and CSCs [123]. Paclitaxel combined with salinomycin was able to significantly inhibit the growth of CSC population of OVCAR3 ovarian cancer cell line [124]. Polymeric nanoparticles of SAL and paclitaxel were able to coeradicate breast cancer cells and CSCs [125].

Embryonic pathways such as Wnt, Hedgehog, Notch, and stem cell niche regulate mechanisms of survival by controlling self-renewal and cell fate decisions of stem cells and progenitor cells. These are involved in CSC maintenance and are emerging as targets to selectively eliminate cancer stem cells. Table 15.2 summarizes a list of inhibitors of self-renewal pathways and the CSC niche, some of which are already in clinical use.

The therapeutic efficacies of most CT drugs are severely hampered by toxicity profiles that limit their life-extending potential. Aberrant gene expression profiles long considered hallmarks of malignancy have been re-

TABLE 15.2   Therapeutic Agents Inhibiting Self Renewal Pathways and Niche of Cancer Stem Cells

Target	Therapeutic agent	Proposed mechanism of action	References
Notch Pathway	Gamma Secretase Inhibitors Gamma Secretase ModulatorsNotch mAbs DLL4 mAbs siRNA, miRNA-based therapeutics	γ-secretase γ-secretase Notch receptors Delta-4 ligand	[148–150]
Hedgehog Pathway	Vismodegib (GDC-0449) Saridegib (IPI-926) 5E1 (anti-Hedgehog monoclonal antibodies)	PTCH and/or SMO inhibitor SMO inhibitor Block receptor–Hh ligand interaction	[151–153]
Wnt Pathway	Aspirin, Sulindac, Celecoxib PKF115-584 FJ9 IWR OMP-18R5 (Anti-Frizzled monoclonal antibodies)	COX-dependent and – independent mechanisms β-catenin/TCF interaction inhibitor Dvl Axin stabilizer Block formation of active receptor signaling complex	[154–157]
mTOR/PI3K/ Akt	Everolimus (RAD-001) Perifosine (KRX-0401,D21266) GDC-0941 Metformin	mTORC1 inhibitor Akt inhibitor PI3K inhibitor Inhibits mTOR activation via AMPK	[158–161]
NF-κB	Dexamethasone Parthenolide	Induce expression of IκBα NF-κB inhibitor	[162, 163]
Niche	Plerixafor (AMD3100) Bevacizumab (Avastin) Obatoclax (GX15-070) Anti-CD44 monoclonal antibodies	CXCR4 antagonist Block VEGF-A / VEGFR binding Pan-Bcl2 inhibitor CD44 activation	[164–167]

evaluated in the context of the CSC with emphasis on genes that regulate self-renewal processes and differentiation programs which are normally tightly regulated in the non-cancerous somatic stem cells. As a result, there is an urgent need to identify compounds that strike targets involved in CSC self-renewal and differentiation programs. The use of chemopreventive natural product (NP) compounds to target CSC self-renewal and differentiation has the potential to guard against malignant transformation of cells. The dietary compounds, including curcumin [126], sulforaphane [127], soy isoflavone [128], epigallocatechin-3-gallate [129], resveratrol [130], lycopene [131], piperine [132], and vitamin D3 [133], have direct or indirect effect on the self-renewal pathways. Recently, vanillin, a major component in *Vanilla planifolia* seed, was shown to inhibit CSC-like behavior in the human nonsmall cell lung cancer NCI-H460 cells through the induction of Akt-proteasomal degradation and reduction of downstream CSC transcription factors Oct4 and Nanog [134].

15.9   FUTURE PERSPECTIVES

The current knowledge of markers or gene expression signatures is insufficient to identify cancer stem cell populations. A number of genes and signaling pathways like Shh, Bmi-1, Tie-2, Notch and Wnt/β-catenin, regulate stem cells. These genes, however. cannot be regarded as "stemness" genes as they also operate in other cell types. Constant efforts should be made to develop reliable genetic signatures that characterize stem cells. Microarray and genome-wide techniques can be valuable for detecting trends in genetic and epigenetic architecture of CSCs. Results from a mixed population constitute an average and non-specific signature. Therefore, pure populations are required for the identification of true signatures. Even after identifying a cancer stem cell signature from a particular type of tumor, functional assays should be used for validation before claims about "stemness" can be made. This is crucial as the particular signature may not be useful in identifying cancer stem cells in a different tumor type. The putative stem cell populations should be cross-examined by marker analysis, functional assays, and analysis of genetic and epigenetic blueprints. In vitro assays are being developed, and the results obtained must be ultimately validated by in vivo self-renewal assay.

The identification and isolation of genes that are functionally noteworthy for "stemness" would provide valuable targets for drug development. Elimination of stemness by gene inactivation or stimulation of stemness by gene activation would functionally link any marker to stem cell identity.

Another mechanism that is shared by normal as well as cancer stem cells is the process of stem cell mobilization from or homing to the niche. This molecular machinery is inappropriately used by cancer cells for invasion and metastasis. Investigating this process and the underlying molecular mechanisms will facilitate the understanding of cancer cell metastasis and will assist in the development of treatments aimed at destroying cancer stem cells without adversely affecting normal stem cell self-renewal.

These studies will enable us to discover strategies for effectively treating cancer by generating novel targets that could reduce cancer resistance and recurrence and improve patient survival while averting systemic toxicity.

15.10   CONCLUSION

It has now been established that deregulation of stem cell function plays a pivotal role in the development and propagation of some cancers. The phrase "cancer stem cell" implicates that tumorigenic cancer cells and normal stem cells are quite similar. It is therefore a possibility that inhibiting self-renewal pathways that drive cancer propagation may lead to unwarranted toxicity if the same pathways are essential for homeostatic function in normal stem cells. Thus, considering the similarities and differences between normal stem cells and tumorigenic cancer cells is required to maximize the potential of this research. The hunt for markers that distinguish tumorigenic from non-tumorigenic cells should be keenly pursued.

Similarly, some oncogenic mutations play a role in proliferation but are not required for stem cell maintenance. Therapies targeting a mutation that is capable of disrupting a cancer stem cell maintenance pathway should possibly eliminate the tumor-forming cells. Such targeted therapies could be lesser toxic and more effective than the current treatment options.

15.11   SUMMARY

- Cancer stem cells and normal stem cells possess two qualities to perform their natural function: self-renewal (e.g., the ability to produce more stem cells) and differentiation.
- CSCs play a role in cancer progression, its evolution, metastasis, and recurrence.
- The CSC hypothesis predicts that long-lived stem cells are more likely to accumulate the initial mutations leading to cancer than their short-lived differentiated progeny

- The tumor microenvironment, in addition to harboring cancer stem cells, consists of various components like hypoxia, cancer-associated fibroblasts, extracellular matrix, immune cells, cytokines, chemokines and cell adhesion molecules that function to maintain stem cells and have a major role in influencing the outcome of the malignancy.
- Signaling pathways like Wnt, Hedgehog, Notch, NF-Kb, and PI3K/Akt/mTOR, play a chief role in the biology of CSCs and normal stem cells.
- CSC targeting is one of the therapeutic approaches for treating cancer. CSCs can be eradicated by targeting treatment against signaling pathways involved and their microenvironment.

ACKNOWLEDGMENTS

Sonal Srivastava is thankful to Indian Council of Medical Research for the award of Senior Research Fellowship. Divya Tandon is thankful to Council for Scientific and Industrial Research for the award of Senior Research Fellowship. Jayant Dewangan is thankful to University Grant Commission for the award of Senior Research Fellowship. This work was supported by Council of Scientific and Industrial Research network project BSC0103. The CDRI communication No. for this manuscript is 9470.

KEYWORDS

- **cancer stem cells**
- **cell surface markers**
- **microenvironment**
- **self renewal pathways**

REFERENCES

1. Lobo, N. A., Shimono, Y., Qian, D., & Clarke, M. F., (2007). The biology of cancer stem cells. *Annu. Rev. Cell Dev. Biol., 23*, 675–699.

2. Abdullah, L. N., & Chow, E. K. H., (2013). Mechanisms of chemoresistance in cancer stem cells. *Clinical and Translational Medicine, 2*(1), 3.

3. Park, C., Bergsagel, D., & McCulloch, E., (1971). Mouse myeloma tumor stem cells: a primary cell culture assay. *Journal of the National Cancer Institute, 46*, 411–422.

4. Dick, D., (1997). Human acute myeloid leukemia is organized as a hierarchy that originates from a primitive hematopoietic cell. *Nature Med., 3*, 730–737, 1.

5. Southam, C. M., & Brunschwig, A., (1961). Quantitative studies of autotransplantation of human cancer. Preliminary report. *Cancer* 14, 971–978.

6. Hamburger, A. W., & Salmon, S. E., (1977). Primary bioassay of human tumor stem cells. *Science (New York), 197*, 461–463.

7. Singh, S. K., Clarke, I. D., Terasaki, M., Bonn, V. E., Hawkins, C., Squire, J., & Dirks, P. B., (2003). Identification of a cancer stem cell in human brain tumors. *Cancer Research, 63*, 5821–5828.

8. Dick, J. E., (2008). Stem cell concepts renew cancer research. *Blood, 112*(13), 4793–4807.

9. Reya, T., Morrison, S. J., Clarke, M. F., & Weissman, I. L., (2001). Stem cells, cancer, & cancer stem cells. *Nature, 414*, 105–111.

10. Shackleton, M., Quintana, E., Fearon, E. R., & Morrison, S. J., (2009). Heterogeneity in cancer: cancer stem cells versus clonal evolution. *Cell, 138*, 822–829.

11. Nowell, P. C., (1976). The clonal evolution of tumor cell populations. *Science (New York), 194*, 23–28.

12. Lengauer, C., Kinzler, K. W., & Vogelstein, B., (1998). Genetic instabilities in human cancers. *Nature, 396*, 643–649.

13. Takata, M., Morita, R., & Takehara, K., (2000). Clonal heterogeneity in sporadic melanomas as revealed by loss-of-heterozygosity analysis. *International Journal of Cancer, 85*, 492–497.

14. Pinner, S., Jordan, P., Sharrock, K., Bazley, L., Collinson, L., Marais, R., Bonvin, E., Goding, C., & Sahai, E., (2009). Intravital imaging reveals transient changes in pigment production and Brn2 expression during metastatic melanoma dissemination. *Cancer Research, 69*, 7969–7977.

15. Shackleton, M., (2010). In: Normal stem cells and cancer stem cells: similar and different, *Seminars in Cancer Biology*, Elsevier, pp. 85–92.

16. Clarke, M. F., Dick, J. E., Dirks, P. B., Eaves, C. J., Jamieson, C. H., Jones, D. L., Visvader, J., Weissman, I. L., & Wahl, G. M., (2006). Cancer stem cells—perspectives on current status and future directions: AACR Workshop on cancer stem cells. *Cancer Research, 66*, 9339–9344.

17. Chen, L. S., Wang, A. X., Dong, B., Pu, K. F., Yuan, L. H., & Zhu, Y. M., (2012). A new prospect in cancer therapy: targeting cancer stem cells to eradicate cancer. *Chinese Journal of Cancer, 31*, 564.

18. Bomken, S., Fišer, K., Heidenreich, O., & Vormoor, J., (2010). Understanding the cancer stem cell. *British Journal of Cancer, 103*, 439–445.

19. Thompson, D. E., Mabuchi, K., Ron, E., Soda, M., Tokunaga, M., Ochikubo, S., Sugimoto, S., Ikeda, T., Terasaki, M., & Izumi, S., (1994). Cancer incidence in atomic bomb survivors. Part II: Solid tumors, 1958–1987. *Radiation Research, 137*, 2s, S17-S67.

20. Sahin, E., & DePinho, R. A., (2010). Linking functional decline of telomeres, mitochondria and stem cells during ageing. *Nature, 464*, 520–528.

21. Wilson, A., Laurenti, E., Oser, G., van der Wath, R. C., Blanco-Bose, W., Jaworski, M., Offner, S., Dunant, C. F., Eshkind, L., & Bockamp, E., (2008). Hematopoietic stem

cells reversibly switch from dormancy to self-renewal during homeostasis and repair. *Cell, 135*, 1118–1129.

22. Ito, M., Liu, Y., Yang, Z., Nguyen, J., Liang, F., Morris, R. J., & Cotsarelis, G., (2005). Stem cells in the hair follicle bulge contribute to wound repair but not to homeostasis of the epidermis. *Nature Medicine, 11*, 1351–1354.

23. Taylor, G., Lehrer, M. S., Jensen, P. J., Sun, T.-T., & Lavker, R. M., (2000). Involvement of follicular stem cells in forming not only the follicle but also the epidermis. *Cell, 102*, 451–461.

24. Ito, M., Yang, Z., Andl, T., Cui, C., Kim, N., Millar, S. E., & Cotsarelis, G., (2007). Wnt-dependent de novo hair follicle regeneration in adult mouse skin after wounding. *Nature, 447*, 316–320.

25. Saito, Y., Uchida, N., Tanaka, S., Suzuki, N., Tomizawa-Murasawa, M., Sone, A., Najima, Y., Takagi, S., Aoki, Y., & Wake, A., (2010). Induction of cell cycle entry eliminates human leukemia stem cells in a mouse model of AML. *Nature Biotechnology, 28*, 275–280.

26. Gupta, P. B., Onder, T. T., Jiang, G., Tao, K., Kuperwasser, C., Weinberg, R. A., & Lander, E. S., (2009). Identification of selective inhibitors of cancer stem cells by high-throughput screening. *Cell, 138*, 645–659.

27. Sharma, S. V., Lee, D. Y., Li, B., Quinlan, M. P., Takahashi, F., Maheswaran, S., McDermott, U., Azizian, N., Zou, L., & Fischbach, M. A., (2010). A chromatin-mediated reversible drug-tolerant state in cancer cell subpopulations. *Cell, 141*, 69–80.

28. Krause, D. S., Theise, N. D., Collector, M. I., Henegariu, O., Hwang, S., Gardner, R., Neutzel, S., & Sharkis, S. J., (2001). Multi-organ, multi-lineage engraftment by a single bone marrow-derived stem cell. *Cell, 105*, 369–377.

29. Wang, X., Kruithof-de Julio, M., Economides, K. D., Walker, D., Yu, H., Halili, M. V., Hu, Y.-P., Price, S. M., Abate-Shen, C., & Shen, M. M., (2009). A luminal epithelial stem cell that is a cell of origin for prostate cancer. *Nature, 461*, 495–500.

30. Shackleton, M, A.-L. M., Vaillant, F., Visvader, J. E., & Lindeman, G. J., (2007). *Mammary Stem Cells*, World Scientific Publishing, London.

31. Harrison, D. E., Astle, C. M., & Delaittre, J. A., (1978). Loss of proliferative capacity in immunohemopoietic stem cells caused by serial transplantation rather than aging. *The Journal of Experimental Medicine, 147*, 1526–1531.

32. Hoshino, K., & Gardner, W. U., (1967). Transplantability and life span of mammary gland during serial transplantation in mice. *Nature, 213*, 193–194.

33. Horne, G. A., & Copland, M., (2017). Approaches for targeting self-renewal pathways in cancer stem cells: implications for hematological treatments. *Expert Opinion on Drug Discovery*, 1–10.

34. Dou, J., Pan, M., Wen, P., Li, Y., Tang, Q., Chu, L., Zhao, F., Jiang, C., Hu, W., & Hu, K., (2007). Isolation and identification of cancer stem-like cells from murine melanoma cell lines. *Cell Mol Immunol, 4*, 467–472.

35. Mu, H., Lin, K. X., Zhao, H., Xing, S., Li, C., Liu, F., Lu, H. Z., Zhang, Z., Sun, Y. L., & Yan, X. Y., (2014). Identification of biomarkers for hepatocellular carcinoma by semiquantitative immunocytochemistry. *World Journal of Gastroenterology, 20*, 5826–5838.

36. Singh, S. K., Hawkins, C., Clarke, I. D., Squire, J. A., Bayani, J., Hide, T., Henkelman, R. M., Cusimano, M. D., & Dirks, P. B., (2004). Identification of human brain tumour initiating cells. *Nature, 432*, 396–401.

37. Lapidot, T., Sirard, C., Vormoor, J., Murdoch, B., Hoang, T., Caceres-Cortes, J., Minden, M., Paterson, B., Caligiuri, M. A., & Dick, J. E., (1994). A cell initiating human acute myeloid leukaemia after transplantation into SCID mice. *Nature, 367*, 645.

38. Mannelli, G., & Gallo, O., (2012). Cancer stem cells hypothesis and stem cells in head and neck cancers. *Cancer Treatment Reviews, 38*, 515–539.

39. Sztiller-Sikorska, M., Koprowska, K., Majchrzak, K., Hartman, M., & Czyz, M., (2014). Natural compounds' activity against cancer stem-like or fast-cycling melanoma cells. *PloS One, 9*, 3, e90783.

40. Qiu, X., Wang, Z., Li, Y., Miao, Y., Ren, Y., & Luan, Y., (2012). Characterization of sphere-forming cells with stem-like properties from the small cell lung cancer cell line H446. *Cancer Letters, 323*, 161–170.

41. Ueda, K., Ogasawara, S., Akiba, J., Nakayama, M., Todoroki, K., Ueda, K., Sanada, S., Suekane, S., Noguchi, M., & Matsuoka, K., (2013). Aldehyde dehydrogenase 1 identifies cells with cancer stem cell-like properties in a human renal cell carcinoma cell line. *PloS One, 8* 10, e75463.

42. Kitamura, H., Okudela, K., Yazawa, T., Sato, H., & Shimoyamada, H., (2009). Cancer stem cell: implications in cancer biology and therapy with special reference to lung cancer. *Lung Cancer, 66*, 275–281.

43. Saha, A., Padhi, S. S., Roy, S., & Banerjee, B., (2014). Method of detecting new cancer stem cell-like enrichment in development front assay (dfa). *Journal of Stem Cells, 9*(4), 235.

44. Fuchs, E., Tumbar, T., & Guasch, G., (2004). Socializing with the neighbors: stem cells and their niche. *Cell, 116*, 769–778.

45. Prasetyanti, P. R., & Medema, J. P., (2017). Intra-tumor heterogeneity from a cancer stem cell perspective. *Molecular Cancer, 16*, 41.

46. Ye, J., Wu, D., Wu, P., Chen, Z., & Huang, J., (2014). The cancer stem cell niche: cross talk between cancer stem cells and their microenvironment. *Tumor Biology, 35*, 3945–3951.

47. Chepko, G., Slack, R., Carbott, D., Khan, S., Steadman, L., & Dickson, R., (2005). Differential alteration of stem and other cell populations in ducts and lobules of TGFα and c-Myc transgenic mouse mammary epithelium. *Tissue and Cell, 37*, 393–412.

48. Zhang, J., Niu, C., Ye, L., Huang, H., He, X., Tong, W.-G., Ross, J., Haug, J., Johnson, T., & Feng, J. Q., (2003). Identification of the haematopoietic stem cell niche and control of the niche size. *Nature, 425*, 836–841.

49. Kopp, H.-G., Avecilla, S. T., Hooper, A. T., & Rafii, S., (2005). The bone marrow vascular niche: home of HSC differentiation and mobilization. *Physiology, 20*, 349–356.

50. Crowder, S. W., Balikov, D. A., Hwang, Y.-S., Sung, H.-J., (2014). Cancer stem cells under hypoxia as a chemoresistance factor in the breast and brain. *Current Pathobiology Reports, 2*(1), 33–40.

51. Lin, Q., & Yun, Z., (2010). Impact of the hypoxic tumor microenvironment on the regulation of cancer stem cell characteristics. *Cancer Biology & Therapy, 9*, 949–956.

52. Das, B., Tsuchida, R., Malkin, D., Koren, G., Baruchel, S., & Yeger, H., (2008). Hypoxia enhances tumor stemness by increasing the invasive and tumorigenic side population fraction. *Stem Cells, 26*, 1818–1830.

53. Jögi, A., Øra, I., Nilsson, H., Lindeheim, Å., Makino, Y., Poellinger, L., Axelson, H., & Påhlman, S., (2002). Hypoxia alters gene expression in human neuroblastoma cells toward an immature and neural crest-like phenotype. *Proceedings of the National Academy of Sciences, 99*, 7021–7026.

54. Holmquist-Mengelbier, L., Fredlund, E., Löfstedt, T., Noguera, R., Navarro, S., Nilsson, H., Pietras, A., Vallon-Christersson, J., Borg, A., & Gradin, K., (2006). Recruitment of HIF-1α and HIF-2α to common target genes is differentially regulated in neuroblastoma: HIF-2α promotes an aggressive phenotype. *Cancer Cell, 10*, 413–423.

55. Pietras, A., Hansford, L. M., Johnsson, A. S., Bridges, E., Sjölund, J., Gisselsson, D., Rehn, M., Beckman, S., Noguera, R., & Navarro, S., (2009). HIF-2α maintains an undifferentiated state in neural crest-like human neuroblastoma tumor-initiating cells. *Proceedings of the National Academy of Sciences, 106*, 16805–16810.

56. Lacina, L., Plzak, J., Kodet, O., Szabo, P., Chovanec, M., Dvorankova, B., & Smetana, Jr, K., (2015). Cancer microenvironment: what can we learn from the stem cell niche. *International Journal of Molecular Sciences, 16*, 24094–24110.

57. Xing, F., Saidou, J., & Watabe, K., (2010). Cancer associated fibroblasts (CAFs) in tumor microenvironment. *Frontiers in Bioscience: A Journal and Virtual Library, 15*, 166.

58. Jodele, S., Chantrain, C. F., Blavier, L., Lutzko, C., Crooks, G. M., Shimada, H., Coussens, L. M., & DeClerck, Y. A., (2005). The contribution of bone marrow–derived cells to the tumor vasculature in neuroblastoma is matrix metalloproteinase-9 dependent. *Cancer Research, 65*, 3200–3208.

59. Wee Yong, V., Bernard, C., Metz, L. M., Rewcastle, N. B., & Brundula, V., (2002). Targeting leukocyte MMPs and transmigration Minocycline as a potential therapy for multiple sclerosis.

60. Chantrain, C. F., Shimada, H., Jodele, S., Groshen, S., Ye, W., Shalinsky, D. R., Werb, Z., Coussens, L. M., & DeClerck, Y. A., (2004). Stromal matrix metalloproteinase-9 regulates the vascular architecture in neuroblastoma by promoting pericyte recruitment. *Cancer Research, 64*, 1675–1686.

61. Shigdar, S., Li, Y., Bhattacharya, S., O'Connor, M., Pu, C., Lin, J., Wang, T., Xiang, D., Kong, L., & Wei, M. Q., (2014). Inflammation and cancer stem cells. *Cancer Letters, 345*, 271–278.

62. Zumsteg, A., & Christofori, G., (2009). Corrupt policemen: inflammatory cells promote tumor angiogenesis. *Current Opinion in Oncology, 21*, 60–70.

63. Asgharzadeh, S., Salo, J. A., Ji, L., Oberthuer, A., Fischer, M., Berthold, F., Hadjidaniel, M., Liu, C. W.-Y., Metelitsa, L. S., & Pique-Regi, R., (2012). Clinical significance of tumor-associated inflammatory cells in metastatic neuroblastoma. *Journal of Clinical Oncology, 30*, 3525–3532.

64. Bottino, C., Dondero, A., Bellora, F., Moretta, L., Locatelli, F., Pistoia, V., Moretta, A., & Castriconi, R., (2014). Natural killer cells and neuroblastoma: tumor recognition, escape mechanisms, & possible novel immunotherapeutic approaches.

65. Sivori, S., Parolini, S., Marcenaro, E., Castriconi, R., Pende, D., Millo, R., & Moretta, A., (2000). Involvement of natural cytotoxicity receptors in human natural killer cell-mediated lysis of neuroblastoma and glioblastoma cell lines. *Journal of Neuroimmunology, 107*, 220–225.

66. Castriconi, R., Dondero, A., Cilli, M., Ognio, E., Pezzolo, A., De Giovanni, B., Gambini, C., Pistoia, V., Moretta, L., & Moretta, A., (2007). Human NK cell infusions prolong survival of metastatic human neuroblastoma-bearing NOD/scid mice. *Cancer Immunology, Immunotherapy, 56*, 1733–1742.

67. Heczey, A., Liu, D., Tian, G., Courtney, A. N., Wei, J., Marinova, E., Gao, X., Guo, L., Yvon, E., & Hicks, J., (2014). Invariant NKT cells with chimeric antigen receptor

provide a novel platform for safe and effective cancer immunotherapy. *Blood, 124*, 2824–2833.

68. Xu, Y., Sun, J., Sheard, M. A., Tran, H. C., Wan, Z., Liu, W. Y., Asgharzadeh, S., Sposto, R., Wu, H. W., & Seeger, R. C., (2013). Lenalidomide overcomes suppression of human natural killer cell anti-tumor functions by neuroblastoma microenvironment-associated IL-6 and TGFβ1. *Cancer Immunology Immunotherapy, 62*, 1637–1648.

69. Santilli, G., Piotrowska, I., Cantilena, S., Chayka, O., D'Alicarnasso, M., Morgenstern, D. A., Himoudi, N., Pearson, K., Anderson, J., & Thrasher, A. J., (2013). Polyphenol E enhances the antitumor immune response in neuroblastoma by inactivating myeloid suppressor cells. *Clinical Cancer Research, 19*, 1116–1125.

70. Kucia, M., Reca, R., Miekus, K., Wanzeck, J., Wojakowski, W., Janowska-Wieczorek, A., Ratajczak, J., & Ratajczak, M. Z., (2005). Trafficking of normal stem cells and metastasis of cancer stem cells involve similar mechanisms: Pivotal role of the SDF-1–CXCR4 Axis. *Stem Cells, 23*, 879–894.

71. Metelitsa, L. S., Wu, H.-W., Wang, H., Yang, Y., Warsi, Z., Asgharzadeh, S., Groshen, S., Wilson, S. B., & Seeger, R. C., (2004). Natural killer T cells infiltrate neuroblastomas expressing the chemokine CCL2. *Journal of Experimental Medicine, 199*, 1213–1221.

72. Orimo, A., Gupta, P. B., Sgroi, D. C., Arenzana-Seisdedos, F., Delaunay, T., Naeem, R., Carey, V. J., Richardson, A. L., & Weinberg, R. A., (2005). Stromal fibroblasts present in invasive human breast carcinomas promote tumor growth and angiogenesis through elevated SDF-1/CXCL12 secretion. *Cell, 121*, 335–348.

73. Gottardi, C. J., & Gumbiner, B. M., (2004). Distinct molecular forms of β-catenin are targeted to adhesive or transcriptional complexes. *The Journal of Cell Biology, 167*, 339–349.

74. Song, X., & Xie, T., (2002). DE-cadherin-mediated cell adhesion is essential for maintaining somatic stem cells in the Drosophila ovary. *Proceedings of the National Academy of Sciences, 99*, 14813–14818.

75. He, T. C., Sparks, A. B., Rago, C., Hermeking, H., Zawel, L., Da Costa, L. T., Morin, P. J., Vogelstein, B., & Kinzler, K. W., (1998). Identification of c-MYC as a target of the APC pathway. *Science (New York), 281*, 1509–1512.

76. Yang, S. Z., Kohno, N., Yokoyama, A., Kondo, K., Hamada, H., & Hiwada, K., (2001). Decreased E-cadherin augments b-catenin nuclear localization: Studies in breast cancer cell lines. *International Journal of Oncology, 18*, 541–548.

77. Ysebaert, L., Chicanne, G., Demur, C., De Toni, F., Prade-Houdellier, N., Ruidavets, J., Mansat-De Mas, V., Rigal-Huguet, F., Laurent, G., & Payrastre, B., (2006). Expression of β-catenin by acute myeloid leukemia cells predicts enhanced clonogenic capacities and poor prognosis. *Leukemia, 20*, 1211–1216.

78. Chien, A. J., Moore, E. C., Lonsdorf, A. S., Kulikauskas, R. M., Rothberg, B. G., Berger, A. J., Major, M. B., Hwang, S. T., Rimm, D. L., & Moon, R. T., (2009). Activated Wnt/ß-catenin signaling in melanoma is associated with decreased proliferation in patient tumors and a murine melanoma model. *Proceedings of the National Academy of Sciences, 106*, 1193–1198.

79. Li, Y., Welm, B., Podsypanina, K., Huang, S., Chamorro, M., Zhang, X., Rowlands, T., Egeblad, M., Cowin, P., & Werb, Z., (2003). Evidence that transgenes encoding components of the Wnt signaling pathway preferentially induce mammary cancers from progenitor cells. *Proceedings of the National Academy of Sciences, 100*, 15853–15858.

80. Schulenburg, A., Cech, P., Herbacek, I., Marian, B., Wrba, F., Valent, P., Ulrich-Pur, H., (2007). CD44-positive colorectal adenoma cells express the potential stem cell markers musashi antigen (msi1) and ephrin B2 receptor (EphB2). *The Journal of Pathology, 213*, 152–160.

81. Yang, W., Yan, H. X., Chen, L., Liu, Q., He, Y. Q., Yu, L. X., Zhang, S. H., Huang, D. D., Tang, L., & Kong, X. N., (2008). Wnt/β-catenin signaling contributes to activation of normal and tumorigenic liver progenitor cells. *Cancer Research, 68*, 4287–4295.

82. Teng, Y., Wang, X., Wang, Y., & Ma, D., (2010). Wnt/β-catenin signaling regulates cancer stem cells in lung cancer A549 cells. *Biochemical and Biophysical Research Communications, 392*, 373–379.

83. Nelson, W. J., & Nusse, R., (2004). Convergence of Wnt, ß-catenin, & cadherin pathways. *Science (New York), 303*, 1483–1487.

84. Orsulic, S., Huber, O., Aberle, H., Arnold, S., & Kemler, R., (1999). E-cadherin binding prevents beta-catenin nuclear localization and beta-catenin/LEF-1-mediated transactivation. *Journal of Cell Science, 112*, 1237–1245.

85. Takahashi-Yanaga, F., & Sasaguri, T., (2008). GSK-3β regulates cyclin D1 expression: a new target for chemotherapy. *Cellular Signalling, 20*, 581–589.

86. Bechard, M., Trost, R., Singh, A. M., & Dalton, S., (2012). Frat is a phosphatidylinositol 3-kinase/Akt-regulated determinant of glycogen synthase kinase 3β subcellular localization in pluripotent cells. *Molecular and Cellular Biology, 32*, 288–296.

87. Yeung, J., Esposito, M. T., Gandillet, A., Zeisig, B. B., Griessinger, E., Bonnet, D., & So, C. W. E., (2010). β-Catenin mediates the establishment and drug resistance of MLL leukemic stem cells. *Cancer Cell, 18*, 606–618.

88. di Magliano, M. P., & Hebrok, M., (2003). Hedgehog signalling in cancer formation and maintenance. *Nature Reviews Cancer, 3*, 903–911.

89. Chen, G. L., Yang, L., Rowe, T., Halligan, B. D., Tewey, K. M., & Liu, L. F., (1984). Nonintercalative antitumor drugs interfere with the breakage-reunion reaction of mammalian DNA topoisomerase II. *Journal of Biological Chemistry, 259*, 13560–13566.

90. Cohen, M. M., (2003). The hedgehog signaling network. *American Journal of Medical Genetics Part A., 123*, 5–28.

91. Drenkhahn, S. K., Jackson, G. A., Slusarz, A., Starkey, N. J., & Lubahn, D. B., (2013). Inhibition of hedgehog/Gli signaling by botanicals: a review of compounds with potential hedgehog pathway inhibitory activities. *Current Cancer Drug Targets, 13*, 580–595.

92. Clement, V., Sanchez, P., De Tribolet, N., Radovanovic, I., i Altaba, A. R., (2007). HEDGEHOG-GLI1 signaling regulates human glioma growth, cancer stem cell self-renewal, & tumorigenicity. *Current Biology, 17*, 165–172.

93. Nakashima, H., Nakamura, M., Yamaguchi, H., Yamanaka, N., Akiyoshi, T., Koga, K., Yamaguchi, K., Tsuneyoshi, M., Tanaka, M., & Katano, M., (2006). Nuclear factor-κB contributes to hedgehog signaling pathway activation through sonic hedgehog induction in pancreatic cancer. *Cancer Research, 66*, 7041–7049.

94. Kasperczyk, H., Baumann, B., Debatin, K. M., & Fulda, S., (2009). Characterization of sonic hedgehog as a novel NF-κB target gene that promotes NF-κB-mediated apoptosis resistance and tumor growth in vivo. *The FASEB Journal, 23*, 21–33.

95. Su, W., Meng, F., Huang, L., Zheng, M., Liu, W., & Sun, H., (2012). Sonic hedgehog maintains survival and growth of chronic myeloid leukemia progenitor cells through β-catenin signaling. *Experimental Hematology, 40*, 418–427.

96. Batsaikhan, B. E., Yoshikawa, K., Kurita, N., Iwata, T., Takasu, C., Kashihara, H., & Shimada, M., (2014). Cyclopamine decreased the expression of Sonic Hedgehog and its downstream genes in colon cancer stem cells. *Anticancer Research, 34,* 6339–6344.

97. Kurebayashi, J., Koike, Y., Ohta, Y., Saitoh, W., Yamashita, T., Kanomata, N., & Moriya, T., (2017). Anti-cancer stem cell activity of a hedgehog inhibitor GANT61 in estrogen receptor-positive breast cancer cells. *Cancer Science.*

98. Zhu, J. Y., Yang, X., Chen, Y., Jiang, Y., Wang, S. J., Li, Y., Wang, X. Q., Meng, Y., Zhu, M. M., Ma, X., Huang, C., Wu, R., Xie, C. F., Li, X. T., Geng, S. S., Wu, J. S., Zhong, C. Y., & Han, H. Y., (2017). Curcumin suppresses lung cancer stem cells via inhibiting Wnt/beta-catenin and sonic hedgehog pathways. *Phytotherapy Research: PTR.*

99. Wang, Z., Li, Y., Banerjee, S., & Sarkar, F. H., (2009). Emerging role of notch in stem cells and cancer. *Cancer Letters, 279,* 8–12.

100. Farnie, G., & Clarke, R. B., (2007). Mammary stem cells and breast cancer—role of Notch signalling. *Stem Cell Reviews, 3,* 169–175.

101. Espinosa, L., Cathelin, S., D'Altri, T., Trimarchi, T., Statnikov, A., Guiu, J., Rodilla, V., Inglés-Esteve, J., Nomdedeu, J., & Bellosillo, B., (2010). The Notch/Hes1 pathway sustains NF-κB activation through CYLD repression in T cell leukemia. *Cancer Cell, 18,* 268–281.

102. Wilson, A., & Radtke, F., (2006). Multiple functions of Notch signaling in self-renewing organs and cancer. *FEBS Letters, 58,* 2860–2868.

103. Rangarajan, A., Talora, C., Okuyama, R., Nicolas, M., Mammucari, C., Oh, H., Aster, J. C., Krishna, S., Metzger, D., & Chambon, P., (2001). Notch signaling is a direct determinant of keratinocyte growth arrest and entry into differentiation. *The EMBO Journal, 20,* 3427–3436.

104. Oswald, F., Liptay, S., Adler, G., & Schmid, R. M., (1998). NF-κB2 is a putative target gene of activated Notch-1 via RBP-Jκ. *Molecular and Cellular Biology, 18,* 2077–2088.

105. Jang, M. S., Miao, H., Carlesso, N., Shelly, L., Zlobin, A., Darack, N., Qin, J. Z., Nickoloff, B. J., & Miele, L., (2004). Notch-1 regulates cell death independently of differentiation in murine erythroleukemia cells through multiple apoptosis and cell cycle pathways. *Journal of Cellular Physiology, 199,* 418–433.

106. Garcia-Heredia, J. M., Verdugo Sivianes, E. M., Lucena-Cacace, A., Molina-Pinelo, S., & Carnero, A., (2016). Numb-like (NumbL) downregulation increases tumorigenicity, cancer stem cell-like properties and resistance to chemotherapy. *Oncotarget, 7,* 63611–63628.

107. Garcia-Heredia, J. M., Lucena-Cacace, A., Verdugo-Sivianes, E. M., Perez, M., & Carnero, A., (2017). The cargo protein MAP17 (PDZK1IP1) regulates the cancer stem cell pool activating the Notch pathway by abducting NUMB. *Clinical Cancer Research: an Official Journal of the American Association for Cancer Research.*

108. Courtney, K. D., Corcoran, R. B., & Engelman, J. A., (2010). The PI3K pathway as drug target in human cancer. *Journal of Clinical Oncology, 28,* 1075–1083.

109. Kim, R. J., Bae, E., Hong, Y. K., Hong, J. Y., Kim, N. K., Ahn, H. J., Oh, J. J., & Park, D. S., (2014). PTEN loss-mediated Akt activation increases the properties of cancer stem-like cell populations in prostate cancer. *Oncology, 87,* 270–279.

110. Aksamitiene, E., Kiyatkin, A., & Kholodenko, B. N., (2012). Cross-talk between mitogenic Ras/MAPK and survival PI3K/Akt pathways: a fine balance. Portland Press Limited.

111. Voskas, D., Ling, L. S., & Woodgett, J. R., (2010). Does GSK-3 provide a shortcut for PI3K activation of Wnt signalling. *F1000 Biol. Rep., 2*, 82.

112. Korkaya, H., Paulson, A., Charafe-Jauffret, E., Ginestier, C., Brown, M., Dutcher, J., Clouthier, S. G., & Wicha, M. S., (2009). Regulation of mammary stem/progenitor cells by PTEN/Akt/β-catenin signaling. *PLoS Biology, 7*, 6, e1000121.

113. Biver, E., Thouverey, C., Magne, D., & Caverzasio, J., (2014). Crosstalk between tyrosine kinase receptors, GSK3 and BMP2 signaling during osteoblastic differentiation of human mesenchymal stem cells. *Molecular and Cellular Endocrinology, 382*, 120–130.

114. Ormanns, S., Neumann, J., Horst, D., Kirchner, T., & Jung, A., (2014). WNT signaling and distant metastasis in colon cancer through transcriptional activity of nuclear β-Catenin depend on active PI3K signaling. *Oncotarget, 5*, 2999–3011.

115. Frank, N. Y., Schatton, T., & Frank, M. H., (2010). The therapeutic promise of the cancer stem cell concept. *The Journal of Clinical Investigation, 120*, 41–50.

116. Chen, K., Huang, Y. H., & Chen, J. L., (2013). Understanding and targeting cancer stem cells: therapeutic implications and challenges. *Acta. Pharmacologica. Sinica., 34*, 732–740.

117. Cicenas, J., & Valius, M., (2011). The CDK inhibitors in cancer research and therapy. *Journal of Cancer Research and Clinical Oncology, 137*, 1409.

118. Osuka, S., Sampetrean, O., Shimizu, T., Saga, I., Onishi, N., Sugihara, E., Okubo, J., Fujita, S., Takano, S., & Matsumura, A., (2013). IGF1 receptor signaling regulates adaptive radioprotection in glioma stem cells. *Stem Cells, 31*, 627–640.

119. Shimizu, T., Sugihara, E., Yamaguchi-Iwai, S., Tamaki, S., Koyama, Y., Kamel, W., Ueki, A., Ishikawa, T., Chiyoda, T., & Osuka, S., (2014). IGF2 preserves osteosarcoma cell survival by creating an autophagic state of dormancy that protects cells against chemotherapeutic stress. *Cancer Research, 74*, 6531–6541.

120. Schiffer, C. A., (2007). BCR-ABL tyrosine kinase inhibitors for chronic myelogenous leukemia. *New England Journal of Medicine, 357*, 258–265.

121. Yoshida, G. J., & Saya, H., (2014). Inversed relationship between CD44 variant and c-Myc due to oxidative stress-induced canonical Wnt activation. *Biochemical and Biophysical Research Communications, 443*, 622–627.

122. Chung, S. S., Adekoya, D., Enenmoh, I., Clarke, O., Wang, P., Sarkyssian, M., Wu, Y., & Vadgama, J. V., (2017). Salinomycin Abolished STAT3 and STAT1 Interactions and Reduced Telomerase Activity in Colorectal Cancer Cells. *Anticancer Research, 37*, 445–453.

123. Gong, Z., Chen, D., Xie, F., Liu, J., Zhang, H., Zou, H., Yu, Y., Chen, Y., Sun, Z., Wang, X., Zhang, H., Zhang, G., Yin, C., Gao, J., Zhong, Y., & Lu, Y., (2016). Codelivery of salinomycin and doxorubicin using nanoliposomes for targeting both liver cancer cells and cancer stem cells. *Nanomedicine (London, England), 11*, 2565–2579.

124. Chung, H., Kim, Y. H., Kwon, M., Shin, S. J., Kwon, S. H., Cha, S. D., & Cho, C. H., (2016). The effect of salinomycin on ovarian cancer stem-like cells. *Obstetrics & Gynecology Science, 59*, 261–268.

125. Muntimadugu, E., Kumar, R., Saladi, S., Rafeeqi, T. A., & Khan, W., (2016). CD44 targeted chemotherapy for co-eradication of breast cancer stem cells and cancer cells using polymeric nanoparticles of salinomycin and paclitaxel. *Colloids and Surfaces B. Biointerfaces, 143*, 532–546.

126. Park, C. H., Hahm, E. R., Park, S., Kim, H. K., & Yang, C. H., (2005). The inhibitory mechanism of curcumin and its derivative against β-catenin/Tcf signaling. *FEBS Letters, 579,* 2965–2971.

127. Li, Y., Zhang, T., Korkaya, H., Liu, S., Lee, H.-F., Newman, B., Yu, Y., Clouthier, S. G., Schwartz, S. J., & Wicha, M. S., (2010). Sulforaphane, a dietary component of broccoli/broccoli sprouts, inhibits breast cancer stem cells. *Clinical Cancer Research, 16,* 2580–2590.

128. Sarkar, F. H., Li, Y., Wang, Z., & Kong, D., (2009). Cellular signaling perturbation by natural products. *Cellular Signalling, 21,* 1541–1547.

129. Gödeke, J., Maier, S., Eichenmüller, M., Müller-Höcker, J., von Schweinitz, D., & Kappler, R., (2013). Epigallocatechin-3-gallate inhibits hepatoblastoma growth by reactivating the Wnt inhibitor SFRP1. *Nutrition and Cancer, 65,* 1200–1207.

130. Bishayee, A., (2009). Cancer prevention and treatment with resveratrol: from rodent studies to clinical trials. *Cancer Prevention Research,* 1940–6207. CAPR-08–0160.

131. van Breemen, R. B., & Pajkovic, N., (2008). Multitargeted therapy of cancer by lycopene. *Cancer Letters, 269,* 339–351.

132. Kakarala, M., Brenner, D. E., Korkaya, H., Cheng, C., Tazi, K., Ginestier, C., Liu, S., Dontu, G., & Wicha, M. S., (2010). Targeting breast stem cells with the cancer preventive compounds curcumin and piperine. *Breast Cancer Research and Treatment, 122,* 777–785.

133. Guyton, K. Z., Kensler, T. W., & Posner, G. H., (2003). Vitamin D and vitamin D analogs as cancer chemopreventive agents. *Nutrition Reviews, 61,* 227–238.

134. Srinual, S., Chanvorachote, P., & Pongrakhananon, V., (2017). Suppression of cancer stem-like phenotypes in NCI-H460 lung cancer cells by vanillin through an Akt-dependent pathway. *International Journal of Oncology.*

135. Dick, D., (1997). Human acute myeloid leukemia is organized as a hierarchy that originates from a primitive hematopoietic cell. *Nature Med., 3,* 730–737, 1.

136. Al-Hajj, M., & Wicha, M. S., (2003). Benito-Hernandez, A., Morrison, S. J., Clarke, M. F., Prospective identification of tumorigenic breast cancer cells. *Proceedings of the National Academy of Sciences, 100,* 3983–3988.

137. Ricci-Vitiani, L., Lombardi, D. G., Pilozzi, E., Biffoni, M., Todaro, M., Peschle, C., & De Maria, R., (2007). Identification and expansion of human colon-cancer-initiating cells. *Nature 445,* 111–115.

138. Cammareri, P., Lombardo, Y., Francipane, M. G., Bonventre, S., Todaro, M., & Stassi, G., (2008). Isolation and culture of colon cancer stem cells. *Methods in Cell Biology, 86,* 311–324.

139. Prince, M., Sivanandan, R., Kaczorowski, A., Wolf, G., Kaplan, M., Dalerba, P., Weissman, I., Clarke, M., & Ailles, L., (2007). Identification of a subpopulation of cells with cancer stem cell properties in head and neck squamous cell carcinoma. *Proceedings of the National Academy of Sciences, 104,* 973–978.

140. Singh, S. K., Hawkins, C., Clarke, I. D., Squire, J. A., Bayani, J., Hide, T., Henkelman, R. M., Cusimano, M. D., & Dirks, P. B., (2004). Identification of human brain tumour initiating cells. *Nature, 432,* 396–401.

141. Eramo, A., Lotti, F., Sette, G., Pilozzi, E., Biffoni, M., Di Virgilio, A., Conticello, C., Ruco, L., Peschle, C., & De Maria, R., (2008). Identification and expansion of the tumorigenic lung cancer stem cell population. *Cell Death & Differentiation, 15,* 504–514.

142. Hermann, P. C., Huber, S. L., Herrler, T., Aicher, A., Ellwart, J. W., Guba, M., Bruns, C. J., & Heeschen, C., (2007). Distinct populations of cancer stem cells determine tumor growth and metastatic activity in human pancreatic cancer. *Cell Stem Cell, 1*, 313–323.

143. Li, C., Heidt, D. G., Dalerba, P., Burant, C. F., Zhang, L., Adsay, V., Wicha, M., Clarke, M. F., & Simeone, D. M., (2007). Identification of pancreatic cancer stem cells. *Cancer Research, 67*, 1030–1037.

144. Yang, Z. F., Ho, D. W., Ng, M. N., Lau, C. K., Yu, W. C., Ngai, P., Chu, P. W., Lam, C. T., Poon, R. T., & Fan, S. T., (2008). Significance of CD90+ cancer stem cells in human liver cancer. *Cancer Cell, 13*, 153–166.

145. Collins, F. S., Gray, G. M., & Bucher, J. R., (2008). Transforming environmental health protection. *Science (New York), 319*, 906.

146. Klonisch, T., Wiechec, E., Hombach-Klonisch, S., Ande, S. R., Wesselborg, S., Schulze-Osthoff, K., & Los, M., (2008). Cancer stem cell markers in common cancers–therapeutic implications. *Trends in Molecular Medicine, 14*, 450–460.

147. Fang, D., Nguyen, T. K., Leishear, K., Finko, R., Kulp, A. N., Hotz, S., Van Belle, P. A., Xu, X., Elder, D. E., & Herlyn, M., (2005). A tumorigenic subpopulation with stem cell properties in melanomas. *Cancer Research, 65*, 9328–9337.

148. Pannuti, A., Foreman, K., Rizzo, P., Osipo, C., Golde, T., Osborne, B., & Miele, L., (2010). Targeting Notch to target cancer stem cells. *Clinical Cancer Research, 16*, 3141–3152.

149. Wu, Y., Cain-Hom, C., Choy, L., Hagenbeek, T. J., de Leon, G. P., Chen, Y., Finkle, D., Venook, R., Wu, X., & Ridgway, J., (2010). Therapeutic antibody targeting of individual Notch receptors. *Nature, 464*, 1052–1057.

150. Fan, X., Matsui, W., Khaki, L., Stearns, D., Chun, J., Li, Y.-M., & Eberhart, C. G., (2006). Notch pathway inhibition depletes stem-like cells and blocks engraftment in embryonal brain tumors. *Cancer Research, 66*, 7445–7452.

151. Rudin, C. M., Hann, C. L., Laterra, J., Yauch, R. L., Callahan, C. A., Fu, L., Holcomb, T., Stinson, J., Gould, S. E., & Coleman, B., (2009). Treatment of medulloblastoma with hedgehog pathway inhibitor GDC-0449. *New England Journal of Medicine, 36*, 1173–1178.

152. Merchant, A. A., & Matsui, W., (2010). Targeting Hedgehog—a cancer stem cell pathway. *Clinical Cancer Research, 16*, 3130–3140.

153. Ericson, J., Morton, S., Kawakami, A., Roelink, H., & Jessell, T. M., (1996). Two critical periods of Sonic Hedgehog signaling required for the specification of motor neuron identity. *Cell, 87*, 661–673.

154. Qiu, W., Wang, X., Leibowitz, B., Liu, H., Barker, N., Okada, H., Oue, N., Yasui, W., Clevers, H., & Schoen, R. E., (2010). Chemoprevention by nonsteroidal anti-inflammatory drugs eliminates oncogenic intestinal stem cells via SMAC-dependent apoptosis. *Proceedings of the National Academy of Sciences, 107*, 20027–20032.

155. Lepourcelet, M., Chen, Y.-N. P., France, D. S., Wang, H., Crews, P., Petersen, F., Bruseo, C., Wood, A. W., & Shivdasani, R. A., (2004). Small-molecule antagonists of the oncogenic Tcf/β-catenin protein complex. *Cancer Cell, 5*, 91–102.

156. Takahashi-Yanaga, F., & Kahn, M., (2010). Targeting Wnt signaling: can we safely eradicate cancer stem cells? *Clinical Cancer Research, 16*, 3153–3162.

157. Chen, B., Dodge, M. E., Tang, W., Lu, J., Ma, Z., Fan, C.-W., Wei, S., Hao, W., Kilgore, J., & Williams, N. S., (2009). Small molecule–mediated disruption of Wnt-

dependent signaling in tissue regeneration and cancer. *Nature Chemical Biology, 5,* 100–107.

158. Sedrani, R., Cottens, S., Kallen, J., & Schuler, W., (1998). In Chemical modification of rapamycin: the discovery of SDZ RAD, *Transplantation Proceedings*, Elsevier, pp. 2192–2194.

159. Kondapaka, S. B., Singh, S. S., Dasmahapatra, G. P., Sausville, E. A., & Roy, K. K., (2003). Perifosine, a novel alkylphospholipid, inhibits protein kinase B activation. *Molecular Cancer Therapeutics, 2,* 1093–1103.

160. Folkes, A. J., Ahmadi, K., Alderton, W. K., Alix, S., Baker, S. J., Box, G., Chuckowree, I. S., Clarke, P. A., Depledge, P., & Eccles, S. A., (2008). The identification of 2-(1 H-indazol-4-yl)-6-(4-methanesulfonyl-piperazin-1-ylmethyl)-4-morpholin-4-yl-thieno [3, 2-d] pyrimidine (GDC-0941) as a potent, selective, orally bioavailable inhibitor of class I PI3 kinase for the treatment of cancer. *Journal of Medicinal Chemistry, 51,* 5522–5532.

161. Dowling, R. J., Zakikhani, M., Fantus, I. G., Pollak, M., & Sonenberg, N., (2007). Metformin inhibits mammalian target of rapamycin–dependent translation initiation in breast cancer cells. *Cancer Research, 67,* 10804–10812.

162. Scheinman, R. I., Cogswell, P. C., Lofquist, A. K., Baldwin Jr, A. S., (1995). Role of transcriptional activation of IkappaBalpha in mediation of immunosuppression of glucocorticoids. *Science (New York), 270,* 283.

163. Naugler, W. E., & Karin, M., (2008). NF-κB and cancer—identifying targets and mechanisms. *Current Opinion in Genetics & Development, 18,* 19–26.

164. Donzella, G. A., Schols, D., Lin, S. W., Este, J. A., Nagashima, K. A., Maddon, P. J., Allaway, G. P., Sakmar, T. P., Henson, G., & DeClercq, E., (1998). AMD3100, a small molecule inhibitor of HIV-1 entry via the CXCR4 co-receptor. *Nature Medicine, 4,* 72–77.

165. Friedman, H. S., Prados, M. D., Wen, P. Y., Mikkelsen, T., Schiff, D., Abrey, L. E., Yung, W. A., Paleologos, N., Nicholas, M. K., & Jensen, R., (2009). Bevacizumab alone and in combination with irinotecan in recurrent glioblastoma. *Journal of Clinical Oncology, 27,* 4733–4740.

166. Wang, G., Nikolovska-Coleska, Z., Yang, C.-Y., Wang, R., Tang, G., Guo, J., Shangary, S., Qiu, S., Gao, W., & Yang, D., (2006). Structure-based design of potent small-molecule inhibitors of anti-apoptotic Bcl-2 proteins. *Journal of Medicinal Chemistry, 49,* 6139–6142.

167. Jin, L., Hope, K. J., Zhai, Q., Smadja-Joffe, F., & Dick, J. E., (2006). Targeting of CD44 eradicates human acute myeloid leukemic stem cells. *Nature Medicine, 12,* 1167–1174.

CHAPTER 16

TUMOR MICROENVIRONMENT AND CANCER STEM CELLS: THERAPEUTIC POTENTIAL OF EPIGENETIC INHIBITORS TO TARGET CANCER STEM CELLS

ANUP KUMAR SINGH, PRIYANK CHATURVEDI, and DIPAK DATTA

Biochemistry Division, CSIR-Central Drug Research Institute, Lucknow–226031, India, Tel.: 522-2612411-18 (Extn: 4347/48), Fax: 522-2623405/2623938, E-mail: dipak.datta@cdri.res.in

CONTENTS

ABSTRACT

It is now widely accepted that tumor originates from a normal cell as a result of multiple genetic and epigenetic alterations; however, the major challenges lie in understanding the fact that how clinical tumors sustained themselves in immunogenic and therapeutically grim microenvironment present in their surroundings. Presence of a special but generally minor subpopulation of tumor cells, also called cancer stem cells (CSCs), within the heterogeneous tumor population explains most of the tumor-associated phenotypes. CSCs are thought to be a very dynamic population of cells continuously evolving in a Darwinian fashion to adapt and survive in challenged conditions. Emerging reports are advocating the role of epigenetic alterations in driving drug resistance of CSCs, and epigenetic inhibitors are showing a promising therapeutic strategy in combination with classical drugs to combat late stage aggressive cancers. In the present chapter, we discuss the latest understanding of interrelationship between tumor microenvironment and CSCs and the role of relevant epigenetic alterations in driving CSC-associated phenotypes such as drug resistance. We will also discuss the possibility of new therapeutic opportunities by combining epigenetic inhibitors with classical drugs to target CSCs and their plasticity properties.

16.1   INTRODUCTION

Majority of solid tumors display phenotypic and functional heterogeneity at the population level. Despite significant advances in diagnosis and treatment of at least few types of cancer, a major thrust of cancer biology remains around the understanding of cellular organization of tumor cell population to target them individually as well as their subcellular integrity. Cancer cell resistance to chemotherapies is a heavy burden to the patients as it leads to recurrence and tumor relapse. For instance, although surgical resection is the most effective treatment for solid tumors, postoperative chemotherapy is minimally effective, and often residual presence of drug-resistant stem-like cell population lead to tumor relapse [1]. These stem-like cells, which are popularly known as cancer stem cells (CSCs), have been shown to constitute a primitive cell population capable of self-renewal and differentiation and reside at the center of cellular hierarchy present inside the heterogeneous tumor population [1a, 2]. Drug resistance against conventional chemotherapeutics is believed to be contributed by CSCs in solid tumors, and due to their accumulation in the course of treatment, tumor eventually relapses and metastasizes [3].

Tumor cells are considered to be hierarchically organized population with a characteristics extent of phenotypic heterogeneity [4] contributed by cancer initiating, endothelial, stromal, hematopoietic and other infiltrating cells that communicate with each other in a dynamic fashion [5]. Decades of extensive research endeavors to characterize tumor heterogeneity led to the identification of CSCs. CSCs have been characterized and isolated from the whole tumor mass based on the presence of special surface biomarkers and subsequently found to show high expression drug-resistant properties and deregulated self-renewal machineries indicating its role in cancer initiation, progression, metastasis and recurrence. As an experimental procedure, CSCs are functionally defined on the basis of their tumor seeding ability in animal models, self-renewal, and ability to give rise to differentiated non-CSC progeny [1a, 6]. Therefore, the distributions of CSCs within a population of cancer cells is measured by the number of cells needed, at a given dilution to seed new tumors [7]. In many aspects, CSCs are close to stem cells of normal tissue at least in terms of the self-renewal process, but unlike normal stem cells, the deregulated self-renewal ability of CSCs makes them resistant to conventional chemotherapy [8]. Similar to their normal tissue counterpart, tumors have the same population of stem-like cells, differentiated cells, other stromal cells, and dead cells. These dividing cells have a limited number of division capacities, and finally, they die in normal tissue. In cancer, however, they show immortality and continue to divide and do not die, leading to their accumulation. According to the theory, proposed in early nineteenth century, cancer could arise from stem cells based on the rationale that human body contains remnants of embryonic tissue stem cells [9]. After various changes in the environment or surrounding, tissues would restart dividing to produce cell masses similar to that tissue [10]. Later, in the twentieth century, this theory was replaced by proposing the concept of dedifferentiation. According to this, tumor mass is derived from the unlimited growth of cells that basically regressed from a more differentiated state to a primitive one called pluripotent state. The stochastic developmental pattern suggests that tumors are homogeneous masses of developmentally similar cells arising from any cell present in the bulk population that have accumulated the necessary mutations in the course of time. On the other hand, recent evidence suggest that cancer development follows a hierarchy in its induction where only a few cells are responsible for its origin and generates all cells present in the tumor [11]. A further layer of complexity is added by many subsequent reports which mention that often majority of the tumor cells exhibit CSC-like properties and questions the idea that just like normal stem cells, whether CSCs do exist as rare populations within the tumors or not [3a, 7, 12]. As an explanation to tumor heterogeneity, two different theories are proposed to describe the process of cancer initiation, namely stochastic model and CSC model of tumor heterogeneity. According to the stochastic model of tumor heterogeneity, the cells present within the tumor population are equally endowed, and once they become dysfunctional, any one of them is able to initiate the tumor formation. On the other hand, the CSC model advocates the presence of cellular hierarchy within the tumor and it suggests that only a fraction of heterogeneous tumor cells are sufficient to initiate tumor formation. Tumor heterogeneity within a cancer cell population can be categorized as genetic and epigenetic variations found among different cells of the tumor. Under genetic heterogeneity, it is thought that randomly accumulating mutations caused substantial genetic variations in the populations of cells. These mutations can be either silent in nature, which is called passenger mutations, or can have a functional impact where it is called driver mutations. Here, it is important to understand that accumulating passenger mutations may have functional importance in the suitable circumstances by becoming driver mutation [4c, 6]. In accordance with the CSC concept, the presence or absence of surface markers also provide heterogeneity based on surface expression of the CSC marker. Therefore, understanding the tumor heterogeneity is the major root to understand CSC biology, and molecular feature associated with phenotype variations will help in designing effective treatments. As a result, the primary aim of clinicians worldwide now is to unravel the mechanism and then to therapeutically intervene at initiation and propagation of various tumors [13].

Epigenetic control of gene expressions as a means for response to various internal and environmental cues is shown to play a pivotal role in mediating environmental influence on cancer. Multiple recent studies emphasize the crucial role of epigenetic regulation in CSC attributes including drug resistance [14]. Dynamic regulation of DNA methylation and covalent histone modifications at enhancers and promoters are fundamental to the modulation of stemness-related gene expression and determination of CSC phenotype [14b, 15]. Histone modifications through polycomb group (PcG) proteins have shown to drive CSC biology [16]. PcG proteins mediate gene repression through chromatin remodeling, specifically by catalyzing posttranslational modifications on histone proteins via polycomb repressive complex 1 (PRC1) and PRC2 [17]. Histone methyl transferase enhancer of zeste homologue 2 (EZH2) is the catalytically active component of PRC2, which mediates the transcriptional repression of its target genes by affecting the local heterochromatin state-mediated trimethylation of lysine 27 at histone H3 (H3K27) [18]. Altogether, epigenetic regulators are emerging as a novel target to combat drug resistance and tumor relapse and small molecules that can target them hold promise as neoadjuvant therapy.

16.2   TUMOR MICROENVIRONMENT AND CANCER STEM CELLS (CSCs)

Tumor microenvironment refers to the local environment in the vicinity of tumor cell population, and it includes various nontumor cells, including immune and stromal cells, surrounding vascular endothelial cells, and other components present in the tumor mass except the actual tumor cells. Considering the origin of these cells within the heterogeneous tumor population, various possibilities are proposed. One such possibility is that cancer could be initiated from the stem cells as human body is developed from embryonic tissue. Since this developmental process is affected by environmental factors, there is a strong scope of uncontrolled division to produce an undifferentiated cell mass or tumor in case of any insult from microenvironment. Bailey was the first scientist to propose as early as 1926 that cancer may be started and maintained by a few transformed cells [20]. In recent decades, the pioneering research on this topic was led by the Dick group, who were the first to isolate and characterize the CSC population in leukemia in the late 90s [21]. In subsequent years, this concept has been validated in various solid tumors [22]. Based on its many similarities and certain key differences with normal stem cells, two main hypotheses have emerged about the origin of CSCs: a) there is a possibility that stem cells themselves would undergo a number of mutations and finally become cancer stem cells or b) highly differentiated cells of the corresponding tissue are dedifferentiated to acquire the pluripotent state [23]. There is also a possibility for third option that there may be fusion between normal stem cells and differentiated cells. Based on modern understanding of CSCs, the population of tumor cells is hierarchically organized just like their normal counterpart tissue of origin, and a few CSCs are found at the top most position of cellular hierarchy. Similar to their normal counterpart, CSCs retain their self -renewal and multilineage differentiation potential even during tumor progression [24]. CSC population can be characterized based on the following key characteristics: (1) only a small fraction of total tumor cell population is sufficient to induce tumor into suitable animal models; (2) these special cells express a unique cell surface marker as compared to rest of the tumor cells; (3) tumor induced by CSC transplantation are heterogeneous mixture of CSCs and non-CSCs; and (4) CSCs can be used for serial transplantation up to many generations [25]. Considering the genetic basis of CSC origin and tumor heterogeneity, as discussed earlier, a large number of mutations continuously occur within the tumor cells, and a great majority of them are "passengers," i.e., they are silent in nature. In contrast to these, there are driver mutations that are basically mutations of oncogenes and tumor suppressors and beneficial to cancer cells as they facilitate uncontrolled proliferation and offer other hallmark features of cancer [6]. One fundamental concern to understand about passenger and driver mutations is the time of their incorporation. A subset of these passengers might have occurred well before the cancer initiation, which can be considered as key driver mutation. Driver mutations are necessary to initiate tumor. Once these driver mutations occur, the cells started to expand, and successive clonal expansion accumulating additional passenger mutations form tumor heterogeneity as some of the clones were predominant and generate clonal bottlenecks [26]. Most of the mutational accumulation occurs at the time of clonal expansion of zygotic cell to expand into tissue. After expansion of zygote into tissue cells, which self-renew themselves, most of the passenger mutations randomly accumulate at this time. The average time required for self-renewal depends on the type of cell, and therefore, the total number of somatic mutations accumulated within a tumor might be ideally directly proportional to the age of the diseased person. Pancreatic ductal adenocarcinoma is an exception where pancreatic ductal epithelial cells do not self-renew; thus, there is no correlation between the age of the patient and the number of mutations accumulated at the time of diagnosis [27]. Furthermore, it is also interesting to see that the CSC model is not followed by all tumor types in every aspect. In many cancers, all cells are equally tumorigenic in the implantation experiment in spite of presence of genetic and phenotypic heterogeneity [21, 28]. As an explanation to such exceptional cases, it is proposed that in many tumors, both clonal evolution and CSC model may be mutually inclusive by joining their hands in a cooperative manner and they are not mutually exclusive [29]. In context of various reports about the emerging concept of plasticity of cancer cells, such possibilities are stronger and subsequently push the CSC model from a static hierarchical to a dynamic model to increase its domain for the explanation of most tumors [30].

The putative theory of a possible connection between epithelial-to-mes-enchymal transition and CSCs is very exciting and considered as a paradigm-shift, linking tumor cell invasion and metastasis with drug resistance and tumor relapse. This has also advocated for the possibility of conversion of a fully differentiated non-CSC into CSCs under appropriate environmental conditions. Now, it is clear that tumor cells oscillate into the various states with characteristic degree of competence to differentiate or dedifferentiate in maintaining the tumor propagation [31]. The newly established CSC plastic-ity model is a lucrative way to explain the varying ability of tumor cells, and this model proposes that each of the tumor cell has its stemness potential that can be of varying degree depending upon multiple genetic, epigenetic, and other environmental models (See Figure 16.1). The CSC plasticity model is best fitted for the tumor population where tumor cells are inter-converting between less and high tumorigenic potential and changing their phenotypes independent of stemness. The exact mechanism governing CSC plastic-ity is unknown; however, its conceptual foundation naturally links clonal evolution and CSC models and ask for investigation on the possibility for inclusion of bidirectional CSCs and non-CSCs inter-conversion within the tumor. It appears that plasticity between CSCs and non-CSCs is orchestrated by micro-environmental and genetic factors. Previously discussed reports

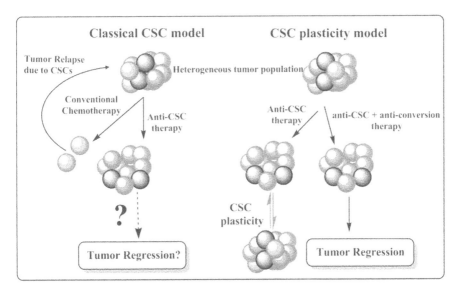

FIGURE 16.1   Classical cancer stem cell model and plasticity model.

based on lineage tracing put forward strong evidence for the differentiation process of CSCs in animal models. However, it is also interesting to note that these reports did not completely exclude the chances that labeled CSCs might have formed from the non-CSCs as a result of plasticity. As nearly all studies on CSC plasticity are based on cell lines and the cell lines were shown to exhibit phenotypic plasticity at higher passages, it is very pivotal to understand and address this possibility [30c]. Verma and coworkers recently showed a landmark support of CSC plasticity in glioma, which is reported to generated from terminally differentiated neurons that later on converted to a stem-like state with the expression of typical CSC markers [32].

16.3   EPIGENETIC REGULATION OF DRUG RESISTANCE IN CSCs

Waddington used the term "Epigenetic" around five decades ago as a discipline that deals with changes in the development of organisms that is independent of changes in DNA sequence [33]. This is largely regulated by local chromatin architecture near the gene promoter that finally determines the accessibility of transcription machineries for their target region on the DNA. These epigenetic modulations can work either through modifications of genetic material such as DNA methylation in CpG islands or local histone modifications that includes histone acetylation/deacetylation and/or histone methylation/demethylation [34]. With the emergence of CSC concepts, it is accepted that nongenetic factors also play their role in driving tumor heterogeneity. According to this concept, heterogeneity at the level of cellular phenotype in tumor cells is a result of hierarchies found within the tumor similar to normal tissue [21]. Here, in this case, varying state of differentiation appears to be dominant over genetic factors-mediated effects on tumor. Furthermore, those phenotypic states that are driven by varying differentiation potential have been shown to be responsible for varying clinical response such as poor prognosis and drug resistance [6]. Non-genetic heterogeneity is the phenotypic differences in cancer cells at the level of differential gene/protein expression governed by factors that are independent of DNA sequence. There are two types of non-genetic heterogeneity of phenotypes, including deterministic and stochastic heterogeneity, which correspond to heterogeneity in normal tissues as tissue-specific differentiation hierarchy and substantial cell-to-cell variability, respectively. Mostly, these fluctuations are transcriptional noise that are likely to involve change in cellular physiology, including the assembly of signaling complexes via translation [35]. A more comprehensive explanation for environmental factors of tumor heterogeneity is provided by the concept of epigenetic landscapes on cell phenotypes where fluctuations in cellular phenotypes are seen as "valleys" corresponding to gene regulatory network with better probability of transcriptional changes [36]. Changes in gene expression profile and the corresponding cellular processes are responsible for shifting the cellular position on the epigenetic landscape, and whenever these fluctuations are larger than a threshold value, the cell will move to a different state of changed phenotypic state corresponding to jumping from one valley to an adjacent one. Epigenetic landscape topology is affected by both intrinsic factors such as genetic makeup and differentiation state as well as by extrinsic factors including various signaling inputs of microenvironment on the cells. These fluctuations in gene regulatory networks can increase the probability that it transfers the cell into a more stable state during cancer that was usually transient in the normal condition [1a, 6]. This also explains the varying response of individual cancers cells against the same chemotherapy as tumor cells accumulate various subclones of different genetic setup and epigenetic landscape within its population. These combinations may also result in the emergence of acquired drug resistant subclones during the course of therapy (See Figure 16.2).

Recent advances in the field of epigenetic have now broadened the basic concept of tumor initiation. Epigenetic abnormalities caused by genome-wide hypomethylation, promoter DNA hypermethylation, mediated suppression of various tumor suppressor genes, and modulation of the expression profiles of histone-modifying enzymes are closely associated with tumorigenesis [34b]. In this case, a crosstalk between genetic and epigenetic factors is prevalent and widely reported in literature [37]. Mutations in several epigenetic modifiers involved in DNA and histone modifications lead to aberrant gene expression patterns that ultimately lead to tumor initiation and progression [38]. Similar to other human malignancies, colon cancer also represents a heterogeneous group of neoplasms driven by multiple genetic and epigenetic aberrations [14a]. For instance, activating mutations in the *KRAS* and *BRAF* genes are shown in nearly 40% and 10% of human colorectal cancers (CRCs), respectively [39]. However, in the past two decades, understanding acquired drug resistance has been a center of attention, and epigenetic mechanisms underlying deregulation of genes resulting in progression and drug resistance of various cancers including colon cancer have

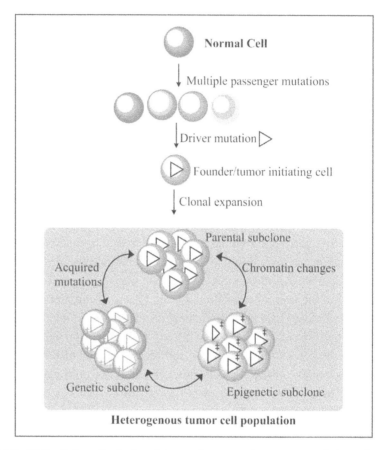

FIGURE 16.2 Epigenetic basis of tumor heterogeneity as accumulation of various subclones in the course of tumor progression.

gained considerable attention. For example, multiple reports have suggested the epigenetic basis of suppression of key proapoptotic genes to develop drug resistance [14a]. Drug resistance has been shown to be associated with loss of death receptor expression from cell surface. However, the basis for their suppression especially in CSCs is largely unknown. Recent studies have revealed that the loss of *DR4* expression can be a result of epigenetic silencing caused by promoter DNA hypermethylation [40]. This is evident from the observation that treatment of TRAIL resistance cancer cells with 5-aza-CdR (DNA methyltranferase inhibitor) increased the expression of the *DR4* gene. Epigenetic mechanisms have also been implicated in the development of acquired resistance to endocrine therapy in breast cancer treatment [41].

16.4   EPIGENETIC INHIBITORS AS A NOVEL THERAPEUTIC STRATEGY AGAINST DRUG-RESISTANT CSCs

Although substantial improvements are being made in cancer treatment strategy, tumor relapse and emergence of therapy resistance remain a big cause of cancer-related death. For cancers that follow the CSC model, tumor relapse is thought to be caused by the presence of highly drug-resistant CSCs in the tumor population which is mainly accumulated or developed during the course of chemotherapy. In this direction, many recent studies have provided the compelling evidence that the presence of CSC population within each cancer type is the key contributor of therapy failure regardless of CSC origin and stability. Therefore, it is clear that a successful treatment strategy will necessarily require complete eradication of the entire CSC population, including stable and transient one. Salinomycin, a carboxylic polyether ionophore, was first isolated from the culture broth of *Streptomyces albus* in 1974 and classically commercialized as anticoccidial for poultry and as a growth ;promoter for ruminants [42]. Later, it was also used as an antibacterial agent, however, real attention was given to salinomycin after the pioneering discovery of Gupta et al. that salinomycin is able to target breast CSCs [43]. In this landmark study, Gupta et al. utilized high throughput approach to screen thousands of chemical compounds including various antibiotics for their potential cytotoxic effect against breast CSCs and discovered salinomycin as most potent compound among all molecules used in the study. Since then, exponentially increasing reports have continuously indicated the anticancer activity of salinomycin in multiple malignancies, however, the exact molecular mechanism of action of salinomycin against CSCs is largely unknown [42a, 44].

Dynamic changes in harmonic balance among various histone markers lead to deregulation in the transcription of certain set of cancer-related genes. Although many other modifications in histone occurs, histone methylation of histone 3 (H3) at lysine (K) residues is the most studied. This modification can lead to either activation or suppression of gene expression; on the other hand, acetylation of lysine residues on H3 and H4, mostly found in the euchromatin region, is transcription permissive [45]. The H3K27me3 form is mediated by the Polycomb group of protein complex (PcG) and associated with repressive markers in the promoter target genes [46]. Actions of the PcG complex PRC2 depend on the activity of its catalytic component EZH2. EZH2 is a histone methyltransferase (HNMT) enzyme (EC 2.1.1.43) that catalyzes the methyl group addition at lysine 27 residue of histone H3 using the cofactor S-adenosyl-L-methionine (SAM). Enzymatic activity of EZH2 leads to the heterochromatin state of local chromatin to cause silencing of gene expression. Highest EZH2 levels are associated with the CSC-like phenotype in breast cancer [47]. All these lines of evidence underscore the cardinal role of epigenetic aberrations in drug resistance and stem-like phenotype. Therapeutic targeting of these epigenetic aberrations for better disease management is increasingly being considered as a viable option [14a].

16.5 CONCLUSION

CSCs have evolved multiple mechanisms that protect them from therapeutic stress and make them relatively resistant to drug-induced apoptosis. Although significant progresses has been made, the presence of residual disease after surgery and chemotherapy is associated with poor survival and tumor relapse. Resistance to therapies is still the most important cause of cancer-related morbidity and mortality, which is now thought to be mediated and sustained by unique landscape of epigenetic modifications present in resistant stem-like population that led it to escape from undergoing apoptosis during chemotherapy [48]. There are plenty of reports in support of the role of epigenetics and CSCs in therapeutic resistance and tumor recurrence [1a, 14b]. While the presence of CSCs in invasive tumors is a well-known player of cancer metastasis and recurrence, knowledge about the molecular mechanisms that regulate the generation and maintenance of CSCs in the tumor remains limited and reports on the involvement of epigenetic factors are rapidly filling this gap. In this regard, we urgently need new therapeutic strategies that can combine conventional cancer therapies with specific epigenetics inhibitors to target CSCs.

16.6 SUMMARY

- Tumors usually consist of mixed populations of malignant cells, some of which are drug-sensitive while others are drug-resistant, where resistant cells have been positively selected in drug-induced stressed micro-environment.
- Both intrinsic and acquired resistance results from the numerous genetic and epigenetic changes occurring in all cancer cells in general and in cancer stem cells (CSCs) in particular.

- Drug resistance against conventional chemotherapeutics is believed to be contributed by CSCs in solid tumors, and due to their accumulation in the course of treatment, tumor eventually relapses and metastasizes.
- Histone modifications through polycomb group (PcG) proteins have shown to drive CSC biology
- Enhancer of zeste homologue 2 (EZH2) is the most important catalytically active component of the PRC2 complex that is involved in transcriptional repression of its target gene by trimethylation of lysine 27 at histone H3 (H3K27)
- Pharmacological inhibition of EHZ2 has shown to reduce hallmarks of CSC properties, like self-renewal, tumorigenic potential, and drug resistance in different tumor types

KEYWORDS

- **cancer stem cell**
- **cancer therapeutics**
- **epigenetics**
- **EZH2**
- **tumor microenvironment**

REFERENCES

1. (a) Singh, A. K., Arya, R. K., Maheshwari, S., Singh, A., Meena, S., Pandey, P., Dormond, O., & Datta, D., (2015). Tumor heterogeneity and cancer stem cell paradigm: Updates in concept, controversies and clinical relevance. *International Journal of Cancer, 136(9)*, 1991–2000. (b) Borst, P., (2012). Cancer drug pan-resistance: pumps, cancer stem cells, quiescence, epithelial to mesenchymal transition, blocked cell death pathways, persisters or what? *Open Biology, 2(5)*, 120066.
2. Pattabiraman, D. R., & Weinberg, R. A., (2014). Tackling the cancer stem cells—what challenges do they pose? *Nature Reviews Drug Discovery, 13(7)*, 497–512.
3. (a) Clarke, M. F., Dick, J. E., Dirks, P. B., Eaves, C. J., Jamieson, C. H., Jones, D. L., Visvader, J., Weissman, I. L., & Wahl, G. M., (2006). Cancer stem cells--perspectives on current status and future directions: AACR Workshop on cancer stem cells. *Cancer Res., 66(19)*, 9339–44. (b) Dean, M., Fojo, T., & Bates, S., (2005). Tumour stem cells and drug resistance. *Nat. Rev. Cancer, 5(4)*, 275–284.
4. (a) Fidler, I. J., (1978). Tumor heterogeneity and the biology of cancer invasion and metastasis. *Cancer Res., 38(9)*, 2651–2660. (b) Heppner, G. H., (1984). Tumor hetero-

geneity. *Cancer Res., 44*(6), 2259–65. (c) Marusyk, A., & Polyak, K., (2010). Tumor heterogeneity: causes and consequences. *Biochim. Biophys. Acta, 1805*(1), 105–117.

5. (a) Shackleton, M., Quintana, E., Fearon, E. R., & Morrison, S. J., (2009). Heterogeneity in cancer: cancer stem cells versus clonal evolution. *Cell, 138*(5), 822–829. (b) Reya, T., Morrison, S. J., Clarke, M. F., & Weissman, I. L., (2001). Stem cells, Cancer, & Cancer Stem Cells. *Nature, 414*(6859), 105–111.

6. Marusyk, A., Almendro, V., & Polyak, K., (2012). Intra-tumour heterogeneity: a looking glass for cancer? *Nat. Rev. Cancer, 12*(5), 323–334.

7. Gupta, P. B., Chaffer, C. L., & Weinberg, R. A., (2009). Cancer stem cells: mirage or reality? *Nat. Med., 15*(9), 1010–1012.

8. Tudoran, O., Soritau, O., Balacescu, L., Visan, S., Barbos, O., Cojocneanu-Petric, R., Balacescu, O., & Berindan-Neagoe, I., (2015). Regulation of stem cells-related signaling pathways in response to doxorubicin treatment in Hs578T triple-negative breast cancer cells. *Molecular and Cellular Biochemistry, 409*(1–2), 163–176.

9. (a) Nguyen, L. V., Vanner, R., Dirks, P., & Eaves, C. J., (2012). Cancer stem cells: an evolving concept. *Nature Reviews Cancer, 12*(2), 133–143. (b) Bailey, H., (1926). The abdominal crises of pernicious anaemia. *Br. Med. J., 2*(3429), 554.

10. Sell, S., (2010). On the stem cell origin of cancer. *The American journal of Pathology, 176*(6), 2584–2594.

11. Ebben, J. D., Treisman, D. M., Zorniak, M., Kutty, R. G., Clark, P. A., & Kuo, J. S., (2010). The cancer stem cell paradigm: a new understanding of tumor development and treatment. *Expert Opinion on Therapeutic Targets, 14*(6), 621–632.

12. (a) Kelly, P. N., Dakic, A., Adams, J. M., Nutt, S. L., & Strasser, A., (2007). Tumor growth need not be driven by rare cancer stem cells. *Science, 317*(5836), 337. (b) Quintana, E., Shackleton, M., Sabel, M. S., Fullen, D. R., Johnson, T. M., & Morrison, S. J., (2008). Efficient tumour formation by single human melanoma cells. *Nature, 456*(7222), 593–598.

13. Abetov, D., Mustapova, Z., Saliev, T., Bulanin, D., Batyrbekov, K., & Gilman, C. P., (2015). Novel small molecule inhibitors of cancer stem cell signaling pathways. *Stem Cell Reviews and Reports, 11*(6), 909–918.

14. (a) Easwaran, H., Tsai, H. C., & Baylin, S. B., (2014). Cancer epigenetics: tumor heterogeneity, plasticity of stem-like states, & drug resistance. *Molecular Cell, 54*(5), 716–727. (b) Munoz, P., Iliou, M. S., & Esteller, M., (2012). Epigenetic alterations involved in cancer stem cell reprogramming. *Molecular Oncology, 6*(6), 620–636.

15. Bock, C., Beerman, I., Lien, W. H., Smith, Z. D., Gu, H., Boyle, P., Gnirke, A., Fuchs, E., Rossi, D. J., & Meissner, A., (2012). DNA methylation dynamics during in vivo differentiation of blood and skin stem cells. *Molecular Cell, 47*(4), 633–647.

16. Vincent, A., & Van Seuningen, I., (2012). On the epigenetic origin of cancer stem cells. *Biochimica et Biophysica Acta (BBA)-Reviews on Cancer, 1826*(1), 83–88.

17. Kahn, T. G., Dorafshan, E., Schultheis, D., Zare, A., Stenberg, P., Reim, I., Pirrotta, V., & Schwartz, Y. B., (2016). Interdependence of PRC1 and PRC2 for recruitment to Polycomb Response Elements. *Nucleic Acids Research, 44*(21), 10132–10149.

18. Di Croce, L., & Helin, K., (2013). Transcriptional regulation by Polycomb group proteins. *Nature Structural & Molecular Biology, 20*(10), 1147–1155.

19. Alvarado, A. S., & Yamanaka, S., (2014). Rethinking differentiation: stem cells, regeneration, & plasticity. *Cell, 157*(1), 110–119.

20. Brucher, B. L., & Jamall, I. S., (2014). Epistemology of the origin of cancer: a new paradigm. *BMC Cancer, 14*(1), 331.

21. Kreso, A., & Dick, J. E., (2014). Evolution of the cancer stem cell model. *Cell Stem Cell, 14*(3), 275–291.
22. Tirino, V., Desiderio, V., Paino, F., De Rosa, A., Papaccio, F., La Noce, M., Laino, L., De Francesco, F., & Papaccio, G., (2013). Cancer stem cells in solid tumors: an over-view and new approaches for their isolation and characterization. *The FASEB Journal, 27*(1), 13–24.
23. Llaguno, S. R. A., Xie, X., & Parada, L. F., (2016). In cell of origin and cancer stem cells in tumor suppressor mouse models of glioblastoma, *Cold Spring Harbor Symposia on Quantitative Biology*, Cold Spring Harbor Laboratory Press, pp. 030973.
24. Beck, B., & Blanpain, C., (2013). Unravelling cancer stem cell potential. *Nature Reviews Cancer, 13*(10), 727–738.
25. (a) Cojoc, M., Mabert, K., Muders, M. H., & Dubrovska, A., (2015). In: A role for cancer stem cells in therapy resistance: cellular and molecular mechanisms, *Seminars in Cancer Biology*, Elsevier: pp. 16–27. (b) Barriere, G., Fici, P., Gallerani, G., Fabbri, F., Zoli, W., & Rigaud, M., (2014). Circulating tumor cells and epithelial, mesenchymal and stemness markers: characterization of cell subpopulations. *Annals of Translational Medicine, 2*(11).
26. Tomasetti, C., Vogelstein, B., & Parmigiani, G., (2013). Half or more of the somatic mutations in cancers of self-renewing tissues originate prior to tumor initiation. *Proceedings of the National Academy of Sciences, 110*(6), 1999–2004.
27. Rhim, A. D., Oberstein, P. E., Thomas, D. H., Mirek, E. T., Palermo, C. F., Sastra, S. A., Dekleva, E. N., Saunders, T., Becerra, C. P., & Tattersall, I. W., (2014). Stromal elements act to restrain, rather than support, pancreatic ductal adenocarcinoma. *Cancer Cell, 25*(6), 735–747.
28. Dosch, J. S., Ziemke, E. K., Shettigar, A., Rehemtulla, A., & Sebolt-Leopold, J. S., (2015). Cancer stem cell marker phenotypes are reversible and functionally homoge-neous in a preclinical model of pancreatic cancer. *Cancer Research, 75*(21), 4582–4592.
29. Zabala, M., Lobo, N., Qian, D., Van Weele, L., Heiser, D., & Clarke, M., (2016). Over-view: Cancer Stem Cell Self-Renewal. *Cancer Stem Cells: Targeting the Roots of Cancer, Seeds of Metastasis, & Sources of Therapy Resistance, 25.*
30. (a) Eun, K., Ham, S., & Kim, H., (2017). Cancer stem cell heterogeneity: Origin and new perspectives on CSC targeting. *BMB reports, 2016.* (b) Prasetyanti, P. R., & Mede-ma, J. P., (2013). Intra-tumor heterogeneity from a cancer stem cell perspective. *Molecular Cancer, 16*(1), 41. (c) Meacham, C. E., & Morrison, S. J. Tumour heterogeneity and cancer cell plasticity. *Nature, 501*(7467), 328–337.
31. (a) Pacini, N., & Borziani, F., (2014). Cancer stem cell theory and the warburg ef-fect, two sides of the same coin? *International Journal of Molecular Sciences, 15*(5), 8893–8930. (b) Csermely, P., Hodsagi, J., Korcsmáros, T., Modos, D., Perez-Lopez, A. R., Szalay, K., Veres, D. V., Lenti, K., Wu, L.-Y., Zhang, X.-S., (2015). In Cancer stem cells display extremely large evolvability: alternating plastic and rigid networks as a potential mechanism: network models, novel therapeutic target strategies, & the contributions of hypoxia, inflammation and cellular senescence, *Seminars in Cancer Biology*, Elsevier: pp. 42–51. (c) Auffinger, B., Tobias, A., Han, Y., Lee, G., Guo, D., Dey, M., Lesniak, M., & Ahmed, A., (2014). Conversion of differentiated cancer cells into cancer stem-like cells in a glioblastoma model after primary chemotherapy. *Cell Death & Differentiation, 21*(7), 1119–1131.

32. Friedmann-Morvinski, D., Bushong, E. A., Ke, E., Soda, Y., Marumoto, T., Singer, O., Ellisman, M. H., & Verma, I. M., (2012). Dedifferentiation of neurons and astrocytes by oncogenes can induce gliomas in mice. *Science, 338*(6110), 1080–1084.

33. Davila-Velderrain, J., Martinez-Garcia, J. C., & Alvarez-Buylla, E. R., (2015). Modeling the epigenetic attractors landscape: toward a post-genomic mechanistic understanding of development. *Frontiers in Genetics, 6*, 160.

34. (a) Deb, G., Singh, A. K., & Gupta, S., (2014). EZH2: not EZHY (easy) to deal. *Molecular Cancer Research, 12*(5), 639–653. (b) Singhal, S. K., Usmani, N., Michiels, S., Metzger-Filho, O., Saini, K. S., Kovalchuk, O., & Parliament, M., (2016). Towards understanding the breast cancer epigenome: a comparison of genome-wide DNA methylation and gene expression data. *Oncotarget, 7*(3), 3002.

35. (a) Veitia, R. A., Govindaraju, D. R., Bottani, S., & Birchler, J. A., (2016). Aging: Somatic mutations, epigenetic drift and gene dosage imbalance. *Trends in Cell Biology.* (b) Chang, A. Y., & Marshall, W. F., (2017). Organelles–understanding noise and heterogeneity in cell biology at an intermediate scale. *J. Cell Sci., 130*(5), 819–826.

36. Moris, N., Pina, C., & Arias, A. M., (2016). Transition states and cell fate decisions in epigenetic landscapes. *Nature Reviews Genetics, 17*(11), 693–703.

37. Lei, J., Levin, S. A., & Nie, Q., (2014). Mathematical model of adult stem cell regeneration with cross-talk between genetic and epigenetic regulation. *Proceedings of the National Academy of Sciences, 111*(10), E880–E887.

38. Plass, C., Pfister, S. M., Lindroth, A. M., Bogatyrova, O., Claus, R., & Lichter, P., (2013). Mutations in regulators of the epigenome and their connections to global chromatin patterns in cancer. *Nature Reviews Genetics, 14*(11), 765–780.

39. Cicenas, J., Tamosaitis, L., Kvederaviciute, K., Tarvydas, R., Staniute, G., Kalyan, K., Meskinyte-Kausiliene, E., Stankevicius, V., & Valius, M., (2017). KRAS, NRAS and BRAF mutations in colorectal cancer and melanoma. *Medical Oncology, 34*(2), 26.

40. Lee, J. C., Lee, W. H., Min, Y. J., Cha, H. J., Han, M. W., Chang, H. W., Kim, S. A., Choi, S. H., Kim, S. W., & Kim, S. Y., (2014). Development of TRAIL resistance by radiation-induced hypermethylation of DR4 CpG island in recurrent laryngeal squamous cell carcinoma. *International Journal of Radiation Oncology* Biology* Physics, 88*(5), 1203–1211.

41. Hiken, J. F., McDonald, J. I., Decker, K. F., Sanchez, C., Hoog, J., VanderKraats, N. D., Jung, K. L., Akinhanmi, M., Rois, L., & Ellis, M., (2016). Epigenetic activation of the prostaglandin receptor EP4 promotes resistance to endocrine therapy for breast cancer. *Oncogene.*

42. (a) Naujokat, C., & Laufer, S., (2016). Salinomycin, a candidate drug for the salinomycin, a candidate drug for the elimination of cancer stem cells elimination of cancer stem cells. *Role of Cancer Stem Cells in Cancer Biology and Therapy, 227.* (b) Steinhart, B., Steinhart, A., Steinhart, R., Muth, K., Muth, M., & Naujokat, C., (2013). Clinical activity of salinomycin in humanadvanced vulvar cancer. *Case Reports in Oncology.*

43. (a) Suntharalingam, K., Lin, W., Johnstone, T. C., Bruno, P. M., Zheng, Y.-R., Hemann, M. T., & Lippard, S. J., (2014). A breast cancer stem cell-selective, mammospheres-potent osmium (VI) nitrido complex. *Journal of the American Chemical Society, 136*(41), 14413–14416. (b) Carmody, L. C., Germain, A., Morgan, B., VerPlank, L., Fernandez, C., Feng, Y., Perez, J. R., Dandapani, S., Munoz, B., & Palmer, M., (2014). Identification of a selective small-molecule inhibitor of breast cancer stem cells—probe, 2.

44. Gupta, P., Onder, T. T., Lander, E. S., Weinberg, R. A., Mani, S., & Lioa, M. J., (2013). Methods for identification and use of agents targeting cancer stem cells. *Google Patents*.

45. Tessarz, P., & Kouzarides, T., (2014). Histone core modifications regulating nucleosome structure and dynamics. *Nature Reviews Molecular Cell biology, 15*(11), 703–708.

46. Wiles, E. T., & Selker, E. U., (2017). H3K27 methylation: a promiscuous repressive chromatin mark. *Current Opinion in Genetics & Development, 43*, 31–37.

47. Volkel, P., Dupret, B., Le Bourhis, X., & Angrand, P. O., (2015). Diverse involvement of EZH2 in cancer epigenetics. *Am. J. Transl. Res., 7*(2), 175–193.

48. Peitzsch, C., Tyutyunnykova, A., Pantel, K., & Dubrovska, A., (2017). In Cancer stem cells: the root of tumor recurrence and metastasis, *Seminars in Cancer Biology*, Elsevier.

CHAPTER 17

NANOPARTICLES IN CANCER THERAPY

MADHUCHANDA BANERJEE

Department of Zoology, Midnapore College (Autonomous), West Bengal, India, E-mail: madhuchanda.banerjee@gmail.com

CONTENTS

ABSTRACT

Recent developments in nanotechnology have opened up numerous opportunities for advancing medical science and disease treatment in human healthcare. These include therapeutic applications of nanomaterial for effective detection and treatment of cancer. The use of nanoparticles (NPs) could be very attractive option for several reasons. They exhibit unique pharmacokinetics and have minimal renal filtration. There is a wide range of NPs such as organic dye-doped NPs, quantum dots, etc., which enable highly sensitive imaging of cancer cells. In totality, the NPs provide unique optical, magnetic, and electrical properties for imaging and remote actuation. This may overcome some limitations associated with conventional cancer diagnosis. Various materials could be used for synthesizing NPs, and their unique physical nature enable them to be modified with various functional groups, which make them suitable to be internalized as well as to encapsulate different therapeutic agents. The internalization of drug-loaded NPs is an important aspect for targeted drug delivery. Introduction of multifunctional NP systems have initiated innovative strategies for cancer therapy. These multifunctional NPs incorporate all the therapeutic as well as imaging molecules inside the NP and on its surface, thus resulting in delivery of both imaging and/or therapeutic agents and specifically targeting them to the affected area.

The chapter will discuss about the use of different types of NPs associated with therapeutic strategies for cancer including both imaging and drug delivery.

17.1   INTRODUCTION

Applications of nanotechnology in medicine are aimed toward diagnosis, followed by treatment of the diseases by working at the nanometer scale where biological macromolecules exist and operate [1, 2]. In the past decade, nanotechnology has proven to be a new and powerful weapon for the detection and treatment of cancer [1, 3–5]. Nanoparticles (NPs) have unique and tunable properties [6, 7]. They exhibit unique pharmacokinetics, which include minimal renal filtration and high surface-to-volume ratios making them flexible to modification, whereby functional moieties could be introduced or combined. This provides them with unique optical, magnetic, and electrical properties for imaging and remote actuation. When these particles are conjugated to biorecognition molecules, they would be recognized by a molecular target (such as a cancer marker) indicating the presence of cancer, thus facilitating cancer detection [8–10] or deliver a cytotoxic agent for use in targeted therapy [11–13]. Certain multifunctional NPs capable of targeting, imaging, and delivering therapeutics are being investigated and could be an upcoming area of research that holds great promise for cancer therapy in the future.

Treatment for cancer is most effective if there could be early detection for the disease, much before it has metastasized or spread beyond the site of the initial tumor. However, this seems challenging because the early stages of cancer are often asymptomatic. Usually, the early detection strategies include imaging techniques to detect physiological and anatomical changes associated with oncogenesis or molecular probes to detect cancer biomarkers such as proteases, antigens, antibodies, proteins and nucleic acid-based markers [14]. In both these strategies, NPs have been reported to be used as contrast agents.

The use of NPs as imaging probes show great advantages when compared to conventional imaging agents. The ability of the NPs to be loaded or loadability is one among these advantages where the concentration of the imaging agent within each NP can be controlled during the process of synthesis. Another advantage is the ability of the NP surface to be tuned such that circulation time of the agent in the blood can be potentially extended. Additionally, surface modification may specifically lead to targeting a particular location within the body.

The contrast agents used in MRI are either made of transition and lanthanide metals or of iron oxide NPs and ferrite NPs. One example of these transition/lanthanide metals would be the ion gadolinium (Gd^{3+}) that has been extensively used. A new array of contrast agents is formed by immobilizing Gd complexes on various nanostructured materials (nanoporoussilicas, dendrimers, perfluorocarbon NPs, and nanotubes) [15]. As MRI contrast agents, superparamagenetic iron oxide nanocrystals are used to detect liver metastases and metastatic lymph nodes. Upon intravenous injection, these nanocrystals are phagocytosed by macrophages and monocytes, which transport them to the liver and lymph nodes. Careful observation with respect to differential accumulation of the NPs in metastatic and inflamed tissue helps in proper diagnosis through MRI [16].

The NPs are also particularly suited for use as molecular probes. One of the earliest demonstrations of NPs in a biomedical application used 13 nm gold colloids as colorimetric DNA sensors. Mirkinet et al. conjugated the gold colloids to oligonucleotides. In the absence of complementary DNA, the solution of colloids remains monodisperse, forming a deep red suspension. When complementary single-stranded DNA sequences are introduced to the solution, they form bridges between the gold colloids, causing them to aggregate. The solution of aggregated gold colloids appears blue. This forms the basis of a simple genomic detection system [17].

As the size of NP is similar to various biological macromolecules and viruses, they can also access molecular markers in situ [8]. Many NPs strongly interact with the electromagnetic radiation and are thereby able to generate a strong signal. Additionally, their optical properties could be tuned, which means that the probes can be made to show desired characteristics (e.g., to have an absorbance or fluorescence peak at a specific wavelength, etc.).

NP-based anti-cancer drug delivery has opened up an array of multidimensional and innovative therapeutic mechanisms that are highly effective, less invasive, and show less toxicity. The use of NP-carrier shows significant advantages over conventional therapeutic techniques [1]. NPs (NPs) have higher water solubility; which makes them suitable carrier of drugs that are otherwise insoluble. Thus, the requirement of toxic organic solvent is eliminated. Nanocarriers can be also be designed so as to adjust the release kinetics of the drug using environmental (pH) or external stimuli (ultrasound, heat). These properties help in controlled release of the therapeutic agent and prevent dissociation of the drug from the nanocarrier before reaching the tumor site. This mechanism also minimizes drug accumulation in other healthy tissues and organs, thus decreasing the systemic toxicity associated with the drug.

In conventional chemotherapy due to non-specific targeting, the cytotoxic drugs affect other healthy dividing cells of the body in addition to the actively dividing cancer cells, which is overcome by the usage of nanosized carriers. The surface area/volume ratio of the NP as well as the introduction of cancer-specific molecules on the NP surface help the nanocarriers to specifically bind to their targets on the cancer cell. The specific attachment leads to internalization of the NP into the tumor cell, thus resulting in increased uptake of the drug by the tumor cells, and finally resulting in higher antitumor activity [2].

In contrast to mono-functional NPs that deliver only a single type of drug or therapeutic agent, multifunctional NPs can integrate various functionalities inside the NP core as well as on the NP surface, thus achieving maximal antitumor activity. Evidence through scientific reports suggests that the NPs whose surface contains a targeting molecule binds to the receptors highly expressed in tumor cells. These NPs may additionally serve as image contrast agents to increase sensitivity and specificity in tumor detection as well as that of therapeutic drug. It is reported that successful therapeutic strategies involve the usage of more than one drug [3, 4]. Clinical trials are being carried out to test the different combinations of treatment to achieve the best results [5, 6]. Such multifunctional nanodevices may significantly improve the current clinical management of cancer patients.

17.2   NPS IN CANCER THERAPY: DEVELOPING DRUG DELIVERY VEHICLES

Once cancer is detected, the most commonly used therapies to treat it are surgery, radiotherapy, and chemotherapy. The challenge in each of these therapies lies in striking the balance between specifically eliminating all the malignant cells, but at the same time, enough care should be taken to avoid damaging surrounding healthy tissue. If a treatment is not aggressive, some malignant cells may survive and grow into a new tumor. If it is too aggressive, it may destroy a large number of healthy tissues thus compromising with normal physiological functions. Conventional treatment procedures such as surgery, radiation, and chemotherapy lack specificity and selectivity. For a therapy to be specific and selective, it should inhibit or suppress the growth of desired cancerous cells at the desired site of action. When cancer treatments harm healthy cells alongside malignant cells, they lack selectivity. Targeted drug delivery aims to increase both the specificity and selectivity of treatment.

Targeting the delivery of a therapeutic to the malignant cells, while avoiding the healthy cells increases the efficacy of the therapeutic and reduce its side effects. Chemotherapeutic drugs conjugated to targeting moieties have been reported to induce tumor regression in tumor-bearing mice in contrast to much reduced activity when nontargeted drug was used. These targeted drugs were also safe at higher doses where free drug was lethal [18]. Thus, this could significantly lower the effective dose, ED, i.e. the dose at which a drug produces an effect.

17.2.1   TARGETING STRATEGIES

To achieve effective drug delivery, the nanocarriers need to fulfill two basic types of requirements. First, drugs should be able to reach the desired tumor sites following administration with minimal loss of their volume and activity in blood circulation. Second, drugs should only kill tumor cells without harmful effects on healthy tissue [19]. These requirements may be facilitated using two strategies: passive and active targeting of drugs [20].

17.2.2 PASSIVE TARGETING

Passive targeting is based on the unique pathophysiological characteristics of tumor vessels, enabling nanodrugs to accumulate around the tumor tissues. Typically, tumor vessels are highly disorganized and show abnormalities of vasculature, namely hypervascularization; aberrant vascular architecture; extensive production of vascular permeability factors, thus stimulating extravasation within tumor tissues; and lack of lymphatic drainage. This "leaky" vascularization leads to the enhanced permeability and retention (EPR) effect, which allows migration of macromolecules up to 400 nm in diameter into the surrounding tumor region [20–23]. As these macromolecules are unable to penetrate through tight endothelial junctions of normal blood vessels, their concentration builds up in the plasma, which increases their plasma half-life. Additionally, they can selectively extravasate into the tumor tissues due to their abnormal vasculature. With passage of time, the tumor concentration builds up reaching up to several folds higher concentration than that of the plasma due to lack of efficient lymphatic drainage in the solid tumor.

Other physiological phenomenon also supports passive targeting. The high metabolic rate of fast-growing tumor cells requires more oxygen and nutrients. This results in the stimulation of glycolysis to obtain extra energy, resulting in an acidic environment [23]. This phenomenon is utilized in designing pH-sensitive liposomes, which are stable at physiological pH 7.4, but degrades to release drug molecules at the acidic pH [24].

Although passive targeting approaches form the basis of clinical therapy, they suffer from several limitations. Passive targeting depends on the degree of tumor vascularization and angiogenesis. Thus, extravasation of nanocarriers will vary with tumor types and anatomical sites. Tumors that do not exhibit EPR effect could be a poor candidate for such type of targeting [24]. For the drugs that cannot diffuse efficiently, there could be further difficulty in controlling the process.

17.2.3 ACTIVE TARGETING

In contrast to passive targeting, where NPs accumulate in the tumor due to EPR, active targeting utilizes biorecognition molecules conjugated to NPs to confer them with the ability to bind to molecular markers. Antibodies [25], antibody fragments [26], proteins [27], aptamers [28], peptides [29], and small molecules [30] have been used as affinity ligands on the surface of the nanocarriers that binds to the specific receptors on cell surface. Nanocarriers recognize and bind to target cells through ligand–receptor interactions by the expression of receptors on the cancer cell surface. The receptors should be uniformly expressed exclusively on the tumor cell to achieve high specificity. Internalization of targeting conjugates may occur by receptor-mediated endocytosis after binding to target cells, thus facilitating drug release inside the cells. The process involves binding of affinity ligands to the receptors followed by internalization of the complex by invagination of the plasma membrane to form endosome. The drug-containing endosome may now be ruptured inside the cell to release the drug due to acidic pH or activity of enzymes.

Designing of such targeted nanocarriers thus involves some constraints which are (1) the need for a nanocarrier of size small enough to fit in through the pores of porous tumor blood vessels, (2) the requirement to direct the drug carrier to its target, and (3) the need to release the drug from the carrier once it reaches the target.

17.3   NP PROPERTIES

The blood supply in the tumor tissue plays an important role in the delivery of therapeutic agents to tumors. The encapsulation of the therapeutic into a particular carrier protects it from degradation caused due to various factors inside the body. These carriers transport the drug into the "leaky" zone (tumor site), where it is released as a result of normal carrier degradation. The size of the permeabilized vasculature can vary depending on the type of tumor, and thus, the size of a drug-carrier should be used such that the efficacy of the spontaneous drug delivery is controlled by utilizing the EPR effect. It has been documented that the pore cut-off size of several tumor models is in the range of 380 and 780 nm [31]. This restricts the distribution of particles larger than 1 µm across the tumor vasculature. Therefore, associating antitumor drugs with colloidal NPs could be an interesting strategy, which would further increase the selectivity of drugs toward cancer cells, while reducing their toxicity toward normal tissues. NPs are defined as submicronic (<500 nm) colloidal system. They can provide a controlled and targeted way to deliver the encapsulated anticancer drugs, resulting in high efficacy and few side effects. Moreover, several parameters in a NP's structure and composition can be programmed to create a targeted drug delivery vehicle. By modifying the physical and chemical properties of NPs, their biological properties such as circulation half-life, immunogenicity, biodistribution, toxicity, biodegradation, method of excretion, etc. can be controlled.

The NP core is synthesized from a wide variety of materials with different geometries and sizes. Materials such as carbon in carbon nanotubes or gold in gold nanorods, etc. have been used to deliver thermal therapy to cancer cells either through cytotoxic application of heat or in association with chemotherapeutics [30]. The poor vascularization of the tumor also makes it more susceptible to damage by heat than normal tissue, a factor that contributes to selectivity. Chemotherapeutic agents may be carried in the cores of hollow or porous NPs (nanocarriers). Liposomes, dendrimers, fullerenes, polymer nanospheres, and mesoporous silica are examples of NPs that have been used to carry drugs. These materials may also be programmed with mechanisms by which the drug may be released. For example, drug release may be triggered by heat, light, ion concentration, ultrasound, radiation or internal triggers like the reduced pH of tumor interstitia or of an endocytosed vesicle.

The geometry of the NP can be altered to modify its overall property. For example, the aspect ratio (i.e., the ratio of the length to the width) of a gold nanorod affects its absorbance spectra, which can be tuned to convert different wavelengths of light to produce heat, thus making it suitable to be used for thermal therapy.

The geometry of the NP also affects the cellular intake of cells. For receptor-mediated endocytosis, when ligand-modified NP attaches to a specific receptor on the cancer cell surface, it has been seen that gold nanorods have less cellular uptake than spherical colloids. This suggests that spherical morphology and spherical objects have a better chance of getting inside a cell than one with a high aspect ratio (nanorods).

NP geometry can also affect its half-life in the blood. The half-life is the amount of time it takes for the concentration of NPs in the blood to be reduced by 50%. Thus, the shape of the NP determines how fast it would be phagocytosed and thereby eliminated from the body.

Reports have documented the effect of shape and geometry with respect to contact of spherical and nonspherical polystyrene microparticles during phagocytosis by alveolar macrophages. It was found that when the macrophage first contacted disc-shaped elliptical particles along the major axis, the particles were rapidly internalized (< 6 minutes). However, when first contact was along the minor axis, even after 12 hours, the particles were not internalized. Interestingly, the spherical particles were rapidly and uniformly internalized because of their symmetry. This effect of shape on particle internalization was found to be independent of particle size.

In another important study, it was found that filamentous micelles (filomicelles) stayed in circulation for over a week, while spherical vesicles were removed from the circulation within days [32]. This shows that having two dimensions on the length scale of nanometers (the diameter of filomicelles is ~20–60 nm and length upto 18μm) helps them reduce the rate of phagocytosis by cells of the mononuclear phagocyte system. Shear forces of blood flow applied to portions of the filomicelle not in contact with the cell exert enough force to pull the carrier away from the cell before internalization [32].

In addition, the NP's surface chemistry can be further modified to increase its half-life. This may again increase its availability to the target cells. The surface chemistry also affects the uptake amount of the therapeutic drug by target and nontarget cells [33].Once it is administered to the body, serum protein is adsorbed onto the surface of the NP, as part of the opsonization process. Opsonization is the process by which a foreign organism or particle becomes covered with nonspecific proteins, thereby making it more visible to phagocytic cells (e.g., monocytes, macrophages, neutrophils, and dendritic cells). The NPs thus decorated with serum proteins are now phagocytosed and removed from the body. The surface chemistry of the NP determines the extent and nature of this adsorption [34] and can be modified so as to minimize opsonization [35, 37]. It has been reported that, without surface modification, NPs have been removed from the bloodstream within seconds of administration by macrophages [37]. The initial adsorption of proteins results in a corona that determines further interactions with other proteins and cells [38]. In general, the primary forces for protein adsorption on NPs are hydrophobic and electrostatic interactions, together with conformational changes and associated changes in entropy [39, 40]. This adsorption could result in formation of a "hard corona," which refers to the proteins that adsorb tightly to the NP, whereas the "soft corona" results from weak adsorption of proteins that are therefore only transiently associated with the NP [34]. The surface-charge of NPs influences the composition of this "hard protein corona," and thus, it is related to its availability to the target cells (Figure 17.1). In this regard, poly (ethylene glycol) (PEG) is the most widely used macromolecule to evade the reticulo-endothelial system

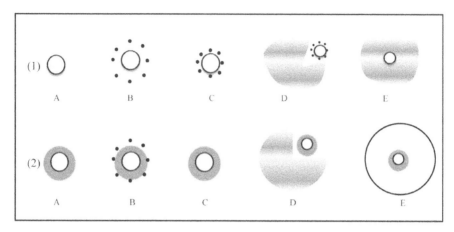

FIGURE 17.1   Pathway of uncoated hydrophobic NP (1) A. NPs in blood circulation, B. opsonins recognize NPs as foreign body due to the hydrophobic surface, C. opsonization of NPs, D & E. Phagocytosis by phagocyte. Pathway of coated hydrophilic NP (2) A. hydrophilic polymer-coated NP, B. repulsion between opsonins and NPs, C. NP still in circulation, D & E. endocytosis by the target cell

and prolong half- life of nanocarriers, thus increasing their chance of reaching its intended target. PEGs have strong effect on NP structure, stabilization, and bio-distribution both *in vitro and in vivo [41–44]*

The overall size of the NP drug delivery system may also be tuned for delivery to the tumor site and then to an intracellular target. It has been seen that maximum cellular uptake is achieved with 50 nm particles [45, 46]. The attachment of several targeting moieties side-by-side on a NP increases the avidity (i.e., the combined strength of multiple bond interactions) compared to free targeting moieties.

17.4   BIORECOGNITION MOLECULES

Biorecognition molecules are necessary to direct NPs to a molecular target. Certain pairs of molecules such as enzymes and substrates, antibodies and antigens, or complementary chains of DNA bind strongly and specifically to each other and not to other molecules in the environment. Biorecognition uses this molecular complementarity, which is found ubiquitously in biological systems.

To give desired targeting capabilities to NP, the NP is conjugated to one member of a molecular complement pair, also known as a targeting or biorecognition molecule. This enables the NP to specifically bind to the other member of the complementary pair, also known as the target. This specificity to a molecular target can be used in diagnosis, where the NP labels a molecular marker. It can also be exploited in targeted therapy, where the NP carries therapeutic elements and releases them at the target site. There are several strategies for identifying new targeting molecules. Some of the most common methods of identifying targeting molecules are polyclonal antibodies, monoclonal antibodies, aptamers, and phage display.

17.4.1   ANTIBODIES

Antibodies are molecules produced by an organism's immune system in response to an immunogenic invader or antigen. Antibodies bind specifically to their target antigen, making them a natural targeting molecule. The population of antibodies produced by an immunized animal is polyclonal in that it recognizes collectively all the antigens an animal has been exposed to in the past. The magnitude of the immune response produced by the antigen determines the proportion of the polyclonal antibody population that is directed against that antigen.

The diversity of the polyclonal antibody population can lead to a lack of specificity toward the target antigen due to antibodies cross-reacting with nontarget antigens. Because the production of polyclonal antibodies occurs in living animals, this technology is limited by the lifespan of the animal and the amount of serum that can be extracted [47].

The major drawbacks associated with polyclonal antibodies were overcome by the production of monoclonal antibodies [48]. Monoclonal antibodies are commonly used in immunofluorescence microscopy to label components of a cell or tissue, affinity chromatography to separate proteins in complex mixtures, and in diagnostic and therapeutic applications [49]. Monoclonal antibodies are used to identify tumor markers in cancer detection, to bind and inactivate toxic proteins, and to interrupt signaling processes in the treatment of cancer [47, 50, 51].

17.4.2   APTAMERS

Aptamers are functional, binding oligonucleotides (nucleic acid chains) that have been identified through a process of in vitro screening [52, 53]. Here, a library of randomized RNA is screened for binding affinity to a protein target. Oligonucleotides that bind to the target are amplified using the poly-merase chain reaction (PCR), and the screening is repeated. Multiple rounds of screening and amplification will yield an aptamer that binds with greatest affinity to the target protein.

17.4.3 PHAGE DISPLAY

Phage display is a powerful tool to find targeting molecules based on their binding affinity. Phage display screens a library of genetically modified bac-teriophage to find a peptide that binds to a target with the greatest affinity [53]. Bacteriophages are viruses that infect bacteria. They are composed of DNA inside a protein coat. The DNA inside the phage encodes the amino acid sequences of the proteins displayed on the protein coat of the phage. Libraries of several million different phages can be created through random mutations of an insert into the phage DNA. Phage display subjects these libraries through a process of panning and amplification that selects for clones that bind most effectively to the target protein.

Through this process, the phage expressing a peptide that binds to the affinity matrix comes to dominate the total phage population and can thereby be selected against a high background of non-specific phage. By expressing random peptides on a library of phage and by using affinity purification and amplification, it is possible to identify peptides that bind to a protein target without any prior knowledge of the nature of the target [55, 56].

17.5   MULTIFUNCTIONAL NPS

Multifunctional NPs/nanocarriers can be defined as nanoscale particles capable of performing at least an additional function to that of carrying a therapeutic or imaging payload. Thus, as previously mentioned, mono-func-tional NPs deliver only a single active agent, whereas multifunctional NP integrates various functionalities within the NP core and on the surface to synergistically achieve maximal anticancer activity [57].

Multifunctional NPs are fabricated using different types of organic and inorganic materials (Figure 17.2) Each of these NPs has unique architecture with attached functionalities, and they demonstrate effective drug delivery to tumors [58]. Organic/ polymeric NPs such as micelles, liposomes, polymer-icnano gels, and dendrimers are useful building blocks for multifunctional

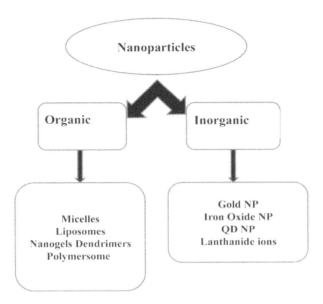

FIGURE 17.2 Multifunctional NPs are synthesized using organic and inorganic types of NPs. Organic NPs include micelles, liposomes, nanogels, dendrimers and polymersome and inorganic NPs include iron oxide NPs, gold NPs, quantum dots (QD), and lanthanide ions.

NPs. They have versatile surface and core chemistry, high biodegradability, effective endocytosis by target cell, and high loading efficiency [59].

17.5.1 NANOMICELLES

Nanomicelles are self-assembling amphiphilic nanosized colloidal dispersions consisting of a hydrophobic core and a hydrophilic shell [60]. These can encapsulate hydrophobic drugs and imaging agents in their core, thus avoiding the need for using toxic organic solvents. (Figure 17.3). Hydrophobicity is considered as a major constraint in formulating clear aqueous solutions with sufficient concentration of therapeutic to be delivered to the tissues. Nanomicelles solubilize hydrophobic drugs by entrapping the drugs within amicellar hydrophobic core with a corona, which is composed of hydrophilic chains extending outwards. The presence of hydrophilic chain outside results in a clear aqueous formulation [60]. Nanomicelles serve as excellent pharmaceutical carriers because of their ability to prevent or minimize drug degradation, have lower adverse side effects, and improve drug bioavailability.

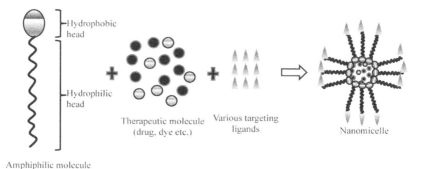

FIGURE.17.3 Formation of nanomicelles is through the assembly of amphiphilic blocks with a hydrophobic head and a hydrophilic outer tail. Therapeutic molecules are encapsulated inside the hydrophobic core. Surface is modified using various targeting ligands.

17.5.2 LIPOSOMES

Lipids are amphiphilic molecules, where one part of the molecule is water-loving (hydrophilic) and the other water-hating (hydrophobic). When lipids are placed in contact with water, the interaction of the hydrophobic part of the molecule with the solvent result in the self -assembly of lipids, often forming liposomes. Liposomes are thus constructed from bilayers of enclosed spherical structures such as phospholipids, cholesterol, and other similar lipid molecules, which consist of an aqueous core surrounded by a lipid bilayer, separating the inner aqueous core from the bulk outside (Figure 17.4) They are highly suitable for the encapsulation in their hydrophilic core of nucleic acid-based components, such as siRNA and plasmid DNA, to be targeted to tumor sites.

17.5.3 POLYMERIC NANOGELS

Nanogels are nanoscale polymeric networks. These are synthesized by cross-linking polymer chains to create an inner porous space that can accommodate a large volume of drug load, and therefore, are highly effective for simultaneous delivery of multiple treatment modalities [62] (Figure 17.5)

The possibility of obtaining a high degree of encapsulation and capability of offering an ideal tridimensional microenvironment for many macromolecules gives them an advantage over the classic NPs. They can also

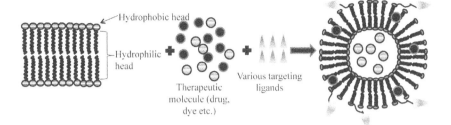

FIGURE 17.4 Liposome NPs are made up of lipid bilayers that act as a drug carrier, with the drug incorporated inside the hydrophobic core or the lipid bilayer.

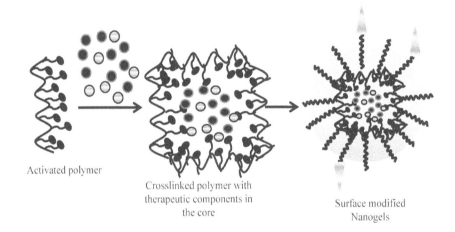

FIGURE 17.5 Polymeric nanogels are synthesized by crosslinking activated polymer chains, thus generating an inner free space that can accommodate therapeutic components.

escape renal clearance owing to their size (100–700 nm), thus enhancing their serum half-life period [63].

17.5.4 DENDRIMERS

Dendrimers are three-dimensional, immensely branched, well-organized organic polymeric NPs that can accommodate multiple functional moieties at their terminal groups. They are synthesized by assembling monomeric subunits to form a highly branched tree-like structure that accommodates the therapeutic drug within the branch-like structure. These branches can be further modified by complexing with various targeting ligands, imaging agents, etc. [64] (Figure 17.6). Some examples of dendritic molecules include polyamidoamine (PAMAM), poly(propylene imine) polyamide, polyglycerol (PG), triazine, etc.

17.5.5 INORGANIC NPS

Inorganic NPs exhibit unique optical and magnetic properties that make them suitable for detection and diagnostic applications. They have a rigid outer surface and an inside core that can be utilized for incorporating a variety of therapeutic agents. Several magnetic NPs have been used widely in image contrast and magnetic resonance to detect the presence of tumors.

By modifying the surface of these molecules with different targeting ligands, they can be used for targeted drug delivery that can enhance the diagnostic capability of these NPs. In this regard, gold NPs have been widely exploited in tumor imaging due to their superior optical and electric properties [65]. Others such as quantum dots, which are semiconductor NPs, have a narrow emission and a broad range of absorption bands and are thus suitable to be used in fabricating imaging probes [66]. Gold NPs and quantum dots have been synthesized along with the organic polymers to form hybrid systems, which can integrate various functionalities such as incorporating

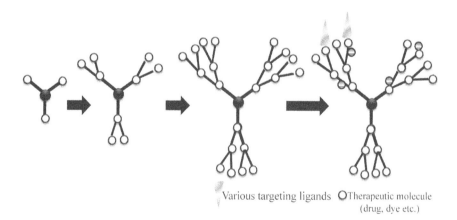

Various targeting ligands ◯ Therapeutic molecule
(drug, dye etc.)

FIGURE 17.6 Dendrimers are highly branched polymers with an inner core and outer branch, both providing multiple points for various treatment modalities.

drug and diagnostic agents for effective drug delivery as well as real-time monitoring of treatment response and tumor activity [67, 68]. Lanthanide-doped NPs have also been used due to their fluorescence properties in various cancer diagnostic trials [69–71].

17.6   NPS IN USE FOR CANCER THERAPY

The nano-encapsulation of traditional chemotherapeutic drugs such as doxorubicin (DOX), paclitaxel(PXL), docetaxel, cis-diamminedichloro-platinum (II) (cisplatin), cytarabine, vincristine (VCR), vinblastine (VLB), vinorelbine (microtubule inhibitor), camptothecin, lurtotecan, and irinote-can has introduced various therapeutic possibilities with respect to cancer treatment. Doxil®, a PEGylated liposomal formulation of doxorubicin, has been successfully used for preclinical and clinical testing in the treatment of ovarian cancer [71]. Currently, PEGylated liposomal doxorubicin is in clinical trials for breast cancer [75], B-cell lymphoma [74], refractory multiple myeloma [75], and melanoma [76]. Trials of metastatic breast cancer with Abraxane® or nab-paclitaxel (nano-albumin-encapsulated paclitaxel) have resulted in a longer time to progression, a higher overall response rate, and a longer overall survival in patients compared to solvent-based paclitaxel. A number of clinical trials are being initiated using these nano-drugs in combination with other biologic and/or cytotoxic agents to treat early and metastatic breast cancer [78], advanced non-small lung cancer in patients who cannot be treated by radiation or surgery [78], and advanced pancreatic cancer [79].

Multifunctional NP have further helped in engineering novel drug com-binations, which could be used in a single drug delivery system for maximal therapeutic efficiency. The combination of hydrophilic (e.g., doxorubicin) or hydrophobic (e.g., paclitaxel) drugs with negatively charged siRNA or DNA can target different metabolic pathways of tumor cells, thus resulting in attaching the tumor cells through multiple pathways [80]. In other reports, an amphiphilic triblock copolymer, poly(N-methyldietheneaminesebacate)-co-[(cholesteryloxocarbonylamido ethyl) methyl bis(ethylene)ammonium bromide] sebacate, or P(MDS-co-CES, was used to deliver paclitaxel and plasmid DNA encoding IL-12 together [81]. In both these systems, the NPs suppressed cancer growth more efficiently when compared to individual delivery of the two components.

Several nanoformulations of siRNA and shRNA inhibitory sequences against genes that suppress the expression of various functional and metabolic pathways of cancer cells have been developed and successfully used to inhibit the growth and progression of cancer. There are reports of successful development of a poly(ethylene glycol)-dioleoylphosphatidyl ethanolamine (PEG-DOPE)-modified G(4)-PAMAM nanocarrier that could deliver a drug-siRNA to tumor cells. The lipid modification of cationic polymers increased the transfection efficiency, and the micellar dendrimer system yielded higher stability and protection of the siRNA against enzymatic degradation [83]. Additionally, siRNA complexes against VEGF and PlK-1 have been reported to be used in combination with paclitaxel, resulting in increased endocytosis in tumor cells and higher tumor suppression [83, 84].

17.6.1 TUMOR-SPECIFIC TARGETING

The aim of nanotherapy involves the capability of nanocarrier to distinguish between cancerous and healthy tissue so as to minimize the systemic toxicity associated with chemotherapy. The unique size and pharmacokinetic properties of the NPs leads to their accumulation at tumor sites. This happens through passive targeting and is dependent on the pathophysiology of the tumor mass as a whole and the uniqueness of the tumor microenvironment. The process of passive delivery can be further increased by modification of the nanomaterials' surface using different hydrophilic moieties.

Active targeting involves targeting of NPs using selective affinity ligands. These ligands are complementary to the overexpressed molecules on tumor cells and thus specifically attach to these cells promoting higher and more sustained drug interactions with the target. These ligands used for surface modifications and recognition of target receptors on tumor cells include antibodies (anti-Her2, anti-CD44, anti-CD24), proteins (transferrins), small bioactive molecules (biotin, folate, galactose, glucose), peptides (like L-arginine, L-aspartic acid (RGD)), and oligonucleotides (aptamers).

A suitable example would be the use of anti-HER2 targeting antibodies conjugated to liposome-grafted PEG chains, which strongly increase the uptake of the NPs in HER2-expressing breast tumors. It was reported that liposomes without the anti-HER2 antibody remain concentrated in the peri-vascular and stromal spaces and are internalized by the cancer-associated macrophages, thus reducing their availability to the tumors [85]. In other drug delivery systems, the overexpression of transferrin receptors by the cancer cells has been utilized. These receptors are targeted using transferrin proteins decorated on the NPs [86]. In the preclinical studies for prostate cancer, transferrin-conjugated paclitaxel encapsulated PLGA NPs showed better antitumor activity when compared to the components used individually without transferrin conjugation.

Other preclinical studies have reported BIND-014 could deliver up to 10-times more docetaxel to tumor sites than nonspecific drug delivery systems [87]. Results showed that BIND-014 had prolonged circulation and retention time in the vasculature as well as five-fold greater antitumor activity compared to clinically administered docetaxel doses [88].

17.6.2   CANCER DIAGNOSTICS AND BIOIMAGING

NP imaging probes show enhanced sensitivity to signal, better spatial resolution, and thus higher capability to probe cellular and molecular information of the tumor mass. The use of magnetic NPs in combination with various functional molecules, such as fluorescent probes etc., may give rise to dual modal imaging probes. Fluorescent dye-doped silica (DySiO2)-encapsulated magnetic NPs have been used to detect neuro-blastoma cancer cells via MRI along with subcellular fluorescence imaging. Coupling of magnetic NPs with radionuclides such as 124I to produce MRI-PET probes that can accurately detect lymph node metastasis have been reported [89].

Multifunctional NPs that have different imaging probes engineered into one NP structure synergistically combine the advantages offered by each specific imaging technique that can lead to faster and more efficient detection of tumors. These can also be used for real-time monitoring of therapeutic efficiency. Studies have shown usage of hybrid NP consisting of an iron oxide NP coated with a PEG-grafted chitosan polymer and conjugated to fluorescent Cy5.5. This tumor targeting moiety accumulates in medulloblastoma tumor tissue in transgenic mice.

Quantum dots have also been successfully used for drug delivery and imaging. A quantum dot-aptamer-doxorubicin (QD-Apt-DOX) conjugate was constructed by surface modification having prostate tumor cell-specific A10RNA aptamer attached to the CdSe-ZnS core of the quantum dot and also having doxorubicin. Upon internalization and release of doxorubicin, optical activation techniques can detect the fluorescence associated with this nanocomplex and can spatially locate the tumor, visualize drug delivery and uptake and detect the real-time response of the tumor cell to the drug [90].

Gold NPs have also been widely used for fabricating multimodal drug delivery system for cancer. They have few advantages ranging from ease of synthesis, presence of negative reactive groups on the surface that can be easily modified for conjugation, and low toxicity [91]. It has been successfully used for a pancreatic cancer model, where gold NPs acted as carrier, gemcitabine was the chemotherapeutic drug, and EGFR served as the target moiety. This combination resulted in a significant inhibition of tumor growth [92].

17.7   SUMMARY

- Use of NPs for cancer therapy includes specifically eliminating the malignant cells without damaging surrounding healthy tissue
- NPs may transport drug to the tumor site through active or passive targeting strategies.
- Several NP characteristics such as size, shape, surface chemistry, etc. are central to their functionality as drug delivery vehicle.
- Biorecognition molecules such as antibodies, aptamers, and phage display direct drug-loaded nanocarriers to the target site.
- Use of multifunctional NP integrates various functionalities inside the core/surface of the NP to synergistically achieve maximal anti-cancer activity.
- Multifunctional nanocarriers are fabricated from organic or polymeric NPs, such as micelles, liposomes, polymeric nanogels, dendrimers, and inorganic NPs
- Various NPs are currently in clinical use for tumor-specific targeting, bioimaging, and cancer diagnostics.

KEYWORDS

- **antibody**
- **aptamer**
- **bioimaging**
- **biorecognition molecule**
- **cancer therapy**
- **dendrimers**
- **liposomes**
- **multifunctional NPs**
- **nanogels**
- **nanomicelles**
- **nanoparticles**
- **phage display**

REFERENCES

1. Wang, M., & Thanou, M., (2010). Targeting nanoparticles to cancer. *Pharmacological Research, 62*, 90–99.
2. Kim, B. Y. S., Rutka, J. T., & Chan, W. C. W., (2010). Nanomedicine. *The New England Journal of Medicine, 365*(25), 2434–2443.
3. Ferrari, M., (2005). Cancer nanotechnology: Opportunities and challenges. *Nature Reviews: Cancer, 5*(3), 161–171.
4. Peer, D., Karp, J. M., Hong, S., Farokhzad, O. C., Margalit, R., & Langer, R., (2007). Nanocarriers as an emerging platform for cancer therapy. *Nature Nanotechnology, 2*, 751–760.
5. Farokhzad, O. C., & Langer, R., (2009). Impact of nanotechnology on drug delivery. *ACS Nano., 3*(1), 16–20.
6. Hirsch, L. R., Stafford, R. J., Bankson, J. A., Sershen, S. R., Rivera, B., Price, R. E., Hazle, J. D., Halas, N. J., & West, J. L., (2003). Nanoshell-mediated near-infrared thermal therapy of tumors under magnetic resonance guidance. *PNAS, 100*(23), 13549–13554.
7. Sun, Y., & Xia, Y., (2003). Gold and silver nanoparticles: A class of chromophores with colors tunable in the range from *400* to *750* nm. *The Analyst., 128*, 686–691.
8. Gao, X., Cui, Y., Levenson, R. M., Chung, L. W. K., & Nie, S., (2004). In vivo cancer targeting and imaging with semiconductor quantum dots. *Nature Biotechnology, 22*(8), 969–976.
9. De, M., Ghosh, P. S., & Rotello, V. M., (2008). Applications of nanoparticles in biology. *Advanced Materials, 20*(22), 4225–4241.

10. Rosi, N. L., & Mirkin, C. A., (2005). Nanostructures in biodiagnostics. *Chemical Reviews., 105*, 1547–1562.

11. Loo, C., Lowery, A., Halas, N., West, J., & Drezek, R., (2005). Immunotargeted nanoshells for integrated cancer imaging and therapy. *Nano Letters, 5*(4), 709–711.

12. Brannon-Peppas, L., & Blanchette, J. O., (2004). Nanoparticle and targeted systems for cancer therapy. *Advanced Drug Delivery Reviews, 56*, 1649–1659.

13. Cheng, J., Teply, B. A., Sheriff, I., Sung, J., Luther, G., Gu, F. X., Levy-Nissenbaum, E., Radovic-Moreno, A. F., Langer, R., & Farokhzad, O. C., (2007). Formulation of functionalized PLGA-PEG nanoparticles for in vivo targeted drug delivery. *Biomaterials, 28*, 869–876.

14. Ullah, M. D., & Aatif, M., (2009). The footprints of cancer development. *Cancer Treatment Reviews, 35*, 193–200.

15. Estelrich, J., Sanchez-Martín, M. J., & Busquets, M. A., (2015). Nanoparticles in magnetic resonance imaging: from simple to dual contrast agents. *Int. J. Nanomedicine, 10*, 1727–1741.

16. Corot, C., Robert, P., Idffee, J. M., & Port, M., (2006). Recent advances in iron oxide nanocrystal technology for medical imaging. *Advanced Drug Delivery Reviews, 58*, 1471–1504.

17. Elghanian, R., Storhoff, J. J., Mucic, R. C., Letsinger, R. L., & Mirkin, C. A., (1997). Selective colorimetric detection of polynucleotides based on the distance-dependent optical properties of gold nanoparticles. *Science, 277*, 1078–1081.

18. Kukowska-Latallo, J. F., Candido, K. A., Cao, Z., Nigavekar, S. S., Majoros, I. J., Thomas, T. P., Balogh, L. P., Khan, M. M., Baker, Jr. J. R., (2005). Nanoparticle targeting of anticancer drug improves therapeutic response in animal model of human epithelial cancer. *Cancer Research, 65*(12), 5317–5324.

19. Cho, K., Wang, X., Nie, S., Chen, Z., & Shin, D. M., (2008). Therapeutic nanoparticles for drug delivery in cancer. *Clin. Cancer Res., 14*, 1310–1316 .

20. Sinha, R., Kim, G. J., Nie, S., & Shin, D. M., (*2006*). Nanotechnology in cancer therapeutics: bioconjugated nanoparticles for drug delivery. *Mol. Cancer Ther., 5*(8), 1909–1917.

21. Smith, A. M., Duan, H., Mohs, A. M., & Nie, S., (*2008*). Bioconjugated quantum dots for *in vivo* molecular and cellular imaging. *Adv. Drug Deliv. Rev., 60*(11), 1226–1240.

22. Matsumura, Y., & Maeda, H., (*1986*). A new concept for macromolecular therapeutics in cancer chemotherapy – mechanism of tumoritropic accumulation of proteins and the antitumor agent smancs. *Cancer Res., 46*(12), 6387–6392.

23. Pelicano, H., Martin, D. S., Xu, R. H., & Huang, P., (2006). Glycolysis inhibition for anticancer treatment. *Oncogene, 25*, 4633–4646.

24. Yatvin, M. B., Kreutz, W., Horwitz, B. A., & Shinitzky, M., (*1980*). pH-sensitive liposomes: possible clinical implications. *Science, 210*(4475), 1253–1255.

25. Jiang, W., Kim, B. Y. S., Rutka, J. T., & Chan, W. C. W., (2008). Nanoparticle-mediated cellular response is size-dependent. *Nature Nanotechnology, 3*, 145–150.

26. Qian, X., Peng, X. H., Ansari, D. O., Yin-Goen, Q., Chen, G. Z., Shin, D. M., Yang, L., Young, A. N., Wang, M. D., & Nie, S., (2008). In vivo tumor targeting and spectroscopic detection with surface-enhanced Raman nanoparticle tags. *Nature Biotechnology, 26*(1), 83–90.

27. Chan, W. C. W., & Nie, S., (1998). Quantum dot bioconjugates for ultrasensitive nonisotopic detection. *Science, 281*, 5385–5390.

28. Farokhzad, O. C., Jon, S., Khademhosseini, A., Tran, T. N. T., LaVan, D. A., & Langer, R., (2004). Nanoparticle-aptamerbioconjugates: A new approach for targeting prostate cancer cells. *Cancer Research, 64*(21), 7668–7672.

29. Cai, W., Shin, D. W., Chen, K., Gheysens, O., Cao, Q., Wang, S. X., Gambhir, S. S., & Chen, X., (2006). Peptide-labeled near-infrared quantum dots for imaging tumor vasculature in living subjects. *Nano Letters, 6*(4), 669–676.

30. Weissleder, R., Kelly, K., Sun, E. Y., Shtatland, T., & Josephson, L., (2005). Cell-specific targeting of nanoparticles by multivalent attachment of small molecules. *Nature Biotechnology, 23*(11), 1418–1423.

31. Lück, M., Paulke, B., Schröder, W., Blunk, T., & Müller, R., (1998). Analysis of plasma protein adsorption on polymeric nanoparticles with different surface characteristics. *J. Biomed. Mater. Res., 39*, 478–485.

32. Champion, J. A., Katare, Y. K., & Mitragotri, S., (2007). Particle shape: a new design parameter for micro- and nanoscale drug delivery carriers. *J. Control. Release, 121*(1–2), 3–9.

33. Geng, Y., Dalhaimer, P., Cai, S., Tsai, R., Tewari, M., Minko, T., & Discher, D. E., (2007). Shape effects of filaments versus spherical particles in flow and drug delivery. *Nature Nanotech., 2*, 249–255.

34. Dobrovolskaia, M. A., & McNeil, S. E., (2007). Immunological properties of engineered nanomaterials. *Nature Nanotechnology, 2*, 469–478.

35. Lundqvist, M., Stigler, J., Elia, G., Lynch, I., Cedervall, T., & Dawson, K. A., (2008). Nanoparticle size and surface properties determine the protein corona with possible implications for biological impacts. *PNAS, 105*(38), 14265–14270.

36. Verma, A., Uzun, O., Hu, Y., Han, H. S., Watson, N., Chen, S., Irvine, D. J., & Stellacci, F., (2008). Surface-structure-regulated cell-membrane penetration by monolayer protected nanoparticles. *Nature Materials, 7*, 588–595.

37. Soo Choi, H., Liu, W., Misra, P., Tanaka, E., Zimmer, J. P., Itty Ipe, B., Bawendi, M. G., & Frangioni, J. V., (2007). Renal clearance of quantum dots. *Nature Biotechnology, 25*(10), 1156–1170.

38. Gref, R., Minamitake, Y., Peracchia, M. T., Trubetskoy, V., Torchilin, V., & Langer, R., (1994). Biodegradable long-circulating polymeric nanospheres. *Science, 263*(5153), 1600–1603.

39. Cedervall, T., Lynch, I., Lindman, S., Berggard, T., Thulin, E., Nilsson, H., Dawson, K. A., & Linse, S., (2007). Understanding the nanoparticle-protein corona using methods to quantify exchange rates and affinities of proteins for nanoparticles. *Proc. Natl. Acad. Sci. USA., 104*, 2050–2055.

40. Gessner, A., Lieske, A., Paulke, B., & Müller, R., (2002). Influence of surface charge density on protein adsorption on polymeric nanoparticles: analysis by two-dimensional electrophoresis. *Eur. J. Pharm. Biopharm., 54*, 165–170.

41. Akerman, M. E., Chan, W. C. W., Laakkonen, P., Bhatia, S. N., & Ruoslahti, E., (2002). Nanocrystal targeting *in vivo*. *Proc. Natl. Acad. Sci. USA., 99*, 12617–12621.

42. Daou, T. J., Li, L., Reiss, P., Josserand, V., & Texier, I., (2009). Effect of poly (ethylene glycol) length on the *in vivo* behavior of coated quantum dots. *Langmuir, 25*, 3040–3044.

43. Boeneman, K., Deschamps, J. R., Buckhout-White, S., Prasuhn, D. E., Blanco-Canosa, J. B., Dawson, P. E., Stewart, M. H., Susumu, K., Goldman, E. R., Ancona, M., & Medintz, I. L., (2010). Quantum dot DNA bioconjugates: attachment chemistry strongly influences the resulting composite architecture. *ACS Nano., 4*, 7253–7266.

44. Maldiney, T., Richard, C., Seguin, J., Wattier, N., Bessodes, M., & Scherman, D., (2011). Effect of core diameter, surface coating, & PEG chain length on the biodistribution of persistent luminescence nanoparticles in mice. *ACS Nano., 5*, 854–862.

45. Chithrani, B. D., & Chan, W. C. W., (2007). Elucidating the mechanism of cellular uptake and removal of protein-coated gold nanoparticles of different sizes and shapes. *Nano Letters, 7*(6), 1542–1550.

46. Chithrani, B. D., Chan, Ghazani, A. A., & W. C. W., (2006). Determining the size and shape dependence of gold nanoparticle uptake into mammalian cells. *Nano. Letters, 6*(4), 662–668.

47. Iqbal, S. S., Mayo, M. W., Bruno, J. G., Bronk, B. V., Batt, C. A., & Chambers, J. P., (2000). A review of molecular recognition technologies for detection of biological threat agents. *Biosensors & Bioelectronics, 15,* 549–578.

48. Abbas, A. K., & Janeway, C. A. J. Jr., (2000). Immunology: Improving on nature in the twenty- first century. *Cell, 100,* 129–138.

49. Lodish, H., Berk, A., Matsudaira, P., Kaiser, C. A., Krieger, M., Scott, M. P., Zipursky, L., & Darnell, J., (2002). *Molecular Cell Biology.* W. H. Freeman and Company, 5th edition.

50. Ross, J. S., Schenkein, D. P., Pietrusko, R., Rolfe, M., Linette, G. P., Stec, J., Stagliano, N. E., Ginsburg, G. S., Symmans, W. F., Pusztai, L., & Hortobagyi, G. N., (2004). Targeted therapies for cancer. *American Journal of Clinical Pathology, 122*(4), 598–560.

51. Nakamura, R. M., Grody, W. W., Wu, J. T., & Nagle, R. B., (2004). (editors) Cancer Di.agnostics: *Current and Future Trends,* Humana Press, Totowa, New Jersey.

52. Ellington, A. D., & Szostak, J. W., (1990). In vitro selection of RNA molecules that bind specific ligands. *Nature, 346*(6287), 818–822.

53. Tuerk, C., & Gold, L., (1990). Systemic evolution of ligands by exponential enrichment: RNA ligands to bacteriophage T4 DNA. *Science, 249*(4968), 505–510.

54. Smith, G. P., (1985). Filamentous fusion phage: Novel expression vectors that display cloned antigens on the virion surface. *Science, 228*(4705), 1315–1317.

55. Cwirla, S. E., Peters, E. A., Barrett, R. W., & Dower, W. J., (1990). Peptides on phage: A vast library of peptides for identifying ligands. *Proc. Natl. Acad. Sci. USA, 87,* 6378–6382.

56. Devlin, J. J., Panganiban, L. C., & Devlin, P. E., (1990). Random peptide libraries: A source of specific protein binding molecules. *Science, 249,* 404–406.

57. Liboiron, B. D., & Mayer, L. D., (2014). Nanoscale particulate systems for multidrug delivery: towards improved combination chemotherapy. *Ther. Deliv., 5*(2), 149–171.

58. Nazir, S., Hussain, T., Ayub, A., Rashid, U., & MacRobert, A. J., (2014). Nanomaterials in combating cancer: Therapeutic applications and developments. *Nanomedicine, 10,* 19–34.

59. Jia, F., Liu, X., Li, L., Mallapragada, S., Narasimhan, B., & Wang, Q., (2013). Multifunctional nanoparticles for targeted delivery of immune activating and cancer therapeutic agents. *J. Control. Release, 172,* 1020–1034.

60. Trivedi, R., & Kompella, U. B., (2010). Nanomicellar formulations for sustained drug delivery: strategies and underlying principles. *Nanomedicine (Lond), 5*(3), 485–505.

61. Velagaleti, P. R., Anglade, E., Khan, I. J., Gilger, B. C., & Mitra, A. K., (2010). Topical delivery of hydrophobic drugs using a novel mixed nanomicellar technology to treat diseases of the anterior and posterior segments of the eye. *Drug Deliv. Technol., 10*(4), 42–47.

62. Chacko, R. T., Ventura, J., Zhuang, J., & Thayumanavan, S., (2012). Polymer nanogels: A versatile nanoscopic drug delivery platform. *Adv. Drug Deliv. Rev., 64,* 836–851.

63. Wilk, K. A., Zielinska, K., Pietkiewicz, J., & Saczko, J., (2009). Loaded nanoparticles with cyanine-tipephotosensizers:preparation, characterization and encapsulation. *Chemical Engineering Transactions, 17,* 987–992.

64. Kojima, C., Kono, K., Maruyama, K., & Takagishi, T., (2000). Synthesis of polyamidoaminedendrimers having poly(ethylene glycol) grafts and their ability to encapsulate anticancer drugs. *Bioconjug. Chem., 11,* 910–917.

65. Kim, D., & Jon. S., (2012). Gold nanoparticles in image-guided cancer therapy. *Inorg. Chim. Acta., 393,* 154–164.

66. Huang, H. C., Barua, S., Sharma, G., Dey, S. K., & Rege, K., (2011). Inorganic nanoparticles for cancer imaging and therapy. *J. Control Release, 155,* 344–357.

67. Bao, Q. Y., Zhang, N., Geng, D. D., Xue, J. W., Merritt, M., Zhang, C., & Ding, Y., (2014). The enhanced longevity and liver targetability of paclitaxel by hybrid liposomes encapsulating paclitaxel-conjugated gold nanoparticles. *Int. J. Pharm., 477,* 408–415.

68. Liang, R., Wang, J., Wu, X., Dong, L., Deng, R., Wang, K., Sullivan, M., Liu, S., Wu, M., Tao, J., et al., (2013). Multifunctional biodegradable polymer nanoparticles with uniform sizes: Generation and *in vitro* anti-melanoma activity. *Nanotechnology, 24,* 455302.

69. Coll, J. L., (2011). Cancer optical imaging using fluorescent nanoparticles. *Nanomedicine, 6,* 7–10.

70. Naccache, R., Rodriguez, E. M., Bogdan, N., Sanz-Rodriguez, F., Cruz Mdel, C., Fuente, A. J., Vetrone, F., Jaque, D., Sole, J. G., & Capobianco, J. A., (2012). High resolution fluorescence imaging of cancers using lanthanide ion-doped upconvertingnanocrystals. *Cancers, 4,* 1067–1105.

71. Cheng, L., Yang, K., Li, Y., Zeng, X., Shao, M., Lee, S. T., & Liu, Z., (2012). Multifunctional nanoparticles for upconversion luminescence/MR multimodal imaging and magnetically targeted photothermal therapy. *Biomaterials, 33,* 2215–2222.

72. Lawrie, T. A., Bryant, A., Cameron, A., Gray, E., & Morrison, J., (2013). Pegylated liposomal doxorubicin for relapsed epithelial ovarian cancer. *Cochrane Database Syst. Rev., 7,* CD006910.

73. Lien, M. Y., Liu, L. C., Wang, H. C., Yeh, M. H., Chen, C. J., Yeh, S. P., Bai, L. Y., Liao, Y. M., Lin, C. Y., Hsieh, C. Y., et al., (2014). Safety and efficacy of pegylated liposomal doxorubicin-based adjuvant chemotherapy in patients with stage I–III triple-negative breast cancer. *Anticancer Res., 34,* 7319–7326.

74. Oki, Y., Ewer, M. S., Lenihan, D. J., Fisch, M. J., Hagemeister, F. B., Fanale, M., Romaguera, J., Pro, B., Fowler, N., Younes, A., et al., (2015). Pegylated liposomal doxorubicin replacing conventional doxorubicin in standard R-CHOP chemotherapy for elderly patients with diffuse large B-Cell lymphoma: An open label, single arm, phase II trial. Clin. *Lymphoma Myeloma Leuk., 15,* 152–158.

75. Usmani, S. Z., & Lonial, S., (2014). Novel drug combinations for the management of elapsed/refractory multiple myeloma. *Clin. Lymphoma Myeloma Leuk., 14S.,* S71–S77.

76. Mei, L., Liu, Y., Zhang, Q., Gao, H., Zhang, Z., & He, Q., (2014). Enhanced antitumor andanti-metastasis efficiency via combined treatment with CXCR4 antagonist and liposomaldoxorubicin. *J. Control Release, 196,* 324–331.

77. Gluck, S., (2014). Nab-paclitaxel for the treatment of aggressive metastatic breast cancer. Clin. *Breast Cancer, 14,* 221–227.

78. Socinski, M. A., Bondarenko, I., Karaseva, N. A., Makhson, A. M., Vynnychenko, I., Okamoto, I., Hon, J. K., Hirsh, V., Bhar, P., Zhang, H., et al., (2012). Weekly nab-paclitaxel in combination with carboplatin *versus* solvent-based paclitaxel plus carboplatin as first-line therapy in patients with advanced non-small-cell lung cancer: Final results of a phase III trial. *J. Clin. Oncol., 30,* 2055–2062.

79. Von Hoff, D. D., Ervin, T., Arena, F. P., Chiorean, E. G., Infante, J., Moore, M., Seay, T., Tjulandin, S. A., Ma, W. W., Saleh, M. N., et al., (2013). Increased survival in pancreatic cancer withnab-paclitaxel plus gemcitabine. *N. Engl. J. Med., 369,* 1691–1703.

80. Creixell, M., & Peppas, N. A., (2012). Co-delivery of siRNA and therapeutic agents using nanocarriers to overcome cancer resistance. *Nano Today, 7,* 367–379.

81. Wang, Y., Gao, S., Ye, W. H., Yoon, H. S., & Yang, Y. Y., (2006). Co-delivery of drugs and DNA from cationic core-shell nanoparticles self-assembled from a biodegradable copolymer. *Nat. Mater., 5,* 791–796.

82. Biswas, S., Deshpande, P. P., Navarro, G., Dodwadkar, N. S., & Torchilin, V. P., (2013). Lipid modified triblockpamam-based nanocarriers for siRNA drug co-delivery. *Biomaterials, 34,* 1289–1301.

83. Zhu, C., Jung, S., Luo, S., Meng, F., Zhu, X., Park, T. G., & Zhong, Z., (2010). Co-delivery of siRNA and paclitaxel into cancer cells by biodegradable cationic micelles based on PDMAEMA-PCL-PDMAEMA triblock copolymers. *Biomaterials, 31,* 2408–2416.

84. Sun, T. M., Du, J. Z., Yao, Y. D., Mao, C. Q., Dou, S., Huang, S. Y., Zhang, P. Z., Leong, K. W., Song, E. W., & Wang, J., (2011). Simultaneous delivery of siRNA and paclitaxel via a "two-in-one"micelleplex promotes synergistic tumor suppression. *ACS Nano., 5,* 1483–1494.

85. Kirpotin, D. B., Drummond, D. C., Shao, Y., Shalaby, M. R., Hong, K., Nielsen, U. B., Marks, J. D., Benz, C. C., & Park, J. W., (2006). Antibody targeting of long-circulating lipidic nanoparticles does not increase tumor localization but does increase internalization in animal models. *Cancer Res., 66,* 6732–6740.

86. Sahoo, S. K., Ma, W., & Labhasetwar, V., (2004). Efficacy of transferrin-conjugated paclitaxel-loaded nanoparticles in a murine model of prostate cancer. *Int. J. Cancer, 112,* 335–340.

87. Hrkach, J., Von Hoff, D., Mukkaram Ali, M., Andrianova, E., Auer, J., Campbell, T., De Witt, D., Figa, M., Figueiredo, M., Horhota, A., et al., (2012). Preclinical development and clinical translation of a PSMA-targeted docetaxel nanoparticle with a differentiated pharmacological profile. *Sci. Transl. Med., 4,* 128–139.

88. Sanna, V., Siddiqui, I. A., Sechi, M., & Mukhtar, H., (2013). Nanoformulation of natural products for prevention and therapy of prostate cancer. *Cancer Lett., 334,* 142–151.

89. Cheon, J., & Lee, J. H., (2008). Synergistically integrated nanoparticles as multimodal probes fornanobiotechnology. *Acc. Chem. Res., 41,* 1630–1640.

90. Bagalkot, V., Zhang, L., Levy-Nissenbaum, E., Jon, S., Kantoff, P. W., Langer, R., & Farokhzad, O. C., (2007). Quantum dot-aptamer conjugates for synchronous cancer imaging, therapy, & sensing of drug delivery based on bi-fluorescence resonance energy transfer. *Nano Lett., 7,* 3065–3070.

91. Patra, C. R., Bhattacharya, R., Mukhopadhyay, D., & Mukherjee, P., (2010). Fabrication of gold nanoparticles for targeted therapy in pancreatic cancer. *Adv. Drug Deliv. Rev., 62,* 346–361.

92. Patra, C. R., Bhattacharya, R., Wang, E., Katarya, A., Lau, J. S., Dutta, S., Muders, M., Wang, S., Buhrow, S. A., Safgren, S. L., et al., (2008). Targeted delivery of gemcitabine to pancreatic adenocarcinoma using cetuximab as a targeting agent. *Cancer Res., 68,* 1970–1978.

CHAPTER 18

CANCER IMMUNOTHERAPY: EXTENDING NEW HORIZONS IN CANCER TREATMENT

DEBA PRASAD MANDAL

Department of Zoology, West Bengal State University, Berunanpukuria, Malikapur, North-24 Parganas, Barasat, Kolkata–700126, West Bengal, India, E-mail: dpmandal1972@gmail.com

CONTENTS

ABSTRACT

Rejuvenating the immune system for healthier life has been an age-old practice. Immunotherapy is referred to a treatment that involves the use of certain parts of the hosts (patient's) immune system to fight diseases such as cancer. Dr William Bradley Coley, father of Cancer Immunotherapy, would have been delighted to see the phenomenal progress of what he initiated

125 years ago. During the past three decades, anticancer immunotherapy has evolved rapidly leading to the approval of various immunotherapeutic regimens by US Food and Drug Administration and the European Medicines Agency. The various therapeutics engaged in this form of treatment can be broadly divided into "passive" and "active" based on their ability to engage the host immune system against cancer. Diverse forms of immunotherapies range from specifically targeting one (or a few) defined tumor-associated antigen(s) to others that operate in a relatively non-specific manner and boost natural or therapy-elicited anticancer immune responses. The myriad therapeutics that are employed ranges from highly specific monoclonal antibodies to the use of an attenuated variant of *Mycobacterium bovis* (Bacille Calmette-Guérin). Interestingly, metronomic doses of conventional chemotherapeutic drugs like doxorubicin and cyclophosphamide are being envisaged in cancer immunotherapy. Characterization of hundreds of antigens and antigenic epitopes expressed on cancer cells recognized by the immune system paved way for a myriad of clinical trials assessing immunization with peptides, proteins, dendritic cells, recombinant viruses, whole cells, and plasmid DNA. This chapter makes an attempt to begin with the historical perspective of this therapy and then to introduce the world of immunotherapy by visiting the recent classification of the agents used.

18.1   HISTORICAL PERSPECTIVE

Immunotherapy, sometimes called biologic therapy or biotherapy, is referred to a treatment that involves the use of certain parts of the hosts (patient's) immune system to fight diseases such as cancer. This therapy broadly can be divided into two procedures. The first one involves stimulating the patient's own immune system to work harder or smarter to attack the transformed cells. The second way is by the administration of immune system components, such as man-made immune system proteins.

The importance of rejuvenating the immune system for healthier life has been an age-old practice. Our ancestors had included immunostimulatory and immunoprotective substances in both regular diet and ancient medicine. Ayurveda along with many ancient texts records the use of numerous plants and herbs with immunomodulatory properties in the treatment of various ailments. It is said that Greek historian Thucydides as long ago as 429 BC had observed that those who survived the smallpox plague in Athens did not become re-infected with the disease. However, the Chinese were credited with the discovery and use of the primitive form of vaccination, called variolation way back between the 14th and 17th centuries. This technology spread to Turkey and arrived in England in the early 18th century by which time smallpox was the most infectious disease in Europe. Finally, British physician, Dr Edward Jenner, in 1796, discovered vaccination in its modern form as we know it today.

William Bradley Coley, MD, is recorded in making the first attempt to harness the immune system in the treatment of cancer as early as in the late 19th century and is coined as the Father of Immunotherapy. Dr. Coley had observed in a number of cases that patients with cancer went into spontaneous remission after developing erysipelas, a bacterial skin infection caused by Group A *Streptococcus* bacterium. He began injecting mixtures of live and inactivated *Streptococcus pyogenes* and *Serratia marcescens* into patients' tumors in 1891. It caused tumor shrinkage in many patients, while it did not in others; this led the Food and Drug Administration (FDA) to assign Coley's Toxins as a "new drug" in 1963, making it illegal to prescribe this kind of therapy outside of clinical trials in the US. Many patients were blessed with Coley's toxins as it achieved responses such as durable complete remission in several types of malignancies, including sarcoma, lymphoma, and testicular carcinoma. The lack of a known mechanism of action for "Coley's toxins" and the risks of deliberately infecting cancer patients with pathogenic bacteria coupled with the exactness of strains used leading to mixed clinical outcome caused oncologists to adopt surgery and radiotherapy as standard treatments early in the 20th century [1]. Dr. Coley's concept of using attenuated bacteria to treat malignancies was revived in 1976 when a trial was conducted to test the use of the tuberculosis vaccine Bacille Calmette-Guérin (BCG) as a means of preventing the recurrence of nonmuscle invasive bladder cancer [2]. Unlike the fate of Coley's toxin, BCG therapy was very effective and continues to be used today.

With the quantitative accounts about antibodies in the 1880s, studies related to the humoral wing of the immune system dominated immunology over the cellular component until the 1940s. In fact, works of Landsteiner and Chase (1942), and Gross (1943) heralded the future development of cellular and cancer immunology [3, 4]. In 1942, Landsteiner and Chase demonstrated that delayed hypersensitivity could be transferred between mice by using immune cells obtained from sensitized donors [3]. Gross reported syngeneic mice immunized against tumors in the same inbred strain could reject a subsequent tumor challenge [4]. The concept that the immune system can be used against cancer was fortified by a series of work published by Professor Frank Macfarlane Burnet. Burnet published his theory of acquired immunological tolerance which proposed that lymphocytes that were able to respond to self-tissues were deleted in prenatal life during the development of the immune system [5]. This work along with the concept of immunosurveillance brought into light that malignant cells can be eliminated by the immune system. Scientist by then had acknowledged the importance of cellular immunology as a mediator of allograft rejection as well as protection against the transferred tumor in mice. The studies were principally pounded with the challenge to manipulate lymphocytes and sustain their survival outside the body. The next important discovery in cancer immunotherapy could be assigned to the identification of a T-cell growth factor (IL-2) in 1976, which provided, for the first time, a means to grow T lymphocytes in vitro. However, small amount of IL2 recovered from culture systems damped hopes of its use in immunotherapy. With the identification of the DNA sequence of the gene encoding IL-2 and its subsequent expression in *Escherichia coli* along with the biological characterization of recombinant IL-2 provided new hopes and opportunities for cancer immunotherapy [6–8].

Immunotherapy against cancer probably received its first clinical momentum with the regression of large, established, invasive human cancers upon IL-2 administration [9]. This was the first manipulation of the human immune system with recombinant immune product to counter tumor progression and led the US FDA to approve IL-2 for the treatment of metastatic renal cell carcinoma in 1992 and for metastatic melanoma in 1998. Another important cytokine to be used in cancer therapy was interferons, and its application as an immunotherapeutic agent against cancer is an increasing prospect in recent times [10].

The use of monoclonal antibodies in cancer immunotherapy became a possibility with the discovery of hybridoma technology in 1975 by two scientists, Georges Kohler and Cesar Milstein, who jointly with Niels Jerne were awarded the 1984 Noble prize for physiology and medicine [11]. Antibodies for tagging, neutralizing, or blocking have made their entry successfully in the anticancer treatment regimes. Sometimes, when they are co-administered along with a chemotherapeutic drug or with a radioactive particle, they are called as *conjugated monoclonal antibodies.*

With the characterization of first human cancer antigen in 1991, hundreds of antigens and antigenic epitopes expressed on cancer cells recognized by the immune system were described [12–14]. These advances paved way for a myriad of clinical trials assessing immunization with peptides, proteins, dendritic cells, recombinant viruses, whole cells, and plasmid DNA. However, a vast majority of these vaccination/immunization in cancer therapy have failed to demonstrate significant clinical benefit. In recent time, a dendritic cell vaccine has claimed to prolong the survival of patients with prostate cancer by about 4 months, although there were no reports of tumor regressions or prolongation of progression-free survival in treated patients [15].

Failure of this immunotherapy is principally assigned to the inability to generate large numbers of antitumor cells with high affinity for tumor antigen, principally due to the immunosuppressive microenvironment at the tumor site that suppresses potent effector mechanisms[16]. Research directed to overcome the causes of failure led to the use of adoptive cell transfer of antitumor immune cells—this treatment approach, referred to as adoptive cell therapy (ACT), provides the best direct evidence that the immune system is capable of curing patients with metastatic cancer [17-19]. The extraordinary success of immunotherapy led the editorial of the journal *Science* to designate it as "Breakthrough of the Year 2013" [20].

18.2 GENERATING AN EFFECTIVE ANTITUMOR RESPONSE

Generation of an effective antitumor immune response involves a series of interrelated sequential steps. Tumor immune evasion principally involves interfering with this crucial interplay. Functional steps to mount an effective antitumor response primarily involves A) the availability of proper tumor antigens; B) antigen presenting cells (APCs) must be able to uptake these antigens and become activated; C) antigen cross-presentation between APCs and T cells should occur; D) these antigen-presented T cells should be able to infiltrate the tumor mileu; E) minimal suppressive activity from myeloid-derived suppressor cells (MDSC) and regulatory T cells (Tregs); and F) prolonged cytotoxic activity of T cells against tumor cells without depletion or deactivation induced by negative regulatory checkpoints [21]. The purpose of immunotherapy is to overcome the resistance imposed by the developing tumor in any (one or many) of the multiple steps mentioned above in a targeted way. The ground reality involves the treatment of diversity of "similar cancers" where the clinician is unaware of the exactness of the immune bottle necked situation, thus making each cancer in a patient unique in its own way. The situation can get even more complicated with multiple lesions occurring in a single patient. All these factors and more have now incited clinicians to initiate multimodality approaches (including chemotherapy, radiotherapy, and surgery) to maximize the potential of immunotherapy.

18.3   CLASSIFICATION OF ANTICANCER IMMUNOTHERAPY

Anticancer immunotherapies are generally broadly classified as "passive" or "active" based on their ability to (re-)activate the host immune system against malignant cells [22]. Passive form of immunotherapy refers to tumor-targeting monoclonal antibodies (mAbs) and adoptively transferred T cells as they are designed to target the various antineoplastic activity [23–26]. The "active" arm is dedicated for those therapeutic agents that exerts its effects only upon the engagement of the host immune system with the developing neoplasia or its components [27]. These "active" forms refer mainly to the anticancer vaccines and checkpoint inhibitors. An alternative classification of immunotherapeutic anticancer regimens by the American Cancer Society broadly divides immunotherapeutic interventions in cancer as a) monoclonal antibodies (mAbs), b) Immune checkpoint inhibitors, c) cancer vaccines, and d) other non-specific immunotherapies [27, 28]. An attempt to classify cancer immunotherapy was recently revisited by Galluzzi and Kroemer along with other scientists [27]. This work was based on contribution by 88 scientists worldwide having affiliation to more than 100 institutes.

18.3.1   PASSIVE IMMUNOTHERAPY

18.3.1.1   Tumor-Targeting Monoclonal Antibodies

Tumor-targeting mAbs is probably the most commonly used immunotherapy by clinicians' worldwide [29]. The targets can be again divided as: (1) tumor cell receptors on which the mAbs binds to and specifically alter the signaling optimized by the tumor cells to enhance the malignant situation; (2) signaling molecules, e.g., VEGF, produced by malignant cells or by stromal components of neoplastic lesions; (3) "tumor-associated antigen" (TAA), an antigen specifically or predominantly expressed by transformed cells that enable selective marking of cancer cells in vivo [27, 30–32].

18.3.1.2 Types of Monoclonal Antibodies

Galluzzi divided the different types of monoclonal antibodies into five groups against the three mentioned in the American Cancer Society. The detailed classification uses functionality of the mAbs in its discrimination

18.3.1.2.1 Naked mAbs that inhibit abnormal signaling

The term "naked" is basically used to mean it is not tagged and are the most common of all types of antibodies that are used to treat cancer. These mAbs target the abnormal signaling pathways that cancer cells harness for survival or progression. Cetuximab, a mAb against epidermal growth factor receptor (EGFR), is approved by the US FDA for the treatment of head and neck cancer (HNC) and colorectal carcinoma (CRC) [33].

18.3.1.2.2 Naked mAbs that serve as death ligand

Naked mAbs can also be used to activate potentially lethal receptors expressed on the surface of malignant cells, which are absent in non-transformed counterparts. Tigatuzumab (CS-1008), a mAb specific for tumor necrosis factor receptor superfamily, member 10B, (TNFRSF10B, best known as TRAILR2 or DR5) is currently under clinical development [32].

18.3.1.2.3 Conjugated mAbs

mAbs may be associated with a chemotherapeutic drug or with a radioactive particle and are called conjugated monoclonal antibodies; also referred to as labeled or loaded antibodies. The specificity of the mAb is based on their ability to recognize TAA and is used as a homing device to enhance targeted delivery. Once the mAb attaches to its target, it then delivers the toxic substance to that specific cell (http:// cancer.org). Ibritumomab tiuxetan (Zevalin) is an example of a radiolabeled mAb (also called radioimmunotherapy or RIT). This is an antibody against the CD20 antigen, which is found on B lymphocytes and is used to treat some types of non-Hodgkin lymphoma. Antibodies labeled with chemotherapeutic agents are also referred to as antibody-drug conjugates (ADCs) that principally lowers the side effect to the toxic drug by inducing specificity. Brentuximab vedotin (Adcetris), an anti-body that targets the CD30 antigen (found on lymphocytes), attached to a chemo drug called MMAE and is used to treat Hodgkin lymphoma and ana-plastic large cell lymphoma. Ado-trastuzumab emtansine (Kadcyla®, also called TDM-1), an antibody that targets the HER2 protein, is attached to a chemo drug called DM1and used to treat breast cancer patients with HER2 overexpression. Gemtuzumab ozogamicin, an anti-CD33 calicheamicin con-jugate, is currently approved for use in acute myeloid leukemia patients [34].

18.3.1.2.4   TAA-labeling mAbs

These naked mAbs opsonize cancer cells and hence activate antibody-dependent cell-mediated cytotoxicity (ADCC), antibody-dependent cellular phagocytosis, and complement-dependent cytotoxicity; an example is the CD20-specific mAb rituximab, which is currently approved for the treat-ment of chronic lymphocytic leukemia (CLL) and non-Hodgkin lymphoma [35–37].

18.3.1.2.5   Bispecific monoclonal antibodies

These are also called "bispecific T-cell engagers" (BiTEs), i.e., chimeric pro-teins consisting of two single-chain variable fragments from two distinctly different mAbs, one targeting a TAA and one specific for a T-cell surface receptor (e.g., blinatumomab, a CD19- and CD3 BiTE recently approved for the therapy of Philadelphia chromosome-negative precursor B-cell acute lymphoblastic leukemia) [38].

These classifications are truly based on the researchers' targeted aim rather than what happens in vivo. This is to bring to light that through an immunotherapy may be designed to act in a particular way, but in reality, it may operate in antineoplastic activity in more than a single attributed dimen-sion.

It may be understood that cetuximab not only inhibits EGFR signaling but also promotes ADCC and mediates immunostimulatory effects at the same time [39, 40]. Again bevacizumab, a vascular endothelial growth fac-tor A (VEGFA)-neutralizing mAb, not only exerts antitumorigenic effects by inhibition of angiogenesis but also by other myriad ways. Bevacizumab has been reported to enhance tumor infiltration by B and T lymphocytes

[41]. This mAb is also active in inhibiting CD4+CD25+FOXP3+ regulatory T cells (Tregs), thereby countering tumor-induced immunosuppression [41]. In general, polymorphisms in the genes coding for the receptors mainly responsible for ADCC, i.e., Fc fragment of IgG, low affinity IIa, receptor (FCGR2A, also known as CD32), and FCGR3A (also known as CD16a), have been shown to influence the response of cancer patients to most tumor-targeting mAbs [42].

18.3.1.3 Adoptive Cell Transfer

"Adoptive cell transfer" (ACT) refers to a particular immunotherapy against cancer involving the following sequential steps - (1) Collection of circulating or tumor-infiltrating lymphocytes (TIL), (2) selection/activation/modification/expansion of these TIL ex vivo, and (3) (re-)administration of these activated immune cells to the same patient, after lymphodepletion pre-conditioning and in combination with immunostimulatory agents [27, 43]. This technique, unlike the dendritic cell (DC)-based interventions, is included in the passive wing of immunotherapy as it involves intrinsic anticancer activity and not like enhanced vaccination such as that in dendritic therapy [27].

With the advent of the modern techniques in molecular biology and biotechnology, it is now possible to manipulate the immune cells ex vivo to render them more competent immunologically. Genetic engineering has made it possible to empower these cells with features like unique antigen specificity, increased and persistence proliferative potential in vivo. Genetically modified features like TAA-specific T-cell receptor (TCR), or "chimeric antigen receptor" (CAR), i.e., a transmembrane protein comprising the TAA-binding domain of an immunoglobulin linked to one or more immunostimulatory domains, adds advantage in T-cell recognition and elimination of cancer cells [44, 45]. Furthermore, these cells can have improved secretory profile and elevated tumor-infiltratory capacity coupled with superior cytotoxicity. The specificity of tumoricidal activity is the most warranted feature in cancer therapy as it lowers side effects and increases patients' compliance along with greater reduction of tumor load. The survival, expansion, migration, and cytotoxic activity of adoptively transferred T cells rely on several cytokines, some of which are supplied by the host immune system; however, all forms of the ACT protocols involve the administration of exogenous interleukins (ILs), including IL-2, IL-15, or IL-21 [27]. Adoptive transfer of natural killer cells (NK cells) or purified activated B lymphocytes does not confer any therapeutic advantage [27].

18.3.1.4   Oncolytic Viruses

Though both oncolytic viruses and oncotropic viruses show preferential tropism for malignant cells, the former is more cytotoxic for malignant cells than the latter [27]. Oncolytic viruses can simply impart cytopathic effect by overload of cellular metabolism resulting from a productive viral infection [46]. Due to the advent of modern breakthroughs in biotechnology, the cytopathic onslaught can be delivered to the cancer cells irrespective of the proliferative potential of the viruses. These viruses can be just a mechanism of delivery of lethal genes (hence their products) specifically to the cancer cells coupled with the fact that their reproduction will be limited only in these transformed cells. Cytotoxicity can be imparted by sequences coding for (1) enzymes that convert an innocuous pro-drug into a cytotoxic agent; (2) proteins that trigger lethal signaling cascades in cancer cells alone; or (3) short-hairpin RNAs that target factors that are strictly required for the survival of transformed cells, but not normal cells [27]. Though the use of such viruses for the treatment of cancer patients has not been approved by US FDA, the regulatory authorities of the People's Republic of China has approved the use of such treatments in combination with chemotherapy for HNC.

   The principal problem of this mode of therapy is the patient's own immune system. These viruses are ready targets for phagocytic activity of the innate immune system of the host, and coupled with the compliment system and preexisting antibodies, these viruses have difficulty in establishing themselves in the patient [27]. This is evident from the fact that large amounts of oncolytic viruses reach the liver and spleen upon injection [47]. The major success of these oncolytic viruses is that they promote the release of TAAs in an immunostimulatory mechanism [27].

18.3.2   ACTIVE IMMUNOTHERAPY

18.3.2.1   DC-Based Immunotherapies

Dendritic cells (DC) form the link between the innate and adaptive immune systems. Being tagged as the most competent among the APCs, they are endowed with the capability to present TAAs to immune cells and initi-ate the tumor-specific immune response. The concept of using autologous DCs in immunotherapies is similar to ACT, which has been elaborated earlier. Autologous or donor-derived DCs proliferated/activated/differ-entiated with TAAs/genetically modified are re-introduced in the host to facilitate tumor-specific immune response. The ex vivo stimulation with agents like granulocyte macrophage colony-stimulating factor (GM-CSF) for DC maturation is particularly important because immature DCs exert immunosuppressive, rather than immunostimulatory, functions [48]. The ex vivo stimulations include (1) TAA-derived peptides; (2) mRNAs cod-ing for one or more specific TAAs; (3) expression vectors coding for one or more specific TAAs; (4) bulk cancer cell lysates (either autologous or of heterologous derivation); and (5) bulk cancer cell-derived mRNA [27]. Regardless of the procedure, the rationale is to load the DCs, ex vivo, with TAAs or TAA-coding molecules, so that upon reinfusion they are able to prime TAA-targeting immune responses. To achieve this objective, inac-tivated cancer cells are also fused with Dcs ex vivo, generating so-called dendritomes [49]. In other version of the said concept, DC-derived exo-somes could be used to stimulate ex-vivo amplified re-introduced DCs *in vivo* [50]. However, these therapeutic procedures are very expensive; in fact, one cellular product containing a significant proportion of (partially immature) DCs is currently licensed for use in cancer patients, namely sipuleucel-T (also known as Provenge). This was developed and marketed by Dendreon Co. (Seattle, WA, US). Dendreon Co. filed its bankruptcy in November 2014, signifying that the product was not able to gain momen-tum in the pharma market due to the end product being too costly for suf-ficient consumption [27].

18.3.2.2 Peptide- and DNA-Based Anticancer Vaccines

Probably vaccination was the first form of immunotherapy to be used in modern times. In this process, DCs and other APCs are targeted with pep-tides or DNA-based stimulations. In peptide-based vaccine, full-length TAAs or peptides derived from such sources are injected through intramus-cular, subcutaneous, or intradermal route, together with one or more immu-nostimulatory agents commonly known as adjuvants. The efficiency of these peptide-based vaccines depends partially on the length of the peptide. While smaller peptides (8–12 amino acids) are believed to directly bind to MHC molecules expressed on the surface of APCs, synthetic long peptides (25–30 residues) must be taken up, processed (cut into small pieces), and presented by APCs for immune sensitization [27]. It has been observed that synthetic long peptides elicit superior immune stimulation than their shorter versions especially when they include epitopes that are recognized by both cytotoxic and helper T cells [51]. The choice of adjuvants in vaccination is of great importance. Freund's adjuvant (IFA), a popular adjuvant in vaccination, has recently been shown to limit the efficacy of peptide-based anticancer vaccination [52]. Autologous tumor lysates complexed with immunostimulatory chaperones, members of the heat-shock protein (HSP) family, has the advantage of multiple TAAs that bind to HSPs and has superior therapeutic outcome but is too expensive.

In a DNA-based anticancer vaccine, the antigen is delivered as DNA construct of the TAA, which serves as a template for the peptide synthesis. Such constructs are either naked or vectored by viral particles/non-pathogenic bacteria/yeasts. If vectored by bacteria or yeast, it becomes the source of the TAA, thereby stimulating the DCs. In case of naked DNA vaccines, they make their way into APCs or muscle cells and express the TAA. "Oncolytic vaccines," i.e., oncolytic viruses genetically altered to code for a TAA, are also used for TAA presentation [53]. Encouraging results were achieved with live-attenuated bacteria expressing a full-length TAA, which was taken up by APCs of the intestinal mucosa, resulting in the priming of a robust, TAA-specific immune response in the so-called "mucosa-associated lymphoid tissue" [54]. A peptide-based vaccine against human papillomavirus type 16 (HPV-16) proteins E6 and E7 has been shown to promote long-lasting responses in the majority of treated patients with vulvar intraepithelial neoplasia [55]. The administration of a multipeptide vaccine after single-dose cyclophosphamide (an alkylating chemotherapeutic agent) has been shown to prolong overall survival in a cohort of renal cell carcinoma (RCC) patients [56].

Despite such advances and success, no peptide- or DNA-based anticancer vaccine is currently approved by the US FDA and EMA for use in humans [27]. A heat shock protein 90-kDa beta (Grp94), member 1 (HSP90B1)-based anticancer vaccine has been approved in Russia for the treatment of RCC patients.

18.3.2.3 Immunostimulatory Cytokines

Cytokines are a family of biological molecules that regulate via autocrine, paracrine, or endocrine circuits thereby modifying various biological functions [57]. However, the use of immunostimulatory cytokines as a solitary treatment in cancer has yielded little or almost no results. These cytokines are generally used alongside other therapeutic regimes. There are exception to this, such as interferon (IFN)-α2b (Intron A) and IL-2 (Aldesleukin and Proleukin), which are used as single agent therapy in patients with melanoma [58]. The US FDA has approved the use of IFN- α2b for the therapy of hairy cell leukemia (HCL), follicular lymphoma, AIDS-related Kaposi's sarcoma, multiple myeloma, melanoma, external genital/perianal warts, and cervical intraepithelial neoplasms. IL-2 is approved for the treatment of metastatic forms of melanoma and RCC. IFN-α2a (Roferon-A) is approved for use in subjects with HCL and chronic phase, Philadelphia chromosome-positive chronic myeloid leukemia, upon minimal pretreatment and it is also approved for the treatment of melanoma. US FDA and EMA also approves the use of GM-CSF (also known as Molgramostim, Sargramostim, Leukomax, Mielogen, or Leukine) and granulocyte colony-stimulating factor (G-CSF, Filgrastim, Lenograstim, or Neupogen) for use in humans, but not as part of anticancer regimens [59]. Recombinant tumor necrosis factor α (TNFα) is approved by several regulatory agencies worldwide (but not by the US FDA) for the administration in combination with melphalan (an alkylating agent) to increase the local concentration of the drug and to promote the selective destruction of the tumor vasculature [60]. The antineoplastic activity of immunostimulatory cytokines has not yet been fully explored, and its success depends on the host immune systems' exact condition; thus, they should be employed with caution to avoid unwarranted, potentially lethal effects.

18.3.2.4 Immunomodulatory mAbs And Checkpoint Inhibitors

Immunomodulatory mAbs function by interacting with and altering the function of soluble or cellular components of the immune system, and thus elicit a fresh or restore an existing anticancer immune response [61, 62]. There are four general ways in which these mAbs work: (1) inhibition of immunosuppressive receptors expressed by activated T lymphocytes, such as cytotoxic T lymphocyte-associated protein 4 (CTLA4) and programmed cell death 1 (PDCD1, best known as PD-1), (2) inhibition of the principal ligands of these receptors, such as the PD-1 ligand CD274 (best known as PD-L1 or B7-H1), (3) activation of co-stimulatory receptors expressed on the surface of immune effector cells such as tumor necrosis factor receptor superfamily, member 4 (TNFRSF4, best known as OX40), TNFRSF9 (best known as CD137 or 4-1BB), and TNFRSF18 (best known as GITR), and (4) neutralization of immunosuppressive factors released in the tumor microenvironment, such as transforming growth factor-β1 (TGF-β1) [27].

The first of these approaches, which is commonly referred to as "checkpoint blockade," has been shown to induce robust and durable responses in a variety of solid tumors. It is important for the immune system to differentiate between self and foreign antigens and is the pivotal theme on which it functions. To ensure this process, the immune system uses "checkpoints" – molecules on certain immune cells that need to be activated (or inactivated) to start an immune response. Cancer cells utilize these checkpoints to evade the immune system. To counter this tumor induced immune modulations, mAbs designed to act as Immune checkpoint inhibitors are used.

PD-1 is a checkpoint protein on T cells which normally acts as an "off switch" when it attaches to another protein (on a different cell of the same host-self cell), namely PD-L1; this keeps the T cells from attacking other cells in the body (self-cells). Some cancer cells have large amounts of PD-L1, which helps them evade immune attack. Monoclonal antibody treatments that target either PD-1 or PD-L1 can boost the immune response against cancer cells and have shown a great deal of promise in treating certain cancers. Based on the results of a recently completed phase III clinical trial demonstrating that nivolumab significantly improves the progression-free and overall survival of patients with BRAFWT melanoma, this monoclonal antibody was approved by the US FDA in 2015. Pembrolizumab (Keytruda) and Nivolumab (Opdivo) are designed antibodies that bind to PD-1.These treatments have also been shown to be helpful against non-small cell lung cancer in large studies and in treating melanoma of the skin. However, these treatments allow the immune system to attack some normal organs in the body, which can lead to serious side effects in some people.

CTLA-4 is another protein on T cells that acts as a type of "off switch" to keep the immune system from attacking self-cells. Ipilimumab (Yervoy) is a monoclonal antibody that attaches to CTLA-4 and prevent it from rendering the cancer cells susceptible to immune onslaught. Co-stimulatory mAbs including urelumab and PF-0582566 (both of which target CD137) are also under clinical development, and the data suggest that combining checkpoint blockers with co-stimulatory mAb mediates superior antineoplastic effects [63]. Few clinical trials testing checkpoint blockers in combination with urelumab or lirilumab (a KIR-inhibiting mAb) have just been initiated [27]. Despite their non-specific mechanism of action, the clinical efficacy of immunomodulatory mAbs (and in particular checkpoint blockers) may be profoundly influenced by the panel of (neo-)TAAs specific to each neoplasm [64].

18.3.2.5 Inhibitors of Immunosuppressive Metabolism

Indoleamine 2,3-dioxigenase 1 (IDO1) catalyzes the first, rate-limiting step in the so-called "kynurenine pathway," a catabolic cascade that converts L-tryptophan (Trp) into L-kynurenine (Kyn) [27].

This depletes cells of Trp, resulting in irresponsiveness to immunological challenges; furthermore, the accumulation of Kyn and some of its derivatives exert cytotoxic effects on immune effector cells while promoting the differentiation of Tregs [65, 66]. These robust immunosuppressive effects may also be through various indirect mechanisms mediated by IDO1-expressing DCs [67]. The immunosuppressive nature is more exemplified by the fact both 1-methyltryptophan (an inhibitor of IDO1 and IDO2) and genetic interventions targeting IDO1 mediate antineoplastic effects while eliciting novel or rejuvenating existing anticancer immune responses [68]. Though no IDO1 inhibitor is currently approved by the US FDA, positive responses of mediators such as INCB024360 (blockers of IDO1) and IDO1-targeting vaccines are accumulating in their clinical trials [27].

Extracellular ATP recruits and activates APCs via purinergic receptor family named P1 receptors and P2 receptors which are further subdivided into into P2Y (G protein coupled) and P2X (intrinsic ion channels) [69]. Furthermore, the degraded products of ATP, e.g., AMP and adenosine, upon binding to adenosine A2a receptor (ADORA2A) and ADORA2B have negative effect on immunostimulation [70].

Extracellular ATP is degraded by two enzymes, namely ectonucleoside triphosphate diphosphohydrolase 1 (ENTPD1 or CD39), which converts ATP into ADP and AMP [71], and ecto-5'-nucleotidase (NT5E, or CD73), which transforms AMP into adenosine [72]. A section of human cancers express increased amounts of CD39 and/or CD73 [73] thereby attenuating

ATP induced activation of APCs and increasing AMP and adenosine induced immune-suppression. mAbs directed against CD39 and/or CD73 exert anti-neoplastic effects in both standalone or combination treatment [74].

18.3.2.6 Pattern Recognition Receptors (PRR) Agonists

Pattern recognition receptors (PRRs) are evolutionarily conserved proteins involved in the recognition of danger signals and include toll-like receptors (TLRs) and nucleotide-binding oligomerization domain containing (NOD)-like receptors (NLRs) [27]. TLRs are transmembrane proteins expressed by most APCs, including monocytes, macrophages and DCs, as well as by some types of epithelial cells [75]. NLRs are expressed by a variety of cell types, including various components of the innate and adaptive immune system [76]. The activation of various PRRs stimulates pro-inflammatory signal transduction cascade and activation of NF-κB, coupled with secretion of immunostimulatory cytokines like type I IFNs and TNFα [27]. PRR signaling also promotes the maturation of DCs as well as the activation of macrophages and NK cells [77]. Some PRRs play important role in the (re)activation of anticancer immune responses by chemo-, radio-, and immunotherapeutic interventions [78].

Currently, three TLR agonists are approved by the US FDA for use in cancer patients: (1) Bacillus Calmette-Guérin (BCG), an attenuated variant of *Mycobacterium bovis* that presumably operates as a mixed TLR2/TLR4 agonist, which is currently used as a standalone immunotherapeutic agent in subjects with noninvasive transitional cell carcinoma of the bladder (2) monophosphoryl lipid A (MPL), a TLR2/TLR4-activating derivative of *Salmonella minnesota* lipopolysaccharide (LPS) currently utilized as adjuvant in Cervarix®, a vaccine for the prevention of HPV-16 and -18 infection, and (3) imiquimod, an imidazoquinoline derivative that triggers TLR7 signaling, currently employed for the treatment of actinic keratosis, superficial basal cell carcinoma, and condylomata acuminata. Picibanil, lyophilized preparation of *Streptococcus pyogenes*, activates TLR2/TLR4, while mifamurtide (a synthetic lipophilic glycopeptide that activates NOD2) has been approved by the EMA for the treatment of osteosarcoma in 2009 [27, 79]. Safety and efficacy of several other PRR agonists are currently being evaluated in clinical trials; these include agatolimod (CpG-7909, PF-3512676, Promune), an unmethylated CpG oligodeoxynucleotide that activates TLR9; polyriboinosinic polyribocytidylic acid (polyI:C, Ampligen, Rintatolimod), a synthetic double-strand RNA that signals via TLR3;

and Hiltonol, a particular formulation of polyI:C that contains carboxy-methylcellulose and poly-L-lysine [27].

18.3.2.7 Immunogenic Cell Death Inducers

Some conventional chemotherapeutics, administered at small doses given over a long period, as well as some forms of radiation therapy, can kill malignant cells while stimulating them to release specific damage-associated molecular pattern (DAMPs). DAMPs bind to receptors expressed on the surface of APCs (including TLR4), which not only boost their ability to engulf particulate material (including TAAs) but also trigger their maturation and activation [27]. Thus, the APCs acquire the ability to elicit a cancer-specific immune response that is associated with the development of immunological memory. Functionally atypical form of apoptosis dubbed as "immunogenic cell death" (ICD) has been reported to have optimal antineoplastic effects in immunocompetent mice [80]. A few FDA-approved therapies have been shown to have inherent ICD-inducing properties, such as doxorubicin, mitoxantrone, and epirubicin (three anthracyclines currently employed against various carcinomas), bleomycin (a glycopeptide antibiotic endowed with antineoplastic properties), oxaliplatin (a platinum derivative agent generally used for the therapy of colorectal carcinoma), cyclophosphamide (an alkylating agent employed against neoplastic and autoimmune conditions), specific forms of radiation therapy, photodynamic therapy (an intervention that relies on the administration of a photosensitizing agent coupled to light irradiation), and bortezomib (a proteasomal inhibitor used for the treatment of multiple myeloma) [27].

18.3.3 NON-SPECIFIC IMMUNOTHERAPY

Lenalidomide (Revlimid, also known as CC- 5013) and pomalidomide (Pomalyst, also known as CC- 4047) are two derivatives of thalidomide that are found to have teratogenic effects. Thalidomide received renewed interest after its ban in 1950s as an inhibitor of TNFα secretion in the 1990s and was approved by the US FDA (under a strictly controlled distribution program) for the therapy of erythema nodosum leprosum (a complication of leprosy etiologically linked to TNFα) in 1998 [81, 82]. Thalidomide in combination with dexamethasone (a glucocorticoid) yielded impressive clinical results in hematological malignancies and received approval by the US FDA [83]. Although thalidomide, lenalidomide, and pomalido-mide, were collectively referred to as "immunomodulatory drugs" (IMiDs) for a long time, their underlying molecular mechanism of action were not properly known till recent times [84]. Recent findings indicate that the therapeutic activity of IMiDs depend, at least in part, on their ability to bind the E3 ubiquitin ligase cereblon (CRBN) and CRBN and regulate the abundance of interferon regulatory factor 4, which perhaps accounts for the immunomodulatory functions of IMiDs. Galluzzi and his co-authors argue "Although endowed with intrinsic antineoplastic activity, IMiDs should be considered active immunotherapeutics" [27].

Denileukin diftitox (also known as Ontak®) is a recombinant variant of IL-2 associated with the diphtheria toxin. Owing to its selective cytotoxicity for cells expressing IL-2 receptor α (IL2RA, best known as CD25), denileu-kin diftitox has been approved by the US FDA and EMA for the treatment of CD25+ cutaneous, T-cell lymphoma and has been accessed to have been successful in improving the efficacy of various immunotherapies by effi-ciently depleting Tregs (which also express CD25) [85].

High numbers of tumor associated macrophages (TAMs) has been cor-related with the various aspects of tumorigenesis namely, invasion, angio-genesis, hypoxia and early occurrence of metastasis. TAMs are broadly classified into two phenotypes M1 and M2. M1 macrophage are responsible for increasing prognosis of cancer patients as they are involved in expression of IL-1, IL-12, TNF-a, and inducible nitric oxide synthase (iNOS). Contrary to this M2 macrophages are correlated with tumor initiation and progres-sion and are known to secrete as IL-10 and reduce the expression of iNOS, inhibit antigen presentation and T cell proliferation. Therapeutic molecules that exert antineoplastic effects by altering the ratio between M2 and M1 TAMs in favoring the latter are being developed.

(1) a second-generation orally active quinoline-3-carboxamide analog initially developed as an antiangiogenic agent, tasquinimod,
(2) a marine-derived antineoplastic agent currently approved in Europe, Russia, and South Korea for the treatment of soft tissue sarcoma and ovarian carcinoma, trabectedin (Yondelis),
(3) inhibitors of chemokine (C-C motif) ligand 2/chemokine (C-C motif) receptor 2 (CCL2/ CCR2) signaling,
(4) mAbs specific for chemokine (C-X-C motif) receptor 4 (CXCR4),
(5) small molecule inhibitors and mAbs that suppress colony stimulating factor 1/colony stimulating factor 1 receptor (CSF1/CSFR1) signaling

18.4 CONCLUSION

Cancer therapy, in the recent past, has seen revolutionary changes both in terms of newer molecules as well as advanced techniques. The immunotherapeutic drugs (Table 18.1) have successfully been implemented to yield selective killing as well as maximize in terms of tumor load reduction. Clinicians now have numerous options to choose the appropriate regime from. He is not left with a few cytotoxic drugs which themselves are proven to be carcinogens. Life expectancy of patients suffering from cancer has extended considerably. With newer drugs in the horizon, things do not seem that bleak anymore.

Despite all these, one must keep in mind that cancer is still by and large an incurable disease. With its incidence rising, it is progressing toward being the most common life-threatening disease. The major hurdle with immunotherapy is that cancer causes rapid immunosuppression. The depleted immune system hardly has the arsenal or the mercenaries to fight the rapidly growing cells. Active players of immunotherapy cannot act that well under such immunosuppressed condition. With the tumor microenvironment being typically harsh for the immune system, passive immunotherapies also face little success toward the final stages of the disease.

More concerning issue is the monetary aspect of the disease. The cost of immunotherapy is very high and in countries where medical insurance/civic healthcare is not generous, patients will not be able to afford these treatments. Another aspect of the cost is the mileage that a patient gets is often meager to the costs incurred. Although much has been accomplished, much remains to be done. A therapy that should be effective and yet affordable by the vast majority is still a major challenge in cancer immunotherapy.

18.5 SUMMARY

- Dr William Bradley Coley, father of cancer immunotherapy, initiated immunotherapy against cancer 125 years ago.
- Humoral wing of the immune system dominated immunology over the cellular component until the 1940s
- Works from Landsteiner and Chase (1942), and Gross (1943) heralded the future development of cellular and cancer immunology.
- Concept that the immune system can be used against cancer was fortified by a series of work published by Professor Frank Macfarlane Burnet in 1949.

TABLE 18.1 Anticancer Immunotherapy Approved by Regulatory Agencies

Nature	Subclass	Agent	Year of approval	Indications	Proposed mechanism of action
Passive forms of immuno-therapy	Tumor targeting monoclonal antibodies	Naked mAbs that inhibit abnormal signaling	Trastuzumab	1998	Breast carcinoma	Inhibition of HER2 signaling
		Bevacizumab	2004	Gastric or gastroesophageal junction adenocarcinoma	
				Colorectal carcinoma	VEGFA neutralization
				Glioblastoma multiforme	
				Cervical carcinoma	
				Lung carcinoma	
				Renal cell carcinoma	
		Cetuximab	2004	Head and neck cancer	Inhibition of EGFR signaling
				Colorectal carcinoma	
		Panitumumab	2006	Colorectal carcinoma	Inhibition of EGFR signaling
		Denosumab	2011	Breast carcinoma	Inhibition of RANKL signal-ing
				Prostate carcinoma	
				Bone giant cell tumors	
		Pertuzumab	2012	Breast carcinoma	Inhibition of HER2 signaling
		Ramucirumab	2014	Gastric or gastroesophageal junction adenocarcinoma	Inhibition of KDR signaling
		Siltuximab	2014	Multicentric Castleman's disease	IL-6 neutralization

Nature	Subclass	Agent	Year of approval	Indications	Proposed mechanism of action
	mAbs as death ligand	Tigatuzumab (CS-1008)	In Clinical Phase Trial	Unresectable or metastatic pancreatic cancer	monoclonal antibody targeting death receptor 5
	Conjugated mAbs	Gemtuzumab ozogamicin	2000	Acute myeloid leukemia	Selective delivery of calicheamicin to CD33+ neoplastic cells
		Ibritumomab tiuxetan	2002	Non-Hodgkin lymphoma	Selective delivery of radioactive isotope to CD20+ neoplastic cells
		Iodine I 131 Tositumomab	2005	Rlapsed or chemotherapy/rituxan-refractory Non-Hodgkin lymphoma	monoclonal antibody directed against the CD20 antigen, combined with radioisotope iodine 131
		Brentuximab vedotin	2011	Anaplastic large cell lymphoma Hodgkin's lymphoma	Selective delivery of MMAE to CD30+ neoplastic cells
		Ado-trastuzumab emtansine	2013	To treat HER2-positive, metastatic breast cancer	Anti-HER2 monoclonal antibody combined with a microtubular inhibitor

TABLE 18.1 (Continued)

Nature	Subclass	Agent	Year of approval	Indications	Proposed mechanism of action
Passive forms of immuno-therapy	Tumor targeting monoclonal antibodies	TAA-label-ling mAbs	Rituximab	1997	Chronic lymphocytic leukemia Non-Hodgkin lymphoma	Selective recognition/opso-nization of CD20+ neoplastic cells
		Alemtuzumab	2001	Chronic lymphocytic leukemia	Selective recognition/ opso-nization of CD52+ neoplastic cells
		Ofatumumab	2009	Chronic lymphocytic leukemia	Selective recognition/opso-nization of CD20+ neoplastic cells
		Obinutuzumab	2013	Chronic lymphocytic leukemia	Selective recognition/opso-nization of CD20+ neoplastic cells
	Bispecific mAbs anti-bodies	Catumaxomab	2009	Malignant ascites in patients with EPCAM+ cancer	CD3- and EPCAM-specific BiTE
		Blinatumumab	2014	Acute lymphoblastic leukemia	CD3- and CD19-specific BiTE
	Oncolytic viruses	Oncorine H101	2005	Head and neck cancer	Selective lysis of malignant cells
Active immuno-therapy	Dendritic cell-based im-mumotherapies	Sipuleucel-T	2010	Prostate carcinoma	Priming of a PAP-specific immune response
	Peptide-based vaccines	Vitespen	2008	Renal cell carcinoma	Activation of a tumor-specific immune response

TABLE 18.1 (Continued)

Nature	Subclass	Agent	Year of approval	Indications	Proposed mechanism of action
Active immuno-therapy	Immunostimulatory cytokines	IL-2	<1995	Melanoma Renal cell carcinoma	Non-specific immunostimulation
		IFN-α2b	<1995	Multiple hematological and solid tumors	Non-specific immunostimulation
		IFN-α2a	1999	Chronic myeloid leukemia Hairy cell leukemia Melanoma	Non-specific immunostimulation
	Immunomodulatory mAbs and Checkpoint inhibitors	Ipilimumab	2011	Melanoma	Blockage of CTLA4-dependent immunological checkpoints
		Nivolumab	2014	Melanoma	Blockage of PDCD1-dependent immunological checkpoints
		Pembrolizumab	2014	Melanoma	Blockage of PDCD1-dependent immunological checkpoints

[Source: Adapted from Ref. 22]

- Cancer immunotherapy can be broadly classified under two major heads "passive" and "active" based on their ability to engage the host immune system against cancer.
- Passive immunotherapy consists of using monoclonal antibodies, adoptive transfer of modified/activated lymphocytes, and Oncolytic viruses
- Monoclonal antibodies (mAbs) can be further subdivided into naked mAbs that inhibit abnormal signaling, naked mAbs that serve as death ligand, conjugated mAbs, TAA-labeled mAbs, bispecific mAbs
- Active immunotherapy includes DC-based immunotherapies, peptide/DNA-based vaccines, immunostimulatory cytokines, immunomodulatory mAbs, Inhibitors of immunosuppressive metabolism, PPR agonists, immunogenic cell death inducers, and metronomic use of conventional chemotherapy.

KEYWORDS

- adoptive cell transfer
- cancer immunotherapy
- checkpoint blockers
- dendritic cell-based interventions
- DNA-based vaccines
- immunostimulatory cytokines
- oncolytic viruses
- peptide-based vaccines
- therapeutic monoclonal antibodies
- toll-like receptor agonists.

REFERENCES

1. Decker, W. K., & Safdar, A., (2009). Bioimmunoadjuvants for the treatment of neoplastic and infectious disease: Coley's legacy revisited. *Cytokine Growth Factor Rev., 20,* 271–281.
2. Kucerova, P., & Cervinkova, M., (2016). Spontaneous regression of tumour and the role of microbial infection--possibilities for cancer treatment. *Anticancer Drugs, 27,* 269–277.

3. Wissler, J. H., Wissler, J. E., & Logemann, E., (2008). Extracellular functional noncoding nucleic acid bioaptamers and angiotropin RNP ribokines in vascularization and self-tolerance. *Ann. New York Acad. Sci., 1137*, 316–342.

4. Morse, M. A., Clay, T. M., & Lyerly, H. K., (2004). *Biology of the Cancer Vaccine Immune Response.* In: *Handbook of Cancer Vaccines*, Morse, M. A., Clay, T. M., Lyerly, H. K., Ed, Springer Science & Business Media, New York, pp. 3–11.

5. Ribatti, D., (2015). Peter Brian Medawar and the discovery of acquired immunological tolerance. *Immunol. Lett., 167*, 63–66.

6. Kim, H. P., Imbert, J., & Leonard, W. J., (2006). Both integrated and differential regulation of components of the IL-2/IL-2 receptor system. *Cytokine Growth Factor Rev., 17*, 349–366.

7. Taniguchi, T., Matsui, H., & Fujita, T., (1983). Structure and expression of a cloned cDNA for human interleukin-2. *Nature, 302*, 305–307.

8. Rosenberg, S. A., Grimm, E. A., McGrogan, M., Doyle, M., Kawasaki, E., Koths, K., & Mark, D. F., (1984). Biological activity of recombinant human interleukin-2 produced in *E. coli. Science, 223*, 1412–1414.

9. Jiang, T., Zhou, C., & Ren, S., (2016). Role of IL-2 in cancer immunotherapy. *Oncoimmunology* [Online] 5, e1163462. http://dx.doi.org/10. 1080/2162402X. 1163462.

10. Razaghi, A., Owens, L., & Heimann, K., (2016). Review of the recombinant human interferon gamma as an immunotherapeutic: Impacts of production platforms and glycosylation. *J. Biotechnol., 240*, 48–60.

11. Gavilondo, J. V., & Larrick, J. W., (2000). Antibody engineering at the millennium. *Bechnique, 29*, 128–32, 134–6, *138* passim.

12. Kawakami, Y., Fujita, T., Matsuzaki, Y., Sakurai, T., Tsukamoto, M., Toda, M., & Sumimoto, H., (2004). Identification of human tumor antigens and its implications for diagnosis and treatment of cancer. *Cancer Sci., 95*, 784–791.

13. Schultze, J. L., & Vonderheide, R. H., (2001). From cancer genomics to cancer immunotherapy: toward second-generation tumor antigens. *Trends Immunol., 22*, 516–523.

14. Robbins, I. F., Wang, R. F., & Rosenberg, S. A., (2000). Tumor antigens recognized by cytotoxic lymphocytes in *Cytotoxic Cells: Basic Mechanisms and Medical Applications*, Sitkovsky, M. V. & Henkart, P A. Eds, J. B. Lippincott, Philadelphia, 363–383.

15. Kantoff, P. W., Higano, C. S., Shore, N. D., Berger, E. R., Small, E. J., Penson, D. F., Redfern, C. H., Ferrari, A. C., Dreicer, R., Sims, R. B., Xu Y., Frohlich, M. W., & Schellhammer, P. F., (2010). Sipuleucel-T immunotherapy for castration-resistant prostrate cancer. *N. Engl. J. Med., 363*, 411–422.

16. Rosenberg, S. A., Sherry, R. M., Morton, K. E., Scharfman, W. J., Yang, J. C., *Topalian, S. L., Royal, R. E., Kammula, U., Restifo, N. P., Hughes, M. S., Schwartzentruber, D., Berman, D. M., Schwarz, S. L., Ngo, L. T., Mavroukakis, S. A., White, D. E., & Steinberg, S. M., (*2005). Tumor progression can occur despite the induction of very high levels of self/tumor antigen-specific CD8+ T cells in patients with melanoma. *J. Immunol., 175*, 6169–6176.

17. Dudley, M. E., Wunderlich, J. R., Robbins, P. F., Yang, J. C., Hwu, P., *Schwartzentruber, D. J., Topalian, S. L., Sherry, R., Restifo, N. P., Hubicki, A. M., Robinson, M. R., Raffeld, M., Duray, P., Seipp, C. A., Rogers-Freezer, L., Morton, K. E., Mavroukakis, S. A., White, D. E., & Rosenberg, S. A., (*2002). Cancer regression and autoimmunity in patients after clonal repopulation with anti-tumor lymphocytes. *Science, 298*, 850–854.

18. Dudley, M. E., Yang, J. C., Sherry, R., Hughes, M. S., Royal, R, Kammula, U., Robbins, P. F., Huang, J., Citrin, D. E., Leitman, S. F., Wunderlich, J., Restifo, N. P., Thomasian,

A., Downey, S. G., Smith, F. O., Klapper, J., Morton, K., Laurencot, C., White, D. E., & Rosenberg, S. A., (2008). Adoptive cell therapy for patients with metastatic melanoma: evaluation of intensive myeloablative chemoradiation preparative regimens. *J. Clin. Oncol., 26*, 5233–5239.

19. Rosenberg, S. A., & Dudley, M. E., (2009). Adoptive cell therapy for the treatment of patients with metastatic melanoma. *Curr. Opin. Immunol., 21*, 233–240.

20. Couzin-Frankel, J., (2013). Breakthrough of the year 2013. Cancer immunotherapy. *Science, 342*, 1432–1433.

21. Pardoll, D., (2015). Cancer and the immune system: basic concepts and targets for intervention. *Semin. Oncol., 42*, 523–538.

22. Lesterhuis, W. J., Haanen, J. B., & Punt, C. J., (2011). Cancer immunotherapy--revisited. *Nat. Rev. Drug. Discov., 10*, 591–600.

23. Humphries, C., (2013). Adoptive cell therapy: Honing that killer instinct. *Nature, 504*, 13–15.

24. Maus, M. V., Fraietta, J. A., Levine, B. L., Kalos, M., Zhao, Y., & June, C. H., (2014). Adoptive immunotherapy for cancer or viruses. *Annu. Rev. Immunol., 32*, 189–225.

25. Weiner, L. M., (2007). Building better magic bullets--improving unconjugated monoclonal antibody therapy for cancer. *Nat. Rev. Cancer, 7*, 701–706.

26. Strebhardt, K., & Ullrich, A., (2008). Paul Ehrlich's magic bullet concept: *100* years of progress. *Nat. Rev. Cancer, 8*, 473–480.

27. Galluzzi, L., Vacchelli, E., Bravo-San Pedro, J. M., Buqué, A., Senovilla, L., et.al., (2014). Classification of current anticancer immunotherapies. *Oncotarget, 5*, 12472–12508.

28. Cancer Immunotherapy http://www.cancer.org/treatment/treatmentsandsideeffects/ treatmenttypes /immunotherapy.

29. Weiner, L. M., Surana, R., & Wang, S., (2010). Monoclonal antibodies: versatile platforms for cancer immunotherapy. *Nat. Rev. Immunol., 10*, 317–327.

30. Kaplan-Lefko, P. J., Graves, J. D., Zoog, S. J., Pan, Y., Wall, J., Branstetter, D. G., Moriguchi, J., Coxon, A., Huard, J. N., Xu, R., Peach, M. L., Juan, G., Kaufman, S., Chen, Q., Bianchi, A., Kordich, J. J., Ma, M., Foltz, I. N., & Gliniak, B. C., (2010). Conatumumab, a fully human agonist antibody to death receptor 5, induces apoptosis via caspase activation in multiple tumor types. *Cancer Biol. Ther., 9*, 618–631.

31. Ferrara, N., Hillan, K. J., Gerber, H. P., & Novotny, W., (2004). Discovery and development of bevacizumab, an anti-VEGF antibody for treating cancer. *Nat. Rev. Drug Discov., 3*, 391–400.

32. Cavallo, F., Calogero, R. A., & Forni, G., (2007). Are oncoantigens suitable targets for anti-tumour therapy? *Nat. Rev. Drug Discov., 7*, 707–713.

33. Ming, L. C., Stephenson, R., Salazar, A. M., & Ferris, R. L., (2013). TLR3 agonists improve the immunostimulatory potential of cetuximab against EGFR head and neck cancer cells. *Oncoimmunology, 2*, e24677 http://www.tandfonline.com/doi/pdf/10. 4161/ onci. 24677.

34. Hughes, B., (2010). Antibody-drug conjugates for cancer: poised to deliver? *Nat. Rev. Drug Discov., 9*, 665–667.

35. Hubert, P., & Amigorena, S., (2012). Antibody-dependent cell cytotoxicity in monoclonal antibody-mediated tumor immunotherapy. *Oncoimmunology, 1*, 103–105.

36. Winiarska, M., Glodkowska-Mrowka, E., Bil, J., & Golab, J., (2011). Molecular mechanisms of the antitumor effects of anti- CD20 antibodies. *Front. Biosci. (Landmark Ed), 16*, 277–306.

37. Jones, B., (2013). Haematological cancer: rituximab maintenance improves the outcome of elderly patients with FL. *Nat. Rev. Clin. Oncol., 10*, 607.

38. Armeanu-Ebinger, S., Hoh, A., Wenz, J., & Fuchs, J., (2013). Targeting EpCAM (CD326) for immunotherapy in hepatoblastoma. *Oncoimmunology, 2*, e22620 http://www.ncbi.nlm.nih.gov/pmc/articles/PMC3583930/pdf/onci-2-e22620.pdf.

39. Kawaguchi, Y., Kono, K., Mimura, K., Sugai, H., Akaike, H., & Fujii, H., (2007). Cetuximab induce antibody-dependent cellular cytotoxicity against EGFR-expressing esophageal squamous cell carcinoma. *Int. J. Cancer, 120*, 781–787.

40. Srivastava, R. M., Lee, S. C., Andrade, F. P. A., Lord, C. A., Jie, H. B., Davidson, H. C., Lopez-Albaitero, A., Gibson, S. P., Gooding, W. E., Ferrone, S., & Ferris, R. L., (2013). Cetuximab-activated natural killer and dendritic cells collaborate to trigger tumor antigen-specific T-cell immunity in head and neck cancer patients. *Clin. Cancer Res., 19*, 1858–1872.

41. Terme, M., Pernot, S., Marcheteau, E., Sandoval, F., Benhamouda, N., Colussi, O., Dubreuil, O., Carpentier, A. F., Tartour, E., & Taieb, J., (2013). VEGFA-VEGFR pathway blockade inhibits tumor-induced regulatory T-cell proliferation in colorectal cancer. *Cancer Res., 73*, 539–549.

42. Mellor, J. D., Brown, M. P., Irving, H. R., Zalcberg, J. R., & Dobrovic, A., (2013). A critical review of the role of Fc gamma receptor polymorphisms in the response to monoclonal antibodies in cancer. *J. Hematol. Oncol., 6*, 1, http://www.ncbi.nlm.nih.gov/pmc/articles/PMC3549734/pdf/1756-8722-6-1.pdf.

43. Galluzzi, L., Vacchelli, E., Eggermont, A., Fridman, W. H., Galon, J., Sautes-Fridman, C., Tartour, E., Zitvogel, L., & Kroemer, G., (2012). Trial Watch: Adoptive cell transfer immunotherapy. *Oncoimmunology, 1*, 306–315.

44. Ray, S., Chhabra, A., Chakraborty, N. G., Hegde, U., Dorsky, D. I., Chodon, T., Von Euw, E., Comin-Anduix, B., Koya, R. C., Ribas, A., Economou, J. S., Rosenberg, S. A., & Mukherji, B., (2010). MHC-I-restricted melanoma antigen specific TCR-engineered human CD4+ T cells exhibit multifunctional effector and helper responses, *in vitro*. *Clin. Immunol., 136*, 338–347.

45. Dotti, G., Gottschalk, S., Savoldo, B., & Brenner, M. K., (2014). Design and development of therapies using chimeric antigen receptor-expressing T cells. *Immunol. Rev., 257*, 107–126.

46. Boisgerault, N., Guillerme, J. B., Pouliquen, D., Mesel-Lemoine, M., Achard, C., Combredet, C., Fonteneau, J. F., Tangy, F., & Gregoire, M., (2013). Natural oncolytic activity of live-attenuated measles virus against human lung and colorectal adenocarcinomas. *Biomed. Res. Int., 387362*, http://dx.doi.org/10. 1155/2013/387362.

47. Bernt, K. M., Ni, S., Gaggar, A., Li, Z. Y., Shayakhmetov, D. M., & Lieber, A., (2003). The effect of sequestration by nontarget tissues on anti-tumor efficacy of systemically applied, conditionally replicating adenovirus vectors. *Mol. Ther., 8*, 746–755.

48. Bonifaz, L., Bonnyay, D., Mahnke, K., Rivera, M., Nussenzweig, M. C., & Steinman, R. M., (2002). Efficient targeting of protein antigen to the dendritic cell receptor DEC-205 in the steady state leads to antigen presentation on major histocompatibility complex class I products and peripheral CD8+ T cell tolerance. *J. Exp. Med., 196*, 1627–1638.

49. Koido, S., Homma, S., Okamoto, M., Namiki, Y., Kan, S., Takakura, K., Kajihara, M., Uchiyama, K., Hara, E., Ohkusa, T., Gong, J., & Tajiri, H., (2013). Improved immunogenicity of fusions between ethanol-treated cancer cells and dendritic cells exposed to dual TLR stimulation. *Oncoimmunology, 2*, e25375, http://dx.doi.org/10. 4161/onci. 25375.

50. Garcia-Vallejo, J. J., Unger, W. W., Kalay, H., & Van Kooyk, Y., (2013). Glycan-based DC-SIGN targeting to enhance antigen cross-presentation in anticancer vaccines. *Oncoimmunology, 2,* e23040 http://www.ncbi.nlm.nih.gov/pmc/articles/PMC4570108/pdf/koni-04-08-970462.pdf.

51. Bijker, M. S., Van den Eeden, S. J., Franken, K. L., Melief, C. J., Offringa, R., Van der Burg, S. H., (2007). CD8+ CTL priming by exact peptide epitopes in incomplete Freund's adjuvant induces a vanishing CTL response, whereas long peptides induce sustained CTL reactivity. *J. Immunol., 179,* 5033–5040.

52. Hailemichael, Y., Dai, Z., Jaffarzad, N., Ye, Y., Medina, M. A., Huang, X. F., Dorta-Estremera, S. M., Greeley, N. R., Nitti, G., Peng, W., Liu, C., Lou, Y., Wang, Z., Ma, W., Rabinovich, B., Sowell, R. T., Schluns, K. S., Davis, R. E., Hwu, P., & Overwijk, W. W., (2013). Persistent antigen at vaccination sites induces tumor-specific CD8(+) T cell sequestration, dysfunction and deletion. *Nat. Med., 19,* 465–472.

53. Pol, J. G., Zhang, L., Bridle, B. W., Stephenson, K. B., Resseguier, J., Hanson, S., Chen, L., Kazdhan, N., Bramson, J. L., Stojdl, D. F., Wan, Y., & Lichty, B. D., (2014). Maraba virus as a potent oncolytic vaccine vector. *Mol. Ther., 22,* 420–429.

54. Bolhassani, A., & Zahedifard, F., (2012). Therapeutic live vaccines as a potential anti-cancer strategy. *Int. J. Cancer, 131,* 1733-1743.

55. Kenter, G. G., Welters, M. J., Valentijn, A. R., Lowik, M. J., Berends-van der Meer, D. M., Vloon, A. P., Essahsah, F., Fathers, L. M., Offringa, R., Drijfhout, J. W., Wafelman, A. R., Oostendorp, J., Fleuren, G. J., Van der Burg, S. H., & Melief, C. J., (2009). Vaccination against HPV-16 oncoproteins for vulvar intraepithelial neoplasia. *N. Engl. J. Med., 361,* 1838–1847.

56. Walter, S., Weinschenk, T., Stenzl, A., Zdrojowy, R., Pluzanska, A., Szczylik, C., Staehler, M., Brugger, W., Dietrich, P. Y., Mendrzyk, R., Hilf, N, Schoor, O., Fritsche, J., Mahr, A., Maurer, D., Vass, V., Trautwein, C., Lewandrowski, P., Flohr, C., Pohla, H., Stanczak, J. J., Bronte, V., Mandruzzato, S., Biedermann, T., Pawelec, G., Derhovanessian, E., Yamagishi, H., Miki, T., Hongo, F., Takaha, N., Hirakawa, K., Tanaka, H., Stevanovic, S., Frisch, J., Mayer-Mokler, A., Kirner, A., Rammensee, H. G., Reinhardt, C., & Singh-Jasuja, H., (2012). Multipeptide immune response to cancer vaccine IMA901 after single-dose cyclophosphamide associates with longer patient survival. *Nat. Med., 18,* 1254–1261.

57. Tato, C. M., & Cua, D. J., (2008). SnapShot: Cytokines IV. *Cell, 132,* 1062-e1061–1062.

58. Sim, G. C., Martin-Orozco, N., Jin, L., Yang, Y., Wu, S., Washington, E., Sanders, D., Lacey, C., Wang, Y., Vence, L., Hwu, P., & Radvanyi, L., (2014). IL-2 therapy promotes suppressive ICOS+ Treg expansion in melanoma patients. *J. Clin. Invest., 124,* 99–110.

59. Arellano, M., & Lonial, S., (2008). Clinical uses of GM-CSF, a critical appraisal and update. *Biologics., 2,* 13–27.

60. Van Horssen, R., Ten Hagen, T. L., & Eggermont, A. M., (2006). TNF-alpha in cancer treatment: molecular insights, antitumor effects, & clinical utility. *Oncologist, 11,* 397–408.

61. Melero, I., Grimaldi, A. M., Perez-Gracia, J. L., & Ascierto, P. A., (2013). Clinical development of immunostimulatory monoclonal antibodies and opportunities for combination. *Clin. Cancer Res., 19,* 997–1008.

62. Nowak, A. K., (2013). Immunological checkpoint inhibitors enter adolescence. *Lancet Oncol., 14,* 1035–1037.

63. Wei, H., Zhao, L., Hellstrom, I., Hellstrom, K. E., & Guo, Y., (2014). Dual targeting of CD137 co-stimulatory and PD-1 co-inhibitory molecules for ovarian cancer immunotherapy. *Oncoimmunology, 3*, e28248 http://www.ncbi.nlm.nih.gov/pmc/articles/PMC4063147/pdf/onci-3-e28248.pdf.

64. Snyder, A., Makarov, V., Merghoub, T., Yuan, J., Zaretsky, J. M., Desrichard, A., Walsh, L. A., Postow, M. A., Wong, P., Ho, T. S., Hollmann, T. J., Bruggeman, C., Kannan, K., Li, Y., Elipenahli, C., Liu, C., Harbison, C. T., Wang, L., Ribas, A., Wolchok, J. D., & Chan, T. A., (2014). Genetic basis for clinical response to CTLA-4 blockade in melanoma. *N. Engl. J. Med., 371*, 2189–2199.

65. Munn, D. H., Sharma, M. D., Hou, D., Baban, B., Lee, J. R., Antonia, S. J., Messina, J. L., Chandler, P., Koni, P. A., & Mellor, A. L., (2004). Expression of indoleamine 2, 3-dioxygenase by plasmacytoid dendritic cells in tumor-draining lymph nodes. *J. Clin. Invest., 114*, 280–290.

66. Mezrich, J. D., Fechner, J. H., Zhang, X., Johnson, B. P., Burlingham, W. J., & Bradfield, C. A., (2010). An interaction between kynurenine and the aryl hydrocarbon receptor can generate regulatory T cells. *J. Immunol., 185*, 3190–3198.

67. Mellor, A. L., Baban, B., Chandler, P., Marshall, B., Jhaver, K., Hansen, A., Koni, P. A., Iwashima, M., & Munn, D. H., (2003). Cutting edge: induced indoleamine 2, 3 dioxygenase expression in dendritic cell subsets suppresses T cell clonal expansion. *J. Immunol., 171*, 1652–1655.

68. Muller, A. J., DuHadaway, J. B., Donover, P. S., Sutanto-Ward, E., & Prendergast, G. C., (2005). Inhibition of indoleamine 2, 3-dioxygenase, an immunoregulatory target of the cancer suppression gene Bin1, potentiates cancer chemotherapy. *Nat. Med., 11*, 312–319.

69. Aymeric, L., Apetoh, L., Ghiringhelli, F., Tesniere, A., Martins, I., Kroemer, G., Smyth, M. J., & Zitvogel, L., (2010). Tumor cell death and ATP release prime dendritic cells and efficient anticancer immunity. *Cancer Res., 70*, 855–858.

70. Deaglio, S., Dwyer, K. M., Gao, W., Friedman, D., Usheva, A., Erat, A., Chen, J. F., Enjyoji, K., Linden, J., Oukka, M., Kuchroo, V. K., Strom, T. B., & Robson, S. C., (2007). Adenosine generation catalyzed by CD39 and CD73 expressed on regulatory T cells mediates immune suppression. *J. Exp. Med., 204*, 1257–1265.

71. Michaud, M., Sukkurwala, A. Q., Martins, I., Shen, S., Zitvogel, L., & Kroemer, G., (2012). Subversion of the chemotherapy-induced anticancer immune response by the ecto-ATPase CD39. *Oncoimmunology, 1*, 393–395.

72. Zhang, B., (2012). CD73 promotes tumor growth and metastasis. *Oncoimmunology, 1*, 67–70.

73. Aliagas, E., Vidal, A., Texido, L., Ponce, J., Condom, E., & Martin-Satue, M., (2014). High expression of ecto-nucleotidases CD39 and CD73 in human endometrial tumors. *Mediators Inflamm., 2014*, 509027.

74. Young, A., Mittal, D., Stagg, J., & Smyth, M. J., (2014). Targeting cancer-derived adenosine: new therapeutic approaches. *Cancer Discov., 4*, 879–888.

75. Kawai, T., & Akira, S., (2011). Toll-like receptors and their crosstalk with other innate receptors in infection and immunity. *Immunity, 34*, 637–650.

76. Saleh, M., (2011). The machinery of Nod-like receptors: refining the paths to immunity and cell death. *Immunol. Rev., 243*, 235–246.

77. Brennan, T. V., Lin, L., Huang, X., Cardona, D. M., Li, Z., Dredge, K., Chao, N. J., & Yang, Y., (2012). Heparan sulfate, an endogenous TLR4 agonist, promotes acute GVHD after allogeneic stem cell transplantation. *Blood, 120*, 2899–2908.

78. Krysko, D. V., Garg, A. D., Kaczmarek, A., Krysko, O., Agostinis, P., & Vandenabeele, P., (2012). Immunogenic cell death and DAMPs in cancer therapy. *Nat. Rev. Cancer*, *12*, 860–875.

79. Ando, K., Mori, K., Corradini, N., Redini, F., & Heymann, D., (2011). Mifamurtide for the treatment of nonmetastatic osteosarcoma. *Expert Opin. Pharmacother.*, *12*, 285–292.

80. Ma, Y., Adjemian, S., Mattarollo, S. R., Yamazaki, T., Aymeric, L., Yang, H., Portela, C. J. P., Hannani, D., Duret, H., Steegh, K., Martins, I., Schlemmer, F., Michaud, M., Kepp, O., Sukkurwala, A. Q., Menger, L., Vacchelli, E., Droin, N., Galluzzi, L., Krzysiek, R., Gordon, S., Taylor, P. R., Van Endert, P., Solary, E., Smyth, M. J., Zitvogel, L., & Kroemer, G., (2013). Anticancer chemotherapy-induced intratumoral recruitment and differentiation of antigen-presenting cells. *Immunity*, *38*, 729–741.

81. Matthews, S. J., & McCoy, C., (2003). Thalidomide: a review of approved and investigational uses. *Clin. Ther.*, *25*, 342–395.

82. Waldman, A. R., (2000). Thalidomide. *Clin. J. Oncol. Nurs.*, *4*, 99–100.

83. Amato, R. J., (2002). Thalidomide: an antineoplastic agent. *Curr. Oncol. Rep.*, *4*, 56–62.

84. Semeraro, M., & Galluzzi, L., (2014). Novel insights into the mechanism of action of lenalidomide. *Oncoimmunology*, *3*, e28386.

85. Attia, P., Maker, A. V., Haworth, L. R., Rogers-Freezer, L., & Rosenberg, S. A., (2005). Inability of a fusion protein of IL-2 and diphtheria toxin (Denileukin Diftitox, DAB389IL-2, ONTAK) to eliminate regulatory T lymphocytes in patients with melanoma. *J. Immunother.*, *28*, 582–592.

86. Senovilla, L., Aranda, F., Galluzzi, L., & Kroemer, G., (2014). Impact of myeloid cells on the efficacy of anticancer chemotherapy. *Curr. Opin. Immunol.*, *30C*, 24–31.

INDEX

Milton Keynes UK
Ingram Content Group UK Ltd.
UKHW030901141024
449569UK00025B/1291